The Acute Management of Surgical Disease

Martin D. Zielinski
Oscar Guillamondegui
Editors

The Acute Management of Surgical Disease

Springer

Editors
Martin D. Zielinski
Trauma and Acute Care Surgery
Department of Surgery
Baylor College of Medicine
Houston, TX, USA

Oscar Guillamondegui
Trauma and Surgical Care Clinic
Vanderbilt University
Nashville, TN, USA

ISBN 978-3-031-07880-4 ISBN 978-3-031-07881-1 (eBook)
https://doi.org/10.1007/978-3-031-07881-1

This Springer imprint is published by the registered company Springer Nature Switzerland AG
The registered company address is: Gewerbestrasse 11, 6330 Cham, Switzerland

To Dr. Maddaus for believing in me
To Dr. Que for my first opportunity
To Dr. Sarr for being an inspiration
To Dr. Zietlow for giving me a chance
To Dr. Jenkins for launching me
To Dr. Rosengart for letting me prove it
To Mom and Dad for four decades of encouragement
To Grace, Hannah, and Eleanor for bringing unrelenting joy
And most importantly, to Dr. Lorenz for more than 20 years of unwavering love

– Martin D. Zielinski

I would like to acknowledge and dedicate this book to all those individuals who never quench the thirst for knowledge in the surgical profession. Without questioning anecdote and challenging paradigm, it makes it difficult to improve the care of the sick patient. I wish you well on your journey.

I would also like to dedicate this work to the three people who somehow put up with my ridiculous ways—Tarah, Bella, and Gabe.

– Oscar Guillamondegui

Contents

John Kirby, MD Mayo Clinic, Rochester, MN, USA

Clifford Y. Ko, MD, MS, MSHS Department of Surgery, David Geffen School of Medicine, UCLA, Los Angeles, CA, USA

Division of Research and Optimal Patient Care, American College of Surgeons, Chicago, IL, USA

The Healthcare Improvement Studies Institute (THIS Institute), University of Cambridge, Cambridge, UK

Ryan J. Law, DO Division of Gastroenterology and Hepatology, Department of Medicine, Mayo Clinic, Rochester, MN, USA

Amelia Walling Maiga, MD, MPH Division of Trauma and Surgical Critical Care, Department of Surgery, Vanderbilt University Medical Center, Nashville, TN, USA

Rebecca G. Maine, MD, MPH Department of Surgery, Harborview Medical Center, University of Washington, Seattle, Washington, USA

Kellie E. Mathis, MD, FACS Mayo Clinic, Rochester, MN, USA

Addison K. May, MD, MBA Atrium Health, Carolinas Medical Center, University of North Carolina School of Medicine, Charlotte, NC, USA

Andrew Medvecz, MD, MPH Vanderbilt University Medical Center, Medical Arts Building, Nashville, TN, USA

Alicia M. Mohr, MD, FACS, FCCM Department of Surgery, University of Florida College of Medicine, Gainesville, FL, USA

Nathan T. Mowery, MD, FACS Department of Surgery, Wake Forest Baptist Medical Center, Winston Salem, NC, USA

Aussama K. Nassar, MD, MSc, FRCSC, FACS Department of Surgery, Stanford University, Stanford, CA, USA

Kerri A. Ohman, MD Section of Colon and Rectal Surgery, Department of Surgery, Washington University School of Medicine in St. Louis, St. Louis, MO, USA

Brandy Padilla-Jones, MD, FACS Department of Trauma and Acute Care Surgery, Las Vegas Sunrise Memorial Hospital, Las Vegas, NV, USA

Caroline Park, MD, MPH, FACS Division of Burn, Trauma and Acute Care Surgery, Department of Surgery, University of Texas Southwestern Medical Center at Dallas, Dallas, TX, USA

Biomedical Engineering, Graduate School of Biomedical Sciences, University of Texas Southwestern Medical Center, Dallas, TX, USA

Andrew Peitzman, MD Department of Surgery, University of Pittsburgh Medical Center, Pittsburgh, PA, USA

Samuel J. Pera, MD Hiram C. Polk Jr. Department of Surgery, University of Louisville, Louisville, KY, USA

Kevin D. Platt, MD Division of Gastroenterology and Hepatology, Department of Medicine, University of Michigan, Ann Arbor, MI, USA

Jacob A. Quick, MD University of Missouri, Columbia, MO, USA

Mariela Rivera, MD, FACS Department of Surgery, Mayo Clinic, Rochester, MN, USA

Bryce R. H. Robinson, MD, MS, FACS, FCCM Department of Surgery, Harborview Medical Center, University of Washington, Seattle, Washington, USA

Anna N. Romagnoli, MD Division of Vascular and Endovascular Surgery, Massachusetts General Hospital, Boston, MA, USA

Jarrett Santorelli, MD Division of Trauma, Surgical Critical Care, Burns and Acute Care Surgery, Department of Surgery, UC San Diego School of Medicine, San Diego, CA, USA

Stephanie A. Savage, MD, MS Acute Care & Regional General Surgery, University of Wisconsin School of Medicine & Public Health, Madison, WI, USA

Robert G. Sawyer, MD, FACS, FCCM, FIDSA Department of Surgery, Western Michigan University Homer Stryker M.D. School of Medicine, Kalamazoo, MI, USA

Department of Engineering, Western Michigan University College of Engineering and Applied Sciences, Kalamazoo, MI, USA

Jessica E. Schucht, MD, PhD Hiram C. Polk Jr. Department of Surgery, University of Louisville, Louisville, KY, USA

Anupamaa Seshadri, MD Department of Surgery, University of Pittsburgh Medical Center, Pittsburgh, PA, USA

Department of Surgery, Beth Israel Deaconess Medical Center, Boston, MA, USA

Myrick C. Shinall Jr, MD, PhD Surgery and Medicine, Vanderbilt University Medical Center, Nashville, TN, USA

Alison A. Smith, MD, PhD Division of Trauma/Critical Care/Acute Care, Clinical Surgery, Department of Surgery, Louisiana State University, New Orleans, LA, USA

Jason W. Smith, MD, PhD, MBA Hiram C. Polk Jr. Department of Surgery, University of Louisville, Louisville, KY, USA

Michael C. Smith, MD Division of Acute Care Surgery, Vanderbilt University Medical Center, Nashville, TN, USA

David A. Spain, MD, FACS Department of Surgery, Stanford University, Stanford, CA, USA

Audrey L. Spencer, MD Department of Surgery, Wake Forest Baptist Medical Center, Winston Salem, NC, USA

Eric Strand, MD Division of General Obstetrics and Gynecology, Department of Obstetrics and Gynecology, Washington University School of Medicine, St. Louis, MO, USA

Isabelle A. Struve, MD Department of Surgery, University of California Davis Health, Sacramento, CA, USA

Erin L. Vanzant, MD Department of Surgery, University of Florida College of Medicine, Gainesville, FL, USA

Michael W. Wandling, MD, MS Division of Acute Care Surgery, McGovern Medical School, The University of Texas Health Science Center—Houston, Houston, TX, USA

Hunter Wessells, MD, FACS Department of Urology, University of Washington School of Medicine, Seattle, WA, USA

Paul E. Wise, MD Section of Colon and Rectal Surgery, Department of Surgery, Washington University School of Medicine in St. Louis, St. Louis, MO, USA

Jeanette Zhang, MD Department of Surgery, Division of Acute Care Surgery, University of Florida College of Medicine Jacksonville, Jacksonville, FL, USA

John Zietlow, MD Department of Surgery, Mayo Clinic, Rochester, MN, USA

Martin D. Zielinski, MD, FACS Professor and Chief, Trauma and Acute Care Surgery, Department of Surgery, Baylor College of Medicine, Houston, TX, USA

Scott Zietlow, MD, FACS Department of Surgery, Mayo Clinic, Rochester, MN, USA

1 Emergency General Surgery: A Paradigm Shift to Meet the Demands of an Evolving Discipline

Mira H. Ghneim and Jose J. Diaz

The Changing Role of the General Surgeon

General surgery is defined by the American Board of Surgery (ABS) as "a discipline that requires a knowledge of and familiarity with a broad spectrum of diseases that may require surgical treatment." By necessity, the breadth and depth of this knowledge varies based on disease category. In most areas, the surgeon is expected to be competent in diagnosing and treating the full spectrum of disease [1]. To achieve such comprehensive knowledge and experience, the ABS established nine principal components that govern general surgery training which include alimentary tract surgery, abdominal surgery, breast/soft tissue/skin surgery, head/neck surgery, vascular surgery, surgical oncology, and trauma and surgical critical care [2].

General surgeons have always been a crucial component of the healthcare system in the United States. They provided comprehensive elective, emergent, and trauma care in rural and urban environments [2]. Prior to the development of surgical fellowships in the 1980s, the general surgeons not only managed the emergency general surgery and trauma patients but often also performed obstetric, gynecological, vascular, endoscopic, and orthopedic procedures. However, within the last two decades, the repertoire of operations performed by general surgeons, and the way in which these operations are performed, has changed drastically. This change was driven by the evolution of surgical disease management and the advent of technological advancement. As a result, there has been a slow and steady extinction of the "omnipotent general surgeon" resulting in a shift of the practice of general surgery [3]. While the general surgery training programs have evolved to focus on quality and range of education and clinical acumen, few surgeons provide in practice the breadth of core components required for training and certification. Today, more graduating chiefs aim for more specialized training and prefer to practice at larger institutions and in urban environments [3].

In 2014, the Resident Education Committee of the Society for Surgery of the Alimentary Tract (SSAT) published an article that discussed how the general surgery many "grew up" with is a shadow of its former self [4]. While the general surgery training remains committed to the principle that general surgeons should have exposure and experience in a wide range of surgical conditions, the complexity of surgical disease and the evolution of disease management have led to specialization and subspecialization. This shift created a tangible shortage in the general surgery

M. H. Ghneim (✉) · J. J. Diaz
Department of Surgery, Program in Trauma, R Adams Cowley Shock Trauma Center, University of Maryland Medical Center, Baltimore, MD, USA
e-mail: mira.ghneim@som.umaryland.edu; jose.diaz@som.umaryland.edu

M. D. Zielinski, O. Guillamondegui (eds.), *The Acute Management of Surgical Disease*,
https://doi.org/10.1007/978-3-031-07881-1_1

workforce in the United States [5, 6]. With the advent and increased popularity of subspecialties such as colorectal surgery, minimally invasive surgery, surgical oncology, and bariatric, breast, vascular, and thoracic surgery, the once broad elective general surgery scope has become severely restricted. This led to a shortage in general surgeon availability and subsequent increasing need for general surgical emergencies and trauma coverage [7]. The number of general surgeons needed to adequately serve the population is estimated to be 7.5 per 100,000 people. Currently, there are 5 per 100,000 people, and in some areas, it drops as low as 0.1–0.46 per 100,00 people. Over the last 25 years, the ratio of general surgeon per 100,000 population has dropped by 25% [8].

Multiple studies have focused on attempting to identify the factors that contributed to the pursuit of fellowship training and general surgeon shortage in the workplace from practicing surgeons and residents [4, 9, 10]. Decreased salaries and reimbursements, lifestyle barriers, burnout due to demanding call schedules, and the need for further training due to the sense that higher expertise leads to better job offers in urban areas were the most commonly cited reason for post-graduate fellowship training (Fig. 1.1).

Several approaches have been suggested to address this decline. The Balanced Budget Act of 1997 has maintained a constant number of newly graduating allopathic surgeons with a modest increase in the number from 1000 to 1050 per year [11], an increase that is insufficient to mitigate the shortage. Some longer-term solutions include building new medical schools, expanding enrollment in existing schools, and persuading the federal government to reduce or eliminate the Medicare cap on funding graduate education with the aim of increasing recruitment [4, 12]. Short-term solutions such as enhanced reimbursement of the general surgeon, employment

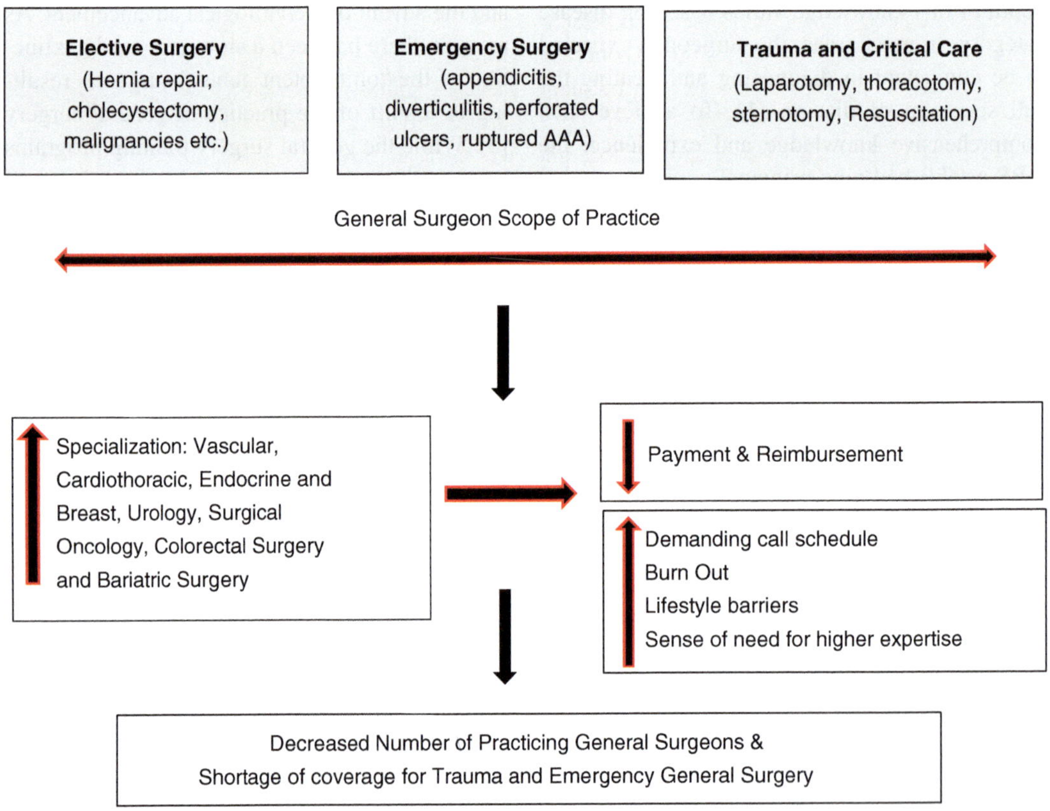

Fig. 1.1 Factors leading to increased specialization

of part-time surgeons to cover call deficiencies, promotion of acute care fellowships, and recruitment of acute care surgeons may alleviate some of the shortage [4]. Acute care surgeons, given the breadth of expertise in trauma, emergency general surgery, and critical care, are equipped to manage emergent and nonemergent surgical disease in smaller facilities where surgical expertise is lacking due to the shortage of general surgeons.

While the role of the general surgeon in the current ultra-specialized world of general surgery may still exist in certain settings such as rural areas, the reality is that general surgery is expansive and cannot be sufficiently taught or mastered by one individual. With the resultant proliferation of the surgical specialties and the public demand for specific expertise, the extinction of the multitalented general surgeon will continue.

The Crucial Role of the Rural Surgeon

While the terms "general surgeon" and "rural surgeon" are not always synonymous, rural surgery is a component of the general surgery practice that remains essentially inaccessible in remote areas [13]. The term "rural surgery" refers to the practice of surgery serving people in rural communities and geographically remote areas [14]. While estimates vary, 15%–25% of the US population reside in rural areas, while only 10%–15% of physicians practice in these areas [15, 16] (Fig. 1.2). Rural patients are often older, have lower income, have major comorbidities, live long distances from tertiary care centers, and desire surgical care closer to home.

Those attracted to a career in rural surgery often come from a rural background. Practicing

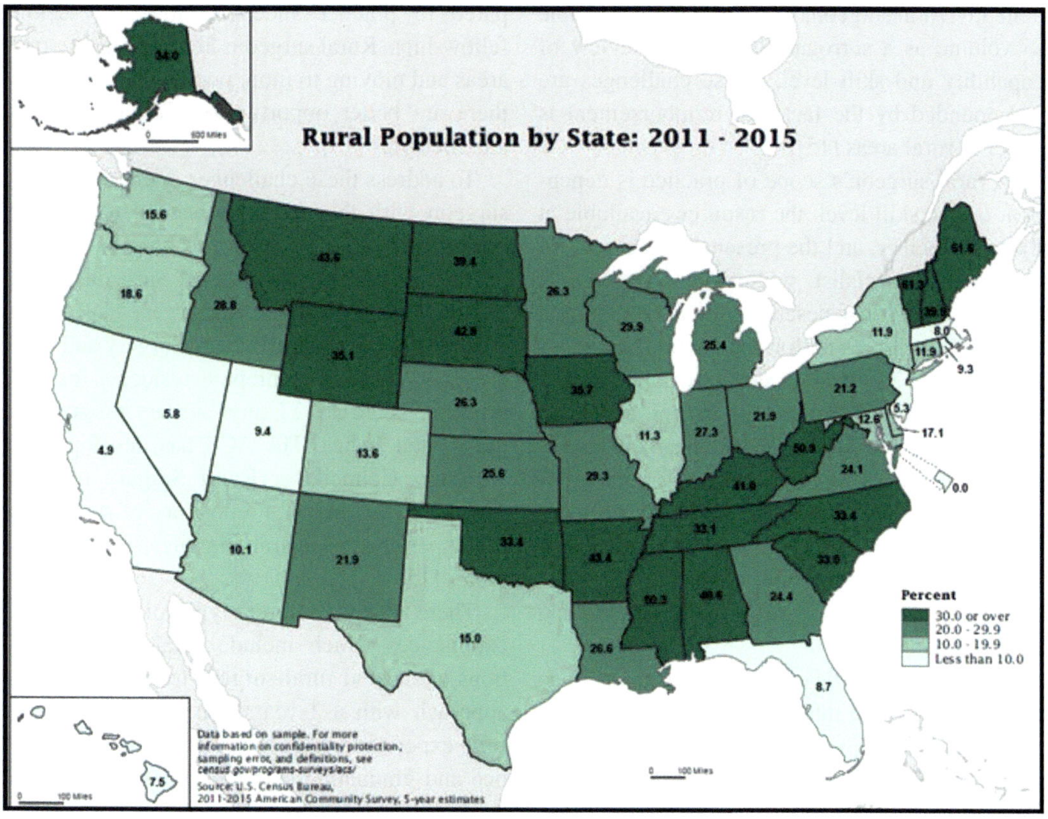

Fig. 1.2 Percentage of the rural population by state (www.census.gov/content/dam/Census/newsroom/blogs/2016/12/ruralamerica/fig02 ruralpopulation-state.jpg)

in a rural environment allows them unparalleled independence, a broad scope of practice, the ability to participate in leadership roles within the hospital and community, and the ability to develop close and longitudinal relationships with their patients [17, 18]. Nonetheless, rural surgeons are also in short supply, particularly in small or isolated towns. This is exacerbated by increased surgical specialization and preference to practice in an urban setting.

Those who pursue a career in rural surgery are faced by many challenges due to "professional isolation" that is attributed to the geographic location of their practice. In some instances, the rural surgeon is the only surgeon in the hospital and lacks the opportunity to discuss difficult cases and operative strategies with other colleagues. The rigorous call schedule and lack of coverage make it challenging to travel for continuing medical education. Additionally, due to small numbers of certain procedures performed annually, rural surgeons are extremely vulnerable to volume as a surrogate for quality review of capability and skill level. These challenges are compounded by the fact that reimbursement is lower in rural areas [15].

A rural surgeon's scope of practice is dependent on the skill level, the resources available at the rural facility, and the presence or absence of surgical subspecialist within the community. Several studies have described the most common types of procedures performed by rural surgeons [19–23] and include open and laparoscopic abdominal (biliary tract, small bowel, and large bowel), vascular, thoracic, and head and neck procedures. Rural surgeons also perform a larger volume of obstetric and gynecological, orthopedic, and urologic procedure than general surgeons. Finally, endoscopy makes up a larger proportion of a rural surgeon's practice than urban surgeons.

Trauma and critical care in rural areas has also continued to be an integral part of the rural surgeon's practice. Coordinating trauma care, performing urgent procedures, triaging and prioritizing transfers to tertiary care centers, and providing definitive care for patients who do not require any surgical specialist interventions are just a few of the tasks that fall upon the rural surgeon [24]. In some hospitals, the surgeon is also the surgical intensivist and is expected to manage difficult airways, hemodynamic instability, sepsis, and other procedures (arterial line, central venous catheter, and tube thoracostomy placements) [15]. Given that rural surgery is very broad-based, some of the skills required to practice are not even Accreditation Council for Graduate Medical Education (ACGME)-required rotations for board certification in surgery, and therefore more surgical experience is crucial [15].

In similar fashion to the general surgery workforce shortage, there currently is a national shortage of rural surgeons leaving the discipline in severe crisis [18, 25–29]. Rural surgeons are aging, and new recruits are not expected to fill the deficit as fewer general surgeons go into rural surgery [15, 27]. Instead, general surgery residents, due to the perception that they are not prepared to practice independently, are seeking fellowships. Rural surgeons are also leaving rural areas and moving to more populated areas where there are better opportunities, reimbursements, and lifestyles [15].

To address these challenges and arm the rural surgeon with the skills set needed to succeed, rural surgery training programs have been developed. The American College of Surgeons (ACS) and the American Board of Surgery have recognized the need for rural general surgery and made a concerted effort to prepare residents for rural practice. There are 11 rural surgery programs in the United States. The ACS has developed the Advisory Council for Rural Surgery (ACRS). The ACRS maintains a repository of rural training experiences and training sites in the United States [15].

There are five different types of rural training experiences which include rural surgery rotations, dedicated rural surgery tracks, immersion approach with a 1-year high operative volume rural experience, fellowships for surgeon in practice and graduating surgeons to enhance endoscopy skills, and transition to practice programs. Overall, the goal is to provide broad experiences in rural general surgery, surgical subspecialties, and endoscopic and laparoscopic procedures [15, 30]. Those training in rural programs have more autonomy in both decision-making and surgical management [15, 31]. Additionally, the rural preceptors serve as proctors, role models, and long-term mentors for participating surgery residents [15].

The impact of trauma on mortality in the rural community is substantial given that only 24% of those who live in rural communities have access to a level I or II trauma center within 1 h of injury [32–34]. As a result, while only 15%–25% of the population lives in rural community, 50% of all motor vehicle collisions and 60% of trauma-related mortality occur in the rural setting [33–37].

The development and strengthening of critical access hospitals in rural areas have been shown to not only save lives and improve patient outcomes but also improve upon the cost burden of trauma care and improve upon the quality of life for trauma survivors [34].

The Rural Trauma Team Development Course (RTTDC) was created by the Rural Trauma Committee of ACS-COT 1998. This is an interactive 1-day course that promotes the development of a rural trauma team at critical access hospitals—with the goal of cultivating relationships between rural trauma facilities and the regional trauma center and developing a rapport based on common communication [38]. Lectures prepare the members of the rural facility to care for critically injured patients and understand the resources and limitations of their individual rural facility [34, 35, 38, 39]. Ultimately, the course optimizes a team-based approach to trauma management and promotes recognition of the need for early patient transfer to the nearest trauma center [34, 35, 38, 39].

While a career in rural surgery can be rewarding, there is a need to enhance the quality of life for rural surgeons to enhance recruitment. As the rural population continues to constitute a considerable portion of the population, reversing the current trends in workforce shortages becomes essential. Innovative and thoughtful solutions are necessary. Expanding the workforce, preparing residents for rural practice, recruitment of general surgeons to rural areas, establishing incentives, and improving reimbursement to increase retention of rural surgeons represent a few.

The Emergence of the Modern Acute Care Surgeon

With the increasing need for coverage of general surgical emergencies, the decreasing number of general surgeons capable and willing to provide on-call services, and the disinterest among trainees in trauma as a career due to a shift to nonoperative management of previously operative blunt injuries, the role of an acute care surgeon emerged [40, 41].

Acute care surgery is a distinct surgical specialty, established by the American Association for the Surgery of Trauma (AAST) between 2005 and 2007, and encompasses three areas of surgical practice: trauma surgery, emergency general surgery, and surgical critical care (Fig. 1.3) [40, 41]. An acute care surgeon is a fellowship trained surgeon equipped with the knowledge and technical skills that allow for the time-sensitive care of both the trauma and the non-trauma emergency general surgery patient population (Fig. 1.4).

The acute care patient population present multiple treatment challenges, including around-the-clock readiness for the provision of comprehensive care across a spectrum of disciplines, the constrained time for preoperative optimization of the patient, and the greater potential for intraoperative and postoperative complications due to the often-emergent, high-complexity, and high-acuity nature of care, the intraoperative and postoperative challenges, and the lack of evidence-based guidelines [42].

If specialization is defined by disease process in addition to procedure and technology, the generalist crisis led to the emergence of the discipline of acute care surgery as a specialty. The acute care surgeon is the specialist of "emergency surgical and critical illnesses" of traumatic and non-traumatic nature with expertise in understanding the acute physiology, resuscitation, and

2003	Joint meeting of ACS, AAST, WEST and EAST addressing problems of access to emergency surgical care and the future of trauma surgery. AAST forms Ad hoc committee to develop the reorganized specialty of Trauma, Surgical Critical Care and Emergency Surgery.
2005	ACEP survey nearly 75% emergency departments identify inadequate on-call specialty coverage. AAST renames previous ad hoc committee - Acute Care Surgery Committee
2006	IOM report- Future of Emergency Care, confirms shortage of on call specialists.
2007	AAST retreat; Development of curriculum, competency tools, case registry, certification criteria, site visits
2008	First formal AAST Acute Care Surgery Fellowship program begins.
2014	Refinement of operative case requirements
2018	Shift from a rotation-based curriculum to a longitudinal/experiential model with case minimum requirements.

Fig. 1.3 Historical timeline for the development of acute care surgery as a specialty (https://www.aast.org/acute-care-surgery-overview)

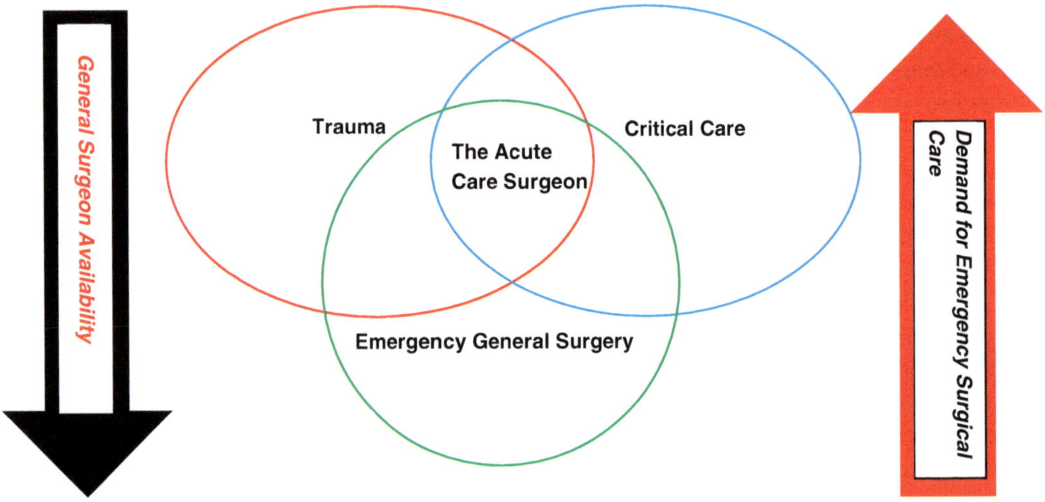

Fig. 1.4 The concept of an acute care surgeon

surgical intervention and coordinating complex patient care in a multidisciplinary fashion.

The Evolution of Trauma Care

Trauma is a leading cause of death in individuals ≤45 years and is the fourth cause of death overall for all ages [43]. Traumatic injury is associated with devastating effects on public health measures including increased healthcare costs, decreased quality of life, increased disability and physical impairment, and loss of potential work years [44]. As a result, over the last few decades, the ACS-COT has concentrated its efforts on creating an emergency surgical care system that decreases mortality and maximizes favorable outcomes. To achieve this goal, the ACS-COT's focus has been on developing a strong knowledge of the pathophysiology of the injured patient, improving screening and diagnostic modalities, and supporting advancements in both operative and nonoperative available therapeutic modalities.

The modern trauma system that exists today is a byproduct of the long-standing civilian-military collaboration and the lessons learned from the US involvement in armed conflict date back to the Wars in Korea and Vietnam [45, 46]. Rapid evacuation and transfer of injured soldiers via helicopter to treatment centers decreased the transfer time by 2.5 h in Korea and 3.5 h in Vietnam when compared to transfer times in World War II. As a result, the mortality decreased from 4.5% in World War II to 1.9% in Vietnam [46]. In addition to rapid transport, the military experience led to the identification of a number of additional factors that contributed to the reduction in mortality. These included rapid availability of blood products, better-organized medical teams, and more effective triage and allocation of medical resources [44]. Ultimately, the most critical lesson learned was that the "correct patient" needed to reach the place for definitive care in the shortest amount of time possible.

Figure 1.5 is a brief timeline of the evolution of trauma care. In 1966, the National Research Council and the US National Academy of Sciences published *Accidental Death and Disability: The Neglected Disease of Modern Society* [47]. This report defined the scope of the healthcare crisis in trauma care at the time. Additionally, it enforced the need to establish a national trauma association, organize community councils on emergency medical services, form a national council on injury prevention, and create a national institute of trauma. This revolutionized the way that trauma is managed in the United States and led to the development of the civilian trauma system. In 1966, the first two trauma centers were developed in the United States: John H. Stroger, Jr. Hospital of Cook County (Chicago) and San Francisco General Hospital. In 1969, the first statewide trauma center was initiated in the State of Maryland by R Adams Cowley.

In 1976, the ACS-COT published the First Optimal Hospital Resources for Care of the Injured Patient [48, 49]. The document focused on improving the care of injured patients, optimizing hospital resources, optimizing care in the setting of limited available resources, establishing trauma as a surgical disease, and emphasizing the need for surgical leadership. This document has been renamed to reflect the evolution and philosophy set forth by the ACS-COT and is now known as the Resources for Optimal Care of the Injured Patient. In it, the main mission of the ACS-COT focused on propagating the establishment of an ideal trauma system. This system focuses on injury prevention, access, prehospital care and transportation, acute hospital care, rehabilitation, and research activities [49]. The ASC-COT also published the criteria and the resources required to provide various levels of care for trauma patients. Based on these criteria, hospitals and trauma centers are classified into different

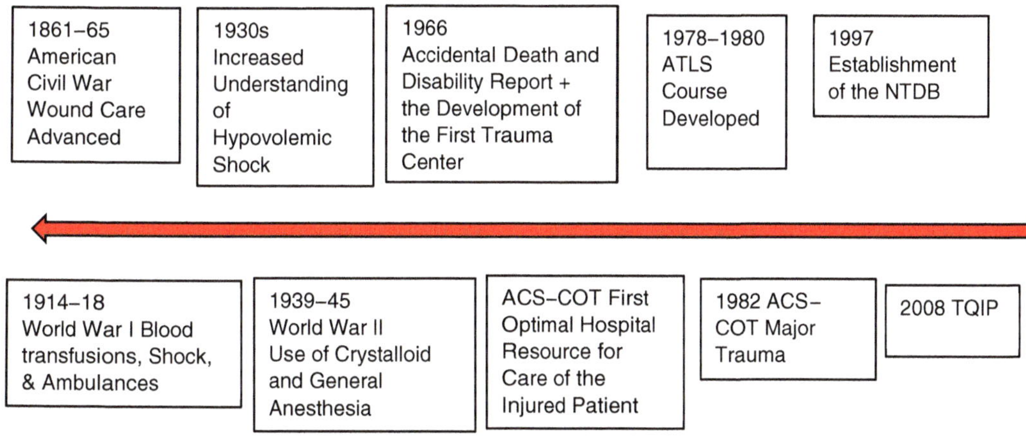

Fig. 1.5 A brief trauma timeline

Table 2.1 Differential diagnosis of the abdominal pain not requiring urgent surgical intervention

Extra-abdominal cavity	Cardiovascular	Acute coronary syndrome, pericarditis, myocarditis, aortic dissection
	Pulmonary	Pneumonia, pleuritis, empyema, pneumothorax, pulmonary embolus
	Gastrointestinal	Esophageal spasm, esophagitis
Intra-abdominal cavity	Genitourinary	Renal colic, pyelonephritis, ovarian torsion, extrauterine pregnancy, endometriosis, ovarian cyst rupture, testicular torsion, pelvic inflammatory disease, epididymitis
	Gastrointestinal	Cholelithiasis, pancreatitis, hepatitis
Systemic diseases	Musculoskeletal	Rectus sheath or retroperitoneal hematomas, radiculopathy, costochondritis, diskitis, herniated disc
	Hematologic	Leukemia, hemolytic anemia, sickle cell disease, lymphoma, connective tissue diseases
	Endocrine	Acute adrenal insufficiency, diabetic ketoacidosis
	Poisoning	Lead, arsenic
	Infectious	Herpes zoster, varicella, osteomyelitis, typhoid, tuberculosis, brucellosis, toxic shock syndrome

Adapted from Mayumi T, Yoshida M, Tazuma S et al. The practice guidelines for primary care of acute abdomen 2015. *Jpn J Radiol* 2016;34:80–115

department (ED) to decrease healthcare provider exposure; this has proven to be especially relevant in the COVID-19 era [4, 5].

Initial Evaluation

The acuity of presentation determines the extent of preoperative evaluation and assessment. All patients with abdominal pain should have an orderly and systematic evaluation. Patients who present with sudden, severe abdominal pain and unstable vital signs or who are thought to have a life-threatening condition may require an operation after only a brief history and physical exam by an experienced surgeon. In general, these patients may have ongoing intraperitoneal bleeding with shock state, perforated hollow viscus with peritonitis and septic shock, or acute transmural bowel ischemia [2].

Given all that, all patients with acute abdomen need to be assessed on urgent bases. When receiving a consult for an acute abdomen, it is important to ask about the initial and current vital signs to assess for hemodynamic normalcy. Upon bedside assessment, clinicians will need to attend to the "ABC" (airway, breathing, and circulation). Depending upon the above information, the patient is conceptually categorized to "sick" or "non-sick" (Fig. 2.1). Patients with an acute abdomen that belong to the "sick" category usually require prompt resuscitation starting at the emergency department (ED). In contrast, patients who are "non-sick" follow the traditional management pathway that includes a detailed history and physical exam, proper workup with labs, and imaging to be followed by definitive management. For the "sick" patient category, once airway and breathing are dealt with, special attention is given to circulation. Intravenous access (IV) is of prime importance ideally with a 16–18-gauge IV access in both antecubital veins with rapid infusions of physiologically balanced warm crystalloid solution to restore tissue perfusion and maintain hemodynamic normalcy. If bleeding is evident or suspected, the patient should be volume resuscitated with balanced blood products. A focused history and physical exam are concur-

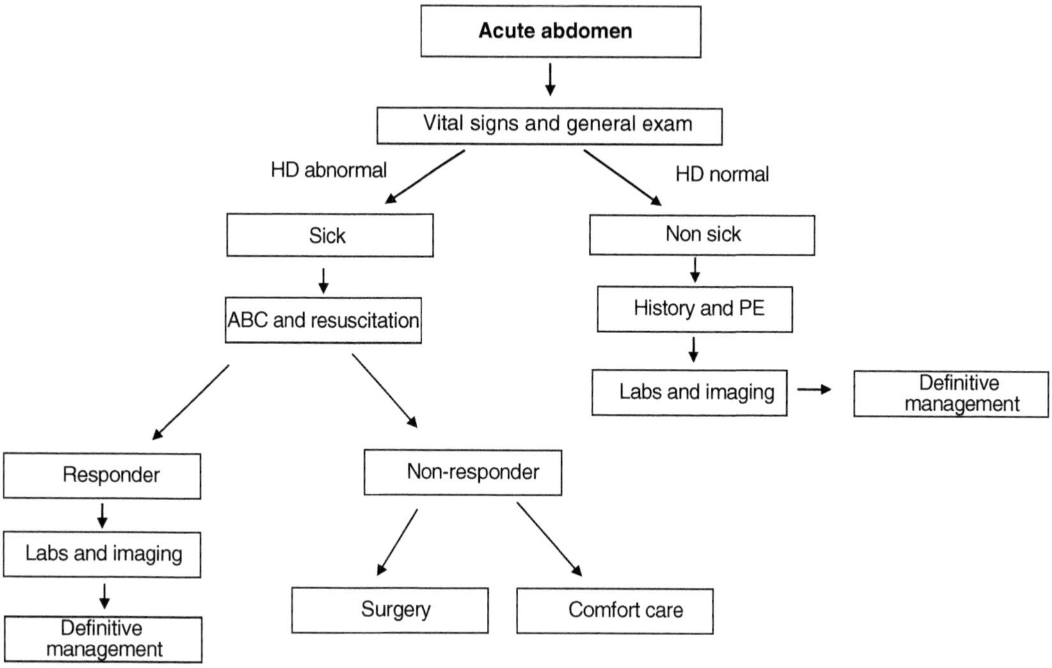

Fig. 2.1 Algorithm for triaging with acute abdomen

rently performed during resuscitation. After restoring hemodynamic normalcy in responders, a detailed assessment follows. For nonresponders, a rapid decision should be made to perform an operative intervention versus comfort care if surgery is not in line with the patient's goals of care.

While assessing patients with acute abdomen, it is important to apply the communication principles of relationship-centered care while responding to the patient and family's emotions using the PEARLS (partnership, empathy, apology/acknowledgment, respect, legitimation, and support) mnemonic [6].

History

History remains one of the essential elements in assessing a patient presenting with an acute abdomen. A thorough, detailed history should only be completed after adequate resuscitation and attending to the patient's airway, breathing, and circulation (ABC). History usually starts with the chief complaint and duration, followed by a detailed history of present illness (HPI) with a review of systems, past medical history, past surgical history, medications and allergy, social history, and family history. On HPI, abdominal pain should be thoroughly analyzed using the widely used acronym OPQRST-AAA (onset, position, quality, radiation, severity, timing, aggravation factors, alleviating factors, associated symptoms such as fever, chills, nausea, vomiting, or change in bowel habits). To help narrow down the differential, it is important to briefly review the pathophysiology and embryologic origin of abdominal pain. Clinical presentation of acute abdominal pain is due to irritation of the sensory-rich visceral and parietal peritoneum. This irritation presents as abdominal pain on history, tenderness, and guarding on physical examination. When only the visceral peritoneum is involved with the disease process, the initial pain is sometimes referred to as visceral pain which is the stretch of the visceral peritoneum and the activation of parasympathetic fibers. Visceral pain is often characterized by dull and poorly localized pain and is referred to along the embryologic origins of the structures involved, easily remembered by their associated blood supply.

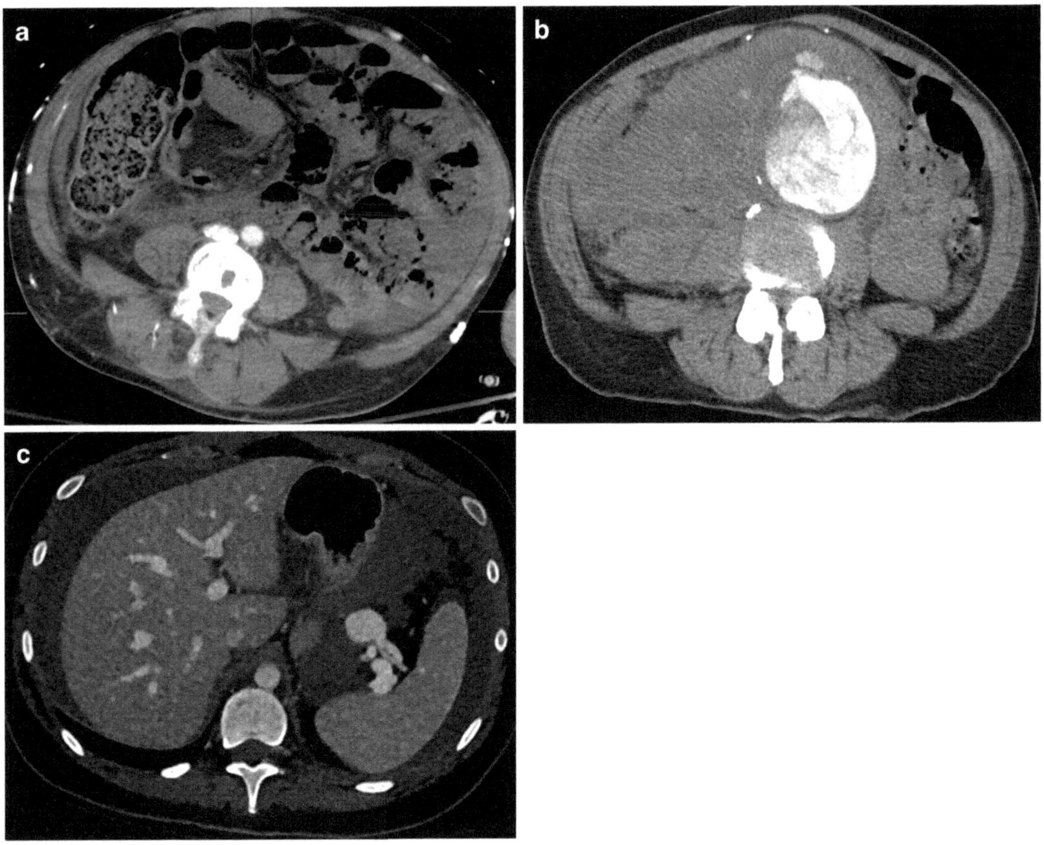

Fig. 2.3 (**a**) Mesenteric ischemia of the small bowel and right colon. (**b**) Ruptured abdominal aortic aneurysm with intravenous contrast. (**c**) Ruptured splenic artery aneurysm with hemoperitoneum

References

1. National Hospital Ambulatory Medical Care Survey: 2015 Emergency department summary tables 2015;34.
2. Langell JT, Mulvihill SJ. Gastrointestinal perforation and the acute abdomen. Med Clin North Am. 2008;92(3):599–625.
3. van Duren BH, Moghul M, Appleton SG, Boxel GI, v. The acute abdomen. BMJ. 2013;346:f2549.
4. Nassar AK, Lin DT, Spain DA, Knowlton LM. Using a virtual platform for personal protective equipment education and training. Med Educ. 2020; https://doi.org/10.1111/medu.14321.
5. Stewart CL, Thornblade LW, Diamond DJ, Fong Y, Melstrom LG. Personal protective equipment and COVID-19. Ann Surg. 2020;272(2):e132–8.
6. Beach MC, Inui T. The relationship-centered care research network. Relationship-centered care J Gen Intern Med. 2006;21(1):3–8.
7. Pinto A, Miele V, Laura Schillirò M, Nasuto M, Chiaese V, Romano L, et al. Spectrum of signs of pneumoperitoneum. Semin Ultrasound CT MRI. 2016;37(1):3–9.
8. Smith JK, Lobo DN. Investigation of the acute abdomen. Surg Oxf. 2012;30(6):296–305.
9. Felder S, Margel D, Murrell Z, Fleshner P. Usefulness of bowel sound auscultation: a prospective evaluation. J Surg Educ. 2014;71(5):768–73.
10. Golledge J, Toms AP, Franklin IJ, Scriven MW, Galland RB. Assessment of peritonism in appendicitis. Ann R Coll Surg Engl. 1996;78(1):11–4.
11. Paulson EK, Kalady MF, Pappas TN. Suspected appendicitis. N Engl J Med. 2003 Jan;348(3):236–42.
12. Alvarado A. A practical score for the early diagnosis of acute appendicitis. Ann Emerg Med. 1986;15(5):557–64.
13. Quinn J, Zeleny T, Rajaratnam V, Ghiurluc D-L, Bencko V. Debate: the per rectal/digital rectal examination exam in the emergency department, still best practice? Int J Emerg Med. 2018;11(1):20.
14. Kessler C. Assessing the utility of digital rectal exams in the ED. Acad Emerg Med Off J Soc Acad Emerg Med. 2012;19(6):693.

15. Adedeji OA, McAdam WA. Murphy's sign, acute cholecystitis and elderly people. J R Coll Surg Edinb. 1996;41(2):88–9.
16. Yeh B. Does this adult patient have appendicitis? Ann Emerg Med. 2008;52(3):301–3.
17. Nagurney JT, Brown DFM, Chang Y, Sane S, Wang AC, Weiner JB. Use of diagnostic testing in the emergency department for patients presenting with non-traumatic abdominal pain. J Emerg Med. 2003;25(4):363–71.
18. Sakka V, Tsiodras S, Giamarellos-Bourboulis EJ, Giamarellou H. An update on the etiology and diagnostic evaluation of a leukemoid reaction. Eur J Intern Med. 2006;17(6):394–8.
19. Little P, Turner S, Rumsby K, Warner G, Moore M, Lowes JA, et al. Developing clinical rules to predict urinary tract infection in primary care settings: sensitivity and specificity of near patient tests (dipsticks) and clinical scores. Br J Gen Pract. 2006;56(529):606–12.
20. Keim V, Teich N, Fiedler F, Hartig W, Thiele G, Mössner J. A comparison of lipase and amylase in the diagnosis of acute pancreatitis in patients with abdominal pain. Pancreas. 1998;16(1):45–9.
21. Ismail OZ, Bhayana V. Lipase or amylase for the diagnosis of acute pancreatitis? Clin Biochem. 2017;50(18):1275–80.
22. Yu C-W, Juan L-I, Wu M-H, Shen C-J, Wu J-Y, Lee C-C. Systematic review and meta-analysis of the diagnostic accuracy of procalcitonin, C-reactive protein and white blood cell count for suspected acute appendicitis. Br J Surg. 2013;100(3):322–9.
23. Liu Z, Meng Z, Li Y, Zhao J, Wu S, Gou S, et al. Prognostic accuracy of the serum lactate level, the SOFA score and the qSOFA score for mortality among adults with sepsis. Scand J Trauma Resusc Emerg Med. 2019;27(1):51.
24. Kruse O, Grunnet N, Barfod C. Blood lactate as a predictor for in-hospital mortality in patients admitted acutely to hospital: a systematic review. Scand J Trauma Resusc Emerg Med. 2011;19(1):74.
25. Eisenberg RL, Heineken P, Hedgcock MW, Federle M, Goldberg HI. Evaluation of plain abdominal radiographs in the diagnosis of abdominal pain. Ann Surg. 1983;197(4):464–9.
26. Mayumi T, Yoshida M, Tazuma S, Furukawa A, Nishii O, Shigematsu K, et al. The practice guidelines for primary care of acute abdomen 2015. Jpn J Radiol. 2016;34(1):80–115.
27. MacKersie AB, Lane MJ, Gerhardt RT, Claypool HA, Keenan S, Katz DS, et al. Nontraumatic acute abdominal pain: unenhanced helical CT compared with three-view acute abdominal series. Radiology. 2005;237(1):114–22.
28. Rosen MP, Sands DZ, Longmaid HE, Reynolds KF, Wagner M, Raptopoulos V. Impact of abdominal CT on the management of patients presenting to the emergency department with acute abdominal pain. Am J Roentgenol. 2000;174(5):1391–6.
29. O'Malley RG, Al-Hawary MM, Kaza RK, Wasnik AP, Platt JF, Francis IR. MDCT findings in small bowel obstruction: implications of the cause and presence of complications on treatment decisions. Abdom Imaging. 2015;40(7):2248–62.
30. Hayakawa K, Tanikake M, Yoshida S, Yamamoto A, Yamamoto E, Morimoto T. CT findings of small bowel strangulation: the importance of contrast enhancement. Emerg Radiol. 2013;20(1):3–9.
31. Missiroli C, Singh AK. Nontraumatic emergencies of abdominal aorta. Semin Ultrasound CT MRI. 2008;29(5):369–77.

The Clinical Pulmonary Infection Score (CPIS) is used to aid in the diagnosis of ventilator-associated pneumonia (VAP). It consists of a six-point clinical score that consists of body temperature, white blood cell count, volume and character of tracheal secretions, arterial oxygenation, chest X-ray characteristics, gram stain of tracheal aspirate, and culture of tracheal aspirate. CPIS greater than six has been correlated with risk of mortality, with arterial oxygenation being the strongest predictor [6, 7]. Its high interrater variability, however, significantly limits its use as a diagnostic tool.

The Pulmonary Embolism Severity Index (PESI) is based on 10 physiologic and diagnostic data points and estimates a patient's risk of mortality following diagnosis of an acute pulmonary embolism [8]. There is also a simplified version, sPESI, which is based on five variables (age greater than 80 years, cancer history, previous diagnosis of cardiopulmonary disease, heart rate >110 beats per minute, arterial oxygen saturation less than 90%). Both PESI and sPESI have been found to have good sensitivity following diagnosis of pulmonary embolism but exhibit specificities of less than 50% [9, 10].

The RIFLE Index is a set of criteria based on consensus definitions for analyzing the severity of acute kidney injury (AKI). The criteria include risk, injury, failure, loss of function, and end stage [11]. The Kidney Disease: Improving Global Outcomes (KDIGO) Staging System of AKI combines previously described classification systems, including RIFLE and Acute Kidney Injury Network (AKIN), with the aim of classifying severity of AKI and to offer corresponding management guidelines [12]. It evaluates changes in serum creatinine, hourly urine output, and glomerular filtration rate (GFR) to stage degree of AKI [13]. KDIGO scoring has been shown to be predictive of in-hospital mortality in both adult and pediatric populations [14–16].

Two commonly used scoring systems for hepatic function are the Child-Turcotte-Pugh (CTP) and the Model for End-Stage Liver Disease (MELD) score. The original version of the CTP, based on the presence of ascites, encephalopathy, nutritional status, serum bilirubin, and albumin, was introduced as a predictive score for operative mortality after portosystemic shunting for variceal bleeding [17]. It was later revised, replacing nutritional status with international normalized ratio (INR) as a measure of coagulopathy [18]. The original MELD score was derived to predict 3-month mortality in patients undergoing transjugular intrahepatic portosystemic shunt (TIPS) placement. It has been validated as a strong predictor of mortality due to hepatic derangement and is used as the primary rank scoring methodology for the United Network for Organ Sharing (UNOS) liver transplant list [19, 20]. A meta-analysis comparing CTP to MELD for patients admitted to the ICU suggested MELD may have better discriminatory capacity to predict endpoint events [20]. MELD score has also been shown to predict mortality in EGS patients [21].

Multi-organ Scoring Systems.

Several systems have been devised that incorporate a broad range of physiologic data points to estimate the severity of global physiologic derangement for the most critically ill patients. The Acute Physiology and Chronic Health Evaluation (APACHE) score was developed to stratify mortality risk in patients admitted to the ICU. It was originally based on 34 points of acute physiologic data collected in the first 24 hours of ICU admission along with health status prior to hospital admission [22]. In single-center reviews, the original APACHE score showed promising predictive reliability, though its use was limited because it was rather cumbersome to calculate. The APACHE II is a simplified version using 12 acute physiologic factors, age, and preexisting health status [23–28]. APACHE III expanded on the second version by incorporating a broader range of pre-admission data, including human immunodeficiency virus (HIV) status and diagnosis of hematological malignancy [29]. APACHE IV expands to a total of 142 variables [30]. Despite incorporating more data points, APACHE III and IV have not been shown to be superior to APACHE II in the clinical setting and therefore are not widely used due to relative complexity of their calculations.

The Simplified Acute Physiology Score (SAPS) incorporates the most severe values of 14 physiologic data point, plus age, collected in the first hour of ICU admission to predict likelihood of mortality. A second generation of the score, SAPS II, added prehospital health, specifically AIDS status, metastatic carcinoma, and hematologic malignancy [31]. In large, multicenter evaluations, SAPS II was found to have good discrimination but only mediocre model calibration [31]. SAPS III was derived from large, international databases, with improved model discrimination compared to SAPS II. However, the SAPS III models continue to require population-specific calibration, especially in comparison to its APACHE contemporaries, which overshadows its advantage of calculation [32, 33].

The Multiple Organ Dysfunction Score (MODS), Logistic Organ Dysfunction Score (LODS), and Sequential Organ Failure Assessment (SOFA) were all devised to predict mortality based on severity of multiple organ dysfunction [34–36]. MODS is based on severity of functional derangement of six organ systems (respiratory, renal, hepatic, cardiovascular, hematological, and central nervous system) at the time of ICU admission and again at any following 24-h interval, allowing for evaluation of the disease progression or effectiveness of treatment [34]. The calculated difference between subsequent scores and those scores obtained on the first day, the delta MODS (dMODS), has been strongly associated with ICU and in-hospital mortality [23, 34]. In contrast, a single LODS score calculated from the worst physiologic data from the same six organ systems during the first day of ICU admission has been validated as a predictor of ICU mortality [35, 37, 38].

The SOFA score was developed with the aim of evaluating the risk of morbidity, as compared to mortality, in patients diagnosed with sepsis after ICU admission. Derived from data collected from the European Society of Intensive Care Medicine, the SOFA score is calculated from physiologic data from the same six organ systems, but certain data points differ for ease of calculation. For example, the cardiovascular component for SOFA is focused on basic requirements for adrenergic support, while MODS requires an adjusted calculation for pressure adjusted heart rate [36]. The SOFA score is calculated 24 h after admission and then in 48-h intervals and has been validated as a predictor for both morbidity and mortality in septic patients as well as those with other etiologies of critical illness [36, 39–41]. The quick SOFA (qSOFA) is an abbreviated version based on three readily available clinical data points (respiratory rate, altered mentation, and systolic blood pressure). It has been validated for use in the emergency department setting for the purpose of early identification of non-ICU patients at risk of sepsis [42]. Further study is needed before use of this simplified score is generalizable to other patient populations [43, 44]. Studies comparing these organ dysfunction-based scoring systems directly to each other have yielded mixed results, indicating no one system is best and that the choice of these systems may be based upon patient population and available data [45–49].

The mortality prediction model (MPM) was developed for use at multiple time points to more accurately evaluate the probability of in-hospital death of ICU patients. MPM0 includes 15 physiologic variables, reflective of both acute and chronic status at the time of admission, and the MPM24 adds 8 additional variables, which can be repeated in 24-h intervals up to 72 h after ICU admission [50, 51]. A modified version described as MPM II is found to predict morbidity and mortality after 24 h of ICU admission and for changes in a patient's risk of mortality over time [50, 51]. Second and third generations of the score have been tailored toward further ease of calculation and improved calibration [52, 53].

Evolution of Scoring Systems for Emergency General Surgery

Definition and Burden of Emergency General Surgery Diseases

Prior to developing its own scoring system, the scope and burden of EGS diseases first had to be clearly delineated. In 2011, the AAST Committee on Severity Assessment and Patient Outcomes set out to do just that using a data-driven approach.

Unique International Classification of Diseases ninth Rev. (ICD-9) diagnosis codes were identified using billing data from seven large academic medical centers. The codes were then reviewed using a modified Delphi methodology and consensus achieved to identify primary EGS diagnoses [54]. Four hundred eight-five unique ICD-9 codes were identified, and clinically, they can be summarized into several areas: resuscitation, general abdominal conditions, intestinal obstruction, upper gastrointestinal tract, hepatic-pancreatic-biliary, colorectal, hernias, soft tissue, vascular, cardiothoracic, and others.

Taking this EGS diagnosis list, the Committee then used data from the National Inpatient Sample (NIS) to estimate the burden of EGS disease in the United States. They estimated over 4 million encounters occurred nationwide in the year 2009 for EGS diagnoses [54]. Furthermore, an estimated incidence of over 2.3 million patients required emergency admission. These findings served as important first steps in understanding the significance of EGS diseases and in standardizing the definition and subsequent management of these diseases.

Disease-Specific Scoring Systems

Prior to the work of the AAST Committee on Severity Assessment and Patient Outcomes, several scoring systems already existed for specific EGS diseases. The Ranson criteria is one of the best known scoring systems for measuring severity of acute pancreatitis [55]. Various demographic and physiologic variables are used to calculate the score at admission and at 48 hours after admission to help predict outcomes. Despite its wide use in clinical practice, other scores, like the Atlanta classification [56] and determinant-based classification [57], have been shown to be more accurate than Ranson criteria in predicting outcomes [58].

The Hinchey classification has been widely used as a severity of acute diverticulitis for risk adjustment in research and operative planning [59]. It defines Stage 1 as pericolonic or mesenteric abscess, Stage 2 as pelvic or retroperitoneal abscess, Stage 3 as purulent peritonitis, and Stage 4 as feculent peritonitis.

The Laboratory Risk Indicator for Necrotizing Fasciitis (LRINEC) score incorporates six laboratory values to create a score correlating to the likelihood of having a necrotizing soft tissue infection [60]. It has been shown to have a positive predictive value of 92% and a negative predictive value of 96%, which is useful for screening. It does not, however, incorporate any other anatomic or physiologic data.

Numerous additional disease-specific scores exist: the Alvarado score for acute appendicitis [61], the Tokyo classification of acute cholecystitis [62], and the Boey score for perforated duodenal ulcers [63]. They have each been shown to be helpful in outcome prediction in clinical practice and risk stratification in research studies. However, they all utilize a combination of demographic characteristics, anatomic, physiologic, and laboratory markers, making it difficult to determine the impact of anatomic severity of illness from other measurements. Furthermore, they each use different nomenclature and unique scales, with little transferability from one disease to another. These flaws all demonstrate the need for a simplified, uniform staging approach to measure and report severity of EGS diseases.

Development of AAST EGS Anatomic Grading Scales

In 2014, the AAST Committee on Patient Assessment and Outcomes introduced a novel grading system to describe the anatomic severity of EGS diseases [64]. Analogous to the already existing AAST Injury Scoring Scales for traumatic organ injuries and modeled after the TNM staging system for cancers, the aim was to provide reproducible anatomic descriptions of disease. Grading ranges from grade I for mild disease limited to the organ itself through grade V which describes severe widespread disease (Table 3.1). Noticeably, operative intervention is not included in grading, as the purpose of the scale is to measure severity of disease at presentation, regardless of the decision to operate. Furthermore, several EGS diseases can be managed nonoperatively.

The grading scale was then applied to eight commonly encountered gastrointestinal EGS conditions: appendicitis, perforated peptic ulcer, acute diverticulitis of the colon, acute cholecystitis, intestinal obstruction, arterial ischemic bowel, hernias, and acute pancreatitis [64]. An example of the application of the AAST anatomic grading scale to acute appendicitis is shown in Table 3.1. To further expand the standardization of describing severity of EGS diseases, the AAST anatomic grading scale was applied to eight additional EGS conditions [65]. The grading system now encompassed breast abscess, esophageal perforation, infectious colitis, pelvic inflammatory disease, perirectal abscess, pleural space infections, soft tissue infections, and surgical site infections. Anatomic severity tables for each of these disease entities are readily accessible to clinicians and researchers through the AAST [66].

Using similar methodologies, a mirror grading system was devised to standardize description of anatomic severity of hemorrhagic surgical diseases [67]. Scores again range from grade I to grade V, progressing from potential for hemorrhage to large-volume hemorrhage (Table 3.2). This was applied to four surgical bleeding diseases: bleeding esophageal varices, colonic diverticular hemorrhage, bleeding peptic ulcer disease, and ruptured abdominal aortic aneurysm. Similar to the scales developed for inflammatory/infectious surgical diseases, this system focuses on anatomic severity and excludes precise amount of hemorrhage, as patient responses

Table 3.1 Description of grading system for anatomic severity of disease in EGS

Grade	Description	Acute appendicitis
I	Local disease confined to the organ with minimal abnormality	Acutely inflamed appendix, intact
II	Local disease confined to the organ with severe abnormality	Gangrenous appendix, intact
III	Local extension beyond the organ	Perforated appendix with local contamination
IV	Regional extension beyond the organ	Perforated appendix with periappendiceal phlegmon or abscess
V	Widespread extension beyond the organ	Perforated appendix with generalized peritonitis

From Shafi S, Aboutanos M, Brown CVR, Ciesla D, Cohen MJ, Crandall ML, et al. Measuring anatomic severity of disease in emergency general surgery. J Trauma. 2014;76 (3):884–7. Used with permission from Wolters Kluwer Health Inc.

Table 3.2 Grading for surgical bleeding diseases

Grade	Anatomic severity of disease template	Bleeding esophageal varices
I	No hemorrhage but potential for hemorrhage	Visible varices on endoscopy with heme-positive gastric aspirate
II	Minimal volume of hemorrhage, no active bleeding	Visible varices with no active bleeding plus blood clot, red wale, or cherry-red spots on endoscopy
III	Limited volume of hemorrhage with no active bleeding or small amount of active bleed	First episode of limited active hemorrhage on endoscopy
IV	Moderate volume of hemorrhage or active bleeding	Recurrent (within 72 h) episode of limited active bleeding on endoscopy
V	Large volume of hemorrhage	Varices with massive, uncontrolled hemorrhage

From Tominaga GT, Brown CVR, Schulz, JT, Barbosa RR, Agarwal S, McQuay N, et al. The American Association for the Surgery of Trauma uniform grading of hemorrhagic emergency general surgery diseases. J Trauma. 2018;84 (4):670–3. Used with permission from Wolters Kluwer Health Inc.

can vary based on premorbid conditions. A more detailed description of the grading system and an example of its application are provided in Table 3.2.

Disease-Specific Data Dictionaries

In order to effectively use the AAST anatomic severity grading scale, reliable uniform definitions need to be achieved in order to, for example, risk stratify or compare outcomes. To promote this goal, data dictionaries with explicit definitions for each of the 16 EGS diseases were created [68]. Loosely based on the previously mentioned cancer staging system and trauma organ injury scale, the definitions use descriptions and grading in four categories: clinical, imaging, operative, and pathologic criteria. If the grade differs between the four categories, the highest grade is applied to the patient. Using these four distinct criteria also accounts for the fact that not all EGS diseases require operative intervention, and therefore grading does not rely solely on operative or pathologic findings. An example of the full data dictionary for acute cholecystitis is given in Table 3.3. Available data dictionaries for the

Table 3.3 Data dictionary for AAST grading system for acute cholecystitis

AAST grade	Description	Clinical criteria	Imaging criteria	Operative criteria	Pathologic criteria
I	Acute cholecystitis	RUQ or epigastric pain, Murphy sign, leukocytosis	Wall thickening, distention, gallstones or sludge, pericholecystic fluid, nonvisualization of the gallbladder on HIDA scan	Inflammatory changes localized to GB, wall thickening, distention, gallstones	Acute inflammatory changes in the GB wall without necrosis or pus
II	GB empyema or gangrenous cholecystitis or emphysematous cholecystitis	RUQ or epigastric pain, Murphy sign, leukocytosis	Above, plus air in GB lumen, wall, or biliary tree, focal mucosal defects without frank perforation	Distended GB with pus or hydrops, necrosis or gangrene of the wall, not perforated	Above, plus pus in the GB lumen, necrosis of GB wall, intramural abscess, epithelial sloughing, no perforation
III	GB perforation with local contamination	Localized peritonitis in RUQ	HIDA with focal transmural defect, extraluminal fluid collection or radiotracer but limited to RUQ	Perforated GB wall (noniatrogenic) with bile outside the GB but limited to RUQ	Necrosis with perforation of the GB wall (noniatrogenic)
IV	GB perforation with pericholecystic abscess or gastrointestinal fistula	Localized peritonitis at multiple locations, abdominal distention with symptoms of bowel obstruction	Abscess in RUQ outside GB, bilioenteric fistula, gallstone ileus	Pericholecystic abscess, bilioenteric fistula, gallstone ileus	Necrosis with perforation of the GB wall (noniatrogenic)
V	GB perforation with generalized peritonitis	Above, with generalized peritonitis	Free intraperitoneal bile	Above, plus generalized peritonitis	Necrosis with perforation of the GB wall (noniatrogenic)

From Tominaga GT, Staudenmayer KL, Shafi S, Schuster KM, Savage SA, Ross S, et al. The American Association for the Surgery of Trauma grading scale for 16 emergency general surgery conditions: Disease-specific criteria characterizing anatomic severity grading. J Trauma. 2016;81 (3):593–602. Used with permission from Wolters Kluwer Health Inc.

remaining EGS diseases are easily accessed through the AAST [66].

Validation of the AAST Anatomic Grading Scales

The AAST EGS grading system was developed based on expert opinion rather than evidence; therefore, validation studies were needed prior to its application to the clinical setting. Numerous such studies have been completed and have supported the grading scale's association with patient outcomes as well as its interrater reliability. Both single-institution and multicenter studies have supported the correlation of AAST EGS grade with patient outcomes in acute appendicitis. In a single-center retrospective cohort study, Hernandez et al. found that of 394 adult patients admitted with acute appendicitis over a 2-year period, increasing AAST EGS grade was associated with increased complications, need for open procedure, and increased length of stay [69]. Patients assigned with higher AAST grades were also more likely to be managed nonoperatively. They also found that AAST EGS grade based on preoperative imaging correlated well with grading based on operative findings.

To determine whether the grading scale can be applied outside the United States and in developing nations, data was retrospectively reviewed from multiple institutions within South Africa between 2010 and 2016 [70]. The group found that in this population, increasing AAST EGS grade was also associated with increased risk of postoperative complication. Several characteristics of the South African cohort should be noted, though. The included patients tended to present with more severe disease than what has been reported in the US cohort, with only 17.4% of the 1415 included patients with grade I disease and just over 38% presenting with grade V acute appendicitis based on intraoperative findings. Furthermore, 63.5% of appendectomies were completed via a midline laparotomy, 31.8% via a limited McBurney incision, and only 4.7% via laparoscopy. Despite these differences, the authors' ability to correlate grade with their cohort's outcomes supports the utility of the AAST EGS grading scale in a variety of populations.

The EAST Appendicitis Study included prospectively collected data from 27 centers [71]. Grading was assigned using the data dictionary for acute appendicitis, using the highest of the subscales in either clinical, radiographic, operative, or pathologic criteria. The authors found that of 2909 cases included, increasing AAST grade at the index hospitalization was associated with infectious complications, Clavien-Dindo class, hospital length of stay, and secondary interventions [71]. This again supported the AAST EGS grading scale as a valid tool to define anatomic severity of disease and to help predict clinical outcomes.

The AAST grading system for acute colonic diverticulitis has also been validated in single-center and multicenter studies [72, 73]. Increasing grade was independently associated with adverse events and increased length of stay, adjusting for factors such as age, comorbidities, and physiology.

The AAST EGS grading system for breast infections was studied both at an academic medical center in the United States and at an institution in South Africa [74]. They found increasing grade correlated with the type of treatment received at both locations, with milder infections receiving more oral antibiotics and more severe disease receiving more intravenous antibiotics. Grade also correlated with the need for procedural intervention to treat the infection and the need for multiple interventions. More severe infections by AAST grade were also more likely to experience complications with higher Clavien-Dindo class. This study not only was able to link AAST grading for breast infections with patient outcomes but also recommended initial treatment.

Another multinational study evaluated the AAST EGS grading scale for adhesive small bowel disease by retrospectively reviewing data from four countries: the United States, Italy, South Africa, and Romania [75]. Using imaging and operative findings to assign grade, they found that lower-grade disease was more likely to undergo successful nonoperative management and higher grades were associated with the need for small bowel resection, creation of an ileostomy, and need for temporary abdominal closure. Higher-grade disease was also associated with longer operative times. Disease grade was also incrementally associated with complications, specifically incidence of pneumonia, higher Clavien-Dindo class, need for ICU admission, and longer hospital length of stay. AAST EGS grade was also independently associated with 30-day mortality. Here, again, the applicability of the AAST EGS grading scale in predicting patient outcomes and also in potentially informing early management decisions in a global patient population was demonstrated.

A multicenter validation study associated patient outcomes with EGS grading scale for skin and soft tissue infections (STI) [76]. Data from 1170 patients at 12 institutions were retrospectively reviewed. Higher STI grade was associated with increased need for vasopressor support, recurrent infection at original STI site, general complications, total number of surgeries, ICU and total length of stay, and likelihood of discharge to someplace other than home. Severity of disease was also correlated with mortality, though this was a bimodal rather than linear relationship, with peaks in grade 2 and grade 5 disease. To provide context of the new grading scale with existing scoring systems, LRINEC scores were calculated for all patients and found to increase with increasing AAST grade. Interestingly, though, the predictive threshold appears to be lower, with median LRINEC scores of 4 for AAST grade 4 and grade 5 STI, whereas LRINEC score 6 has been the traditionally used threshold.

Since the introduction of the AAST EGS anatomic severity grading scale, validation studies for many more EGS diseases have been completed, including acute pancreatitis and acute cholecystitis [77, 78]. Taken together, they demonstrate that EGS grading scales can easily be used in disparate EGS disease processes and can be predictive of patient outcomes.

The breast infection grading system had disparate interrater reliability when applied to different populations [74]. When applied at a large academic medical center, 100 percent agreement was achieved. However, when the same group evaluated a cohort from South Africa, poor reliability was found, with greatest discrepancy in scoring involving grades 2 and 3 breast infections. The authors posited that it largely stemmed from the availability of ultrasonography to distinguish between the two. However, the poor interrater reliability in a more diverse, resource-limited setting highlights the potential for improvement to support more global application of the grading scale. In its application to STI, there was moderate interrater reliability observed [76]. The highest concordance was seen when grading based on operative criteria, and more variability was noted when using clinical, radiologic, or pathologic criteria. Given the mixed findings in interrater reliability, as the grading scales for various EGS diseases are refined, there is potential for improvement to achieve a global, standardized definition.

Limitations of Solely Anatomic-Based Grading

While the AAST EGS grading scale has found success in providing a uniform language to describe severity of surgical disease, there are several limitations to applying a solely anatomic definition to clinical practice. First, regarding the design of the AAST EGS grading scales themselves, several components, specifically the operative findings and pathologic criteria, are available only after treatment, limiting its use to a retrospective role. An ideal scoring system would allow for early risk stratification, prediction of outcomes, and guidance on management at the time of presentation.

It is widely acknowledged that many other patient factors outside of anatomic severity of disease influence clinical outcomes. Frailty has been associated with increased perioperative morbidity and mortality in elective procedures and more recently in emergency general surgery operations [79, 80]. Comorbid medical conditions also impact long-term expected survival, as originally described by the Charlson Comorbidity Index [81], and are prominent in tools such as the

American College of Surgeons National Surgical Quality Improvement Program (ACS NSQIP) Risk Calculator, which has become central in preoperative preparations and patient counseling [82]. Combinations of comorbidities have also been demonstrated to portend increased morbidity compared to single comorbidities specifically in EGS diseases [83].

Physiologic derangement can also play an important role in influencing patient outcomes. When physiology scores, specifically markers of systemic inflammatory response syndrome, and comorbidity were added to AAST EGS grade, the new scoring system improved upon the AAST anatomic grade alone in predicting in-hospital mortality, in-hospital complications, and extended hospital stay [84]. The ideal scoring system will likely build upon the AAST anatomic grading system and incorporate physiology at presentation, preexisting comorbidities, and frailty to provide a well-rounded evaluation of patients and allow for prediction of outcomes and guidance of early management strategies.

Applications of the AAST EGS Grading Scales

The availability and easy application of the AAST EGS grading scales make it a useful tool for clinicians and researchers alike. The data dictionaries for each EGS disease provide detailed criteria, many of which are readily available at the time of admission. With increasing regionalization and multidisciplinary approach to patient care, the AAST EGS grading scales allow for standardization across institutions and providers. It provides a common language for more effective handoffs between care teams.

The implications for improving research and quality of care benchmarks in EGS diseases are plentiful. The data dictionaries provide explicit guidance in creating data registries for EGS diseases, which can be particularly useful in relatively rare diseases. There is the potential for large-scale projects akin to ACS NSQIP or Trauma Quality Improvement Program (TQIP). Using standardized definitions also improves accuracy of research and potential for multicenter and multinational investigations.

The AAST EGS grading scales can benefit surgical education as we train future generations of surgeons. Residents learn precision in how they describe and define commonly encountered EGS conditions and the implications it can have on their patients' expected clinical course and outcomes. It also allows for evaluation and comparison of experiences between trainees and training programs.

Conclusions

The AAST EGS anatomic grading scale provides a standardized language to describe the severity of common EGS diseases. Grade of anatomic severity has been shown to correlate with outcomes in validation studies. Its application provides opportunities to inform patient management, to create data registries, and to improve the quality of research on EGS diseases.

References

1. Antman EMCM, Bernick PJ, McCabe CH, Horacek T, Papuchis G, Mautner B, Corbalan R, Radley D, Braunwald E. The TIMI risk score for unstable angina/non-ST elevation MI: a method for prognostication decision making. JAMA. 2000;248(7):835.
2. Hess EPAD, Chandara S, Murad MH, Erwin PJ, Hollander JE, Montori VM, Stiell IG. Diagnostic accuracy of the TIMI risk score in patients with chest pain in the emergency department: a meta-analysis. CMAJ. 2010;182(10):1039–44.
3. Morrow DAAE, Charlesworth A, Cairns R, Murphy SA, de Lemons JA, Giugliano RP, McCabe CH, Braunwald E. TIMI risk score for ST-elevation myocardial infarction: a convenient, bedside, clinical score for risk assessment at presentation. Circulation. 2000;102:2031–7.
4. Fox KADO, Goldberg RJ, Pieper KS, Eagle KA, Van de Werf F, Avezum A, Goodman SG, Flather MD, Anderson FA Jr, Granger CB. Prediction of risk of death and myocardial infarction in the six months after presentation with acute coronary syndrome: prospective multinational observational study (GRACE). BMJ. 2006;333(7578):1098.
5. Tang EWWC, Herbison P. Global registry of acute coronary events (GRACE) hospital discharge risk score

accurately predicts long-term mortality post acute coronary syndrome. Am Heart J. 2007;153(1):29–35.
6. Schurink CAVNC, Jacobs JA, Rozenberg-Arska M, Joore HC, Buskens E, Hoepelman AI, Bonten MJ. Clinical pulmonary infections score for ventilator-assisted pneumonia: accuracy and inter-observer variability. Intensive Care Med. 2004;30(2):217–24.
7. Luna CMBD, Niederman MS, Matarucco W, Baredes NC, Desmery P, Palizas F, Menga G, Rios F, Apezteguia C. Resolution of ventilator associated pneumonia: prospective evaluation of the clinical pulmonary infection score as an early clinical predictor of outcome. Crit Care Med. 2003;31:676–82.
8. Aujesky DOD, Stone RA, Auble TE, Perrier A, Cornuz J, Roy PM, Fine MJ. Derivation and validation of a prognostic model for pulmonary embolism. Am J Respir Crit Care Med. 2005;172(8):1041.
9. Jimenez DAD, Moores L, Gomez V, Lobo JL, Uresandi F, Otero R, Monreal M, Muiriel A, Yusen RD, RIETE Investigators. Simplification of the pulmonary embolism severity index for prognostication in patients with acute symptomatic pulmonary embolism. Arch Intern Med. 2010;170(15):1383.
10. Kohn CGME, Parker MW, Hernandez AV, Coleman CI. Prognostic accuracy of clinical prediction rules for early post-pulmonary embolism in all-cause mortality: a bivariate meta-analysis. Chest. 2015;147(4):1043.
11. Bellomo RRC, Kellum JA, Mehta RL, Palevsky PM, the Acute Dialysis Quality Initiative Workgroup. Acute renal failure—definition, outcome measures, animal models, fluid therapy and informational technology needs: the Second International Consensus Conference of the Acute Dialysis Quality (ADQI) Group. Crit Care. 2004;8:R204–12.
12. Lopes JA, et al. The RIFLE and AKIN classifications for acute kidney injury: a critical and comprehensive review. Clin Kidney J. 2013;6(1):8–14.
13. Group KDIGOKAKIW. KDIGO clinical practice guideline for acute kidney injury. Kidney Int. 2012:1–138.
14. Fuji TUS, Takinami M, Bellomo R. Validation of the kidney disease improving global outcomes criteria for AKI and comparison of three criteria in hospitalized patients. Clin J Am Soc Nephrol. 2014;9(5):848–54.
15. Selewski DTCT, Heung M, Troost JP, Ehrmann BJ, Lombel RM, Blatt NB, Luckritz K, Hieber S, Gajarksi R, Kershaw DB, Shanley TP, Gipson DS. Validation of KDIGO acute kidney injury criteria in a pediatric critical care population. Intensive Care Med. 2014;40(10):1481–8.
16. Jha VKV. Acute kidney injury: validating the KDIGO definition and staging—one step at a time. Nat Rev Nephrol. 2014;10:550–1.
17. Child CTJ. The liver and portal hypertension. In: Child C, editor. Surgery and portal hypertension. Philadelphia, WB Saunders; 1964. p. 50–8.
18. Pugh RNM-LI, Dawson JL. Transection of the oesophagus for bleeding oesophageal varicies. Br J Surg. 1973;60:646–9.
19. Kamath PSKW. The model for end-stage liver disease (MELD). Hepatology. 2007;45(3):797–805.
20. Peng YXQ, Guo X. Child-Pugh versus MELD score for the assessment of prognosis in liver cirrhosis. A systematic review and meta-analysis of observational studies. Medicine. 2016;95(8):e2877.
21. Havens JMCA, Olufajo OA, Askari R, Salim A, Christopher KB. Association of model for end-stage liver disease score with mortality in emergency general surgery patients. JAMA Surg. 2016;151(7):e160789.
22. Knauss WAZJ, Wagner DP, Draper EA, Lawrence DE. APACHE—acute physiology and chronic health evaluation: a physiologically based classification system. Crit Care Med. 1981;9(8):591–7.
23. Bouch DCTJ. Severity scoring systems in the critically ill. Contin Educ Anaesth Crit Care Pain. 2008;8(5):181–5.
24. Larvin MMM. APACHE-II score for assessment and monitoring of acute pancreatitis. Lancet. 1989;2(8656):201–5.
25. Capuzzo MVV, Sgarbi A, Bortolazzi S, Pavroni V, Gilli G, Gritti G, Alvisi R. Validation of severity scoring systems SAPS II and APACHE II in a single center population. Intensive Care Med. 2000;26(12):1779–85.
26. Headley JTR, Smith TL. Independent validation of APACHE II severity illness score for predicting mortality in patients with breast cancer admitted to the intensive care unit. Cancer. 1992;70(2):497–503.
27. Sanchez-Hurtaldo LAA-VA, Tejeda-Huezo BC, Garcia-Cruz JC, Juarez-Cedillo T. Validation of a prognostic score for mortality in elderly patients admitted to intensive care unit. Indian J Crit Care Med. 2016;20(12):695–700.
28. Knaus WADE, Wagner DP, Zimmerman JE. APACHE II: a severity of disease classification system. Crit Care Med. 1985;13(10):818–29.
29. Knaus WAWD, Draper EA, Zimmerman JE, Bergner M, Bastos PG, Sirio CA, Murphy DJ, Lotring T, Damiano A. The APACHE III prognostic system. Risk prediction of hospital mortality for critically ill hospitalized adults. Chest. 1991;100(6):1619–36.
30. Zimmerman JEKA, McNair DS, Malila FM. Acute physiology and chronic health evaluation (APACHE) IV: hospital mortality assessment for today's critically ill patients. Crit Care Med. 2006;34(5):12977–1310.
31. Le Gall J-R, Saulnier F. A new simplified acute physiology score (SAPS II) based on a European/North American multicenter study. JAMA. 1993;270:2957–63.
32. Metnitz PGMR, Almeida E, Jordan B, Bauer P, Campos RA, Iapichino G, Edbrooke D, Capuzzo M, Le Gall JR, SAPS 3 Investigators. SAPS 3—from evaluation of the patient to evaluation of the intensive care

unit. Part 1: objectives, methods, and cohort description. Intensive Care Med. 2005;31(10):1336–44.
33. Poole DRC, Anghileri A, Giardino M, Latronico N, Radrizzani D, Langer M, Bertolini G. External validation of the simplified acute physiology score (SAPS) 3 in a cohort of 28, 357 patients from 147 Italian intensive care units. Intensive Care Med. 2009;35(11):1916.
34. Marhsall JCCD, Christou NV, Bernard GR, Sprung CL, Sibbald WJ. Multiple organ dysfunction score: a reliable descriptor of a complex clinical outcome. Crit Care Med. 1995;23(10):1638–52.
35. Le Gall J-RKJ, Lemeshow S, Saulnier F, Alberty C, Artigas A, Teres D. The logistic organ dysfunction system: a new way to assess organ dysfunction in the intensive care unit. JAMA. 1996;276(10):802–10.
36. Vincent JLMR, Takala J, Willatts S, De Mendonca A, Bruining H, Reinhart CK, Suter PM, Thijs LG. The SOFA (sepsis-related organ failure assessment) score to describe organ dysfunction/failure. On behalf of the working group on sepsis-related problems of the European society of intensive care medicine. Intensive Care Med. 1996;22(7):707–10.
37. Metnitz PGHLGJ-R, Steltzer H, Krenn CG, Lang T, Valentin A. Evaluation of the logistic organ dysfunction system for the assessment of organ dysfunction and mortality in critically ill patients. Intensive Care Med. 2001;27:992–8.
38. Kim TKYJ. Comparison of the predictive power of the LODS and APACHE ii scoring systems in a neurological intensive care unit. J Int Med Res. 2012;40:777–86.
39. Namendys-Silva SAT-BJ, Herrera-Gomez A. Application of the sequential organ failure assessment score to patients with cancer admitted to the intensive care unit. Am J Hosp Palliat Care. 2009;26(5):341–6.
40. Badreldin AMDF, Ismail MM, Heldwein MB, Lehmann T, Bayer O, Doesnst T, Hekmat K. Comparison between the sequential organ failure assessment score (SOFA) and cardiac surgery score (CASUS) for mortality prediction after cardiac surgery. Thorac Cardiovasc Surg. 2012;60(1):35–42.
41. Craig DGRT, Wright EC, Martin KG, Davidson JS, Haves PC, Simpson KJ. The sequential organ failure assessment (SOFA) score is prognostically superior to the model for end-stage liver disease (MELD) and MELD variants following paracetamol (acetaminophen) overdose. Aliment Pharmacol Ther. 2012;35(6):705–13.
42. Raith EPUA, Bailey M, McGloughlin S, MacIsaac C, Bellomo R, Pilcher DV. Australian and new Zealand Intensive Care Society (ANZICS) Centre for Outcomes and Resource Evaluation (CORE). Prognostic accuracy of the SOFA score, SIRS criteria, and qSOFA score for in-hospital mortality among adults with suspected infection admitted to the intensive care unit. JAMA. 2017;317(3):290–300.
43. Seymour CWLV, Iwashyna TJ, Brunkhorst FM, Rea TD, Scherag A, Rubenfeld G, Kahn JM, Shanker-HAri M, Singer M, DEutschman CS, Escobar GJ, Angus DC. Assessment of clinical criteria for sepsis: for the third international consensus definitions for sepsis and septic shock (sepsis-3). JAMA. 2016;315(8):762–74.
44. Freund YLN, Krastinova E, Van Laer M, Claessens YE, Avondo A, Occelli C, Feral-Pierssens AL, Truchot J, Ortega M, Carnerio B, Pernet J, Claret PG, Dami F, Bloom B, Riou B, Beaune S, French Society of Emergency Medicine Collaborators Group. Prognostic accuracy of sepsis-3 criteria for in-hospital mortality among patients with suspected infection presenting to the emergency department. JAMA. 2017;31(3):301–8.
45. Peres Bota DMC, Lopes Ferreira F, Nguyen Ba V, Vincent JL. The multiple organ dysfunction score (MODS) versus the sequential organ failure assessment (SOFA) score in outcome prediction. Intensive Care Med. 2002;28(11):1619–24.
46. B K. A comparison of three organ dysfunction scores: MODS, SOFA, and LOD for predicting ICU mortality in critically ill patients. J Med Assoc Thail. 2007;90(6):1074–81.
47. Johnson SSA. Comparison of different scoring systems used in the intensive care unit. J Pulm Respir Med. 2015;5(276)
48. Pettila VPM, Sarna S. Comparison of multiple organ dysfunction scores in the prediction of hospital mortality in the critically ill. Crit Care Med. 2002;30(8):1705–11.
49. Salluh JISM. ICU severity of illness scores: APACHE, SAPS, and MPM. Curr Opin Crit Care. 2014;20(5):557–65.
50. Lemeshow SKJ, Teres D, Avrunin JS, Gelbah SH, Rappoport J, Rue M. Mortality probability models for patients in the intensive care unit for 48 or 72 hours: a prospective multicenter study. Crit Care Med. 1994;22(9):1351–8.
51. Lemeshow STD, Klar J, Avrunin JS, Gehlbach SH, Rapoport J. Mortality probability models (MPM II) based on an international cohort of intensive care unit patients. JAMA. 1993;270(20):2478–86.
52. Higgins TLKA, Nathanson BH, Copes W, Stark M, Teres D. Prospective validation of the intensive care unity mortality prediction model (MPM). Crit Care Med. 2009;37(5):1619.
53. Higgins TLTD, Copes WS, Nathanson BH, Stark M, Kramer AA. Assessing contemporary intensive care unit outcome: an updated mortality probability admission model (MPMM0-III). Crit Care Med. 2007;35(3):827–35.
54. Shafi S, Aboutanos MB, Agarwal S, Brown CVR, Crandall M, Feliciano DV, et al. Emergency general

surgery: definition and estimated burden of disease. J Trauma. 2013;74(4):1092–7.
55. Ranson JH, Rifkind KM, Roses DF, et al. Prognostic signs and the role of operative management in acute pancreatitis. Surg Gynecol Obstet. 1974;139(1):69–81.
56. Bradley EL 3rd. A clinically based classification system for acute pancreatitis. Summary of the international symposium on acute pancreatitis, Atlanta, Ga, September 11 through 13, 1992. Arch Surg. 1993;128(5):586–90.
57. Dellinger EP, Forsmark CE, Layer P, et al. Determinant-based classification of acute pancreatitis severity: an international multidisciplinary consultation. Ann Surg. 2012;256(6):875–80.
58. Kadiyala V, Suleiman SL, McNabb-Baltar J, et al. The Atlanta classification, revised Atlanta classification, and determinant-based classification of acute pancreatitis: which is best at stratifying outcomes? Pancreas. 2016;45(4):510–5.
59. Hinchey EJ, Schaal PG, Richards GK. Treatment of perforated diverticular disease of the colon. Adv Surg. 1978;12:85–109.
60. Wong CH, Khin LW, Heng KS, et al. The LRINEC (laboratory risk indicator for necrotizing fasciitis) score: a tool for distinguishing necrotizing fasciitis from other soft tissue infections. Crit Care Med. 2004;32(7):1535–41.
61. Alvarado A. A practical score for the early diagnosis of acute appendicitis. Ann Emerg Med. 1986;15(5):557–64.
62. Hirota M, Takada T, Kawarada Y, et al. Diagnostic criteria and severity assessment of acute cholecystitis: Tokyo guidelines. J Hepato-Biliary-Pancreat Surg. 2007;14(1):78–82.
63. Boey J, Choi SK, Poon A, et al. Risk stratification in perforated duodenal ulcers. A prospective validation of predictive factors. Ann Surg. 1987;205(1):22–6.
64. Shafi S, Aboutanos M, Brown CVR, Ciesla D, Cohen MJ, Crandall ML, et al. Measuring anatomic severity of disease in emergency general surgery. J Trauma. 2014;76(3):884–7.
65. Crandall ML, Agarwal S, Muskat P, Ross S, Savage S, Schuster K, et al. Application of a uniform anatomic grading system to measure disease severity in eight emergency general surgical illnesses. J Trauma. 2014;77(5):705–8.
66. American Association for the Surgery of Trauma. Data dictionaries for AAST grading system for EGS conditions. http://www.aast.org/emergency-general-surgery-anatomic-grading-scales. Accessed 9 July 2020.
67. Tominaga GT, Brown CVR, Schulz JT, Barbosa RR, Agarwal S, McQuay N, et al. The American Association for the Surgery of Trauma uniform grading of hemorrhagic emergency general surgery diseases. J Trauma. 2018;84(4):670–3.
68. Tominaga GT, Staudenmayer KL, Shafi S, Schuster KM, Savage SA, Ross S, et al. The American Association for the Surgery of Trauma grading scale for 16 emergency general surgery conditions: disease-specific criteria characterizing anatomic severity grading. J Trauma. 2016;81(3):593–602.
69. Hernandez MC, Aho JM, Habermann EB, Choudhry AJ, Morris DS, Zielinski MD. Increased anatomic severity predicts outcomes: validation of the American Association for the Surgery of Trauma's emergency general surgery score in appendicitis. J Trauma. 2017;82(1):73–9.
70. Hernandez MC, Kong VY, Aho JM, Bruce JL, Polites SF, Laing GL, et al. Increased anatomic severity in appendicitis is associated with outcomes in a South African population. J Trauma. 2017;83(1):175–81.
71. Vasileiou G, Ray-Zack M, Zielinski M, Qian S, Yeh DD, Crandall M. Validation of the American Association for the Surgery of Trauma emergency general surgery score for appendicitis—an EAST multicenter study. J Trauma. 2019;87(1):134–9.
72. Savage SA, Klekar CS, Priest EL, Crandall ML, Rodriguez BC, Shafi S. Validating a new grading scale for emergency general surgery. J Surg Research. 2015;196:264–9.
73. Shafi S, Priest EL, Crandall ML, Klekar CS, Nazim A, Aboutanos M, et al. Multicenter validation of American Association for the Surgery of Trauma grading system for acute colonic diverticulitis and its use for emergency general surgery quality improvement program. J Trauma. 2016;80(3):405–11.
74. Murphy BL, Hernandez MC, Naik ND, Glasgow AE, Kong VY, Clarke DL, et al. Validation of the American Association for the Surgery of Trauma's emergency general surgery breast infection grading system. J Surg Res. 2018;228:263–70.
75. Hernandez MC, Birindelli A, Bruce JL, Buitendag JJP, Kong VY, Beuran M, et al. Application of the AAST EGS grade for adhesive small bowel obstruction to a multi-national patient population. World J Surg. 2018;42:3581–8.
76. Savage SA, Li SW, Utter GH, Cox JA, Wydo SM, Cahill K, et al. The EGS grading scale for skin and soft-tissue infections is predictive of poor outcomes: a multicenter validation study. J Trauma. 2019;86(4):601–8.
77. Younis M, Hernandez M, Ray-Zack M, Haddad NN, Choudhry A, Reddy P, Zielinski MD. Validation of AAST EGS grade for acute pancreatitis. J Gastrointest Surg. 2018;22(3):430–7.
78. Hernandez M, Murphy B, Aho JM, Haddad NN, Saleem H, Zeb M, et al. Validation of the AAST EGS acute cholecystitis grade and comparison with the Tokyo guidelines. Surgery. 2018;163(4):739–46.
79. Joseph G, Zangbar B, Pandit V, Fain M, Mohler MJ, Kulvatunyou N, et al. Emergency general surgery in the elderly: too old or too frail? J Am Coll Surg. 2016;222(5):805–13.
80. Murphy PB, Savage SA, Zarzaur BL. Impact of patient frailty on morbidity and mortality after com-

mon emergency general surgery operations. J Surg Res. 2020;247:95–102.
81. Charlson ME, Pompei P, Ales KL, MacKenzie CR. A new method of classifying prognostic comorbidity in longitudinal studies: development and validation. J Chronic Dis. 1987;40(5):373–83.
82. American College of Surgeons. NSQIP Surgical Risk Calculator. http://www.riskcalculator.facs.org/RiskCalculator. Accessed 9 July 2020.
83. Ho VP, Schiltz NK, Reimer AP, Madigan EA, Koroukian SM. High-risk comorbidity combinations in older patients undergoing emergency general surgery. JAGS. 2019;67:503–10.
84. Baghdadi YMK, Morris DS, Choudhry AJ, Thiels CA, Khasawneh MA, Polites SF, et al. Validation of the anatomic severity score developed by the American Association for the Surgery of Trauma in small bowel obstruction. J Surg Res. 2016;204(2):428–34.

Infectious Disease Considerations

4

Brittany Bankhead and Haytham M. A. Kaafarani

Introduction

A 45-year-old female with a past medical history of morbid obesity, diabetes mellitus (type II), hypertension, and hypercholesterolemia presents to the emergency department with a 3-day history of subjective fever, fatigue, and perineal discomfort. Initial vital signs reveal she is normotensive and mildly tachycardic. Physical exam demonstrates subtle erythema at the perineum and left labia with associated tenderness but is otherwise unremarkable. Computed tomography imaging in the emergency department demonstrates extensive subcutaneous emphysema and inflammatory stranding in the perineum and perirectal area, as well as cephalad to the mons pubis. Laboratory findings reveal hyponatremia, a moderate leukocytosis, hyperglycemia, and a mild elevation in an arterial lactic acid. Broad-spectrum antibiotics were administered, and she is booked emergently for an incision and drainage with wide excisional debridement in the operating room. After an appropriate 30 cc/kg bolus of crystalloid, norepinephrine is initiated intraoperatively to maintain an adequate mean arterial pressure. Perioperatively, an insulin drip is initiated in the intensive care unit for improved glycemic control, and cultures are followed to tailor her postoperative antibiotic therapy.

The acute care surgeon encounters a wide variety of surgical infections and perioperative infectious complications throughout their career. The emergency surgery patient population often presents for urgent and emergent surgical management while not medically optimized. Surgical literature is clear that when compared to elective surgery, emergent surgery has significantly higher risks of mortality and complications, up to eightfold higher, including infectious complications.

Many acute care surgical diseases present as infections, often with resultant sepsis. For example, necrotizing soft tissue infections (NSTIs) and toxic megacolon from *Clostridium difficile* infections often present not only with sepsis but also with hemodynamic failure, shock, and evidence of dysfunction of one or more organ systems. When emergency surgical disease presents without infection (e.g., an incarcerated incisional hernia or a closed-loop obstruction necessitating bowel resection), the surgeon should keep in mind all efforts at prevention of postoperative

B. Bankhead (✉)
Department of Surgery, Division of Trauma, Burns, and Critical Care, Texas Tech University Health Sciences Center, Lubbock, TX, USA
e-mail: Brittany.K.Bankhead@ttuhsc.edu

H. M. A. Kaafarani
Department of Surgery, Division of Trauma, Emergency Surgery and Surgical Critical Care, Harvard Medical School and Massachusetts General Hospital, Boston, MA, USA
e-mail: HKAAFARANI@mgh.harvard.edu

M. D. Zielinski, O. Guillamondegui (eds.), *The Acute Management of Surgical Disease*,
https://doi.org/10.1007/978-3-031-07881-1_4

infections in this high-risk patient population that simply cannot be preoperatively well-optimized due to the time-sensitive nature of their procedure. Optimization in the emergency setting should still include, for example, timely administration of appropriate perioperative antibiotics, maintaining normothermia, and optimizing postoperative glucose levels. In this chapter, we will discuss infections resulting from emergency surgery (i.e., surgical site infections ("SSIs")), visit key principles of antimicrobial management in the emergency surgery patient, and then highlight an example of infection resulting from other disease processes but requiring acute surgical management, NSTIs.

Surgical Site Infections (SSIs) in Acute Care Surgery

According to the Centers for Disease Control and Prevention (CDC), an SSI is defined as (1) superficial incisional, (2) deep incisional, or (3) organ/space SSI (Table 4.1). For most surgical procedures, the diagnosis of SSI is encompassed within 30 days of surgery, but in certain specific procedures (e.g., implantation of prosthesis), that time frame is extended to a total of 90 days from surgery. From an acute care surgery perspective, an infection that occurs due to a traumatic wound and following a traumatic injury is not an SSI, but rather a skin and skin structure infection.

Table 4.1 Surgical site infection definitions and criteria

Superficial surgical site infection (SSI)
Must meet the following criteria:
Date of event for infection occurs within 30 days after any NHSN operative procedure (where day 1 = the procedure date) **AND** Involves only skin and subcutaneous tissue of the incision **AND** patient has at least one of the following: (a) Purulent drainage from the superficial incision. (b) Organisms identified from an aseptically obtained specimen from the superficial incision or subcutaneous tissue by a culture or nonculture-based microbiologic testing method, which is performed for purposes of clinical diagnosis or treatment (e.g., not active surveillance culture/testing (ASC/AST). (c) Superficial incision that is deliberately opened by a surgeon, attending physician[a], or other designees **AND** Culture or nonculture-based testing is not performed **AND** Patient has *at least one* of the following signs or symptoms: Pain or tenderness Localized swelling Erythema Heat
(d) Diagnosis of a superficial incisional SSI by the surgeon or attending physician[a] or other designees.

[a]The term attending physician for the purposes of application of the NHSN SSI criteria may be interpreted to mean the surgeon(s), infectious disease, other physicians on the case, emergency physician, or physician's designee (nurse practitioner or physician's assistant)

Comments:

There are two specific types of superficial incisional SSIs:

1. Superficial incisional primary {SIP)—a superficial incisional SSI that is identified in the primary incision in a patient that has had an operation with one or more incisions (e.g., C-section incision or chest incision for CBGB)
2. Superficial incisional secondary {SIS)—a superficial incisional SSI that is identified in the secondary incision in a patient that has had an operation with more than one incision (e.g., donor site incision for CBGB)

Table 4.1 (continued)

Reporting instructions for superficial SSI:
The following do not qualify as criteria for meeting the NHSN definition of superficial SSI:

- Diagnosis/treatment of cellulitis (redness/warmth/swelling), by itself, does not meet criterion "d" for superficial incisional SSI. Conversely, an incision that is draining or that has organisms identified by culture or nonculture-based testing is not considered a cellulitis
- A stitch abscess alone (minimal inflammation and discharge confined to the points of suture penetration)
- A localized stab wound or pin site infection – Such an infection might be considered either a SKIN (SKIN) or soft tissue (ST) infection, depending on its depth, but not an SSI
  Note: A laparoscopic trocar site for an NHSN operative procedure is not considered a stab wound
- Circumcision is not an NHSN operative procedure. An infected circumcision site in newborns is classified as CIRC and is not an SSI

An infected burn wound is classified as *burn* and is not an SSI

Deep incisional SSI

Must meet the following criteria:

Date of event for infection occurs within 30 or 90 days after the NHSN operative procedure (where day 1 = the procedure date)

AND

Involves deep soft tissues of the incision (e.g., fascial and muscle layers)

AND patient has at least *one* of the following:

(a) Purulent drainage from the deep incision

(b) A deep incision that spontaneously dehisces or is deliberately opened or aspirated by a surgeon, attending physician[a], or other designees

AND

Organism is identified by a culture or nonculture-based microbiologic testing method which is performed for purposes of clinical diagnosis or treatment (e.g., not active surveillance culture/testing (ASC/AST) *or* culture or nonculture-based microbiologic testing method is not performed

AND

Patient has *at least one* of the following signs or symptoms:

Fever (>38 °C)

Localized pain or tenderness

Note: A culture or nonculture-based test that has a negative finding does not meet this criterion

(c) An abscess or other evidence of infection involving the deep incision that is detected on gross anatomical or histopathologic exam or imaging test

[a] The term attending physician for the purposes of application of the NHSN SSI criteria may be interpreted to mean the surgeon(s), infectious disease, other physicians on the case, emergency physician, or physician's designee (nurse practitioner or physician's assistant)

Comments:

There are two specific types of deep incisional SSIs:

1. Deep incisional primary (DIP)—a deep incisional SSI that is identified in a primary incision in a patient that has had an operation with one or more incisions (e.g., section incision or chest incision for CBGB)
2. Deep incisional secondary (DIS)—a deep incisional SSI that is identified in the secondary incision in a patient that has had an operation with more than one incision (e.g., donor site incision for CBGB)

Organ/space SSI

Must meet the following criteria:

Date of event for infection occurs within 30 or 90 days after the NHSN operative procedure {where day 1 = the procedure date) according to the list in Table 4.2 (see below)

AND

Infection involves any part of the body deeper than the fascial/muscle layers, which is opened or manipulated during the operative procedure

AND patient has at least *one* of the following:

1. Purulent drainage from a drain that is placed into the organ/space {e.g., closed suction drainage system, open drain, T-tube drain, CT-guided drainage)

(continued)

Table 4.1 (continued)

2. Organisms are identified from fluid or tissue in the organ/space by a culture or nonculture-based microbiologic testing method which is performed for purposes of clinical diagnosis or treatment {e.g., not active surveillance culture/testing {ASC/AST}
3. An abscess or other evidence of infection involving the organ/space that is detected on gross anatomical or histopathologic exam or imaging test evidence suggestive of infection

AND

Meets at least *one* criterion for a specific organ/space infection site listed in Table 4.3 (see below). These criteria are found in the surveillance definitions for specific types of infections chapter

Table 4.2 The sequential [sepsis-related] organ failure assessment (SOFA) score. The score if calculating the total number of points accrued in each system

System	0	1	2	3	4
Respiration (PaO_2/ FiO_2, mmHg)	≥400	<400	<300	<200 with respiratory support	<100 with respiratory support
Coagulation (platelets, × 10^3/uL)	≥150	<150	<100	<50	<20
Liver (bilirubin, mg/dL)	<1.2	1.2–1.9	2.0–5.9	6.0–11.9	>12
Cardiovascular	MAP ≥70 mmHg	MAP <70 mmHg	Dopamine <5 or dobutamine (any dose)	Dopamine 5.1–15 or epinephrine ≤0.1 or norepinephrine ≤0.1 (micrograms/minute)	Dopamine >15 or epinephrine >0.1 or norepinephrine >0.1
CNS (GCS score)	15	13–14	10–12	6–9	<6
Renal (creatinine, mg/dL, urine output, mL/d)	<1.2	1.2–1.9	2.0–3.4	3.5–4.9; <500	>5; <200

When all surgeries are considered, the incidence of SSIs is reported to be as high as 2–5%. Still, SSIs account for nearly a third of all hospital-acquired infections and are thus considered the second most common nosocomial infection after pneumonia. The degree of contamination plays a large role in the risk of SSI. This risk has been shown in multiple studies to be the highest for contaminated and dirty procedures compared to clean or clean-contaminated wounds. For emergency surgery, the risk of SSI is the highest both because of the contamination often present in emergency surgery (e.g., perforated colon) and because patients often have multiple comorbidities that cannot be optimized due to the time sensitivity of the procedure.

When they occur postoperatively, SSIs result in serious morbidity, decreased quality of life, and cost to the patient and healthcare system [1]. This often results from the need for (1) additional diagnostic and surgical procedures (e.g., incision and drainage or debridement of infected wound, hernia occurrence, and need for repair, skin flaps, and grafts), (2) additional treatment with antibiotics, (3) increased hospital length of stay and readmissions, (4) need for wound care supplies, and (5) home-visiting nurse care. One study using patient-centered surveys and large administrative databases suggested almost a threefold increase in the total cost for patients diagnosed with SSI following discharge from the hospital compared to those who do not develop SSI.

Table 4.3 The "Quick" Sequential Organ Failure Assessment (qSOFA) Score

Assessment	Point(s)
Hypotension (systolic blood pressure ≤100 mmHg)	1
Tachypnea (≥ 22 breaths/min)	1
Altered mentation (GCS ≤ 14)	1

It is well-established that most SSIs are directly caused by the patient's endogenous flora at the time of surgery. For example, SSIs after clean wounds are often caused by skin-related *Staphylococcus aureus* or coagulase-negative *Staphylococcus*, while SSIs after intestinal surgery often 1 intestinal bacteria. However, newer data continues to emerge that SSIs are occasionally caused by non-endogenous pathogens. Specifically, failure to preserve surgical field sterility (e.g., instrument contamination, surgical glove perforation), operating room air contamination (e.g., increased personnel traffic, suboptimal air flow, and ventilation), and even surgical techniques (e.g., excessive tissue injury or tension) can increase the risk of SSIs.

Patient comorbidities, often present in the acute care surgery patient, also contribute significantly to the risk of developing an SSI [2]. These include advanced age, immunosuppression, malnutrition, smoking, diabetes mellitus, and obesity. In most patients requiring emergency surgery, the time sensitivity of the procedure does not allow enough time to optimize the risk factors as in elective surgery (e.g., smoking cessation, glucose-level control). However, even in the setting of emergency surgery, several systems-related risk factors should be recognized as contributors to the increased risk of SSIs, and efforts should be made each time to mitigate their effects, as we will discuss in the below sections.

Optimal Choice and Timing of Perioperative Prophylactic Antibiotics

Only half the patients undergoing surgery receive their prophylactic antibiotics within 60 min of the incision as recommended, and even a smaller percentage of patients achieve it in emergency surgery. Administering perioperative prophylactic antibiotics within 60 min from the incision is essential to decrease the risk of SSIs as it helps achieve peak bactericidal concentrations at the skin level at the time of incision [3]. Notably, less than 20% of patients receive an appropriate antibiotic that covers the likely pathogens causing their SSI. Proper antibiotic dosing based on the patient's weight and redosing during surgery based on the specific antibiotic's half-life and the amount of fluid resuscitation the patient is receiving are two other important considerations in antibiotic prophylaxis.

Respecting Sterility

Even in high-risk surgery such as emergency surgery, all the operating room staff should feel comfortable to bring up any patient safety issues related to inadvertent breaching of the sterile field (e.g., insufficient skin preparation, instrument or equipment contamination, surgical team's glove perforation [4, 5]). In observational studies, glove perforations occur in most major surgical procedures, but the rate of SSIs only increases if that occurs in the absence of appropriate antibiotic prophylaxis.

Optimizing the Operating Room Environment

The quality of air and the concentration of airborne particles (and bacteria) depend on (1) the density and traffic of people in that closed space such as the operating room and (2) the quality of air flow design [6–8]. In surgery, the link between air flow and SSIs has only been suggested so far in the orthopedic field, but it likely applies to all types of surgery. In emergency surgery, it is crucial that the traffic of individuals in and out of the operating room is minimized, when possible.

Skin Preparation

It is well established that preoperative shaving increases the rate of SSI. A recent Cochrane review suggests that the risk of SSIs doubles with skin shaving [9]. While the relationship with hair clipping is not as clear, acute care surgeons should refrain from hair removal of the surgical site, when possible. When faced with the choice of skin preparation, level one evidence suggests that alcohol-based solutions are superior to Betadine and should be adopted in emergency surgery, except with open wounds or exposed mucosa. There is no strong evidence suggesting a protective role for adhesive tapes, and their use is currently not routinely recommended.

Perioperative Glucose, Temperature, and Oxygen Optimization

Following emergency surgery, perioperative normoglycemia (glucose levels below 200 mg/dL) can decrease the risk of SSIs not only in diabetic but also in nondiabetic patients. The use of supplemental oxygen for the immediate few hours after surgery may also be useful to decrease the risk of SSI, but the value of such an intervention beyond 6 h postoperatively is less evident. Maintenance of normothermia can also decrease the risk of SSIs. The evidence for the use of antibacterial-coated sutures, antimicrobial irrigants, and antibacterial dressings is not sufficient to recommend their use.

Antimicrobial Management in Emergency Surgery

Infection induces a local tissue inflammatory response. In severe infections, the body also initiates a systemic inflammatory reaction with occasional unintended remote tissue damage and diminished tissue perfusion [10]. Sepsis is defined as a syndrome with clinical, physiologic, and biochemical abnormalities caused by a dysregulated host response to infection. The specific definition of sepsis has rapidly evolved over the past few years but is best thought of as a continuum ranging from infection to early sepsis to severe sepsis, septic shock, and finally septic shock with multisystem organ dysfunction.

The Sequential Organ Failure Assessment (SOFA) and its abbreviated "quick" version qSOFA are the most commonly used scores to diagnose and screen for sepsis (Tables 4.2 and 4.3). In general, septic shock occurs when severe sepsis is associated with decreased end-organ tissue perfusion and is often associated with hypotension or hemodynamic instability [11–14]. Septic shock can manifest as dysfunction of diverse organs such as the brain (agitation, encephalopathy, delirium), lungs (dyspnea, hypoxia, respiratory failure), heart (hypotension, dysrhythmias, pulmonary edema), and kidneys (acidosis, renal insufficiency, renal failure) [15–17].

Localizing the source of the suspected infection or sepsis is key. A comprehensive physical examination can often identify possible sources of infection (e.g., soft tissue changes, abdominal tenderness) [18]. Laboratory examination often shows leukocytosis and/or acidosis. If initially elevated, lactate and base deficit levels can be used as laboratory indices of the effectiveness of resuscitation. For the acute care surgeon, computed tomography or ultrasound are often essential for diagnosing sources of abdominal, thoracic, or deep skin and soft tissue infection.

Once a source of infection is found or suspected, culturing the site and testing the pathogen's sensitivity to antimicrobial agents are essential, so empiric antibiotics can be promptly narrowed to avoid unintended consequences of broad-spectrum antibiotic coverage.

Adequate treatment relies on two major steps: (1) adequate source control and (2) appropriate (choice, dose, duration) antimicrobial therapy. The "Surviving Sepsis" campaign intermittently publishes evidence-based guidelines that can assist the acute care surgeon treating the septic surgical patient. Several prospective observational studies suggest that delay in the initiation of antibiotics worsens mortality and that early empiric antibiotic therapy improves outcomes. The initial selection of empiric antibiotics should be determined both by the likely type of infection, the likely causative pathogen, the antibiotic penetration to the site of infection, the acuity (acute vs. chronic) of the infection, the severity (signs of systemic toxicity, shock) of the infection, as well as any relevant patient-specific factors and prior history of drug-resistant organisms. The local regional resistance rates and the specific hospital antibiograms should also play an important role in the choice of both the empiric and the tailored antibiotic therapy. Once cultures show the specific organisms, narrowing antibiotic coverage is essential.

In emergency surgery, the importance of prompt and adequate source control of the infection cannot be underestimated. For example, the mortality of an NSTI without surgical debridement is 100%, and the mortality and morbidity of patients with necrotic or perforated hollow viscus approach unacceptable levels. Source control can be obtained by surgical, radiologic, or endoscopic approaches, depending on the nature and location of the infection as well as the patient's comorbidities and hospital resources. While surgical infections are discussed across different chapters of this book, we will highlight a few concepts that are key in the management of the emergency surgery patient.

Duration of Antibiotic Therapy

The duration of antibiotic therapy should be dictated by patient factors, infection characteristics, and the severity of disease. Most surgeons continue to treat patients until past the resolution of signs of infection (e.g., leukocytosis, fever), often extending antibiotic courses up to 10 or even 14 days after source control. In the last few decades, evidence has emerged that prolonged antibiotic courses are not only unnecessary but often harmful, with unintended consequences such as *Clostridium difficile* infections or multidrug resistance organisms.

For intra-abdominal infections (IAI), which the acute care surgeon often encounters, the STOP-IT trial recently randomized more than 500 patients with IAI who underwent surgical or percutaneous infection source control to receive the "standard of care" of antibiotics until 2 days after the resolution of signs of infection or to receive a fixed 4-day course of antibiotics [19]. The standard care group received on average 8 days of antibiotics. The fixed course group received on average of 4 days of antibiotics. The rate of SSIs, recurrent intra-abdominal infection, and mortality was similar between the two groups (21.8% and 22.3%, $p = 0.92$). Based on these study results, as well as subsequent ad hoc and observational studies confirming the findings, we recommend that that emergency surgery patients with IAI receive a short-fixed course of 4 days of antibiotics after adequate infection source control. In patients with unusual circumstances (e.g., suspicion of inadequate source control, immunosuppression, refractory critical illness), the surgeon may consider longer courses.

Antibiotics in Patients with Organ Failure

Antibiotics can have severe side effects, can cause other infections such as *Clostridium difficile* colitis, and can occasionally cause fever mimicking infections [20]. Caution must especially be exercised in the use of antibiotics in patients with preexisting organ dysfunction, especially renal or hepatic failure. Aminoglycosides, for example, can cause or exacerbate renal failure. The acute care surgeon in particular should acknowledge that decreased creatinine clearance, whether acute or chronic, requires adjusting all antimicrobial drug dosage, as most of them are excreted, at least partially, by the kidneys. As such, many antibiotics, including the commonly prescribed vancomycin and penicillin, require adjustments in dosage or frequency of administration in the presence of renal insufficiency to prevent toxicity.

Special Consideration: Necrotizing Soft Tissue Infection (NSTI)

NSTIs are skin and soft tissue infections characterized by life-threatening, widespread, and severe tissue infection and necrosis. NSTIs are sometimes reported in the literature as gas gangrene, necrotizing fasciitis, Fournier's gangrene (perineum), and Ludwig's angina (floor of the mouth). One of the earliest descriptions of NSTIs comes from Roman times describing the fatal disease of Emperor Galerius: "A malignant ulcer formed itself low down in his secret parts and spread by degrees. Gangrene seized all the neighboring parts. It diffused itself the wider the more the corrupted flesh was cut away. His bowels came out, and his whole seat putrefied. The stench was so foul as to pervade not only the palace, but even the whole city. His body was dissolved into one mass of corruption."

Type 1 NSTIs are monomicrobial—most caused by *Streptococcus* and *Clostridium* species—while type 2 NSTIs are polymicrobial (e.g., *Staphylococcus*, gram-negative organisms, anaerobic organisms). Much less common type 3 NSTIs are caused by the saltwater organism *Vibrio vulnificus*. Among the pathogens that can cause NSTIs, *Clostridium perfringens* secrete exotoxins, specifically lecithinases, collagenases, and proteases that result in thrombosis of the soft tissue small vessels, which subsequently results in the widespread tissue necrosis along deep tissue planes. Group A *Streptococcus* can also cause life-threatening toxic shock syndrome.

Immunocompromised, malnourished, obese, and diabetic patients, as well as intravenous drug users, are at a particularly high risk for developing NSTIs. Early suspicion and diagnosis of NSTIs and prompt surgical debridement are essential steps to decrease morbidity and mortality. A recent study suggested that initial admission of these patients to non-acute care surgery or medical services significantly delays the time to source control and likely increases mortality. The most worrisome finding in many of these patients, in addition to erythema (Fig. 4.1) or skin changes (e.g., bullae, grayish discoloration) (Fig. 4.2), is pain out of proportion and far from the area of concern on physical examination. "Dishwater-like" fluid (Fig. 4.2) or crepitus are other uncommon findings that should alert the examining surgeon, when found.

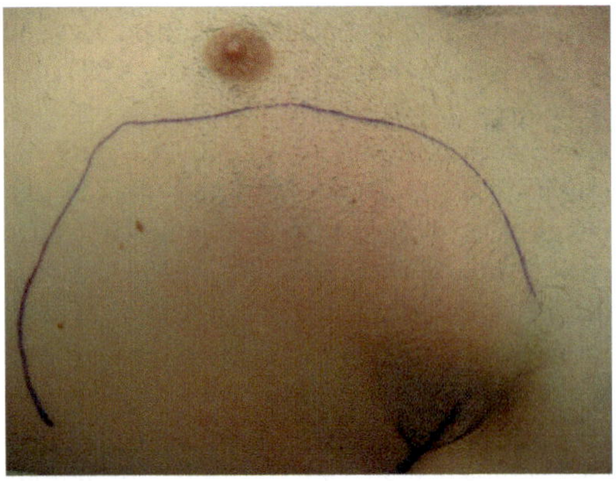

Fig. 4.1 An example of how the skin changes in deep necrotizing skin and soft tissue infections could be subtle

A soft tissue infection with systemic signs of toxicity such as hypotension or altered mental status is alarming, even in the absence of impressive skin findings, and should always alert the surgeon to the possibility or even likelihood of NSTI [21–24]. Laboratory workup typically

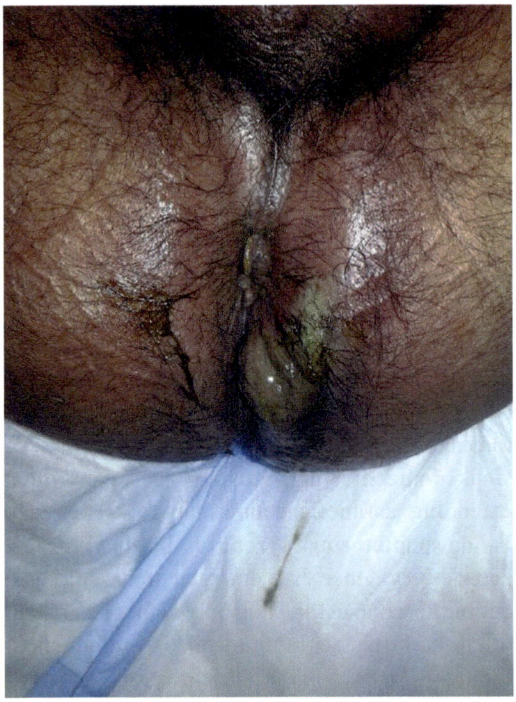

Fig. 4.2 An example of necrotic skin changes associated with necrotizing skin and soft tissue infection of the perineum

Table 4.4 Laboratory Risk Indicator for Necrotizing Fasciitis (LRINEC) score

LRINEC Score variable	Points
C-reactive protein (mg/L) >150	4
WBC count (× 10^6 per mm^3)	
<15	0
15–25	1
>25	2
Hemoglobin (g/dL)	
>13.5	0
11–13.5	1
<11	2
Sodium (mmol/L) <135	2
Creatinine (umol/L) >141	2
Glucose (mmol/L) >10	1

shows leukocytosis, hyponatremia, elevated C-reactive protein levels, and acidosis. The Laboratory Risk Indicator for Necrotizing Fasciitis (LRINEC) Score assigns different point scores to six laboratory values (Table 4.4). While the original study suggested an LRINEC Score of six or more diagnoses of NSTI with an accuracy as high as 92–96%, later studies have not confirmed that high degree of correlation [25, 26]. As such, we do not recommend that LRINEC be used alone to diagnose NSTIs. Computed tomography scans typically show soft tissue stranding and edema at the deeper fascial or muscular layers, non-homogenous enhancement of muscle tissue with intravenous contrast, and/or multiple noncontiguous fluid collections (chain of lakes signs). The presence of deep tissue air (subcutaneous emphysema) has a high specificity but low sensitivity. Operative findings suggestive of NSTIs include necrotic, nonadherent, non-bleeding deep tissue (i.e., tissue separating easily with finger dissection), "dishwater" discharge, and thrombosed small vessels.

NSTIs require prompt wide surgical debridement, broad-spectrum antibiotics, and hemodynamic support (Fig. 4.3). The initial debridement should be aggressive and continue until remaining tissue is clearly healthy, viable, and bleeding briskly. The debridement should always include the overlying skin irrespective of its appearance, and a second look (and more, if needed) with further debridement should be planned 12–24 h after the initial one(s) to ensure infection source control. In extremity NSTIs, amputation might be indicated, and in Fournier's gangrene, diverting ostomies might be temporarily needed.

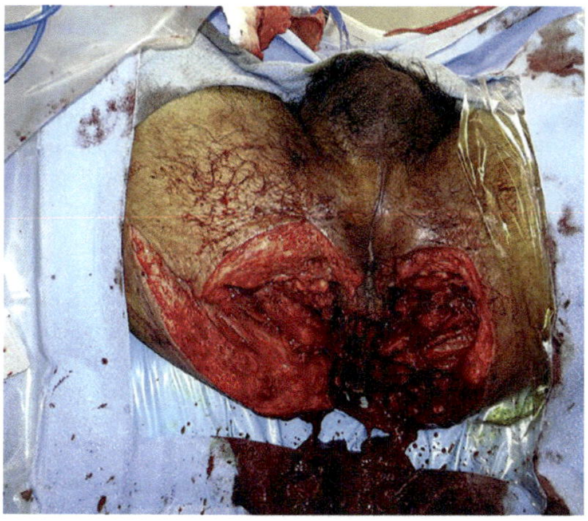

Fig. 4.3 An example of how wide and extensive debridement is often needed in necrotizing skin and soft tissue infection

In addition to prompt and aggressive surgical debridement, broad-spectrum antibiotics should be started as soon as NSTI is suspected. The antibiotic coverage should cover gram-positive, gram-negative, and anaerobic organisms, until cultures specify the inciting organism. In addition, clindamycin has been shown by in vitro studies to have anti-inflammatory and toxin-neutralizing effects and should be used as part of the initial antibiotic treatment. There is no convincing data on how long of a course of antibiotic course should be after source control in NSTIs, but most experts recommend 10–14 days. The usefulness of hyperbaric oxygen in the treatment of NSTIs remains controversial. Despite one cohort observational studies suggesting lower mortality of NSTI patient with hyperbaric oxygen, most surgeons and intensivists hesitate to offer that therapy due to the logistical barriers that might interfere with the continuous intense surgical and critical care needs of the patient. A small randomized controlled trial suggested that immunoglobulins can slightly improve survival. Finally, AB103 is a peptide mimetic of the T-lymphocyte receptor, CD28, who has been recently suggested to limit the inflammatory responses to bacterial toxins and decrease the incidence of organ failure in NSTI patients.

NSTI mortality ranges between 11% and 35%, with prompt diagnosis and shorter to first and adequate debridement significantly improving survival. In a review from the American Association for the Surgery of Trauma (AAST), the overall mortality rate over 6 studies involving 341 patients was lower for those managed with early compared with late debridement (14% versus 26%).

References

1. Boltz MM, Hollenbeak CS, Julian KG, Ortenzi G, Dillon PW. Hospital costs associated with surgical site infections in general and vascular surgery patients. Surgery. 2011;150(5):934–42.
2. Ortega G, Rhee DS, Papandria DJ, Yang J, Ibrahim AM, Shore AD, Makary MA, Abdullah F. An evaluation of surgical site infections by wound classification system using the ACS-NSQIP. J Surg Res. 2012;174(1):33–8.
3. Keely Boyle K, Rachala S, Nodzo SR. Centers for Disease Control and Prevention 2017 guidelines for prevention of surgical site infections: review and relevant recommendations. Curr Rev Musculoskelet Med. 2018;11:357–69.
4. Manjunath AP, Shepherd JH, Barton DP, Bridges JE, Ind TE. Glove perforations during open surgery for gynaecological malignancies. BJOG. 2008;115(8):1015–9.
5. Misteli H, Weber WP, Reck S, Rosenthal R, Zwahlen M, Fueglistaler P, Bolli MK, Oertli D, Widmer AF, Marti WR. Surgical glove perforation and the risk of surgical site infection. Arch Surg. 2009;144(6):553–8; discussion 558.
6. Panahi P, Stroh M, Casper DS, Parvizi J, Austin MS. Operating room traffic is a major concern during Total joint arthroplasty. Clin Orthop Relat Res. 2012;470:2690–4.
7. Darouiche RO, Wall MJ Jr, Itani KM, Otterson MF, Webb AL, Carrick MM, Miller HJ, Awad SS, Crosby CT, Mosier MC, Alsharif A, Berger DH. Chlorhexidine-alcohol versus povidone-iodine for surgical-site antisepsis. N Engl J Med. 2010;362(1):18–26.
8. Swenson BR, Hedrick TL, Metzger R, Bonatti H, Pruett TL, Sawyer RG. Effects of preoperative skin preparation on postoperative wound infection rates: a prospective study of 3 skin preparation protocols. Infect Control Hosp Epidemiol. 2009 Oct;30(10):964–71.
9. Tanner J, Norrie P, Melen K. Preoperative hair removal to reduce surgical site infection. Cochrane Database Systematic Rev. 2011:CD004122.
10. Kaafarani HA, Itani KF. Inflammation, infection, & antimicrobial therapy in surgery. In: Doherty GM, editor. Current diagnosis & treatment: surgery. 15ed. McGraw Hill; 2020. Accessed July 14, 2022. https://accessmedicine.mhmedical.com/content.aspx?bookid=2859§ionid=242153833.
11. Singer M, Deutschman CS, Seymour CW, et al. The third international consensus definitions for sepsis and septic shock (Sepsis-3). JAMA. 2016;315:801.
12. Ho VP, Kaafarani H, Rattan R, Namias N, Evans H, Zakrison TL. Sepsis 2019: what surgeons need to know. Surg Infect. 2020;21(3):195–204.
13. Shankar-Hari M, Phillips GS, Levy ML, et al. Developing a new definition and assessing new clinical criteria for septic shock: for the third international consensus definitions for sepsis and septic shock (Sepsis-3). JAMA. 2016;315:775.
14. Seymour CW, Liu VX, Iwashyna TJ, et al. Assessment of clinical criteria for sepsis: for the third international consensus definitions for sepsis and septic shock (Sepsis-3). JAMA. 2016;315:762.
15. Seetharaman S, Wilson C, Landrum M, et al. Does use of electronic alerts for systemic inflammatory response syndrome (SIRS) to identify patients with sepsis improve mortality? Am J Med. 2019;132:862.
16. Freund Y, Lemachatti N, Krastinova E, et al. Prognostic accuracy of Sepsis-3 criteria for in-hospital mortality among patients with suspected infection presenting to the emergency department. JAMA. 2017;317:301.
17. Mele TS, Kaafarani HMA, Guidry CA, Loor MM, Machado-Aranda D, Mendoza AE, Morris-Stiff G, Rattan R, Schubl SD, Barie PS. Surgical infection society research priorities: a narrative review of fourteen years of progress. Surg Infect. 2021;22:568–82.
18. Darenberg J, Ihendyane N, Sjölin J, et al. Intravenous immunoglobulin G therapy in streptococcal toxic shock syndrome: a European randomized, double-blind, placebo-controlled trial. Clin Infect Dis. 2003;37(3):333–40.
19. Sawyer RG, Claridge JA, Nathens AB, et al. Trial of short-course antimicrobial therapy for intraabdominal infection. N Engl J Med. 2015;372(21):1996–2005.
20. van Nood E, Vrieze A, Nieuwdorp M, et al. Duodenal infusion of donor feces for recurrent Clostridium difficile. N Engl J Med. 2013;368(5):407–15.
21. Kaafarani HM, King DR. Necrotizing skin and soft tissue infections. Surg Clin North Am. 2014;94(1):155–63.
22. Martinez M, Peponis T, Hage A, et al. The role of computed tomography in the diagnosis of necrotizing soft tissue infections. World J Surg. 2018;42(1):82–7.
23. Soh CR, Pietrobon R, Freiberger JJ, et al. Hyperbaric oxygen therapy in necrotising soft tissue infections: a study of patients in the United States Nationwide inpatient sample. Intensive Care Med. 2012;38(7):1143–51.
24. Kongkaewpaisan N, Hwabejire J, Lee JM, Narueponjirakul N, Meier K, Mendoza A, Saillant N, Rosenthal M, King D, Fagenholz P, Velmahos G, Kaafarani HMA. Necrotizing soft tissue infection: time is crucial, and the admitting service matters. Surg Infect. 2020;21(10):828–33.
25. Wong CH, Khin LW, Heng KS, Tan KC, Low CO. The LRINEC (Laboratory Risk Indicator for Necrotizing Fasciitis) score: a tool for distinguishing necrotizing fasciitis from other soft tissue infections. Crit Care Med. 2004;32(7):1535–41.
26. Abdullah M, McWilliams B, Khan SU. Reliability of the laboratory risk indicator in Necrotising fasciitis (LRINEC) score. Surgeon. 2019;17(5):309–18. https://doi.org/10.1016/j.surge.2018.08.001.

5 Damage Control Surgery

Jessica E. Schucht, Samuel J. Pera,
and Jason W. Smith

Most surgeons can think of a case that required the application of damage control principles. These patients appear "sick" and need quick decision-making both before and in the surgical team's operating room. Surgeons need to know how to properly care for these patients as they present equally to academic centers and community hospitals.

Case Presentation

A 65-year-old patient presents to the emergency department febrile, tachycardic with severe hypotension. The ED physician calls the surgeon stating the patient has severe abdominal pain and labile vital signs transiently responsive to fluids. He has obtained cultures, started antibiotics, and is requesting assistance. Upon examination, the patient is somnolent but responsive with abdominal distension and rebound peritonitis in the left lower quadrant. The patient has leukocytosis, elevated creatinine, lactic acidosis, and a CT scan with a representative image shown in Figs. 5.1 and 5.2.

In the above picture, active contrast extravasation can be seen. With the concern for active hemorrhage and peritonitis, the surgeon consents the patient and family for surgery. What are the critical aspects of consent for this patient? How will this patient tolerate surgery physiologically? Will this patient require multiple operations? How to decide when to do a damage control procedure? These are essential questions that need to be considered for any patient requiring emergent surgery.

After discussion with the family, the patient is taken to the OR. He undergoes successful intubation, arterial line access, central line access, and Foley placement. It is imperative to have invasive lines to monitor the patient's blood pressure and urine output correctly and administer vasoactive medications as needed. Once in the abdomen, the following is found (Fig. 5.3).

Seen are an acute sigmoid volvulus and a descending mesocolon hematoma caused by tension placed on the vascular pedicle. During the resection, anesthesia informs the surgery team of increasing pressor requirements, a base deficit of −11, difficulty keeping the patient warm, and there's been no urine output throughout the case. How should the surgeon proceed now? Is

J. E. Schucht · S. J. Pera · J. W. Smith (✉)
Hiram C. Polk Jr. Department of Surgery, University of Louisville, Louisville, KY, USA
e-mail: jessica.schucht@louisville.edu; samuel.pera@louisville.edu; jasonw.smith@louisville.edu

M. D. Zielinski, O. Guillamondegui (eds.), *The Acute Management of Surgical Disease*,
https://doi.org/10.1007/978-3-031-07881-1_5

this patient appropriate for an anastomosis? Would the patient be best served by definitive care or a damage control procedure?

This case is an excellent example of a patient requiring a damage control procedure. Determining which patient necessitates a damage control procedure requires excellent clinical acumen by the surgical team. Some patients can be identified preoperatively, say if the patient presents in septic shock due to a perforated viscous or hemodynamically unstable due to a ruptured aneurysm or penetrating trauma. At other times, it isn't until the intraoperative setting that the surgeon needs to decide a damage control procedure is warranted and not pursue definitive care. To understand how best to make these decisions, the surgeon needs to understand the patient's physiologic changes under stress, intraoperative findings that merit damage control, and institutional surgical capabilities. A collaborative approach between the primary surgical team, surgical consultants, anesthesiologist, and the intensivist team is necessary to provide high-quality care to patients.

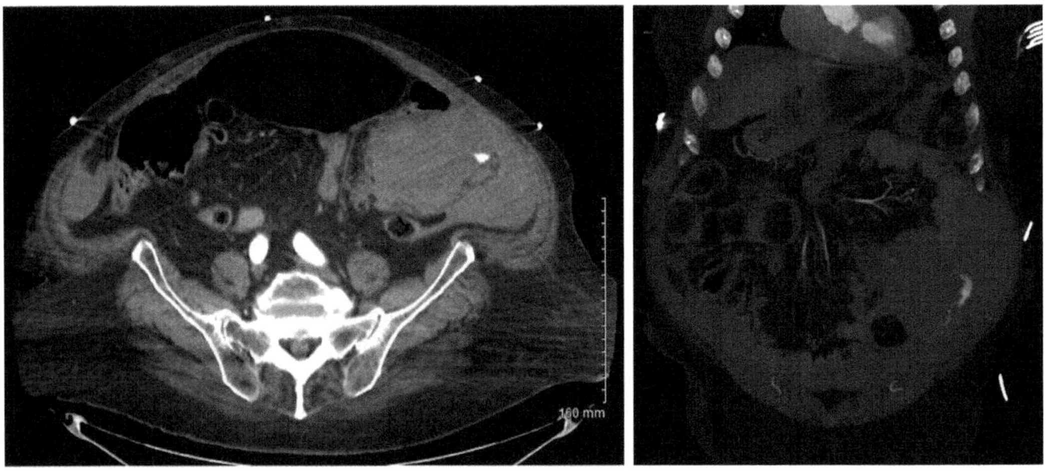

Figs. 5.1 and 5.2 CT scan demonstrating active contrast extravasation in a hemodynamically unstable gentleman

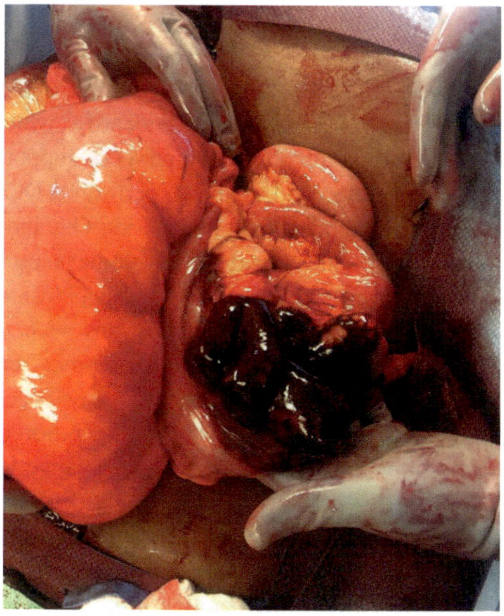

Fig. 5.3 Intraoperative imaging of acute sigmoid volvulus with compromised bowel

Historical Basis

Damage control procedures were initially described for care in critically injured trauma patients. These patients had significant physiological derangements due to hemorrhagic shock, with many succumbing to the disease process. It wasn't until the 1980s that damage control principles were developed and significantly improved patients' morbidity and mortality [1, 2]. These studies ushered in the idea of quick hemorrhage control, intra-abdominal packing, and limited surgical resection to stabilize the patient before definitive repair in the following days. Both were novel in their care of patients and challenged the surgical dogma of the time. In 1993, Rotondo and Schwab coined the term "damage control," defined as initial control of hemorrhage and contamination followed by intraperitoneal packing and rapid closure. They showed that damage control patients with significant vascular injury and two or more visceral injuries had markedly improved survival compared to the definitive care group [3]. These seminal studies forever changed the management of the traumatically injured patient. In the decades since damage control, surgery has become the standard of care in treating injured patients with severe physiological compromise who require surgical intervention.

After demonstrating improved outcomes for the traumatically injured undergoing damage control procedures, it was only natural that the same principles would be applied to various surgical indications. Regardless of the indication, damage control is not a surgical procedure; instead, it is an alternative treatment mode to primary definitive surgical care. During the initial damage control surgery, the goal is not to achieve final repair or control of the surgical pathology but instead to temporize the patient by identifying the greatest mortality threat and alleviating it. In general, the standard practice is to conduct an abbreviated surgery to control blood loss and/or contamination, continue simultaneous resuscitation, and delay definitive surgical management until the patient stabilizes from the initial pathologic insult.

Pathophysiology

As we've improved our care of patients in shock, there has been a dramatic expansion into understanding what occurs on a cellular level. Shock causes hypoperfusion, which leads to derangements in fluid exchange and electrolyte handling, tissue ischemia, and worsening inflammation [4]. Tissue ischemia and inflammation can result in endothelial cellular dysfunction affecting microcirculatory perfusion, hypothesized to contribute to prolonged tissue hypoxia, irreversible cellular injury, multi-organ failure, and death [5]. Ultimately, if damage control can be achieved in a timely fashion, progressive vasoconstriction can be avoided resulting in improved circulation.

Indication for Damage Control Surgery

Identifying which patients require a damage control procedure can be challenging. Many early studies found that trauma patients who were hypothermic, coagulopathic, and acidotic had worse outcomes [6]. When found in conjunction with one another, these three variables were strong predictors of adverse outcomes in patients suffering shock [7]. One of the original studies found an almost 90% mortality in patients with the lethal triad and requiring massive transfusion [8].

It is also important to note the possible overutilization of damage control surgery resulting from the paradigm shift. In one study, Harvin et al. found that they performed damage control laparotomy on approximately 39% of their patients. After performing their quality initiative, damage control laparotomy decreased to 23% over 2 years. They noted no difference in deep space infection, fascial dehiscence, unplanned relaparotomy, or mortality. From this study, four indications for damage control laparotomy were identified: (1) therapeutic packing to control hemorrhage, (2) expedition to interventional radiology for hemorrhage control, (3) hemodynamic instability defined as a continuous vasopressor and/or ongoing transfusion requirement, and (4) abdominal compartment syndrome treatment or prophylaxis [9]. Although these indications are from a quality initiative and not a randomized trial, they provide the foundation for damage control surgery indications.

Avoiding the lethal triad is the driving force behind damage control procedures, goal-directed resuscitation, and adequate temperature maintenance. This has significantly improved the care of trauma patients over the last few decades. The benefits of damage control surgery must always be weighed against the possible complications of leaving the abdomen open, mainly as damage control surgery is applied to an ever more significant patient population.

Damage Control Laparotomy

As damage control laparotomy became widespread, there was a push to identify which patients these techniques would best support. Intraoperatively, the decision to perform a DCL would be based on several indications. One indication is fluid status, as extensive volume resuscitation may prevent a tension-free fascial closure. If closed under tension, complications such as fascial dehiscence, bowel evisceration, and abdominal compartment syndrome may occur. Another indication is the need for reoperation or second-look situations. Complex pancreaticoduodenal injuries, hepatic injuries, or pelvic injuries may require multiple operations to achieve successful results. And lastly, those who have signs of the lethal triad intraoperative need to have a damage control procedure with temporary closure, resuscitation, and rewarming [10].

Unfortunately, there have been no randomized controlled trials determining which patients would benefit most. Expert review panels have investigated the issue identifying over 36 unique prehospital indications and 87 intraoperative indications [11]. While this provides a guide, this issue still lacks appropriate data to answer who is best served with DCL conclusively.

Damage Control Laparotomy for Emergency General Surgery Patients

With the success of DC procedures for trauma patients, the same principles are now applied to EGS patients. While these are two distinct patient populations, they share some similarities. Many present with severe physiological derangement requiring immediate intervention. Most need significant fluid resuscitation to restore the intravascular volume. There are a few critical differences between trauma and EGS patients. EGS patients are typically older with significant medical comorbidities, and for patients that may require

DCL, the cause is septic shock instead of hemorrhagic shock [10, 12]. While randomized controlled trials are lacking, a few studies have looked at which patients would benefit most from DCL. In one of the most extensive studies, Becher et al. looked retrospectively at 215 patients who underwent emergent laparotomy for nontraumatic indications. 53 patients underwent a staged or damage control procedure. Patients who underwent DCL had significantly higher mortality than those who underwent a one-stage operation (45% vs. 20%). As expected, patients who underwent DCL presented with more severe illness, had higher ASA scores, were more likely to be in severe sepsis/septic shock, and had significant lactic acidosis. Interestingly, patients presented with the lethal triad did not discriminate between survivors and non-survivors in multivariable logistic regressions models. The data did suggest that patients who may realize a survivor benefit from DCL are those who present in severe sepsis/septic shock, elevated lactic level (>3), and acidosis (pH <7.25), are elderly (>70) and male, and those with multiple comorbidities [13]. While this study is not without limitations, it does suggest which patients may benefit most from DCL. In a separate retrospective study, Subramanian et al. found that age was not an independent predictor of worse outcomes when investigating elderly patients over 65 who underwent DCL [14]. This showed that despite more significant comorbidities, elderly patients could tolerate DCL physiologically.

Damage Control Laparotomy Operative Sequence

Regardless of the indication for DCL, a similar sequence is followed in both hemorrhagic and septic shock. The sequence can be broken down into preoperative care, damage control operation, damage control resuscitation, second-look laparotomy, and postoperative care [6, 15].

Preoperative: Attempt to identify patients who will need a DCL by using presentation information such as the preoperative base deficit, hypothermia, coagulopathy, hemodynamic instability, patient age, or sex. Another aspect to consider is projected operative time which will be based on the etiology of the patient's illness dictating which procedure will be performed. Definitive repairs that require extensive resection and reanastomosis may be prohibitive. Also, resuscitation should be initiated at the time of assessment. For hemorrhagic shock, a massive transfusion protocol should be activated with appropriate large-bore IV access. Resuscitation should follow a 1:1:1 ratio (packed red blood cells, plasma, and platelets) as this was shown to decrease mortality in large multicenter randomized controlled trials [16, 17]. In septic shock, crystalloid resuscitation and potentially vasopressors may be required to stabilize the patient's hemodynamics. Crystalloid resuscitation should target a CVP of 8–12 mmHg in non-intubated patients or 12–15 mmHg in intubated patients, MAP >65, UOP >0.5 cc/kg/h, or central venous oxygen saturation (ScvO2) of >70%, if able [18]. Cultures should be obtained and antibiotics started expeditiously. Strict volume measurement following fluid replacement and associated output are required but should not delay transport to the operating room.

Damage control operation: When the decision has been made to proceed with DCL, the index operation's objective is to determine the insulting pathology resulting in the physiological deranged state. If the cause is hemorrhage, this should be controlled rapidly. Likewise, if sepsis is the concern, then the goal will be decontamination and source control. Once accomplished, the surgeon should reassess the abdomen and proceed with temporary abdominal closure if the insulting pathology has been addressed. The patient should then be transferred to an ICU setting for ongoing management.

Damage control resuscitation: Resuscitation began at patient arrival and continued during the operation and in the ICU. Throughout the surgical intervention, it is imperative that the surgeon maintain close communication with the anesthesia colleagues. How the patient responds to resuscitation can significantly impact the initial plan of definitive surgery, damage control surgery, or an intraoperative conversion of a definitive repair to damage control. Perioperative resuscitation should aim to optimize patient hemodynamics; correct acidosis, coagulopathy, and electrolyte abnormalities; and ensure adequate end-organ perfusion. Once the damage control operation is complete, multiple open abdomen resuscitation strategies can be followed. In 2010, Smith et al. showed the efficacy of direct peritoneal resuscitation for trauma patients undergoing damage control laparotomy. They found a significantly shorter time to definitive abdominal closure. Direct peritoneal resuscitation allowed for a higher rate of primary fascial closure, lower intra-abdominal complication rate, and a lower ventral hernia formation rate at 6 months [19]. In 2014, Smith et al. applied direct peritoneal resuscitation to EGS patients and again found a higher rate of primary fascial closures performed in a shorter time. While not significant, they found lower overall mortality at 30 days in the direct peritoneal resuscitation group [5]. Another resuscitation strategy investigated by Harvin et al. utilized 3% hypertonic saline while the fascia was open. They showed a decrease in the total amount of fluids given, a decrease in time to fascial closure, and a significant number of patients achieving primary fascial closure on the first take back [20].

Second-look laparotomy: With adequate resuscitation and stabilization, the patient should return to the operating room for a second-look laparotomy, typically with a 24–48-h window of the index operation. The precise timing of return to the OR is patient-specific. If the patient has normalized, then the goal of the second-look laparotomy will be to achieve definitive intra-abdominal repair with primary fascial closure. If definitive repair is not indicated during the second-look procedure, then a thorough evaluation should be completed and a temporizing dressing applied with plan for a third look laparotomy.

Postoperative care: Once definitive repair of abdominal pathology is complete, the patient should be liberated from the ventilator as judiciously as possible. Nutrition needs to be met by enteral means if possible, and if not warranted, parenteral support should be considered. The role of antibiotic use and duration should be case-specific based upon the pathologic situation.

Damage Control Laparotomy Outcomes

Damage control laparotomy has resulted in an overall decreased morbidity and mortality. In the original study describing damage control surgery, the survival rate approached 60% compared to an 11% survival rate in the control group [3]. In another study, Smith et al. compared outcomes following penetrating, blunt, and intraperitoneal sepsis damage control laparotomy. The authors found that the intraperitoneal sepsis group had the lowest primary fascial closure rate, the highest rate of intra-abdominal complications, and the highest 90-day mortality. For all three groups, those whose abdomens were open for over 8 days had nearly twice the risk of death [21]. Based on these two studies, it is likely that trauma patients have better outcomes than the emergency surgery patient population following damage control laparotomy.

Other studies did not show a conclusive benefit of damage control surgery for emergency general surgery patients. Hau et al. showed in a prospective multicenter cohort study that there was no significant difference in mortality when comparing a planned relaparotomy group (aka damage control laparotomy) vs. a relaparotomy when necessary (21% vs. 13%). The stratification of patients into either group was based on surgeon preference at the time of surgery. They found a higher incidence of multi-organ failure and infectious complications in the planned relaparotomy group, which may correlate with why those patients were stratified into the damage control group, to begin with [22]. van Ruler et al. also found no difference in mortality in a randomized controlled trial comparing a planned relaparotomy (aka damage control laparotomy) strategy compared to an on-demand or as-needed laparotomy strategy (12-month mortality 36% vs. 29%). 42% of patients in the as-needed laparotomy group required a second-look laparotomy, with 69% of those patients having significant intra-abdominal findings. Compare that to the planned relaparotomy group, where 94% of those patients underwent second-look laparotomy and only 34% of those were significant for intra-abdominal findings. This study showed that in the properly selected patients, second-look laparotomy would have positive intraoperative findings. Unfortunately, these relaparotomy (either planned or unplanned) subgroups were not analyzed to determine associated mortality [23].

Damage Control Laparotomy Complications

DCL comes with its unique complications due to the abdominal cavity being left open for an extended period. There are fewer complications if the abdominal cavity can be closed by day 7 or 8, after which complications become much more frequent [24, 25]. Those complications include abdominal compartment syndrome, enterocutaneous fistula, intra-abdominal abscess, and the inability to close the abdominal fascia primarily.

Abdominal compartment syndrome can occur following either hemorrhagic shock or septic shock patients. There are several risk factors associated with abdominal compartment syndrome, including abdominal surgery, trauma, hemoperitoneum, intra-abdominal abscess/infection, acidosis, hypothermia, coagulopathy, massive resuscitation, mechanical ventilation, and an open abdomen. These risk factors diminish the abdominal wall compliance, increase the intra-abdominal contents, and cause a capillary leak [26]. Abdominal compartment syndrome can be a resultant effect of a damage control procedure or a by-product of the insinuating event requiring damage control in the first place. Regardless of the inciting event, the abdomen needs to be decompressed, and once done, there will be difficulty in achieving a definitive closure. Occasionally, temporary closure devices can cause compartment syndrome physiology if the closure is tight or the abdominal viscera swells during ICU resuscitation. Overall, these patients need to be monitored closely with judicious use of fluid, closely following urine output, and attempted abdominal closure when able. Adjuncts such as negative pressure wound vacuum, direct peritoneal resuscitation, and hypertonic saline can be used to help decrease the time to fascial closure [19, 20, 27].

Enterocutaneous fistula (ECF) can occur due to increased or excessive manipulation of the viscera. ECFs can also be caused by a prolonged open abdomen that is unable to have primary fascial closure. Intra-abdominal abscesses (IAA) are more likely to occur after damage control surgery due to the temporary closure devices, inciting infection, and any packs left in the abdomen to help with hemostasis. The Open Abdomen Registry did further investigation to identify inciting events in the formation of enterocutaneous fistula, enteroatmospheric fistula, and intra-abdominal abscess formation. Using the Registry, they compared patients with and without these specific complications and found large bowel resection, extensive volume fluid resuscitation, and an increasing number of abdominal explorations were statistically significant predictors [28]. In a separate systematic review, Cristaudo et al. identified that lack of definitive fascial closure, large bowel resection, and >5 to 10 L of intravenous fluids in less than 48 hours were predictors of enteroatmospheric fistula. They also identified large bowel resection, >5 to 10 L, and over 10 L of intravenous fluids in less than 48 hours were predictors of an intra-abdominal abscess [29].

Lastly, a significant source of morbidity and mortality of a damage control laparotomy is the open abdomen and whether the fascia can be re-approximated. The issue of the open abdomen causing the complications or the complication result due to a prolonged open abdomen indicates the importance of achieving fascial closure. Independent predictors associated with the lack of primary fascial closure include IAA, worst base deficit, and higher abdominal explorations [30]. The systematic review performed by Cristaudo et al. identified enteral nutrition, organ dysfunction, local and systemic infection, the number of reexplorations, worsening Injury Severity Score, and the development of a fistula appeared to significantly delay definitive fascial closure [29]. Miller et al. retrospectively evaluated 344 patients who required an open abdomen due to either damage control surgery or abdominal compartment syndrome. Only 276 patients made it to fascial closure, and of those, only 65% achieved primary closure at a mean of 3.5 days and a complication rate of 9%. Of the remaining patients, 29% required prolonged temporary closure, and 6% underwent prosthetic implant closure. The overall mean time to final fascial closure was 45 days. There was fistula formation in each of the three closure groups, the early primary closure had the lowest at 3%, and the highest was temporary closure group of 30% [25]. This study emphasized the importance of primary closure when feasible. If not, there are other options, but they are associated with significantly higher complications. Other options include sequential closure, in-lay or bridging mesh, skin closure with future hernia repair, and temporary abdominal coverage. These techniques are appropriate to use in the acute setting, and after complete recovery, more complex operations, including component separation and permanent mesh, can be considered.

Damage Control Vascular Procedures

Damage control for vascular injuries involves a spectrum of varying pathologies, including vascular trauma of an extremity, ruptured aneurysm, uncontrolled gastrointestinal hemorrhage, tumor invasion into prominent vasculature, or an iatrogenic injury. The similarities between these pathological variants are rapid and profound blood loss resulting in hemodynamic instability. Specific to vascular surgery are the techniques to obtain control as many vessels can be ligated with limited repercussions. For vessels that cannot be ligated, a damage control approach needs to be considered. The same principles apply for damage control vascular procedures as it does for damage control laparotomy—rapid identification of the injury, control of hemorrhage, temporary closure, resuscitation, and lastly definitive repair with appropriate closure. Damage control vascular procedures include balloon tamponade or temporary intravascular shunts (TIVS) [12].

Extremity Vascular Injuries

Major vascular injuries of an extremity represent a subset of patients who present in profound shock and need immediate care addressing the vascular injury. Historically, these patients were managed with a life over limb philosophy, resulting in a large percentage of amputations [31]. The military experience in Iraq and Afghanistan in the early 2000s challenged that philosophy with the advent of temporary surgical shunts. In one of the most extensive studies at the time, Rasmussen et al. identified 126 extremity vascular injuries, of which 30 were managed with the placement of a temporary shunt at a smaller field hospital before transfer to the main Air Force Theater Hospital, where the definitive repair was performed. Twenty-two of the shunts were placed proximally, eight distally, and four of the proximal shunts were venous. None of the patients received systemic heparin. Each of the patients proceeded to definitive repair, with only two patients requiring amputation [32]. Although this was a small sample size with no randomization, this showed the feasibility of limb salvage using intravascular shunts. Ball et al. completed a retrospective review of civilians suffering iliac artery injuries. Before intravascular shunts, management had previously been vessel ligation with possible extra-anatomic bypass if the patient survived. This resulted in mortality ranging from 30 to 90%, frequently secondary to blood loss before arrival. There was a high mortality rate of 45% in their analysis, with the majority dying from refractory shock in the first 24 hours. When they compared ligation to intravascular shunt placement, fewer patients required amputations (47% compared to 0%) and fasciotomies (93% compared to 43%) with lower mortality (73% vs. 43%) [33]. The other injury pattern to mention is a concomitant orthopedic injury and a significant vascular injury. Wlodarczyk et al. addressed this question in 2017. They identified 291 patients who had both an extremity vascular injury and an orthopedic injury. The patients were broken up into three groups—those who were shunted first, those who were not shunted and underwent initial vascular repair, and those who were not shunted and underwent initial orthopedic fixation. They found that the shunted group had a higher Abbreviated Injury Scale and Mangled Extremity Severity Score and with a lower rate of compartment syndrome. The non-shunted orthopedic fixation first group had a significantly longer length of stay and a higher amputation rate [34]. This study emphasized the importance of first addressing the vascular injury before proceeding with orthopedic fixation.

Intra-Abdominal Vascular Damage Control

The management of intra-abdominal vascular control is based on the tenets of a damage control laparotomy. There are a few examples to mention. While the incidence of a ruptured abdominal aortic aneurysm has decreased with imaging and screening advancements, the mortality remains high at nearly 50% [35]. Tadlock et al. applied damage control principles to the surgical management for ruptured abdominal aortic aneurysms to reduce mortality. A small sample size limited the study, but they showed the damage control group received more blood products and less crystalloid infusion, a decrease in mortality, and no graft infections, albeit the latter two findings failed to reach significance [36]. This study suggested that not only was damage control safe in this patient population, but there may also be a survival benefit as well.

Another instance where damage control principles should be applied is for an unstable gastrointestinal bleed. These patients are best served endoscopically or with interventional radiology. However, if the conservative measures are not effective or the patient becomes hemodynamically unstable, the surgeon needs to be prepared to control the bleeding surgically. Whether the bleed is from esophageal varices, peptic ulcers, marginal ulcers, AVM, or postoperative complications, the principles of damage control surgery should be applied [10, 37]. One modality the surgeon should be familiar with is balloon tamponade. These devices have proven helpful in obtaining temporary vascular control in solid organ injuries, challenging to access vascular injuries, cardiac injuries, carotid injuries, and facial artery injuries [38].

Finally, the elective surgeon needs to understand damage control vascular techniques and principles. While uncommon, there are reports of applying damage control surgery in elective pancreas surgery following massive hemorrhage. In one study, 8 patients out of 835 undergoing elective pancreas surgery required damage control principles due to massive hemorrhage. All 8 patients survived [39]. In another study, 6 patients out of 178 undergoing debridement for necrotizing pancreatitis required damage control principles again due to hemorrhage. Four of the six survived [40]. Had these patients been operated on before damage control principles being widely adapted or by surgeons not versed in damage control management, these complications would likely have been uniformly fatal.

Damage Control Thoracotomy

After wide adaption of damage control laparotomy and vascular procedures, trauma surgeons began using the same techniques to manage thoracic trauma. Patients have the same overall physiology following traumatic thoracic injury in which major hemorrhage occurs. These patients require rapid stabilization, resuscitation, and subsequent definitive care. Damage control surgery has been described following cardiac injury, lung injury, intrathoracic vascular injury, tracheobronchial injury, and oro-esophageal injury [41]. One of the earliest studies investigating the efficacy of damage control thoracotomy was by Vargo et al. 11 out of 196 patients undergoing thoracotomy had an abbreviated operation—six due to coagulopathy, three due to planned reexploration, two due to secondary to thoracic compartment syndrome, one due to cardiac compressive shock, and one due to airway hypertension both following rib approximation. Mortality was 36%, with the causes being severe TBI in two patients and uncontrolled coagulopathy in the other two [42]. As one of the preliminary studies, Vargo et al. demonstrated that damage control thoracotomy was safe and may provide a survival benefit to patients. This was further confirmed in 2 more observational studies evaluating 25 patients and 44 patients all undergoing damage control thoracotomy. Their mortality rates were 40% and 23%, respectively [43, 44]. Finally, there was concern regarding the increased risk of infectious and hemorrhagic complications related to the open chest. Lang et al. investigated these findings and found that a damage control thoracotomy compared to traditional definitive closure did not have a higher risk of infectious or hemorrhagic complications and no significant mortality difference [45]. Unfortunately, all of these trials were retrospective and non-randomized. Randomized trials are needed to precisely define indications, expected outcomes, and mortality for the most effective utilization of damage control thoracotomy.

In conclusion, the development of damage control surgery principle has resulted in decreased morbidity and mortality for some of the sickest patients. These principles can be applied to almost all surgical disciplines including trauma, emergency general surgery, and thoracic, vascular, and elective surgery. The basic tenets include an initial, abbreviated surgical intervention, rewarming, and resuscitation in the ICU, followed by definitive care. Further research needs to be conducted in order to identify the optimal patient population who would maximally benefit from a damage control procedure.

References

1. Stone HH, Strom PR, Mullins RJ. Management of the major coagulopathy with onset during laparotomy. Ann Surg. 1983;197(5):532–5.
2. Feliciano DV, Mattox KL, Jordan GL Jr. Intra-abdominal packing for control of hepatic hemorrhage: a reappraisal. J Trauma. 1981;21(4):285–90.
3. Rotondo MF, et al. 'Damage control': an approach for improved survival in exsanguinating penetrating abdominal injury. J Trauma. 1993;35(3):375–82; discussion 382–3.
4. Fruchterman TM, et al. Selective microvascular endothelial cell dysfunction in the small intestine following resuscitated hemorrhagic shock. Shock. 1998;10(6):417–22.
5. Smith JW, et al. Adjunctive treatment of abdominal catastrophes and sepsis with direct peritoneal resuscitation: indications for use in acute care surgery. J Trauma Acute Care Surg. 2014;77(3):393–8; discussion 398–9.
6. Rotondo MF, Zonies DH. The damage control sequence and underlying logic. Surg Clin North Am. 1997;77(4):761–77.
7. Wilson RF, et al. Problems with 20 or more blood transfusions in 24 hours. Am Surg. 1987;53(7):410–7.
8. Ferrara A, et al. Hypothermia and acidosis worsen coagulopathy in the patient requiring massive transfusion. Am J Surg. 1990;160(5):515–8.
9. Harvin JA, et al. Decreasing the use of damage control laparotomy in trauma: a quality improvement project. J Am Coll Surg. 2017;225(2):200–9.
10. Weber DG, Bendinelli C, Balogh ZJ. Damage control surgery for abdominal emergencies. Br J Surg. 2014;101(1):e109–18.
11. Roberts DJ, et al. Indications for use of damage control surgery and damage control interventions in civilian trauma patients: a scoping review. J Trauma Acute Care Surg. 2015;78(6):1187–96.
12. Ball CG. Damage control surgery. Curr Opin Crit Care. 2015;21(6):538–43.
13. Becher RD, et al. Damage control operations in non-trauma patients: defining criteria for the staged rapid source control laparotomy in emergency general surgery. World J Emerg Surg. 2016;11:10.
14. Subramanian A, et al. Outcomes of damage-control celiotomy in elderly nontrauma patients with intra-abdominal catastrophes. Am J Surg. 2010;200(6):783–8; discussion 788–9.
15. Waibel BH, Rotondo MM. Damage control surgery: it's evolution over the last 20 years. Rev Col Bras Cir. 2012;39(4):314–21.
16. Holcomb JB, et al. The prospective, observational, multicenter, major trauma transfusion (PROMMTT) study: comparative effectiveness of a time-varying treatment with competing risks. JAMA Surg. 2013;148(2):127–36.
17. Holcomb JB, et al. Transfusion of plasma, platelets, and red blood cells in a 1:1:1 vs a 1:1:2 ratio and mortality in patients with severe trauma: the PROPPR randomized clinical trial. JAMA. 2015;313(5):471–82.
18. Moore LJ, Moore FA. Early diagnosis and evidence-based care of surgical sepsis. J Intensive Care Med. 2013;28(2):107–17.
19. Smith JW, et al. Direct peritoneal resuscitation accelerates primary abdominal wall closure after damage

control surgery. J Am Coll Surg. 2010;210(5):658–64, 664–7.
20. Harvin JA, et al. Chasing 100%: the use of hypertonic saline to improve early, primary fascial closure after damage control laparotomy. J Trauma Acute Care Surg. 2013;74(2):426–30; discussion 431–2.
21. Smith JW, et al. Not all abdomens are the same: a comparison of damage control surgery for intra-abdominal sepsis versus trauma. Am Surg. 2016;82(5):427–32.
22. Hau T, et al. Planned relaparotomy vs relaparotomy on demand in the treatment of intra-abdominal infections. The peritonitis study Group of the Surgical Infection Society-Europe. Arch Surg. 1995;130(11):1193–6. discussion 1196-7
23. van Ruler O, et al. Comparison of on-demand vs planned relaparotomy strategy in patients with severe peritonitis: a randomized trial. JAMA. 2007;298(8):865–72.
24. Khan A, et al. Damage-control laparotomy in non-trauma patients: review of indications and outcomes. J Trauma Acute Care Surg. 2013;75(3):365–8.
25. Miller RS, et al. Complications after 344 damage-control open celiotomies. J Trauma. 2005;59(6):1365–71. discussion 1371-4
26. Kirkpatrick AW, et al. Intra-abdominal hypertension and the abdominal compartment syndrome: updated consensus definitions and clinical practice guidelines from the world Society of the Abdominal Compartment Syndrome. Intensive Care Med. 2013;39(7):1190–206.
27. Batacchi S, et al. Vacuum-assisted closure device enhances recovery of critically ill patients following emergency surgical procedures. Crit Care. 2009;13(6):R194.
28. Bradley MJ, et al. Independent predictors of enteric fistula and abdominal sepsis after damage control laparotomy: results from the prospective AAST open abdomen registry. JAMA Surg. 2013;148(10):947–54.
29. Cristaudo AT, et al. Treatments and other prognostic factors in the management of the open abdomen: a systematic review. J Trauma Acute Care Surg. 2017;82(2):407–18.
30. Goussous N, Jenkins DH, Zielinski MD. Primary fascial closure after damage control laparotomy: sepsis vs haemorrhage. Injury. 2014;45(1):151–5.
31. Fox CJ, et al. Damage control resuscitation for vascular surgery in a combat support hospital. J Trauma. 2008;65(1):1–9.
32. Rasmussen TE, et al. The use of temporary vascular shunts as a damage control adjunct in the management of wartime vascular injury. J Trauma. 2006;61(1):8–12; discussion 12–5.
33. Ball CG, Feliciano DV. Damage control techniques for common and external iliac artery injuries: have temporary intravascular shunts replaced the need for ligation? J Trauma. 2010;68(5):1117–20.
34. Wlodarczyk JR, et al. To shunt or not to shunt in combined orthopedic and vascular extremity trauma. J Trauma Acute Care Surg. 2018;85(6):1038–42.
35. Bown MJ, et al. A meta-analysis of 50 years of ruptured abdominal aortic aneurysm repair. Br J Surg. 2002;89(6):714–30.
36. Tadlock MD, et al. Damage control in the management of ruptured abdominal aortic aneurysm: preliminary results. Vasc Endovasc Surg. 2010;44(8):638–44.
37. Cortese F, et al. Gastroduodenal major haemorrhages in critical patients: an original surgical technique. Ann Ital Chir. 2013;84(6):671–9.
38. Ball CG, et al. A decade's experience with balloon catheter tamponade for the emergency control of hemorrhage. J Trauma. 2011;70(2):330–3.
39. Morgan K, Mansker D, Adams DB. Not just for trauma patients: damage control laparotomy in pancreatic surgery. J Gastrointest Surg. 2010;14(5):768–72.
40. Ball CG, et al. Damage control principles for pancreatic surgery. J Gastrointest Surg. 2010;14(10):1632–3; author reply 1634.
41. Rotondo MF, Bard MR. Damage control surgery for thoracic injuries. Injury. 2004;35(7):649–54.
42. Vargo DJ, Battistella FD. Abbreviated thoracotomy and temporary chest closure: an application of damage control after thoracic trauma. Arch Surg. 2001;136(1):21–4.
43. Mackowski MJ, et al. Damage control for thoracic trauma. Am Surg. 2014;80(9):910–3.
44. O'Connor JV, DuBose JJ, Scalea TM. Damage-control thoracic surgery: management and outcomes. J Trauma Acute Care Surg. 2014;77(5):660–5.
45. Lang JL, et al. Does temporary chest wall closure with or without chest packing improve survival for trauma patients in shock after emergent thoracotomy? J Trauma. 2011;70(3):705–9.

limited utility in diagnosing acute surgical conditions. When compared with CT, radiography has a lower sensitivity and specificity in most applications [5]. When the clinical suspicion of acute pathology is high, CT will often be performed regardless in addition to radiographs further increasing the radiation, cost, and time to diagnosis.

Ultrasound

Ultrasound (US) is a quick and inexpensive method for evaluating acute abdominal and pelvic pain [6]. The lack of ionizing radiation often makes it the preferred initial modality in the pregnant and pediatric populations. Doppler analysis allows the assessment of blood flow within an organ in cases such as ovarian torsion [7]. Compression with the transducer aids in real-time localization of pain [8]. The ability to perform the exam at the bedside reduces the need to transport critically ill patients. Ultrasound suffers from being operator-dependent with the need for an experienced sonographer [9]. Additionally, large body habitus and/or overlying bowel gas may limit the evaluation of deep organs.

Magnetic Resonance Imaging

Magnetic resonance imaging (MRI) is less commonly used in diagnosing acute surgical conditions. The examination is lengthy, often requiring the patient to remain relatively motionless in an enclosed environment for up to 30 min. Many patients with metal devices or suspected foreign bodies are unable to safely enter the magnetic field. Also, MRI is a limited and costly resource and not always readily available. MRI benefits from the absence of ionizing radiation making it useful in evaluating causes of acute abdominal pain in pregnant or pediatric patients [10]. In fact, at many institutions, MRI is used in the workup of appendicitis in pregnancy when the initial ultrasound is equivocal (Fig. 6.1).

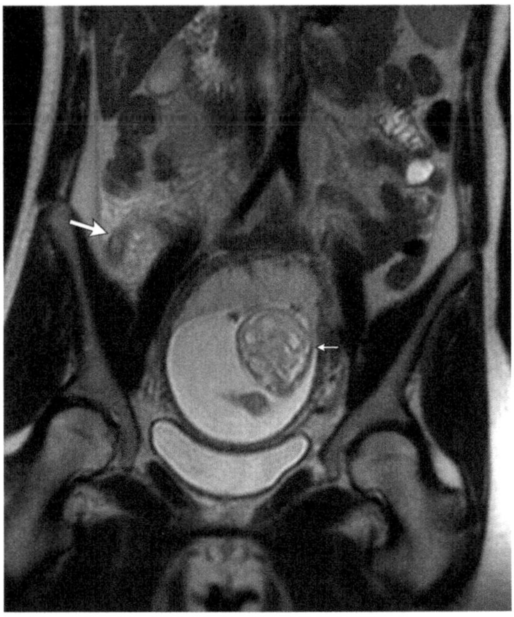

Fig. 6.1 Coronal T2-weighted (SSFSE) MRI in a patient presenting with right lower quadrant pain at 16 weeks gestation. Initial ultrasound was equivocal due to poor visualization. The appendix is enlarged measuring 1 cm (large arrow) with subtle peri-appendiceal hyperintensity suggesting inflammation of the surrounding fat. Findings were consistent with appendicitis, which was confirmed at surgery. Note the intrauterine pregnancy (small arrow)

Computerized Tomography

Advances in computerized tomography (CT) have made it one of the most useful tools in diagnosing acute conditions and ensuring timely surgical intervention [11]. CT has the ability to quickly acquire a large volume of data and post-process it in a variety of manners depending on the clinical question. High spatial resolution and the ability to create three-dimensional multiplanar reformats also assist in complicated evaluations.

Although newer technology has decreased the amount of ionizing radiation, CT still possesses the highest radiation dose of most commonly performed radiology examinations [12]. This is especially important in the pediatric and pregnant population when limiting radiation dose is paramount. The use of low-dose protocols and appropriate shielding can be utilized to ensure the dose is as low as reasonably achievable if CT is required.

Important Principles of CT

A basic understanding of how a CT image is obtained is useful in interpretation. There are several key components on a CT image: air, fat, water, soft tissue, and bone. If a component absorbs radiation, it is considered radiodense and will appear bright. The Hounsfield unit (HU) is a measurement of radiodensity. By definition, pure water is assigned an HU of 0. Air does not effectively absorb radiation and appears dark (negative HU). In contrast, bone/metal absorbs radiation relatively well and appears bright (positive HU). The individual makeup of tissue at a particular location on CT will determine how bright that spot appears. As the CT gantry rotates, it measures these tiny pixels in three dimensions (voxels) which are combined together to create the CT image that we are accustomed to seeing [13].

Appropriate window and leveling settings are important when interpreting to aid in contrast between similar tissues. Commonly used window/level settings include the soft tissue, bone, and lung among many others (Fig. 6.2). Axial, coronal, and sagittal views are typically reconstructed from one data set. Many imaging software packages now include the ability to create multiplanar formats in any orientation at the workstation and manipulate in three dimensions.

Intravenous (IV) iodinated contrast is often useful in detection of pathology. Knowledge of the timing at which a CT scan was performed following administration of IV contrast is important

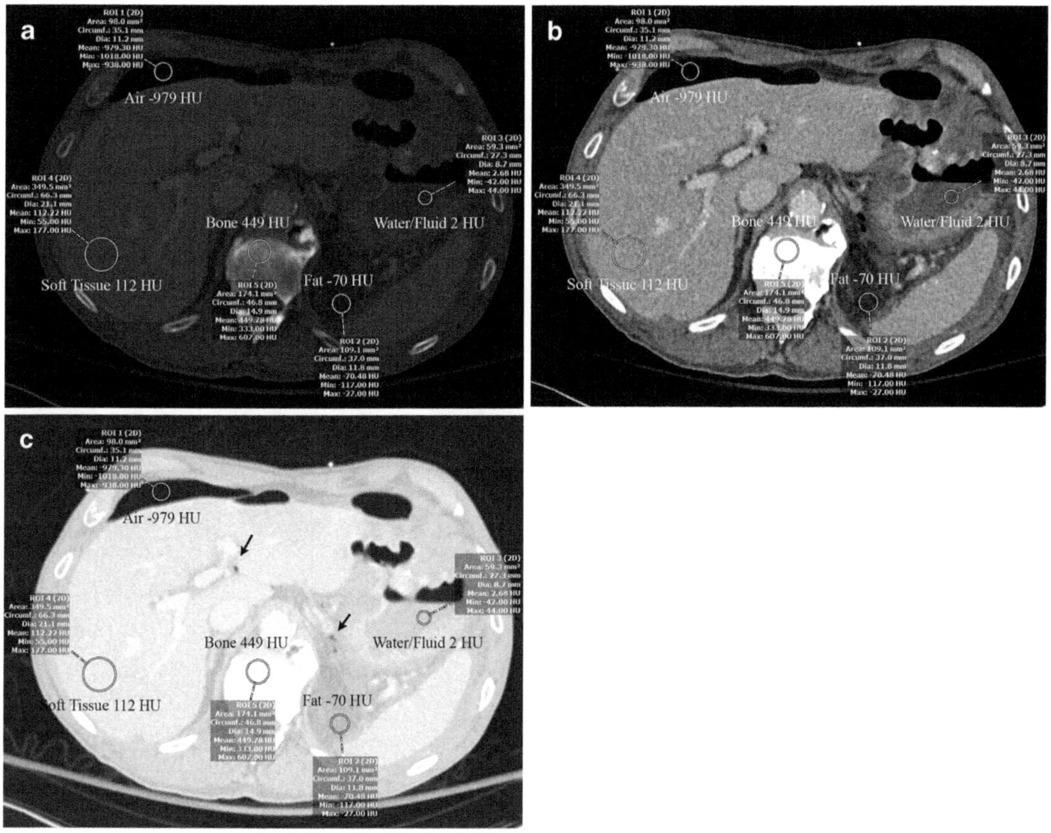

Fig. 6.2 Axial contrast-enhanced CT slice through the abdomen with preset window and level settings demonstrating the range of different tissue densities/attenuation. The major components are air, fat, water, soft tissue, and bone. The selected window and level setting examples include bone (**a**), soft tissue (**b**), and lung (**c**). Note the tissue density (HU) does not change between settings. Additionally, there are several locules of free air within the abdomen that are more apparent when utilizing the lung window (small arrows). This patient had a perforated viscus

when interpreting the results. For example, different timing is used to evaluate the arteries, veins, organs, and urinary collecting system. With the recent improvement in CT scanner resolution, the role of oral contrast is diminished [14]. Oral contrast limits the evaluation of the bowel wall in suspected perforation and ischemia. It is associated with longer wait times due to patient preparation [15]. Oral contrast remains useful when evaluating the bowel wall for subtle implants or peritoneal disease as well as in identifying leak/perforation from hollow viscus. Water or neutral oral contrast can be considered when distention of the bowel is required. Throughout this chapter, contrast-enhanced CT will refer to the use of IV contrast only unless oral contrast is specified.

Critical Findings on CT

Free Air

Free intraperitoneal air on CT or radiography may be the first finding of gastrointestinal perforation. Intraperitoneal air is easiest to detect on CT when utilizing window and level settings typically reserved for viewing the lungs to help differentiate air from mesenteric fat. With larger volume pneumoperitoneum, upright abdominal radiographs can demonstrate crescentic air below the diaphragms (Fig. 6.3). However, radiographs are less sensitive than CT. In 10% of patients, pneumoperitoneum may be related to other causes such as postoperative air, peritoneal dialysis, and entry through the gynecologic tract [16].

Hemorrhage

Active hemorrhage on CT will present as a focal collection of IV contrast outside of the expected course of a blood vessel. On delayed imaging, the pool of extravasated contrast will expand and become less dense as it is diluted by additional blood (Fig. 6.4). Nontraumatic causes of hemoperitoneum include malignancy, gynecologic, vascular, or iatrogenic [17]. Bleeding may also be confined to an organ such as the bowel. In this case, there will be shifting high-density contrast moving through the bowel on delayed imaging. A pseudoaneurysm may mimic active hemorrhage, but the extravasated pool of contrast will not expand on delayed imaging.

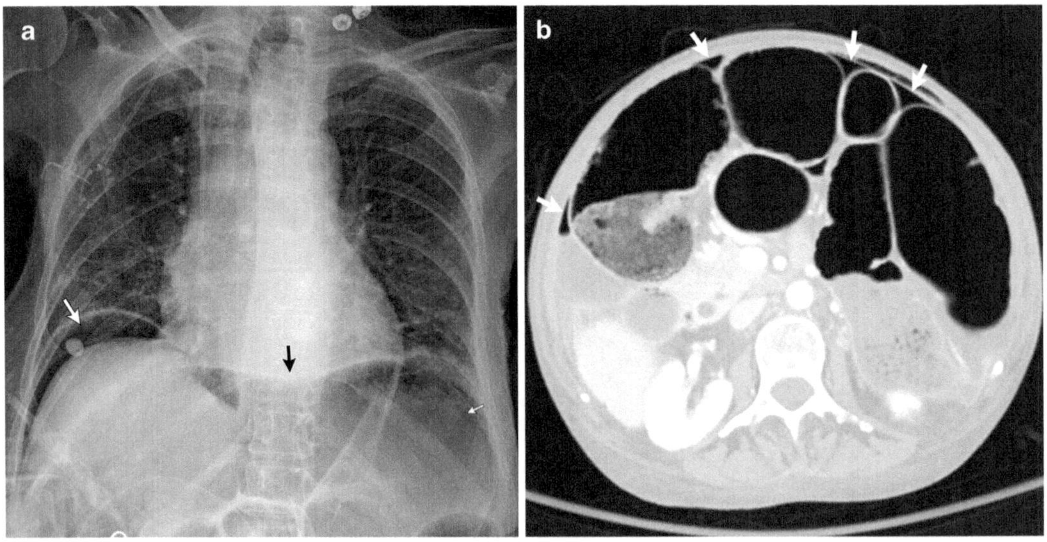

Fig. 6.3 Chest radiograph and contrast-enhanced CT in a patient presenting with peritonitis. Chest radiograph (**a**) demonstrates free air under the diaphragm (large white arrow), a "continuous diaphragm sign" (black arrow), and a density gradient over the upper left abdomen (small white arrow) consistent with pneumoperitoneum. Axial CT (**b**) shows diffusely dilated bowel with free intraperitoneal air (white arrow). Bowel perforation was confirmed during exploratory laparotomy

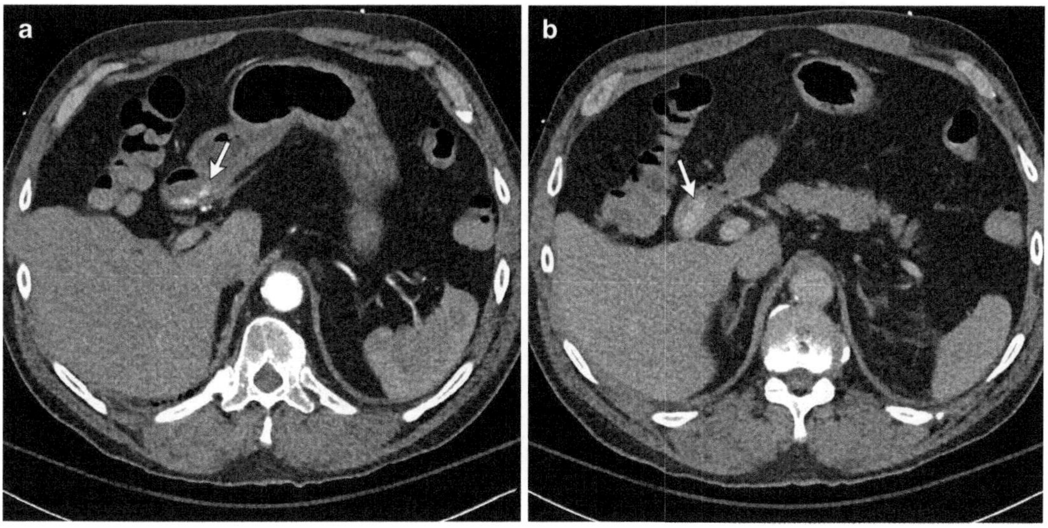

Fig. 6.4 Contrast-enhanced CT in a 61-year-old male presenting with abdominal pain. Arterial phase axial image (**a**) demonstrates a focal collection of contrast in the lumen of the duodenum. On delayed imaging (**b**), the contrast within the duodenum has migrated, expanded, and been diluted. This was subsequently proven to be related to peptic ulcer disease

Tissue Enhancement

Various vascular tissues demonstrate increased uptake of iodinated IV contrast creating enhancement on CT. Increased enhancement in an unexpected location may indicate a neoplastic, infectious, or inflammatory process. Conversely, the absence of enhancement may indicate ischemia such as in acute mesenteric ischemia, small bowel volvulus, or ovarian torsion. Utilization of multiple imaging planes can assist in the evaluation of mucosal integrity and enhancement.

Inflammatory Fat Stranding

On typical CT window/level settings, fat appears darker (less dense/lower HU) than surrounding soft tissue and organs. When there is an adjacent inflammatory process, the mesenteric and retroperitoneal fat becomes edematous and demonstrates increased vascularity. This leads to an increase in density (increased HU), creating the commonly referenced "inflammatory fat stranding" that can be the first clue to a developing pathology (Fig. 6.5). Table 6.1 contains examples of potential etiologies which should be considered when critical findings are present (Table 6.1).

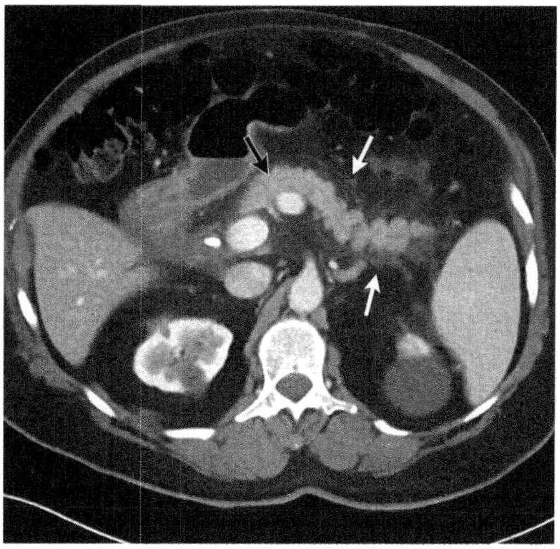

Fig. 6.5 Contrast-enhanced CT in a 75-year-old male with abdominal pain one day after endoscopic retrograde cholangiopancreatography (ERCP) for choledocholithiasis. Increased density of the mesenteric fat and edema ("inflammatory fat stranding" white arrows) surrounding the pancreas (black arrow) consistent with post-ERCP pancreatitis

Table 6.1 Important findings on CT with commonly associated causes

Pneumoperitoneum [18]	
	Perforated viscus (most common)
	Postoperative
	Peritoneal dialysis
	Gynecologic tract
	Increased thoracic pressure
	Pneumatosis cystoides intestinalis
	Trauma
	Iatrogenic
	Idiopathic
Hemorrhage	
	Gastrointestinal bleed
	Hemoperitoneum [19]
	Malignancy/vascular tumor
	Ruptured ovarian cyst
	Ruptured ectopic pregnancy
	Ruptured aneurysm
	Iatrogenic
	Anticoagulation
	Trauma
Tissue enhancement	
	Increased
	Inflammatory reaction
	Infection/abscess
	Neoplasm/tumor
	Decreased
	Ischemia/infarction
Fat stranding [20]	
	Inflammatory
	Infectious
	Infarction/fat necrosis

Table 6.2 Acute abdominal surgical conditions when imaging is essential

Gastrointestinal	
	Esophageal perforation
	Perforated bowel
	Mesenteric ischemia
	Appendicitis
	Diverticulitis
	Volvulus
	Gastric
	Midgut
	Cecal
	Sigmoid
	Obstruction
	Gastric outlet
	Small bowel
	Colonic
	Hemorrhage
Biliary tract	
	Cholecystitis
	Calculus
	Acalculous
	Gangrenous
	Emphysematous
	Perforated
	Acute cholangitis
	Pancreatitis
Genitourinary	
	Urinary obstruction
	Renal abscess
	Pyonephrosis
	Emphysematous pyelonephritis
	Emphysematous cystitis
	Ovarian torsion
	Tubo-ovarian abscess
	Ectopic pregnancy
	Testicular torsion
	Fournier's gangrene

Imaging Examples of Acute Surgical Emergencies

Our goal in the remainder of this chapter is to briefly review findings associated with the most commonly encountered surgical conditions. While this is not an exhaustive list, we hope that many of the principles we review here can be applied to those unique circumstances which are not described. Below are select examples and imaging findings of common acute conditions with which surgeons should be familiar with (Table 6.2).

Gastrointestinal

Gastric and Duodenal Perforation

Despite improved medical therapy, peptic ulcer disease (PUD) remains one of the most common causes of gastric and duodenal perforation. Many ulcers are not visible on CT prior to perforation due to only superficial involvement of the gastric mucosa. Deep and penetrating ulcers may be visible as a focal defect in the gastric wall (Fig. 6.6). A hazy appearance of the inflamed surrounding mesenteric fat can also help localize a penetrating ulcer [21].

Following Roux-en-Y gastric bypass, marginal ulcers can occur at the jejunal side of a gastrojejunal anastomosis and result in perforation [22]. The postoperative nature and location can make these difficult to detect. However, multiplanar reformats can be especially helpful for evaluating the surgical site and should be carefully reviewed.

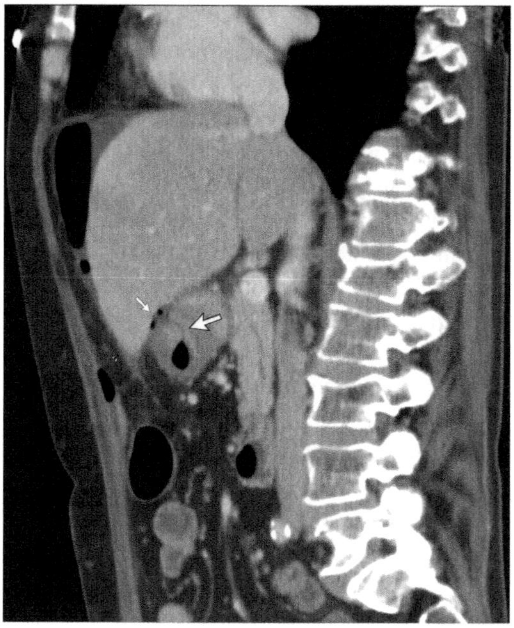

Fig. 6.6 Contrast-enhanced CT in a patient presenting with 1 day of progressive, sharp epigastric pain. Sagittal reformat demonstrates a focal defect along the lesser curvature of the stomach near the antrum (large arrow). Several small adjacent foci of free gas are seen near the liver capsule (small arrow) suggestive of perforation. Surgery confirmed a perforated ulcer and the repair was uncomplicated. Biopsy returned as benign ulceration

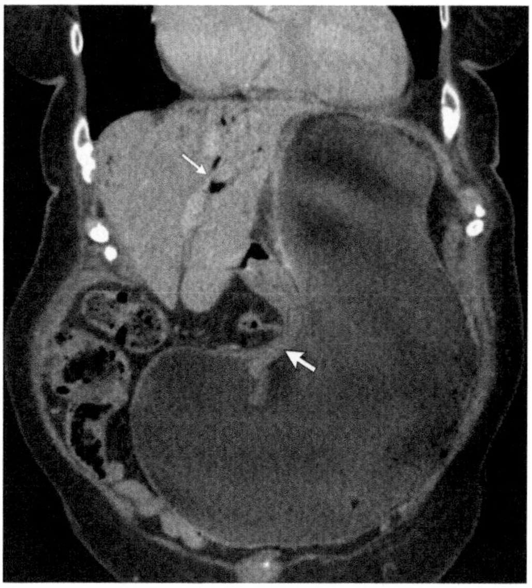

Fig. 6.7 Contrast-enhanced CT in a patient with 4 days of abdominal pain, nausea, and emesis. Coronal reformats demonstrate marked distention of the stomach. The pylorus is thickened and collapsed, consistent with gastric outlet obstruction (large arrows). Gas is present within the portal veins (small arrow), and there is gastric wall pneumatosis (not shown) indicative of ischemia. Endoscopic evaluation revealed a large ulcer extending from the gastric body to the antrum. Subsequent endoscopy demonstrated intermittent volvulus. The ulceration was believed to be due to volvulus related ischemia

The use of positive oral contrast can increase the sensitivity of perforation. However, this obscures the gastric mucosa and reduces the ability to determine the precise location of perforation [23]. Water or neutral contrast is commonly used to distend the stomach without obscuring the gastric wall.

Additional less common nontraumatic causes of gastric perforation include malignancy and postsurgical complications such as gastric banding [24]. Malignancy will present with similar CT findings of focal gastric wall thickening and central ulceration. Often, it is impossible to differentiate between PUD and malignancy using CT alone, and direct visualization/biopsy is required.

Gastric Outlet Obstruction

Patients with gastric outlet obstruction may be initially detected with an abdominal radiograph demonstrating marked distension of the stomach. CT is then useful to further investigate the numerous potential underlying causes (Fig. 6.7). Historically, PUD was the most common etiology of gastric obstruction. However, with advances in the treatment of PUD, malignancy has become the most common [25]. Both can present similarly as previously described and may be difficult to differentiate on imaging alone.

Gastric volvulus is an emergent cause of gastric obstruction. There are two types of gastric volvulus: organoaxial and mesenteroaxial [26]. In organoaxial, the stomach rotates around the long axis with the greater curvature appearing above the lesser curvature. In mesenteroaxial, the stomach rotates about the short axis with the pylorus moving above the gastroesophageal junction. Restriction of blood supply by twisting the vasculature in the mesentery can be seen on contrast-enhanced CT as decreased enhancement of the gastric wall.

Other potential causes of obstruction that can be seen on CT include bezoars, gallstones, and malpositioned gastric bands.

Small Bowel Obstruction

CT is the recommended modality for diagnosing and evaluating the patient with suspected small bowel obstruction (SBO) [27]. Commonly, dilated loops of bowel with air fluid levels seen on radiographs indicate a high-grade obstruction [28]. However, radiographs are less sensitive than CT and cannot evaluate for an underlying etiology. CT findings for SBO include dilated loops of small bowel >2.5 cm, mesenteric edema, and ascites. Additionally, the "small bowel feces" sign (Fig. 6.8) refers to the appearance of fecalized stool in the small bowel indicative of delayed transit and potential obstruction. The location of obstruction can be identified by searching for a focal transition point where the bowel is acutely narrowed. Typically, the small bowel proximal to an obstruction is dilated, while the bowel distal to the obstruction is decompressed (Fig. 6.9).

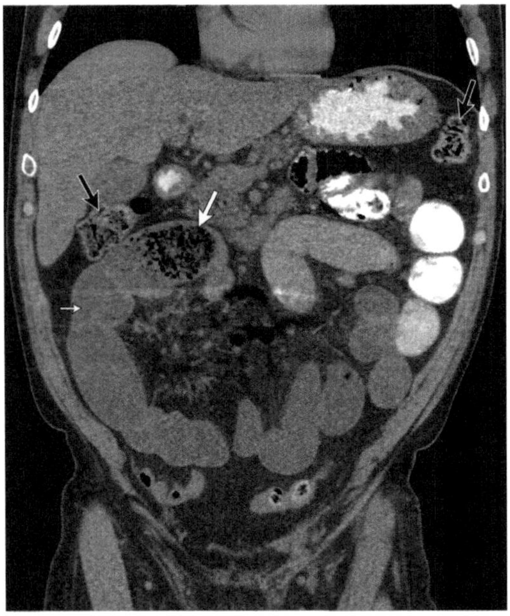

Fig. 6.8 IV and oral contrast-enhanced CT in a 67-year-old male with abdominal pain. Coronal reformat shows dilated loops of fluid filled bowel (small white arrow). A section of small bowel contains air filled stool (large white arrow; "small bowel feces sign") similar in appearance to stool within adjacent colon (black arrows) indicating delayed transit. The patient underwent exploratory laparotomy with lysis of adhesion for small bowel obstruction

Adhesions are the most common cause of SBO [29]. However, they are not typically visible on CT, and often a cause for obstruction cannot be confidently identified. A closed-loop obstruction occurs when two ends of small bowel are simultaneously obstructed, typically by adhesions. A "C" or "U" configuration of the bowel is a common finding when the two points of obstruction are caused by an adhesion in the same location. The vascular strangulation that follows may result in decreased bowel wall enhancement on contrast-enhanced CT and eventually necrosis. Oral contrast impairs visualization of the bowel wall and limits the evaluation for bowel ischemia [23]. For this reason, CT with oral contrast should not be routinely used in the evaluation for SBO. Additionally, slow transit time further decreases utility, and the patient preparation may delay obtaining the results [15].

Appendicitis

In the majority of patients with suspected appendicitis, CT is the best examination with a sensitivity and specificity approaching 100% [30]. Traditionally, the diagnosis was made clinically. However, several studies have shown that imaging can substantially decrease the rate of nega-

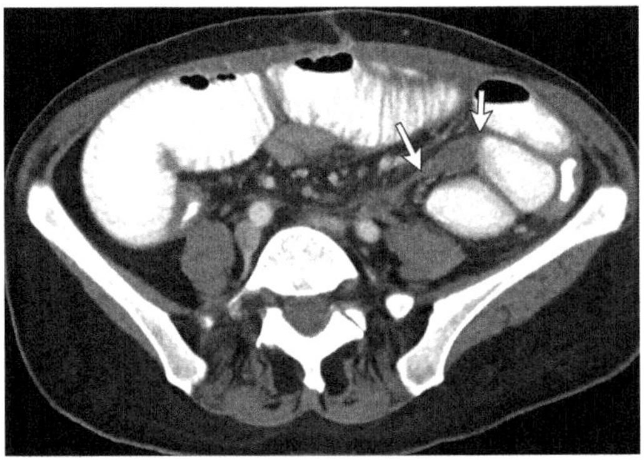

Fig. 6.9 IV and oral contrast-enhanced CT in a patient with history of prior abdominal surgeries now experiencing persistent abdominal pain and bloating. Axial CT slice demonstrates multiple dilated loops of small bowel. There is a focal transition point in the left lower abdomen with decompressed small bowel distally (arrows). No contrast passes into the distal small bowel. Findings are consistent with high-grade small bowel obstruction. Surgery confirmed multiple adhesions along the abdominal wall

tive appendectomies [31]. An enlarged appendix measuring >6 mm with associated inflammatory mesenteric fat stranding is a highly suggestive finding [32]. Appendicoliths can also be seen, although they are not indicative of active inflammation. Ultrasound and MRI are useful in pregnant patients. Sonographic findings include an appendix measuring >6 mm and noncompressibility when using transducer pressure. However, the position of the appendix or overlying bowel gas can obscure fine detail. MRI can be used in equivocal cases. The use of IV contrast is not required to make the diagnosis with MRI [33].

Complications of appendicitis include perforation, peritonitis, and abscess formation. Focal decreased enhancement of the appendiceal wall may indicate necrosis and pending rupture. Using multiplanar reformats, a defect in the wall can often be seen and is the most specific sign of perforation [34] (Fig. 6.10). Other findings include surrounding low-density peri-appendiceal fluid, abscess formation, extraluminal air, and extraluminal appendicolith. The development of a well-defined fluid collection with the surrounding enhancing wall suggests abscess formation.

Bowel Ischemia

Intravenous contrast-enhanced CT angiography is the best examination in cases of suspected mesenteric ischemia [35]. Causes of intestinal ischemia include embolic disease, venous thrombosis, intussusception, closed-loop obstruction, and volvulus [36]. Specific findings on CT include decreased wall enhancement, surrounding mesenteric fat stranding, and free fluid adjacent to the bowel wall regardless of the etiology (Fig. 6.11). Thinning of the bowel wall is specific to arterial embolic occlusion, while thickening and edema of the bowel wall are seen with venous outflow obstruction. Focal involvement of a particular segment of the bowel can aid in localizing where the vascular compromise occurred. In advanced cases, pneumatosis and portal venous gas related to bowel necrosis can be seen. Closed-loop obstruction and volvulus may demonstrate a twisting of the vasculature around the rotation point commonly referred to as the "whirlpool sign" seen on CT and US [37]. As previously discussed, positive oral contrast may obscure the bowel wall and should not be used if specifically evaluating for enhancement.

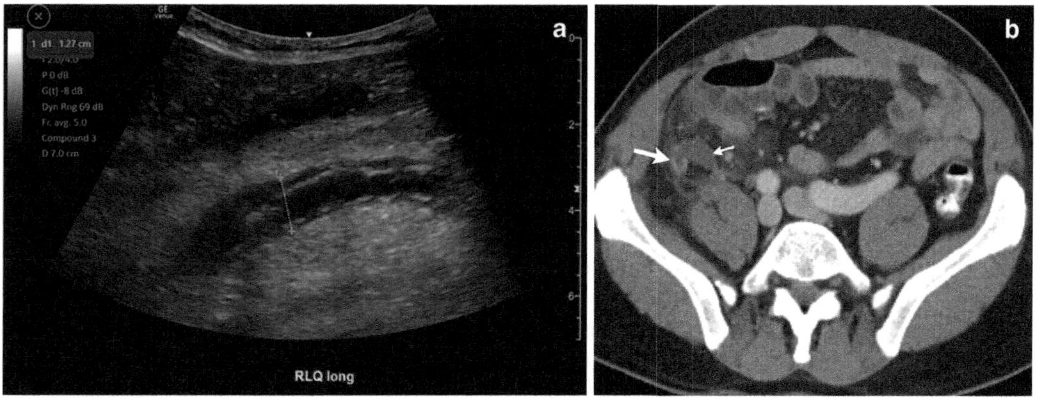

Fig. 6.10 US and contrast-enhanced CT in a patient presenting with 4 days of right lower quadrant pain. US (**a**) demonstrates a blind-ending, dilated tubular structure measuring 1.2 cm. Real-time imaging reveals noncompressibility and surrounding hyperemia (not shown). CT was obtained to assess for complications (**b**). Axial CT reformats demonstrate a focal wall defect along the anterior wall of the appendix consistent with perforation (large arrow). A small amount of free fluid is seen adjacent to the appendix (small arrow). Surgery confirmed a gangrenous and perforated appendix

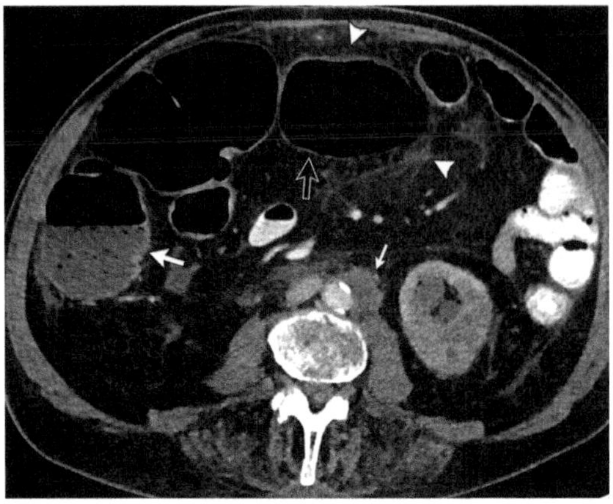

Fig. 6.11 IV and oral contrast-enhanced CT in a patient with metastatic lung cancer presenting with abdominal pain. Axial CT image shows wall thinning and decreased enhancement of the transverse/descending colon (black arrow) when compared with the normal appearing ascending colon (large white arrow). There is mesenteric edema and inflammatory fat stranding along the transverse and descending colon (arrowhead). Additionally, a mass is seen invading the tissues along the anterior aorta in the region of the expected inferior mesenteric artery (IMA) origin (small arrow). The distribution is consistent with mesenteric ischemia from IMA occlusion

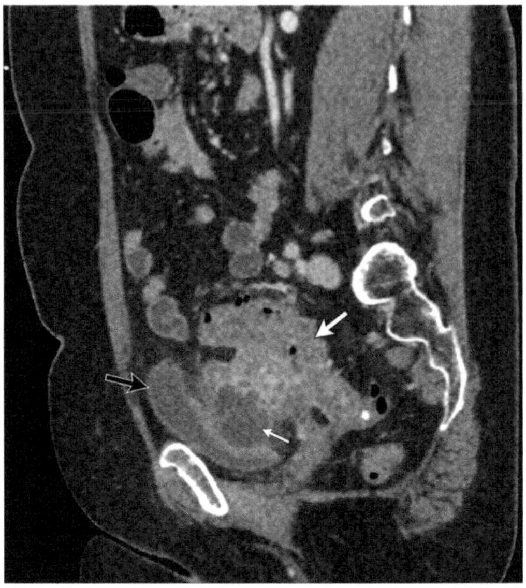

Fig. 6.12 Contrast-enhanced CT in a patient presenting with persistent low-grade abdominal pain. Sagittal reformats demonstrate thickening of the sigmoid colon with surrounding inflammatory fat stranding (large white arrow). There are multiple adjacent colonic diverticula. A pericolonic diverticular abscess (small white arrow) is interposed between the sigmoid colon and urinary bladder (black arrow). This location was not amenable to percutaneous drainage. Conservative management was unsuccessful and surgical intervention was required for definitive treatment

Diverticulitis

Diverticulitis is a commonly encountered condition best diagnosed by CT [38]. Often, the first imaging finding will be mesenteric fat stranding, which can then be used to direct scrutiny to the adjacent bowel. However, the surrounding inflammation can mask diverticula which won't be apparent until follow-up imaging. CT is also useful to look for complications such as perforation, abscess, obstruction, or bleeding [39] (Fig. 6.12). A small amount of intraperitoneal air will be present when perforation has occurred. Most perforations are locally contained. However, 1–2% of patients will have non-contained perforation which can lead to more advanced complications such as abscess and fistula to surrounding structures.

Malignancy can present similarly to diverticulitis with wall thickening and enlargement of surrounding lymph nodes [40]. Signs that favor diverticulitis include segmental involvement >10 cm and surrounding mesenteric inflammation. A follow-up CT scan or endoscopic evaluation should be considered for further evaluation in select patients once symptoms have resolved [40].

Biliary Tract

Cholecystitis

Ultrasound is the recommended initial test in a patient with right upper quadrant pain and suspected cholecystitis [41]. Gallbladder distention, wall thickness >3 mm, hypoechoic pericholecystic fluid, and cholelithiasis are commonly encountered features. Pain with transducer pressure over the right upper abdomen is often reported. However, the sensitivity and specificity of a "sonographic Murphy's sign" may be unreliable if the patient has recently been administered pain medication [42].

When the initial US is equivocal, several advanced options are available. Cholescintigraphy (hepatobiliary iminodiacetic acid (HIDA) scan) has higher sensitivity and specificity than US, but results take longer to obtain, and evaluation for other causes of pain is limited [43]. In a HIDA scan, an injected radiotracer is circulated and excreted into the bile. Failure to visualize radiotracer uptake in the gallbladder at 4 h is essentially diagnostic of acute cholecystitis. CT and MRI are other second-line options with findings that include distention, wall thickening, and surrounding inflammatory changes [41] (Fig. 6.13). Similar imaging findings are also seen in acalculous cholecystitis [44]. CT and MRI are useful in evaluating potential complications of cholecystitis.

Emphysematous Cholecystitis

Proliferation of gas-forming organisms within the gallbladder is a life-threatening condition. CT has the highest sensitivity for demonstrating gas within the gallbladder lumen or wall [45]. US is less sensitive but may show thin echogenic (bright) lines with decreased posterior transmission creating a "dirty shadowing" appearance. A calcified gall bladder wall or gall stones will also appear echogenic and potentially mimic gas. However, the calcium creates a more complete posterior shadow referred to as "clean shadowing." Historically, radiographs were used to stage the degree of disease based on gas location in the lumen, wall, or pericholecystic tissue [46]. However, CT has now largely replaced the use of radiographs and should be obtained if there is a concern (Fig. 6.14).

Gangrenous Cholecystitis and Perforation

Compromise of the gallbladder vascular supply can lead to wall ischemia. On the US, thin echoic lines may be seen within the lumen representing sloughed membranes [47]. In addition, CT may demonstrate decreased enhancement in the necrotic wall [48]. If the compromise continues, the gallbladder wall may progress to perforation with high associated mortality. Perforation typically occurs near the fundus where the vascular supply is weakest. A focal wall defect is the most specific sign and may be seen with CT and less likely with US [49] (Fig. 6.15). Secondary signs include a collapsed gall bladder, fluid collecting in the right hemiabdomen, and inflammatory fat stranding.

Acute Cholangitis

Obstruction and subsequent infection of the biliary system carry a high mortality rate requiring a timely and accurate diagnosis [50]. Dilation and wall thickening of the bile ducts can be seen with all modalities. Specifically, intrahepatic biliary

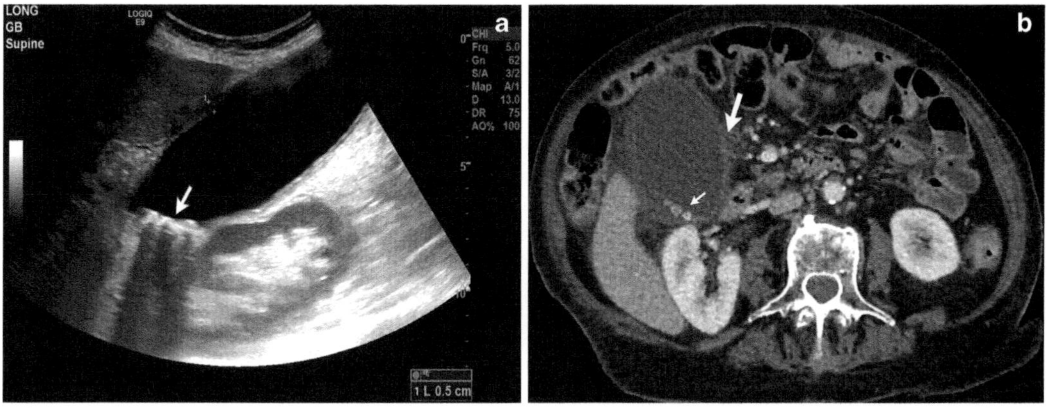

Fig. 6.13 US and contrast-enhanced CT in a patient presenting to the emergency department with abdominal pain, fever, and weakness. US (**a**) shows a gall bladder with a mildly thickened wall (0.5 cm). Multiple layering echogenic gallstones with associated posterior shadowing are seen. Transducer pressure over the right upper quadrant elicited pain. Axial CT (**b**) demonstrates wall thickening with surrounding inflammatory fat stranding (large arrow). The gallstones are partially calcified and visible on CT (small arrow). Findings were confirmed during cholecystectomy

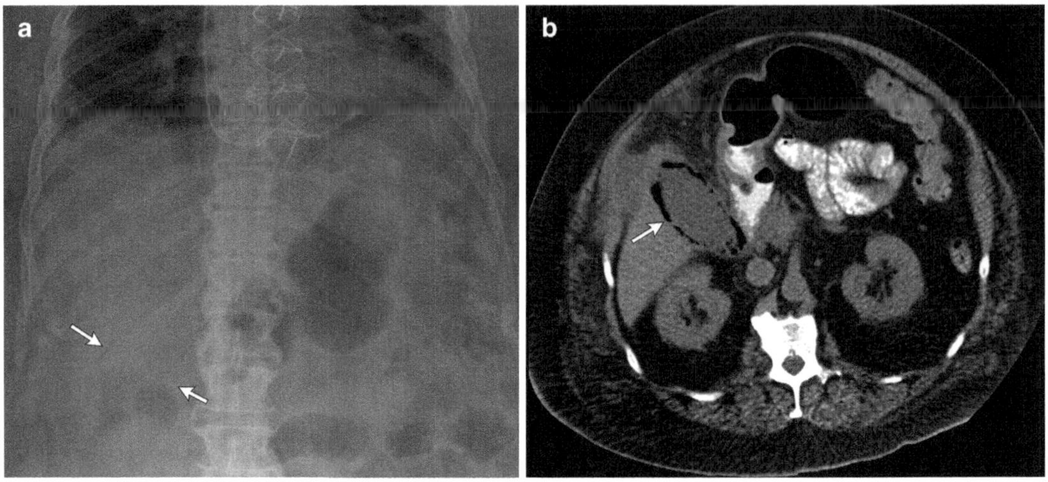

Fig. 6.14 Abdominal radiograph and contrast-enhanced CT in a diabetic patient admitted with chest pain who spiked a fever during evaluation for acute coronary syndrome. Radiograph (**a**) demonstrates a curvilinear area of lucency (arrow) over the right abdomen suspicious for emphysematous cholecystitis. Axial CT (**b**) confirms the diagnosis and shows extensive gas within the gallbladder wall (arrow). Management was initially attempted with percutaneous cholecystostomy due to comorbidities. However, the patient developed hemodynamic instability and was taken to the operating room emergently

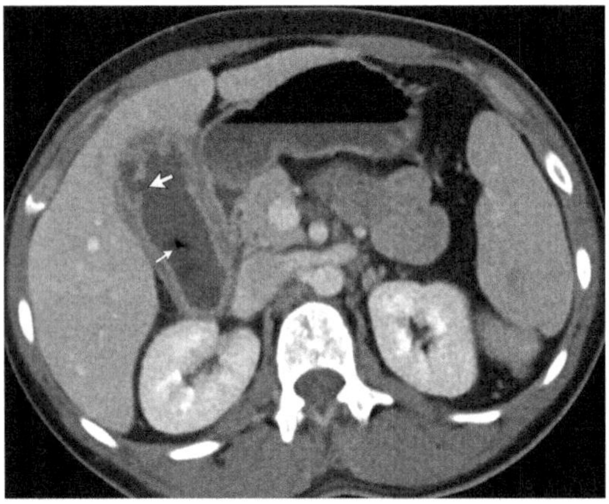

Fig. 6.15 Contrast-enhanced CT performed in a patient with a 1-week history of intermittent abdominal pain. Axial image shows thickening and edema of the gallbladder wall. There is a focal defect near the fundus at the site of perforation (large arrow). Additionally, there are several locules of gas within the lumen (small arrows) consistent with necrosis. Surgery confirmed multifocal perforation with several gallstones having eroded through the wall

ductal dilation is the most common imaging finding [51]. US can demonstrate purulence within the bile ducts as a layering echogenic density.

On CT, inhomogeneous geographic enhancement of the liver has also been described, although it is a nonspecific finding and can be seen in other conditions.

Choledocholithiasis is the most common inciting factor in up to 80% of acute cholangitis [52]. Determining the underlying cause of obstruction may be difficult during acute inflammation. An abrupt cutoff of the common bile duct can be seen with CT, although it may be impossible to differentiate between a gallstone and mass. Overlying bowel gas limits deep sonographic evaluation, and choledocholithiasis is more difficult to detect than cholelithiasis.

Magnetic resonance cholangiopancreatography (MRCP) is an excellent noninvasive option [53]. Gallstones will appear as darkened filling defects within the hyperintense (bright) bile. Excellent spatial resolution allows stones as small as 2 mm to be detected. MRCP does not require the use of radiation of iodinated contrast. However, MRCP is more expensive, less available, and not therapeutic when compared with traditional endoscopic retrograde cholangiopancreatography.

Genitourinary

Acute Renal Obstruction

Both CT and US can be used to evaluate renal obstruction depending on the age of the patient. Unenhanced CT is the initial preferred method of evaluation in most adult patients with suspected renal stones [54]. The use of IV contrast can aid in evaluating perfusion but may obscure stones within the collecting system and is not routinely recommended.

US can also be used to quickly evaluate for renal stones, hydronephrosis, and bladder distension. Calcified stones appear echogenic with posterior shadowing. Using Doppler imaging, stones my demonstrate a colorful "twinkling" artifact which can further aid in detection [55]. US benefits from the absence of radiation, but the entire ureter may not be visualized due to overlying bowel gas.

Signs of acute urinary obstruction include an enlarged, edematous kidney with hydronephrosis [56]. If IV contrast is used, CT will show decreased perfusion of the parenchyma on the ipsilateral side known as a delayed nephrogram [57] (Fig. 6.16). Over time, the decreased perfusion leads to thinning of the renal cortex which is seen in long-standing chronic obstruction. Ureteral dilation will be present depending on the level of obstruction. Common locations of ureteral obstruction include the ureteropelvic junction, the pelvic brim, and the ureterovesical junction [58].

Often, a calcified phlebolith may be in close proximity to the distal ureter simulating a renal stone. If a stone is present, the wall of the ureter will surround the calcification leading to the "soft tissue rim sign" [59] (Fig. 6.17). Urothelial cancers, pelvic masses, or metastatic implants can also result in urinary obstruction.

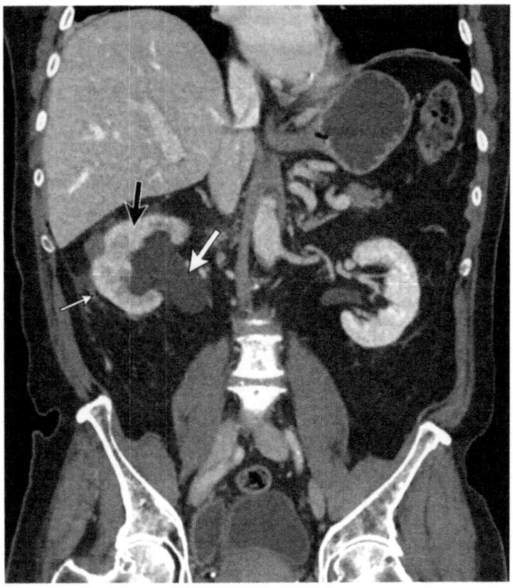

Fig. 6.16 Contrast-enhanced CT of a patient experiencing fever, dysuria, and pelvic pressure undergoing urologic workup for prostate related urinary retention. Coronal reformat demonstrates right hydroureteronephrosis (large white arrow). There is decreased enhancement of the right renal parenchyma when compared with the left (black arrow), resulting in a "delayed nephrogram." Surround perinephric inflammatory fat stranding suggests inflammation and/or infection (small white arrow). There was a 9 mm obstructing distal ureteral stone that is not shown. Due to fever and concern for superimposed infection, the patient received a right ureteral stent followed by stone extraction

Emphysematous Pyelonephritis

Gas within the renal parenchyma is suggestive of a bacterial infection causing emphysematous pyelonephritis [60]. The use of lung window/level settings can aid in detecting air on CT. On US, air will appear as echogenic foci with posterior "dirty shadowing." Radiographs can also detect air, although the sensitivity is much lower than with CT and US.

Ovarian Torsion

Due to its dynamic nature and lack of radiation, US is the preferred method for evaluation of suspected ovarian torsion [61]. An asymmetrically enlarged (>4 cm) and edematous ovary with peripherally displaced follicles is a classic appearance on all modalities. The most specific sign is the visualization of the twisted pedicle known as the "whirlpool sign" [62] (Fig. 6.18). However, the presence of vascular flow does not exclude torsion due to the potential for torsion/detorsion and a dual vascular supply which can mimic normal blood flow. In fact, Doppler flow

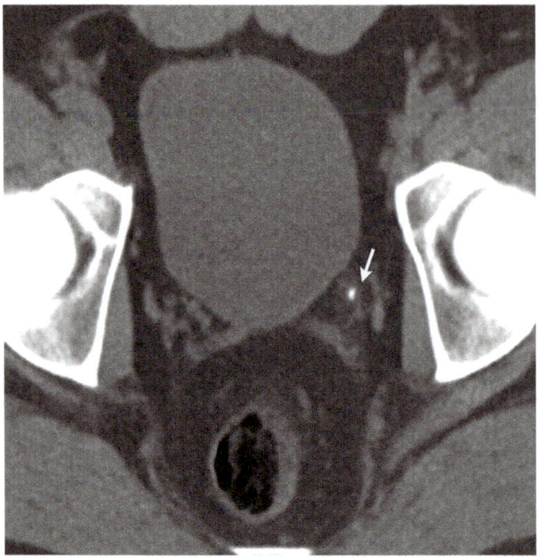

Fig. 6.17 Unenhanced CT of the abdomen and pelvis in a 24-year-old male presenting with several days of left flank pain and hematuria. Axial image at the level of the urinary bladder shows a 4 mm density surrounded by a thin rim of soft tissue representing the distal ureteral wall and periureteral inflammatory fat stranding (soft tissue rim sign). No associated hydronephrosis was present and the patient was managed conservatively

may appear normal in up to 60% of cases [63]. On CT and MRI, the enlarged ovary may display decreased enhancement indicating ischemia and possible infarction [64]. The torsed ovary may appear in the midline or in the contralateral adnexa in more than half the cases [65] (Fig. 6.19). The uterine and ovarian ligaments may appear thickened, and the uterus may be deviated toward the side of torsion. Due to the serious adverse consequences of untreated torsion, a high level of clinical suspicion should be maintained even in the absence of definitive imaging findings.

Tubo-Ovarian Abscess

Tubo-ovarian abscess (TOA) is the end result of untreated pelvic inflammatory disease related to sexually transmitted infections [66]. Because TOA usually occurs in females of reproductive age, they are typically discovered on US first. In the early stages, echogenic layering fluid within the fallopian tube represents purulence and pyosalpinx. As the infection

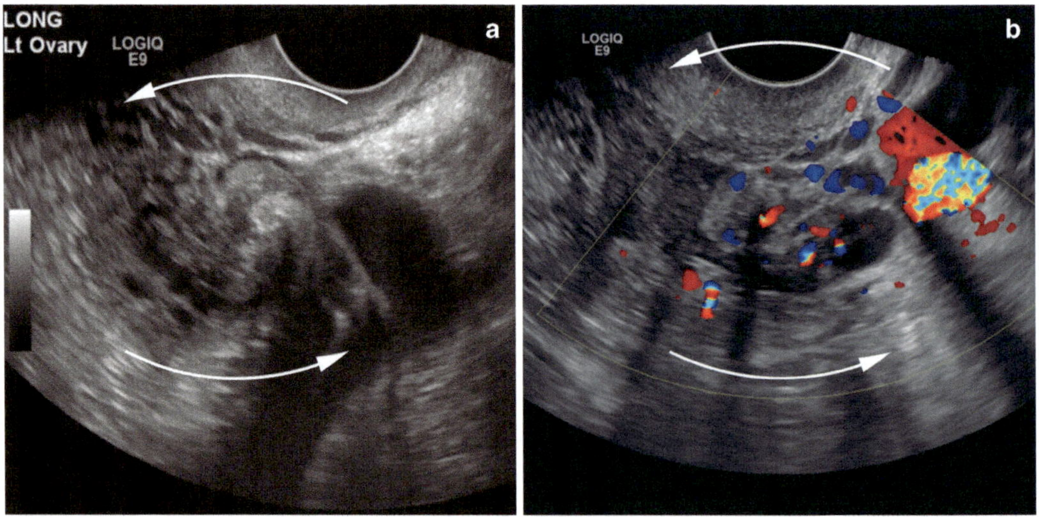

Fig. 6.18 Transvaginal US in a 38-year-old female with acute onset pelvic pain. A single grayscale screen capture from a cine video clip (**a**) in the left adnexa demonstrates a swirling appearance of the vessels leading to the ovary ("whirlpool sign"). Doppler imaging (**b**) confirms the swirling pattern is vascular with small amounts of flow detected. The left ovary was enlarged without vascular flow (not shown). Additionally, a large mass was seen within the left ovary. Surgery confirmed a 1080-degree rotation of the vascular pedicle. A large dermoid cyst was associated with the ovary causing torsion. The cyst was removed and the ovary was found to be viable

progresses, the fallopian tube and ovary become a conglomerate within the surrounding inflammation and can no longer be resolved as separate entities [67]. The most common appearance is a solid and cystic mass on US with internal septations. If a CT is obtained, there will be a multiloculated cystic mass in the adnexa [68] (Fig. 6.20). Rarely gas can be seen within the abscess which essentially confirms the diagnosis [69]. Other findings include thickening of the uterine ligaments and free fluid within the vesicouterine pouch. Perforated TOA presents with peritonitis and can lead to additional intra-abdominal abscesses and potentially fistulas to adjacent structures [69].

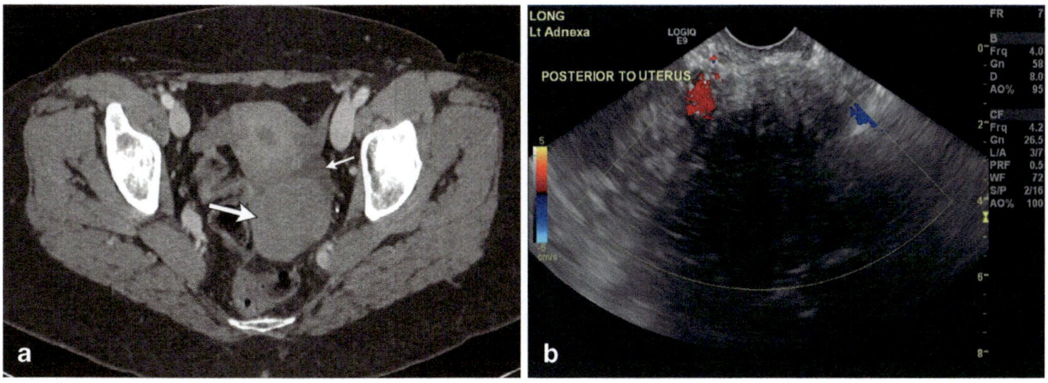

Fig. 6.19 Contrast-enhanced CT and US in a female patient presenting with abdominal pain. Axial CT (**a**) obtained first demonstrates a large adnexal mass (large arrow) posterior to the uterus and left of midline. No left ovary was identified. US (**b**) subsequently obtained demonstrates a similar ill-defined left adnexal mass without vascular flow on Doppler imaging consistent with a torsed ovary. Surgery revealed a 720-degree twist of the left ovarian vascular pedicle. The left ovary and fallopian tube were necrotic and unable to be salvaged

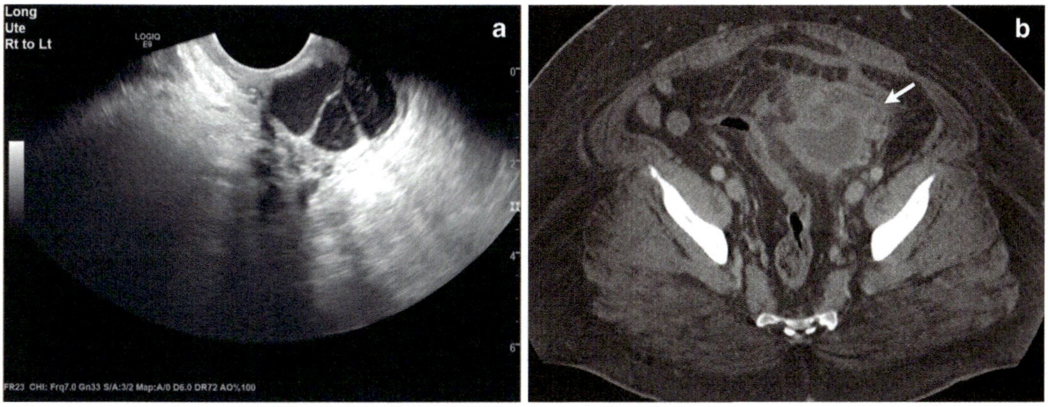

Fig. 6.20 US and CT of a female patient presenting with abdominal pain, fever, and leukocytosis. US (**a**) demonstrates a multilobulated adnexal mass with internal septations and partially complex internal fluid. Axial CT (**b**) shows a complex partially cystic and tubular mass within the left adnexa (arrow). Findings were consistent with tubo-ovarian abscess. The abscess required drain placement, which aspirated 120 mL of purulent material

Ectopic Pregnancy

Patients with a newly positive pregnancy test and pelvic pain should undergo transvaginal pelvic ultrasound to determine the location of pregnancy [61]. A fluid collection in the uterine cavity has a 99.5% chance of representing a intrauterine pregnancy and is normal until proven otherwise [70]. Likewise, close inspection is warranted in the absence of an intrauterine gestational saclike structure. Most ectopic pregnancies occur in the fallopian tube with the majority of those implanting in the ampulla [71]. Other locations include interstitial, cervical, ovarian, or rarely intra-abdominal. The most common finding is an adnexal mass separate from the ovary in the setting of a positive pregnancy test [72]. If the mass is closely adjacent to the ovary, gentle transducer pressure can be applied to attempt and separate the mass from the ovary. A visualized yolk sac or fetal pole is 100% specific for an ectopic pregnancy. CT is not recommended in a potentially pregnant patient. If performed, CT and MRI will demonstrate a cystic mass with surrounding hypervascularity and enhancement [73]. Hemoperitoneum can be seen representing subsequent rupture (Fig. 6.21). Potential mimics include a corpus luteum and other cystic ovarian lesions. As mentioned, transducer pressure with US may help differentiate between an ectopic pregnancy and an ovarian lesion.

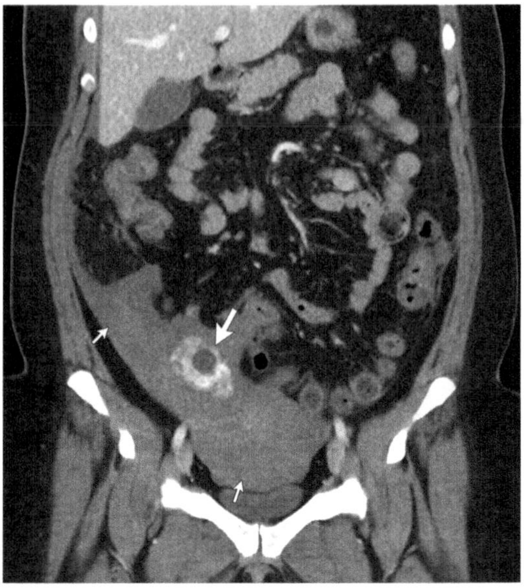

Fig. 6.21 Contrast enhanced CT in a pregnant patient presenting with 5 days of abdominal pain following an equivocal US to determine the location of pregnancy at 12 weeks gestation. Coronal reformat demonstrates a hypodense cystic mass surrounded by hyperdense, hypervascular tissue in the right adnexa consistent with an ectopic pregnancy (large arrow). There is heterogenous, hyperdense fluid layering along the pelvis and right paracolic gutter, indicating rupture and hemoperitoneum (small arrows). Exploratory laparotomy confirmed the rupture of tubal ectopic pregnancy and large hemoperitoneum

Testicular Torsion

Similar to ovarian torsion, male patients presenting with acute scrotal and/or abdominal pain should undergo ultrasound with Doppler [74]. The affected testicle will typically be enlarged due to edema and venous congestion [75]. Doppler typically demonstrates absent arterial flow. However, the presence of blood flow does not entirely exclude intermittent torsion. The most specific sign is direct visualization of the twisted pedicle (whirlpool sign) and a pseudomass just below the external inguinal ring [76]. Other secondary signs include a reactive hydrocele (anechoic fluid) and thickening of the surrounding scrotal skin with hyperemia (Fig. 6.22). A heterogeneous appearance of the testicle is a poor indicator and likely represents necrosis of the testicle [77]. US can also be used to determine the therapeutic success of manual detorsion [78]. Returned presence of blood flow with Doppler should be documented.

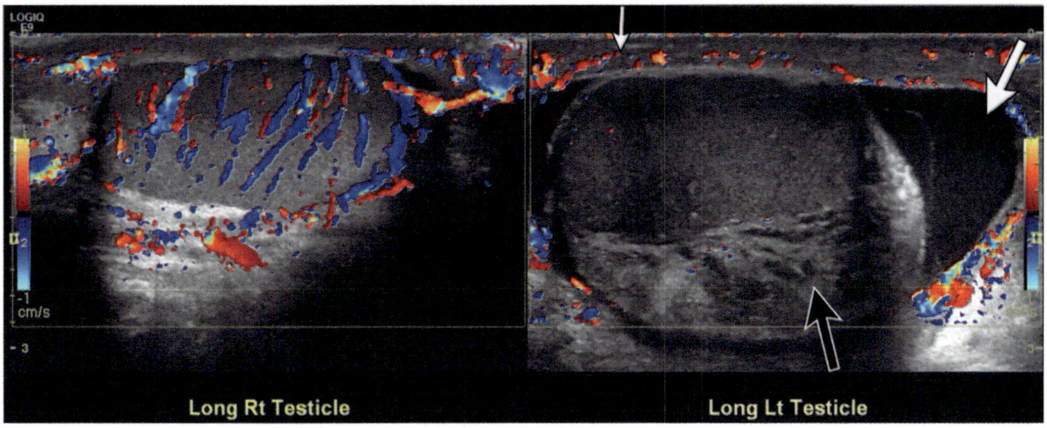

Fig. 6.22 Doppler US of the testicles in a 17-year-old with 3 days of left groin pain demonstrates an enlarged left testicle and epididymis without vascular flow (black arrow). Surrounding the left testicle is a minimally complex fluid collection (reactive hydrocele) and inflammatory thickening with hyperemia of the overlying scrotal skin (small white arrow). At surgery, the testicle was not viable and was subsequently removed

Conclusion

In conclusion, understanding common imaging findings in acute abdominal surgical conditions will help surgeons make timely management decisions. Consultation with the radiologist and a team-based collaborative approach can help improve patient outcomes.

References

1. Valtchinov VI, Ip IK, Khorasani R, Schuur JD, Zurakowski D, Lee J, et al. Use of imaging in the emergency department: do individual physicians contribute to variation? AJR Am J Roentgenol. 2019;213(3):637–43.
2. Selvarajan SK, Levin DC, Parker L. The increasing use of emergency department imaging in the United States: is it appropriate? AJR Am J Roentgenol. 2019;213(4):W180–w4.
3. Mendelson EB. The development and meaning of appropriateness guidelines. Radiol Clin N Am. 1995;33(6):1081–4.
4. van Randen A, Laméris W, Luitse JSK, Gorzeman M, Hesselink EJ, Dolmans DEJGJ, et al. The role of plain radiographs in patients with acute abdominal pain at the ED. Am J Emerg Med. 2011;29(6):582–9.e2.
5. MacKersie AB, Lane MJ, Gerhardt RT, Claypool HA, Keenan S, Katz DS, et al. Nontraumatic acute abdominal pain: unenhanced helical CT compared with three-view acute abdominal series. Radiology. 2005;237(1):114–22.
6. Puylaert JB, van der Zant FM, Rijke AM. Sonography and the acute abdomen: practical considerations. AJR Am J Roentgenol. 1997;168(1):179–86.
7. Gerscovich EO, Corwin MT, Sekhon S, Runner GJ, Gandour-Edwards RF. Sonographic appearance of adnexal torsion, correlation with other imaging modalities, and clinical history. Ultrasound Q. 2014;30(1):49–55.
8. Puylaert JB, Rutgers PH, Lalisang RI, de Vries BC, van der Werf SD, Dörr JP, et al. A prospective study of ultrasonography in the diagnosis of appendicitis. N Engl J Med. 1987;317(11):666–9.
9. Pinto A, Pinto F, Faggian A, Rubini G, Caranci F, Macarini L, et al. Sources of error in emergency ultrasonography. Crit Ultrasound J. 2013;5(Suppl 1):S1.
10. Oto A. MR imaging evaluation of acute abdominal pain during pregnancy. Magn Reson Imaging Clin N Am. 2006;14(4):489–501. vi
11. Rosen MP, Sands DZ, Longmaid HE 3rd, Reynolds KF, Wagner M, Raptopoulos V. Impact of abdominal CT on the management of patients presenting to the emergency department with acute abdominal pain. AJR Am J Roentgenol. 2000;174(5):1391–6.

12. McCollough CH, Primak AN, Braun N, Kofler J, Yu L, Christner J. Strategies for reducing radiation dose in CT. Radiol Clin N Am. 2009;47(1):27–40.
13. Goldman LW. Principles of CT and CT technology. J Nucl Med Technol. 2007;35(3):115–28; quiz 29-30.
14. Kessner R, Barnes S, Halpern P, Makrin V, Blachar A. CT for acute nontraumatic abdominal pain-is Oral contrast really required? Acad Radiol. 2017;24(7):840–5.
15. Razavi SA, Johnson JO, Kassin MT, Applegate KE. The impact of introducing a no oral contrast abdominopelvic CT examination (NOCAPE) pathway on radiology turn around times, emergency department length of stay, and patient safety. Emerg Radiol. 2014;21(6):605–13.
16. Mularski RA, Ciccolo ML, Rappaport WD. Nonsurgical causes of pneumoperitoneum. West J Med. 1999;170(1):41–6.
17. Lubner M, Menias C, Rucker C, Bhalla S, Peterson CM, Wang L, et al. Blood in the belly: CT findings of Hemoperitoneum. Radiographics. 2007;27(1):109–25.
18. Mularski RA, Sippel JM, Osborne ML. Pneumoperitoneum: a review of nonsurgical causes. Crit Care Med. 2000;28(7):2638–44.
19. Furlan A, Fakhran S, Federle MP. Spontaneous abdominal hemorrhage: causes, CT findings, and clinical implications. Am J Roentgenol. 2009;193(4):1077–87.
20. Pereira JM, Sirlin CB, Pinto PS, Jeffrey RB, Stella DL, Casola G. Disproportionate fat stranding: a helpful CT sign in patients with acute abdominal pain. Radiographics. 2004;24(3):703–15.
21. Horton KM, Fishman EK. Current role of CT in imaging of the stomach. Radiographics. 2003;23(1):75–87.
22. Levine MS, Carucci LR. Imaging of bariatric surgery: Normal anatomy and postoperative complications. Radiology. 2014;270(2):327–41.
23. Horton KM, Eng J, Fishman EK. Normal enhancement of the small bowel: evaluation with spiral CT. J Comput Assist Tomogr. 2000;24(1):67–71.
24. Guniganti P, Bradenham CH, Raptis C, Menias CO, Mellnick VM. CT of gastric emergencies. Radiographics. 2015;35(7):1909–21.
25. Shone DN, Nikoomanesh P, Smith-Meek MM, Bender JS. Malignancy is the most common cause of gastric outlet obstruction in the era of H2 blockers. Am J Gastroenterol. 1995;90(10):1769–70.
26. Peterson CM, Anderson JS, Hara AK, Carenza JW, Menias CO. Volvulus of the gastrointestinal tract: appearances at multimodality imaging. Radiographics. 2009;29(5):1281–93.
27. Diamond M, Lee J, LeBedis CA. Small bowel obstruction and ischemia. Radiol Clin N Am. 2019;57(4):689–703.
28. Lappas JC, Reyes BL, Maglinte DD. Abdominal radiography findings in small-bowel obstruction: relevance to triage for additional diagnostic imaging. AJR Am J Roentgenol. 2001;176(1):167–74.
29. Delabrousse E, Destrumelle N, Brunelle S, Clair C, Mantion G, Kastler B. CT of small bowel obstruction in adults. Abdom Imaging. 2003;28(2):0257–66.
30. Garcia EM, Camacho MA, Karolyi DR, Kim DH, Cash BD, Chang KJ, et al. ACR appropriateness criteria(®) right lower quadrant pain-suspected appendicitis. J Am Coll Radiol. 2018;15(11s):S373–s87.
31. Lee CC, Golub R, Singer AJ, Cantu R Jr, Levinson H. Routine versus selective abdominal computed tomography scan in the evaluation of right lower quadrant pain: a randomized controlled trial. Acad Emerg Med. 2007;14(2):117–22.
32. Daly CP, Cohan RH, Francis IR, Caoili EM, Ellis JH, Nan B. Incidence of acute appendicitis in patients with equivocal CT findings. Am J Roentgenol. 2005;184(6):1813–20.
33. Petkovska I, Martin DR, Covington MF, Urbina S, Duke E, Daye ZJ, et al. Accuracy of unenhanced MR imaging in the detection of acute appendicitis: single-institution clinical performance review. Radiology. 2016;279(2):451–60.
34. Pinto Leite N, Pereira JM, Cunha R, Pinto P, Sirlin C. CT evaluation of appendicitis and its complications: imaging techniques and key diagnostic findings. Am J Roentgenol. 2005;185(2):406–17.
35. Ginsburg M, Obara P, Lambert DL, Hanley M, Steigner ML, Camacho MA, et al. ACR appropriateness criteria(®) imaging of mesenteric ischemia. J Am Coll Radiol. 2018;15(11s):S332–s40.
36. Dhatt HS, Behr SC, Miracle A, Wang ZJ, Yeh BM. Radiological evaluation of bowel ischemia. Radiol Clin N Am. 2015;53(6):1241–54.
37. Singh D, Chawla A. The "abdominal whirlpool" sign. Abdom Radiol (NY). 2016;41(7):1437–8.
38. Galgano SJ, McNamara MM, Peterson CM, Kim DH, Fowler KJ, Camacho MA, et al. ACR appropriateness criteria(®) left lower quadrant pain-suspected diverticulitis. J Am Coll Radiol. 2019;16(5s):S141–s9.
39. Onur MR, Akpinar E, Karaosmanoglu AD, Isayev C, Karcaaltincaba M. Diverticulitis: a comprehensive review with usual and unusual complications. Insights Imaging. 2017;8(1):19–27.
40. Lau KC, Spilsbury K, Farooque Y, Kariyawasam SB, Owen RG, Wallace MH, et al. Is colonoscopy still mandatory after a CT diagnosis of left-sided diverticulitis: can colorectal cancer be confidently excluded? Dis Colon Rectum. 2011;54(10)
41. Peterson CM, McNamara MM, Kamel IR, Al-Refaie WB, Arif-Tiwari H, Cash BD, et al. ACR appropriateness criteria(®) right upper quadrant pain. J Am Coll Radiol. 2019;16(5s):S235–s43.
42. Noble VE, Liteplo AS, Nelson BP, Thomas SH. The impact of analgesia on the diagnostic accuracy of the sonographic Murphy's sign. Eur J Emerg Med. 2010;17(2)
43. Kiewiet JJ, Leeuwenburgh MM, Bipat S, Bossuyt PM, Stoker J, Boermeester MA. A systematic review and meta-analysis of diagnostic performance of imaging in acute cholecystitis. Radiology. 2012;264(3):708–20.

44. Mirvis SE, Vainright, Nelson AW, Johnston GS, Shorr R, Rodriguez A, et al. The diagnosis of acute acalculous cholecystitis: a comparison of sonography, scintigraphy, and CT. Am J Roentgenol. 1986;147(6):1171–5.
45. Grayson DE, Abbott RM, Levy AD, Sherman PM. Emphysematous infections of the abdomen and pelvis: a pictorial review. Radiographics. 2002;22(3):543–61.
46. Gill KS, Chapman AH, Weston MJ. The changing face of emphysematous cholecystitis. Br J Radiol. 1997;70(838):986–91.
47. Jeffrey RB, Laing FC, Wong W, Callen PW. Gangrenous cholecystitis: diagnosis by ultrasound. Radiology. 1983;148(1):219–21.
48. Bennett GL, Rusinek H, Lisi V, Israel GM, Krinsky GA, Slywotzky CM, et al. CT findings in acute gangrenous cholecystitis. AJR Am J Roentgenol. 2002;178(2):275–81.
49. Kim PN, Lee KS, Kim IY, Bae WK, Lee BH. Gallbladder perforation: comparison of US findings with CT. Abdom Imaging. 1994;19(3):239–42.
50. Catalano OA, Sahani DV, Forcione DG, Czermak B, Liu C-H, Soricelli A, et al. Biliary infections: spectrum of imaging findings and management. Radiographics. 2009;29(7):2059–80.
51. Bader TR, Braga L, Beavers KL, Semelka RC. MR imaging findings of infectious cholangitis. Magn Reson Imaging. 2001;19(6):781–8.
52. Csendes A, Diaz JC, Burdiles P, Maluenda F, Morales E. Risk factors and classification of acute suppurative cholangitis. Br J Surg. 1992;79(7):655–8.
53. Mandelia A, Gupta AK, Verma DK, Sharma S. The value of magnetic resonance cholangiopancreatography (MRCP) in the detection of choledocholithiasis. J Clin Diagn Res. 2013;7(9):1941–5.
54. Coursey CA, Casalino DD, Remer EM, Arellano RS, Bishoff JT, Dighe M, et al. ACR appropriateness criteria® acute onset flank pain—suspicion of stone disease. Ultrasound Q. 2012;28(3):227–33.
55. Lee JY, Kim SH, Cho JY, Han D. Color and power Doppler twinkling artifacts from urinary stones: clinical observations and phantom studies. AJR Am J Roentgenol. 2001;176(6):1441–5.
56. Reddy S. State of the art trends in imaging renal of colic. Emerg Radiol. 2008;15(4):217–25.
57. Wolin EA, Hartman DS, Olson JR. Nephrographic and pyelographic analysis of CT urography: differential diagnosis. Am J Roentgenol. 2013;200(6):1197–203.
58. Potenta SE, D'Agostino R, Sternberg KM, Tatsumi K, Perusse K. CT urography for evaluation of the ureter. Radiographics. 2015;35(3):709–26.
59. Dyer RB, Chen MY, Zagoria RJ. Classic signs in uroradiology. RadioGraphics. 2004;24(suppl_1):S247–80.
60. Craig WD, Wagner BJ, Travis MD. Pyelonephritis: radiologic-pathologic review. Radiographics. 2008;28:255.
61. Bhosale PR, Javitt MC, Atri M, Harris RD, Kang SK, Meyer BJ, et al. ACR appropriateness criteria® acute pelvic pain in the reproductive age group. Ultrasound Q. 2016;32(2):108–15.
62. Lee EJ, Kwon HC, Joo HJ, Suh JH, Fleischer AC. Diagnosis of ovarian torsion with color Doppler sonography: depiction of twisted vascular pedicle. J Ultrasound Med. 1998;17(2):83–9.
63. Peña JE, Ufberg D, Cooney N, Denis AL. Usefulness of Doppler sonography in the diagnosis of ovarian torsion. Fertil Steril. 2000;73(5):1047–50.
64. Duigenan S, Oliva E, Lee SI. Ovarian torsion: diagnostic features on CT and MRI with pathologic correlation. Am J Roentgenol. 2012;198(2):W122–W31.
65. Hiller N, Appelbaum L, Simanovsky N, Lev-Sagi A, Aharoni D, Sella T. CT features of adnexal torsion. Am J Roentgenol. 2007;189(1):124–9.
66. Munro K, Gharaibeh A, Nagabushanam S, Martin C. Diagnosis and management of tubo-ovarian abscesses. Obstetr Gynaecol. 2018;20(1):11–9.
67. Kaakaji Y, Nghiem HV, Nodell C, Winter TC. Sonography of obstetric and gynecologic emergencies: part II, Gynecologic emergencies. AJR Am J Roentgenol. 2000;174(3):651–6.
68. Wilbur AC, Aizenstein RI, Napp TE. CT findings in tuboovarian abscess. Am J Roentgenol. 1992;158(3):575–9.
69. Revzin MV, Mathur M, Dave HB, Macer ML, Spektor M. Pelvic inflammatory disease: multimodality imaging approach with clinical-pathologic correlation. Radiographics. 2016;36(5):1579–96.
70. Rodgers SK, Chang C, DeBardeleben JT, Horrow MM. Normal and abnormal US findings in early first-trimester pregnancy: review of the Society of Radiologists in ultrasound 2012 consensus panel recommendations. Radiographics. 2015;35(7):2135–48.
71. Bouyer J, Coste J, Fernandez H, Pouly JL, Job-Spira N. Sites of ectopic pregnancy: a 10 year population-based study of 1800 cases. Hum Reprod. 2002;17(12):3224–30.
72. Lin EP, Bhatt S, Dogra VS. Diagnostic clues to ectopic pregnancy. Radiographics. 2008;28(6):1661–71.
73. Kao LY, Scheinfeld MH, Chernyak V, Rozenblit AM, Oh S, Dym RJ. Beyond ultrasound: CT and MRI of ectopic pregnancy. Am J Roentgenol. 2014;202(4):904–11.
74. Avery LL, Scheinfeld MH. Imaging of penile and scrotal emergencies. Radiographics. 2013;33(3):721–40.
75. Bandarkar AN, Blask AR. Testicular torsion with preserved flow: key sonographic features and value-added approach to diagnosis. Pediatr Radiol. 2018;48(5):735–44.
76. Munden MM, Williams JL, Zhang W, Crowe JE, Munden RF, Cisek LJ. Intermittent testicular torsion in the pediatric patient: sonographic indicators of a difficult diagnosis. Am J Roentgenol. 2013;201(4):912–8.
77. Kaye JD, Shapiro EY, Levitt SB, Friedman SC, Gitlin J, Freyle J, et al. Parenchymal echo texture predicts testicular salvage after torsion: potential impact on the need for emergent exploration. J Urol. 2008;180(4S):1733–6.
78. Ringdahl EN, Teague L. Testicular torsion. Am Fam Physician. 2006;74(10):1739–43.

A Primer on Practice Management Guidelines

7

Rebecca G. Maine and Bryce R. H. Robinson

Abbreviations

AAST	American Association for the Surgery of Trauma
ACS	American College of Surgeons
AHCPR	Agency for Health Care Policy and Research
AHRQ	Agency for Healthcare Research and Quality
ATLS	Advance Trauma Life Support
COI	Conflicts of interest (COI)
EAST	Eastern Association for the Surgery of Trauma
GRADE	Grading of Recommendations, Assessment, Development and Evaluation
IOM	National Academy of Sciences Institute of Medicine
MeSH	Medical subject headings
NICE	National Institute for Health and Care Excellence
PICO	Population, intervention, comparator, and outcomes
PMG	Practice management guideline
RCT	Randomized controlled trial

Practice Management Guidelines (PMGs) and Systematic Reviews

A surgeon is asked by her hospital's information technology group to update order sets during the integration phases of a new, electronic health record. Upon review, the surgeon notes that many of the existing order sets for admission, discharge, and common care pathways are over 10 years old. The surgeon begins a PubMed® literature search to update these order sets but becomes quickly overwhelmed. The literature is difficult to evaluate due to the magnitude of the papers written and the unclear strength of evidence being reviewed. The surgeon first focuses on review articles but finds a great deal of expert opinion without transparency regarding conflicts of interest and bias. She also notes that there are few meta-analyses or randomized controlled trials available for surgical topics. Nearly exacerbated and with a deadline fast approaching, the surgeon reaches out to other medical, nonsurgical, leaders asked to update their specific order sets for help and advice. Multiple colleagues suggest a quick review of recently written practice management guidelines, especially those using GRADE methodology, by surgical and medical societies. In the end, she identified several relevant guidelines that enabled her update and presented them for approval at her institutional surgical council prior to the deadline. With the knowledge gained after her review, she was able

R. G. Maine · B. R. H. Robinson (✉)
Department of Surgery, Harborview Medical Center, University of Washington, Seattle, Washington, USA
e-mail: rmaine@uw.edu; brobinso@uw.edu

M. D. Zielinski, O. Guillamondegui (eds.), *The Acute Management of Surgical Disease*, https://doi.org/10.1007/978-3-031-07881-1_7

to confidently describe the evidence and justify her recommendations to the council. All of her order sets were approved, and her surgical colleagues were grateful that she had been able to distill the key information needed to help them integrate best practices into their daily patient care.

Medical knowledge is rapidly changing, and medical practitioners need to consolidate and interpret findings from different, sometimes contradictory, studies to make the best decisions for their individual patients. This is especially true for the acute care surgeon, who regularly treats a wide variety of clinical problems [1]. Systematic reviews consolidate the knowledge and research on a particular topic with the goal of developing a more comprehensive understanding of the "true nature" of the clinical situation [2]. Systematic reviews aim to be thorough, transparent, and unbiased reviews of published information on a particular topic [2, 3]. Transparency comes from using a clearly described and reproducible methodology [2]. The methods of a systematic review depend on the available studies. They range from meta-analyses of randomized controlled trials to descriptive summaries of findings from studies with varied designs [2]. What distinguishes a systematic review from a narrative review is the use of a clear, reproducible methodology to identify articles [2].

Authors of systematic reviews must determine what level of evidence [4] is appropriate to answer their specific research question [2]. Systematic reviews can provide some of the highest levels of evidence to guide clinical understanding, especially if it is a meta-analysis of well-designed randomized controlled trials (RCTs) with similar interventions and outcomes [4–6]. Rigorous approaches to systematic reviews have been proposed by several groups. The Cochrane Collaboration is a leader among these groups, with teams of international researchers who assemble the best evidence in a transparent and unbiased way to write summaries that guide clinician decision-making [3]. It was established in 1993 as organizations and governments around the world expressed growing interest in developing evidence-based guidelines. The collaboration strives to reduce bias by including not only published data but also information about registered trials and the "gray literature" [3]. The types of meta-analyses the collaboration produces represent the highest level of evidence to support clinical decision-making [5].

Of course, clinicians cannot rely on systematic reviews alone to answer clinical questions. First, for many specific clinical questions, no systematic reviews exist. This is especially true for topics where the published literature is limited for fields like surgery where the nature of the treatments and small numbers of patients who need specific procedures make RCTs more challenging. Second, systematic reviews represent a summary of data at a particular point in time. As such, they rely on the researchers' ongoing interest in the topic to write updated systematic reviews when new studies are published.

Practice management guidelines focus on clinical decision-making. Management guidelines have been in use for much of the twentieth century in some form [7] but have grown in their popularity and rigor of approach since the late 1980s. At that time, significant geographic variation in care for different conditions existed without clear scientific basis, which led to substantial differences in the cost and quality of medical care [7, 8]. In 1992, a National Academy of Sciences Institute of Medicine (IOM) report defined clinical practice guidelines or PMGs as "systematically developed statements to assist practitioners and patient decisions about appropriate healthcare for specific circumstances" [4, 9]. Guidelines are typically developed with a specific set of clinical questions in mind, often focused on diagnosis or treatments options for a condition. Guidelines can also focus on treatment options and their associated prognosis, risks and benefits, or costs [9]. Ideally, they are valid and reproducible at different locales [8].

Guidelines are usually developed, in part, from existing literature, but also incorporate other factors including the judgment of guideline developers, expert opinion, patient preference, feasibility, and costs. The Delphi method, which elicits expert opinion through a structured process, was frequently used in the development of initial trauma guidelines [8]. Guidelines should include the reasoning behind their recommendations, thus enabling clinicians to apply the recommendations appropriately to specific patients and/or engage patients in a shared decision-making process [7]. Good PMGs do more than guide clinical decisions. They serve as an educational tool, as well as providing standards against which the quality of care can be measured [1, 10]. This includes helping to assess legal liabilities [1, 7, 10]. PMGs can help guide resource allocation [1, 7, 10]. Guidelines can also serve as a means to rapidly translate research into practice [1].

The Need for PMGs

For more than the past 20 years, it has been impossible for clinicians to stay abreast of all the current literature [8]. Between 1985 and 2001, the number of published randomized controlled trials increased from 5000 a year to 25,000 per year [7]. In 2014, there were 1,039,145 articles indexed in PubMed [11]. The number of systematic reviews and meta-analyses has also grown exponentially in the past few years. PubMed indexed 1023 systematic reviews in 1991 and 28,959 in 2014 [11]. Clinicians are unable to effectively or efficiently distill all of this available data, which hinders their efforts to ensure they are providing the optimal, evidence-based care for their patients.

As mentioned, systematic reviews can play an important role in informing clinician decision-making, but they also fail to address important factors for clinical decisions. These factors include patient preferences and comorbidities, feasibility of broad application of evidence, and costs associated with different options. PMGs are typically developed by a team of experts, ideally multidisciplinary, who summarize the evidence to recommend a course of action for different patient populations. PMGs ideally explain the reasoning behind a recommendation so that guideline users can assess whether a particular treatment option is optimal for their specific patient.

Many governments have established groups to develop and/or compile PMGs. In the United States, the US Department of Health and Human Services created the Agency for Health Care Policy and Research (AHCPR) in 1989 to increase the use of scientific evidence to standardize and improve clinical care. AHCPR was renamed the Agency for Healthcare Research and Quality (AHRQ) in 1999. AHRQ contributed to the early guidelines and methodologies for evaluating literature to formulate clinical guidance in the United States [5]. In the United Kingdom, the National Institute for Health and Care Excellence (NICE) has published over 120 clinical guidelines based on summaries of published evidence [12]. PMGs are supported by many other organizations, including the World Health Organization, and several national and professional societies [1, 10, 12, 13].

Historical Perspectives of PMGs

Surgeons and surgical societies were early adopters of PMGs. The Society for Vascular Surgery and the American College of Surgeons (ACS) were already publishing guidelines for specific conditions as the IOM called for guidelines and more evidence-based standardizations [10]. The ACS published the first edition of the "Resources for the optimal care for the injured patient" in 1990 as a comprehensive guideline for the triage of trauma patients and the establishment of inclusive trauma systems. This was nearly 20 years after the first Advance Trauma Life Support (ATLS) guidelines were developed [10]. In his 1993 presidential address to the Eastern Association for the Surgery of Trauma (EAST), Dr. Michael Rhodes focused on the growth of PMGs and their value to all stages of care for the injured patients, including prehospital transport, initial resuscitation, surgical care, critical care, and rehabilitation [10]. At that time, all three major trauma associations in the United States, EAST, the Western Trauma Association, and the American Association for the Surgery of Trauma (AAST), had developed or were in the process of developing PMGs for the management of injured patients [10]. In 1999, Dr. Tim Fabian in his EAST presidential address highlighted the growth of PMGs and the role of EAST and other professional organizations in that growth [8]. Professional trauma organizations in the United States have continued to develop PMGs, not only for injuries but also for emergency general surgery and surgical critical care [1]. In his 2020 presidential address at EAST, Dr. Elliott Haut argued that the growing success of EAST had been in large part due to their commitment to developing PMGs to support the larger acute care surgery community [1].

As a leader in acute care surgery PMGs, EAST has championed the incorporation of evidence into practice. They have advocated for a rigorous methodology to PMG development that allows for the incorporation of the range of available data. EAST PMGs require intensive work and typically take between 12 and 18 months to complete [8]. EAST PMGs were initially developed using a ten-step methodology (Fig. 7.1) that aligned with the AHCPR and the Brain Trauma Foundation schema to evaluate the quality of the published data [8]. In 2012, EAST adopted the Grading of Recommendations, Assessment, Development and Evaluation (GRADE) methodology for guideline development [1].

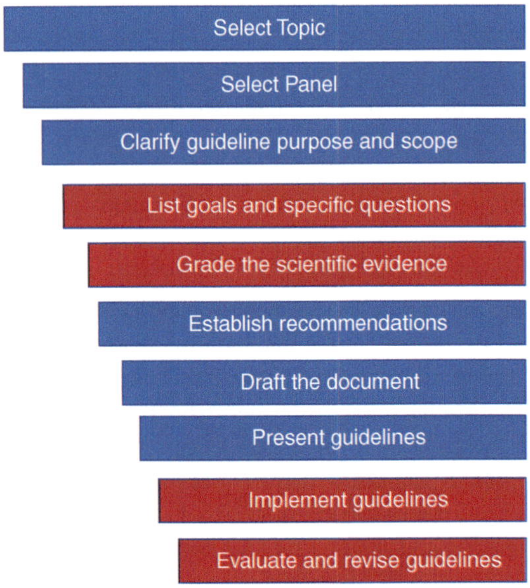

Fig. 7.1 The EAST's initial ten steps for practice management guideline developments [8]

The Role of the Agency for Health Research and Quality

In the late 1980s and the early 1990s, as interest in PMGs grew, AHRQ developed guidance for clinicians and researchers to assess the quality of studies on a particular topic. While many early guidelines were developed from Delphi processes or expert opinion, it was acknowledged that the strongest guidelines were derived from the strongest evidence. In 1990, the IOM published recommendations for PMGs (Table 7.1) [4, 7]. The AHRQ developed a hierarchy of literature that highlighted study designs that have the lowest rate of bias resulting in the strongest sci-

Table 7.1 Key characteristics of clinical guidelines [4, 7]

Characteristic	Explanation
Validity	Following the guidelines leads to the predicted health gains and costs
Reproducibility	Another guideline group would make the same recommendations with the same method and evidence
Reliability	Healthcare professionals in similar clinical situations interpret the guidelines the same way
Representative development	Key stakeholders (including patients) participate in developing the guideline
Clinical applicability	Patient populations for the guidelines are defined derived from scientific evidence and/or best clinical judgment
Clarity	Recommendations are presented with precise, unambiguous language
Meticulous documentation	Explicitly state the methods for developing guidelines, including participants, evidence gathering and interpretation, and recommendation reasoning
Scheduled review	The process and timing of future reviews should be outlined, including triggers for reviews

entific evidence for or against an intervention [5]. The highest-quality evidence is a meta-analysis of well-conducted RCTs that answer a similar, if not identical, question in similar populations [5, 6]. Individual RCTs follow this, with observational studies, case series, and expert opinion representing sequentially weaker evidence for a particular course of action in medical care [5, 6].

High-quality literature alone is insufficient for making PMG recommendations, which must synthesize the evidence for clinical context. While several RCTs may exist on a topic, their results may contradict. Study results may be consistent but find only a small clinical benefit from costly and inconvenience interventions, suggesting that clinicians may reasonably select alternatives [14]. Thus, PMG developers must judge the evidence to create their recommendations and then assess and report the strength of that recommendation. Several systems have been proposed to grade the strength of a recommendation based on the evidence [5, 6, 14] (Fig. 7.2). It is essential to consider the quality, quantity, and consistency of the data, the balance between benefit and harm, how the evidence is put into practice, and inherent baseline risks of different treatments [14, 15].

AHRQ's approach, which is based the strength of the recommendation on the appraisal of the literature quality alone, had shortcomings for guideline development. First, many important clinical topics are not easily evaluated with the "gold standard" RCT, but the AHRQ recommendation scale was not flexible in providing strong recommendations from other types of study design [15]. Furthermore, the AHRQ recommendation scale did not incorporate an assessment of the quality of the studies within the hierarchy of study designs [15]. This failed to address the fact that some non-randomized trials could be designed with minimal bias, while RCTs could be designed with significant bias. A more robust approach to guideline development was needed to allow for the assessment individual study quality based on its risk of bias [15]. The AHRQ approach did not define a way for the application of judgment by guideline developers as they synthesize the evidence [14, 15]. Furthermore, the AHRQ recommendations were not clear about how to incorporate essential components of PMG development, including factors like cost, patient preference, how to address variation in literature quality across specific aspects of a recommendation, how consistent the evidence is, and how decisions may vary for different populations [14].

The Need for High-Quality PMGs

As early guidelines proliferated, it was clear that many PMGs were developed without a rigorous and transparent process [7]. To address this shortcoming, in 2011, the IOM authored a report that proposed standards to develop PMGs. The report's primary goal was to encourage PMG use by ensuring that guideline users could assess the quality of PMGs and determining their trustworthiness. Greater transparency in the entire development process and standard reporting recommendations would facilitate such a recommendation. The committee offered eight core recommendations [7].

Transparency

Any critical evaluation of a manuscript includes an assessment of the methods that the researchers applied to answer their question. No research paper would be published without this methodology section. However, many PMGs in the first decades of publication lacked a similar explanation of methodology [16]. Thus, the IOM called for PMGs to be transparent in their process for developing guidelines [7]. Transparency includes explicitly stating who is part of the guideline development group and how it is funded. Transparency also includes explicit statements of the certainty of recommendations and clear explanations about how the guideline developers arrived at their recommendations [7].

Managing Conflicts of Interest

Ideally, PMGs are developed by a group of experts from different backgrounds/fields who are able to incorporate a range of perspectives, including the patient/public perspective [7]. Conflicts of interest (COI), defined by the IOM as "a set of circumstances that creates a risk that professional judgment or actions regarding a primary interest will be unduly influenced by a secondary interest," are not uncommon in medicine [7]. However, a 2000 study found that two-thirds of guidelines did not include information about the individuals who developed them, let alone

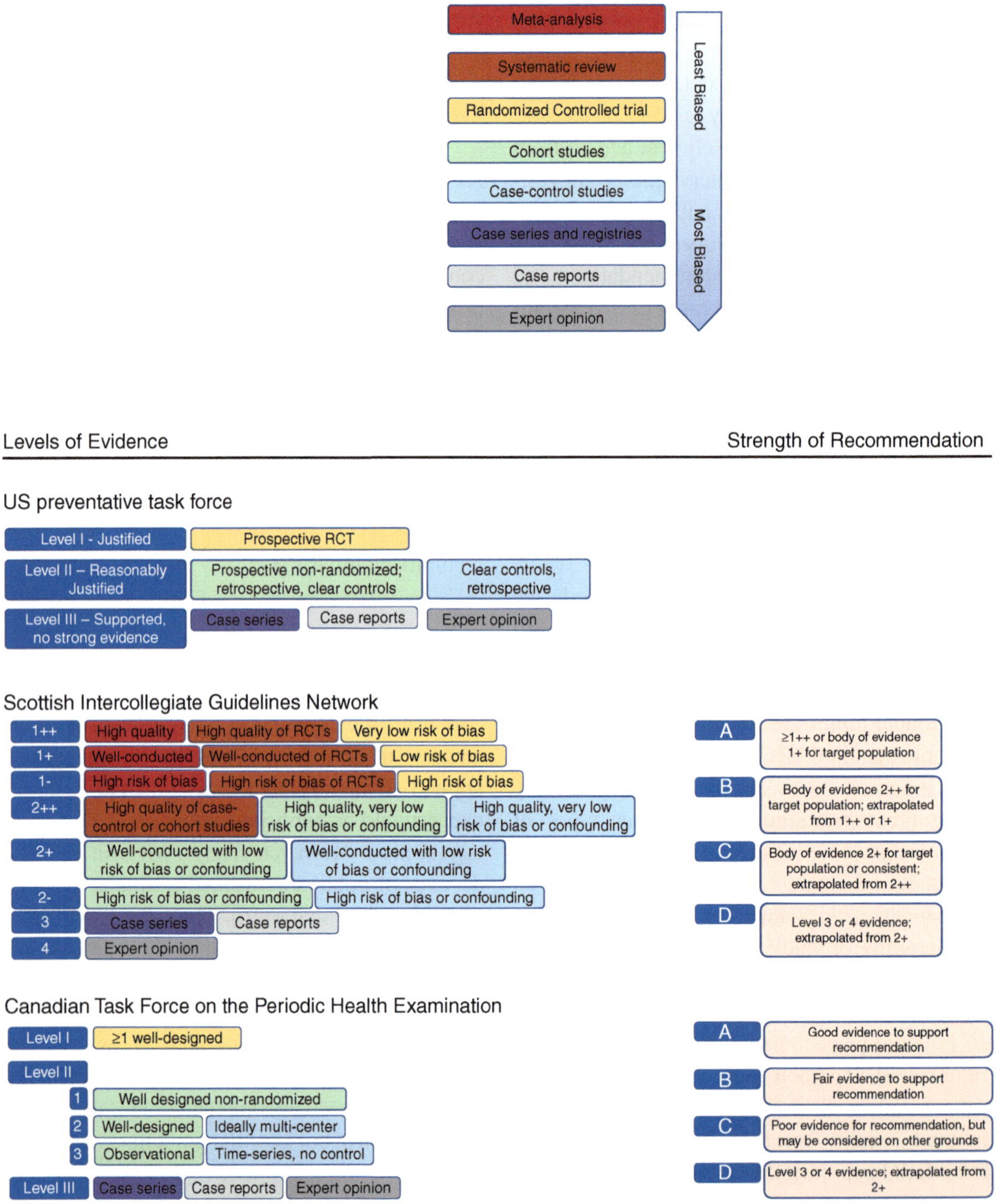

Fig. 7.2 Study designs, levels of evidence, and strength of recommendations [5–8, 15, 20]

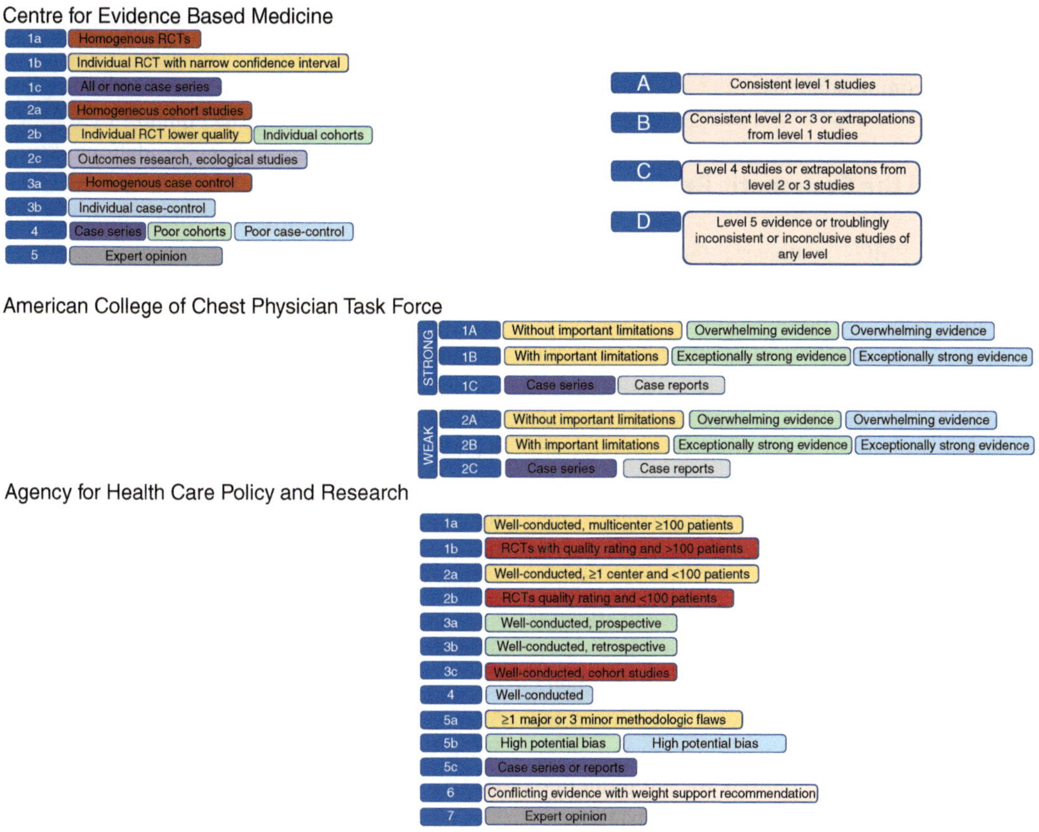

Fig. 7.2 (continued)

specific information about COIs [7, 16]. Conflicts are often financial, rewarding either an individual or their research endeavors [7]. For guideline development, the potential financial impact of a recommendation may be more subtle such as intellectual conflicts of interest. In guideline development, this arises when an individual or professional group stands to benefit or suffer from a recommendation made in a guideline, for example, when pending research funds are related to a guideline recommendation [7]. While some biases are obvious and explicit, many biases that arise from conflicts of interest are unconscious [7].

The ideal PMG development team has no COIs. Some organizations explicitly require this or prevent individuals with potential conflicts from leading a PMG group [7]. However, for some PMGs, this is neither realistic nor desired, as experts in a field can provide valuable insight into a recommendation specifically because they have extensive experience with a particular treatment or technique being considered. Disclosure of COIs is the minimum that PMG development groups must do to ensure guideline users can assess the potential influence of COIs on recommendations. Many groups advocate for individuals with any conflicts to recuse themselves from aspects of the recommendations related to their COI [7]. Another strategy is to have methodology experts lead PMG development groups to minimize the potential bias of context experts [7]. Disclosure of COIs for PMG development teams should be made early in the guideline's development process and should include a description of how the conflict might influence their decision-making. This process can prevent individuals with potentially large conflicts from participating in the process from the beginning and could highlight the divestment opportunities that could minimize conflicts as the process proceeds [7]. Improved reporting of COIs should increase trust in PMG recommendations.

PMGs and the Systematic Review

Optimally, PMGs synthesize the existing evidence in a reliable and reproducible manner to develop their recommendations. Systematic reviews of the existing literature underpin the evidence to inform decisions [1, 7, 14]. The systematic review process is done variably across different groups. In one approach, reviews are done completely within the PMG development group as an integral part of the process. They can also be done completely externally to the group developing the recommendations. Some groups use a mixed interplay between the evidence reviewers and those providing the recommendations [7]. Advantages and disadvantages exist for each type of relationship between the individuals evaluating the evidence and those making the recommendations for the guideline. A completely external panel has an advantage of impartiality but may prevent the guideline developers from deeply understanding the evidence, including nuances about certain studies as they make recommendations. Furthermore, they cannot ensure the review focuses on the critical clinical questions [7]. In contrast, a review conducted completely within the PMG development group risks a biased inclusion and interpretation of the literature [7]. Furthermore, context experts on committees rarely contain the skill set of a systematic review professional versed in the techniques of literature searches, review, and assimilation [7]. The hybrid approach where the PMG developers work closely with an external and expert systematic review group is the ideal approach to developing the needed evidence base for the highest-quality guideline [7]. In an analysis of PMGs for diabetes from around the world, the authors found that less than 20% of the articles were consistently used across guidelines, suggesting that many PMGs could benefit from better literature reviews [7].

Rating the Quality of the Evidence

Just as important as the process of collecting the evidence is determining the quality of the evidence to inform PMG recommendations. Study design and its associated risk of bias are key components of assessing evidence quality [4]. However, not all randomized controlled trials are designed or conducted equally well, nor are they necessarily designed to answer the specific clinical question(s) posed for a PMG [7, 17]. Several tools exist to evaluate the quality and relevance of a set of studies being considered for a PMG, but there are inconsistencies across the tools [6, 7]. The IOM evaluated different approaches to rating the evidence and found that all approaches were incomplete and that inconsistencies in approaches were common. This led to the development of the GRADE methodology, which is discussed in greater detail below [7, 14].

Rate the Strength of the Recommendations

High-quality study designs alone do not drive PMG recommendations. In addition to identifying methodologic and/or applicability problems among with well-designed trials trying to answer a specific clinical question, many other factors contribute to the ultimate recommendation in guidelines. Strong recommendations are possible even when evidence is derived from less rigorous study designs. When the best available evidence, often in the form of observational studies, clearly supports the risk or benefit to a particular treatment strategy, making a recommended course of action is clear [7]. When guideline recommendations are based on this type of data, the authors must also acknowledge that stronger data from higher-quality studies could change the recommendation. High-quality evidence from randomized controlled trials and meta-analyses may not support a strong recommendation for or against a treatment because the RCTs conflict or they are only partially relevant to the clinical questions or to all patient populations considered in the PMGs [7, 17]. The influence of other factors in clinical decision-making can be quite large. A study that evaluated the relationship between evidence and an individual's recommendations for care found that they aligned only 51% of the time [7, 18]. To be trustworthy, PMGs must explicitly state the reason for their recommendations, including clearly noting potential benefits and harms, summarizing the evidence used for recommendations, identifying remaining gaps in the evidence, and acknowledging the other values (patient preference, costs/resource use, etc.) considered for the final decision [7, 14, 15].

Clear Articulation of Recommendation

PMGs do not benefit their users if those users cannot discern a course of action for their patients from the PMG recommendations. Unclear PMG recommendations are half as likely to be followed than clear PMG recommendations [7]. Optimally, PMGs use consistent, clear, precise language to explicitly state the strength of the recommendations while avoiding vague terms like "if indicated" or "if necessary" [7]. Recommendations should start with words that indicate the strength of the recommendation (i.e., "must" or "should" for strong recommendations, "could" or "might" for weaker recommendations). Furthermore, the quality of the evidence supporting the recommendation should be clearly outlined as should the specific population on which the PMGs focus [7]. Clear language and explicit reasoning in PMGs enable guideline users to readily discern if the recommendation is appropriate for each of their patients.

External Review

An external review process can reduce the risk of bias in published guidelines while also providing feedback from important stakeholder groups about the feasibility of implementing them before they are finalized and published. Some organizations, like NICE, employ a review panel, while other guidelines are reviewed by professional organization(s) and/or are subject to peer review through a journal publication process [7]. Ideally, the public provides comments on PMG drafts, prior to publication, either through general comment periods or by leveraging patient advocacy organizations when feasible [7]. Furthermore, the strongest PMG review processes include a planned systematic way to respond to reviewers' comments and maintain the anonymity of external reviewers [7].

Planned Updates

The continually changing landscape of evidence-based medicine requires that PMGs be updated routinely; however, little definitive research defines the optimal frequency for updating PMGs. As such, guidelines should always include the date that it was published and the date that the systematic evidence review was conducted. When review cycles are too short, a PMG group may invest significant time and money for few meaningful changes [7]. There is disagreement about the ideal frequency of PMG updates, with every 2 or 3 years recommended for some topics and much longer for others [7].

Some advocate for a situational approach rather than a time-based schedule to update PMGs. PMGs updated using this approach are updated when there are changes in (1) the evidence about the risks and benefits of an intervention, (2) important outcomes, (3) available interventions, (4) evidence about the value of the current practice, (5) societal values related to specific outcomes, or (6) resources available to provide healthcare [7, 19]. To identify these changes, new literature must be regularly reviewed. This type of ongoing review often incorporates less evidence, which consumes less time and money than repeating a formal large-scale systematic review as part of a PMG revision after too short a time period. This scaled-back process has been found to identify fewer sources of data but rarely misses relevant and important literature [7].

Overall, the IOM advocates for standardization of several aspects of the PMG process which

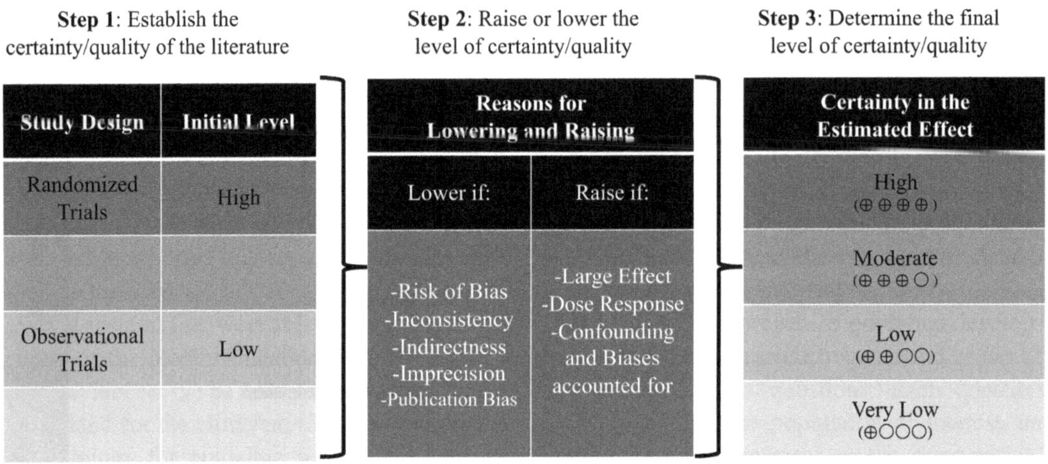

Fig. 7.4 The GRADE approach to determining the quality of the evidence by estimating the certainty of effect

Certainty Assessment							Summary of Findings				
# of participants (studies)	Risk of Bias	Inconsistency	Indirectness	Imprecision	Publication Bias	Overall Certainty of the Evidence	Study Event Rate		Relative Effect (95% CI)	Anticipated Absolute Effects	
							With Intervention	Without Intervention		Risk with Intervention	Risk Difference
Mortality (Critical Outcome)											
588 (8)	No Serious	No Serious	No Serious	No Serious	None	High (⊕⊕⊕⊕)	44/238 (18.6%)	28/350 (7.9%)	RR 0.54 (0.41-0.7)	186 per 1000	86 fewer per 1000
Additional Procedures Needed (Critical Outcome)											
1789 (4)	No Serious	No Serious	Serious	Serious	None	Moderate (⊕⊕⊕○)	15/1301 (1.2%)	12/488 (2.5%)	RR 1.5 (0.67-3.34)	12 per 1000	6 more per 1000
Wound Complications (Important Outcome)											
2061 (6)	No Serious	Serious	Serious	Serious	None	Low (⊕⊕○○)	46/1468 (3.1%)	3/593 (0.51%)	RR 0.35 (0.17-0.7)	31 per 1000	20 fewer per 1000

Fig. 7.5 Example of a GRADE evidence table

ture reviewed. The opposite is true when a very low certainty is assigned.

With the quantitative and qualitative analyses complete, evidence tables are created for each question (Fig. 7.5). The evidence table is a data-rich visual of each PIC and its multiple outcomes (Os). Each outcome is labeled as critical or important from the aforementioned vote of the writing group. The previously defined levels of certainty (quality assessments) are also represented (why certainty was raised or lowered) with the overall certainty listed. Often included in the evidence table is the quantitative effect estimate (relative risk from the meta-analysis) for each outcome. With evidence tables in hand, members of the writing group have a high-level summary of each question, outcome, and literature certainty/quality allowing for discussions to proceed regarding recommendations.

Making Recommendations

Guideline authors now have the difficult task of creating evidence-based recommendations. As stated above, these discussions are enhanced when writing teams include expert, multidisciplinary clinicians, methodologists, and patients. Each PICO question, to include all its reviewed outcomes, has a single recommendation. Guideline panels must integrate multiple domains to make a strong or weak decision for or against an intervention [23]. Domains that panels must consider include the quality of the evidence and outcomes (e.g., the evidence table), balance of benefits and harms of the intervention, resources needed, patient's values and preferences, feasibility, equity, and acceptability (Fig. 7.6). Guideline panels aim to exclude expert opinion in the recommendation process and concurrently take into account possible conflicts and biases of their panelists. For some recommendations, the synthesis of judgments made regarding the domains allows for a straightforward path toward panel consensus. Other times, it is much more elusive. When this occurs, the most popular techniques for obtaining consensus include the Delphi method, the nominal group technique where numeric values are assigned to the spectrum of recommendations possible, or a combination thereof [24].

The strength of the recommendation reflects the extent to which the writing group can be confident that the desirable effects outweigh the negative [25]. A strong recommendation is provided when adherence to a recommendation clearly outweighs the undesirable effect. Active language is used for GRADE recommendations. A strong recommendation would include phrasing such as "we recommend for/against" or "we strongly recommend for/against." A strong recommendation for a patient means that the great majority would want (or not want) the intervention. For clinicians, it means that the recommendation should be implemented for most patients. Importantly for policymakers, a strong recommendation implies a new performance measure or community standard of care. Weak or sometimes called conditional recommendations are less definitive. A weak recommendation for a patient means that most would choose the intervention though a substantial number would not. For clinicians, such a recommendation acknowledges that different choices/interventions are appropriate for different patients. As for policymakers, a weak guideline recommendation denotes that more debate is needed between the various stakeholders prior the implementation of a policy.

Translating Guidelines into Clinical Practice

As stated in their name, PMGs are merely guidelines provided by an expert panel. Assumed in all PMGs is that care at the bedside is individualized

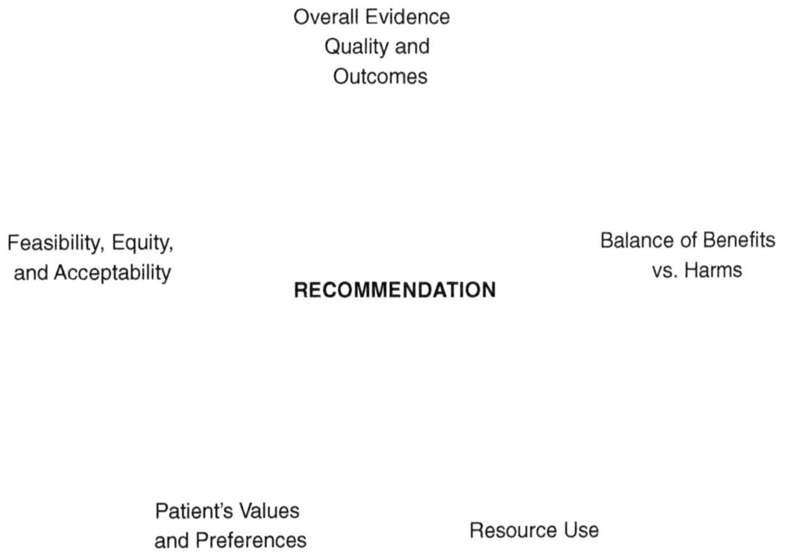

Fig. 7.6 Putting practice management guideline recommendations together with GRADE

for each patient depending on the values and preferences of the patient and the clinical circumstances. Implementing the recommendations of a high-quality, evidenced-based PMG may be challenging as PMGs provide recommendations based only on the available literature. Bedside providers need to carefully compare the PICO addressed to the individual patient situation or population of patients under their care. One needs to consider that the patient's values, resources available, and institutional culture may vary greatly from that presented in the PMG.

Practice management guidelines should be used to strengthen existing institutional care pathways generated by local care leaders. Suffice to say, many clinical situations arise that simply do not have an evidence-based answer. As such, internal and external expert opinion may need to be used in an effort to strengthen hospital-specific algorithms. Multiple societal organizations (e.g., Western Trauma Association, ACS Committee on Trauma) have acknowledged this accepted shortcoming of PMGs and have focused on the generation of "best practice guidelines." Best practice guidelines serve as an amalgamation of GRADE and non-GRADE PMGs as well as expert opinion in an effort to provide clinicians with guidance for commonly encountered scenarios. Patients, clinicians, and policymakers are best served by the continued evolution of guidelines generated with an emphasis on transparency. Taken together, the ultimate goal of any guideline is to reduce patient care variability so that safety and positive outcomes are maximized.

References

1. Haut ER. Eastern Association for the Surgery of trauma (EAST) practice management guidelines and the perpetual quest for excellence. J Trauma Acute Care Surg. 2020;89(1):1–10.
2. Neely JG, Magit AE, Rich JT, Voelker CC, Wang EW, Paniello RC, et al. A practical guide to understanding systematic reviews and meta-analyses. Otolaryngol Head Neck Surg. 2010;142(1):6–14.
3. Cipriani A, Furukawa TA, Barbui C. What is a Cochrane review? Epidemiol Psychiatr Sci. 2011;20(3):231–3.
4. Grimshaw J, Russell I. Achieving health gain through clinical guidelines. I: developing scientifically valid guidelines. Qual Health Care. 1993;2(4):243–8.
5. Hadorn DC, Baker D, Hodges JS, Hicks N. Rating the quality of evidence for clinical practice guidelines. J Clin Epidemiol. 1996;49(7):749–54.
6. Woolf SH, Battista RN, Anderson GM, Logan AG, Wang E. Assessing the clinical effectiveness of preventive maneuvers: analytic principles and systematic methods in reviewing evidence and developing clinical practice recommendations. A report by the Canadian task force on the periodic health examination. J Clin Epidemiol. 1990;43(9):891–905.
7. Institute of Medicine Committee on Standards for Developing Trustworthy Clinical Practice G. In: Graham R, Mancher M, Miller Wolman D, Greenfield S, Steinberg E, editors. Clinical practice guidelines we can trust. Washington (DC): National Academies Press (US) Copyright 2011 by the National Academy of Sciences. All rights reserved; 2011.
8. Fabian TC. Evidence-based medicine in trauma care: whither goest thou? J Trauma. 1999;47(2):225–32.
9. Woolf S, Schunemann HJ, Eccles MP, Grimshaw JM, Shekelle P. Developing clinical practice guidelines: types of evidence and outcomes; values and economics, synthesis, grading, and presentation and deriving recommendations. Implement Sci. 2012;7:61.
10. Rhodes M. Practice management guidelines for trauma care: presidential address, seventh scientific assembly of the eastern Association for the Surgery of trauma. J Trauma. 1994;37(4):635–44.
11. Ioannidis JP. The mass production of redundant, misleading, and conflicted systematic reviews and meta-analyses. Milbank Q. 2016;94(3):485–514.
12. Thornton J, Alderson P, Tan T, Turner C, Latchem S, Shaw E, et al. Introducing GRADE across the NICE clinical guideline program. J Clin Epidemiol. 2013;66(2):124–31.
13. Wang X, Zhou Q, Chen Y, Yang N, Pottie K, Xiao Y, et al. Using RIGHT (reporting items for practice guidelines in healthcare) to evaluate the reporting quality of WHO guidelines. Health Res Policy Syst. 2020;18(1):75.
14. Atkins D, Best D, Briss PA, Eccles M, Falck-Ytter Y, Flottorp S, et al. Grading quality of evidence and strength of recommendations. BMJ. 2004;328(7454):1490.
15. Harbour R, Miller J. A new system for grading recommendations in evidence based guidelines. BMJ. 2001;323(7308):334–6.
16. Grilli R, Magrini N, Penna A, Mura G, Liberati A. Practice guidelines developed by specialty societies: the need for a critical appraisal. Lancet. 2000;355(9198):103–6.
17. Helfand M, Balshem H. AHRQ series paper 2: principles for developing guidance: AHRQ and the effective health-care program. J Clin Epidemiol. 2010;63(5):484–90.
18. Raine R, Sanderson C, Hutchings A, Carter S, Larkin K, Black N. An experimental study of determinants

of group judgments in clinical guideline development. Lancet. 2004;364(9432):429–37.
19. Shekelle P, Eccles MP, Grimshaw JM, Woolf SH. When should clinical guidelines be updated? BMJ. 2001;323(7305):155–7.
20. Guyatt G, Gutterman D, Baumann MH, Addrizzo-Harris D, Hylek EM, Phillips B, et al. Grading strength of recommendations and quality of evidence in clinical guidelines: report from an American college of chest physicians task force. Chest. 2006;129(1):174–81.
21. Guyatt GH, Oxman AD, Schünemann HJ, Tugwell P, Knottnerus A. GRADE guidelines: a new series of articles in the Journal of Clinical Epidemiology. J Clin Epidemiol. 2011;64(4):380–2.
22. Guyatt G, Oxman AD, Akl EA, Kunz R, Vist G, Brozek J, et al. GRADE guidelines: 1. Introduction-GRADE evidence profiles and summary of findings tables. J Clin Epidemiol. 2011;64(4):383–94.
23. Andrews JC, Schünemann HJ, Oxman AD, Pottie K, Meerpohl JJ, Coello PA, et al. GRADE guidelines: 15. Going from evidence to recommendation-determinants of a recommendation's direction and strength. J Clin Epidemiol. 2013;66(7):726–35.
24. Jaeschke R, Guyatt GH, Dellinger P, Schünemann H, Levy MM, Kunz R, et al. Use of GRADE grid to reach decisions on clinical practice guidelines when consensus is elusive. BMJ. 2008;337:a744.
25. Andrews J, Guyatt G, Oxman AD, Alderson P, Dahm P, Falck-Ytter Y, et al. GRADE guidelines: 14. Going from evidence to recommendations: the significance and presentation of recommendations. J Clin Epidemiol. 2013;66(7):719–25.

Quality Assessment in Acute Surgical Disease

8

Michael W. Wandling, Lillian S. Kao, and Clifford Y. Ko

Introduction

The Institute of Medicine's publication of *To Err Is Human: Building a Safer Health System* in 2000 fundamentally changed the American healthcare system [1]. This book highlighted the imperfect system in which healthcare is provided and the need to improve patient safety. In the subsequent years, the delivery of high-quality care has become a top priority of contemporary medicine. Governmental bodies (i.e., Centers for Medicare & Medicaid Services and the Agency for Healthcare Research and Quality), regulatory agencies (i.e., The Joint Commission), professional organizations (i.e., the American College of Surgeons), private sector corporations (i.e., private insurers), and interest groups (i.e., the National Quality Forum) have all made efforts to improve the quality of healthcare in the United States. Organizations such as these are a source of clinical practice guidelines, quality measures, quality improvement (QI) initiatives, and educational campaigns that are valuable resources for patients, physicians, and hospitals. While efforts aimed at improving quality have become ubiquitous in modern healthcare, considerable room for improvement remains.

The meaningful improvement of healthcare quality relies upon the continuous evaluation and modification of current practices in a way that positively influences patient care. Avedis Donabedian created a model for evaluating quality by focusing on (1) the environment in which clinical care is delivered (frequently referred to as "structure"), (2) the processes of providing care to patients, and (3) the resulting patient outcomes (Fig. 8.1) [2]. After more than 50 years, Donabedian's structure, process, and outcome model continues to be the framework upon which quality assessment is performed.

In 2001, the Institute of Medicine published *Crossing the Quality Chasm: A New Health System for the 21st Century*, laying out the factors necessary to create a healthcare system capable of delivering the high-quality care patients deserve. This book identified six domains for a healthcare system that are essential to delivering high-quality care:

M. W. Wandling · L. S. Kao
Division of Acute Care Surgery, McGovern Medical School, The University of Texas Health Science Center—Houston, Houston, TX, USA
e-mail: michael.w.wandling@uth.tmc.edu; lillian.s.kao@uth.tmc.edu

C. Y. Ko (✉)
Department of Surgery, David Geffen School of Medicine, UCLA, Los Angeles, CA, USA

Division of Research and Optimal Patient Care, American College of Surgeons, Chicago, IL, USA

The Healthcare Improvement Studies Institute (THIS Institute), University of Cambridge, Cambridge, UK
e-mail: cko@facs.org

M. D. Zielinski, O. Guillamondegui (eds.), *The Acute Management of Surgical Disease*, https://doi.org/10.1007/978-3-031-07881-1_8

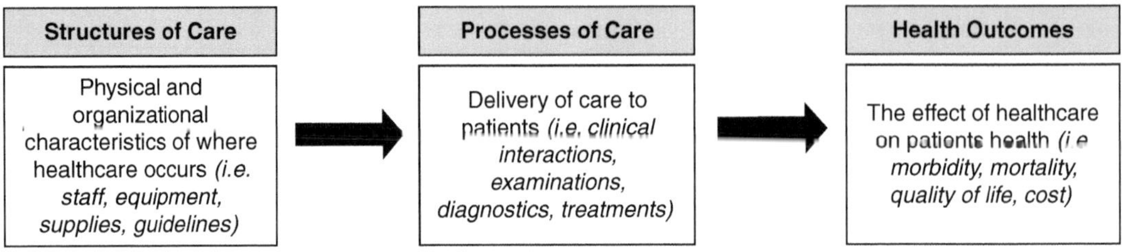

Fig. 8.1 The Donabedian model for assessing quality of care

1. *Safe*: Avoid patient harm while attempting to optimize health.
2. *Effective*: Provide appropriate, evidence-based care to patients who are likely to receive benefit while avoiding doing so for patients unlikely to benefit.
3. *Patient-centered*: Provide care that respects and is consistent with the preferences, needs, and values of individual patients and incorporates these factors into all clinical decisions.
4. *Timely*: Minimize all delays in the delivery of care.
5. *Efficient*: Eliminate waste of resources, including equipment, supplies, ideas, energy, and other contributors to unnecessary financial expenditure.
6. *Equitable*: Provide care that is uniform in quality for all patients, regardless of gender, ethnicity, geographic location, socioeconomic status, or any other characteristic [3].

Prioritizing the improvement of these six domains within a healthcare system enables the delivery of high-quality care that is optimally suited to meet patient needs [3]. Although specifically described in regard to the healthcare system as a whole, these domains are fundamentally important to all quality initiatives within a healthcare system, including those focusing on the delivery of surgical care.

Quality Assessment in Surgery

Surgery has been at the forefront of QI in medicine. The development of clinical data registries has revolutionized the way in which surgical care is evaluated. Professional societies such as the American College of Surgeons (ACS), the Society of Thoracic Surgeons (STS), and the Society for Vascular Surgery (SVS) have all created and maintained clinical data registries aimed at improving the quality of surgical care delivered. For a clinical data registry to effectively facilitate QI, it must contain performance data on a variety of clinically relevant quality metrics. Performance measurement alone, however, does not improve quality. The data collected in clinical registries must be analyzed and interpreted for QI opportunities to be identified.

Clinical data registries are often a component of a larger QI program. While simply monitoring institutional or individual performance over time may be of some benefit, the real strength of a clinical data registry is in its ability to collect standardized clinical and quality metrics from a large number of institutions and use that data to provide risk-adjusted comparative performance feedback to participating hospitals and surgeons. However, like performance measurement, participation in QI programs does not directly improve quality. For meaningful QI to occur, performance assessments must be closely analyzed and correctly interpreted, opportunities for QI must be identified, and local QI projects must be implemented. Many QI programs, like the ACS National Surgical Quality Improvement Program (NSQIP), provide QI education and tools that help both hospitals and surgeons use these data to improve the quality of care delivered at participating hospitals [4–6].

Optimizing clinical outcomes and providing patients with the best possible care are the core focus of surgical QI. However, it is also important to consider the economic implications of the quality of surgical care delivered. This is particularly true in high-risk specialties like emergency general surgery (EGS). In addition to being associated with worse clinical outcomes, complications following surgery are associated with increased healthcare expenditures [7, 8]. The occurrence of one or more postoperative complications has been reported to increase a patient's hospital costs by an average of $10,000 [9]. With nearly 100 million surgeries performed annually in the United States alone, the cumulative patient morbidity and financial burden of surgical complications on the American healthcare system are astonishing. This reality has been a signification motivational force behind the prioritization of the delivery of high-quality surgical care through many ongoing QI efforts.

Currently, several governmental programs financially incentivize the delivery of high-quality surgical care. Pay-for-performance initiatives such as the Merit-Based Incentive Payment System (MIPS) component of the Medicare Access and CHIP Reauthorization Act (MACRA) links reimbursement to clinical outcomes. Public reporting programs like Medicare's Hospital Compare program encourage the delivery of high-quality care by making hospital performance data available to the public. By making these data readily available to the public, patients are empowered to make informed decisions when choosing where to pursue their surgical care. Programs such as these incentivize both surgeons and hospitals to provide the highest possible quality of care, as high performers gain financial and competitive advantage over poor-performing surgeons and hospitals.

Quality Metrics

Given the importance of quality assessment in surgery, it is important for surgeons to be familiar with the quality metrics on which their performance is being measured. Standard quality metrics include process, outcome, and balancing measures. Process measures are those focused on quantifying adherence to a clearly defined protocol, guideline, or clinical pathway. Examples of process measures in surgery include compliance with preoperative bowel regimen prior to elective colon resection, administration of preoperative antibiotics in accordance with the Surgical Care Improvement Project (SCIP) measures, and appropriate utilization of venous thromboembolism (VTE) prophylaxis perioperatively. Outcome measures quantify performance on predefined clinical outcomes. Examples of common outcome measures in surgery include surgical site infection, postoperative venous thromboembolism, and hospital readmission. Balancing measures are quality metrics aimed at evaluating a system from an alternative direction to ensure there are not unanticipated adverse effects of efforts to improve quality [10]. Examples of balancing measures include re-intubation (confirm efforts to minimize ventilator days are not resulting in increased rates of re-intubation) and readmission rates (confirm efforts to decrease length of stay are not leading to increasing readmissions). Quality metrics may vary considerably across specialty, clinical data registry, or hospital. However, their objective of measuring performance in an effort to improve quality remains the same.

The best quality metrics are those that are clearly defined and clinically important. The majority of traditional quality metrics focus on processes of care and clinical outcomes deemed important by clinicians and policy-makers. In recent years, however, there has been an increased emphasis on identifying quality metrics that are most important to patients. Patient-reported outcomes (PROs) are defined as "any report of the status of a patient's health condition that comes directly from the patient, without interpretation of the patient's response by a clinician or anyone else." [11] While the majority of quality metrics currently being used in surgical quality assessment are traditional process and outcome measures, there is increasing interest in incorporating PRO measures into surgical quality initiatives, and it is important for surgeons to be familiar with these metrics as well [12, 13].

Assessing Quality in Acute Care Surgery

Quality assessment in acute care surgery presents a number of unique challenges. Patients who present to hospitals in need for urgent or emergent surgical intervention are fundamentally different from those being taken to the operating room for elective surgeries. In trauma and EGS, patients are rarely able to be medically, nutritionally, or hemodynamically optimized prior to surgery, which is a stark contrast to patients undergoing elective surgical intervention. As a result, patients presenting acutely for urgent and emergent operations experience higher rates of complication than patients undergoing elective procedures [14–16].

Another factor complicating surgical quality assessment in acute care surgery is the significant proportion of patients under the care of a surgical team who do not go on to require surgical intervention. This is particularly true for diagnoses such as low-grade blunt solid organ injury in trauma and small bowel obstruction or acute diverticulitis in EGS. Traditional surgical quality initiatives such as ACS NSQIP were designed to evaluate quality metrics specifically developed for assessing the quality of care provided to patients undergoing surgery. Consequently, specialty-specific quality initiatives are necessary.

Quality Initiatives in Emergency General Surgery

While trauma has a well-established quality program that has been growing since the development of the first version of *Resources for Optimal Care of the Injured Patient* in 1976, no such programs are widely used in EGS. To date, the quality programs available for performance assessment in EGS are limited to those used for elective general surgery. While the presence of urgent or emergent surgical intervention is accounted for in some existing surgical quality initiatives, this delineation is often not enough to account for variability in disease severity and physiologic derangement frequently encountered in EGS. Furthermore, existing surgical quality programs are unable to account for the nonoperative management of surgical disease that plays such an important role in many EGS diagnoses. As acute care surgery has developed into a distinct surgical specialty, there has been an increasing interest in developing an EGS quality program capable of providing meaningful performance assessment while addressing the unique aspects of emergency surgical care.

In recognition of the need for a QI program for EGS, ACS NSQIP created an EGS-specific quality program that was piloted at 16 hospitals across the United States and Canada in 2015. This EGS registry contained all data process and outcome measures collected by ACS NSQIP, as well as an additional 16 EGS-specific variables aimed at addressing the unique characteristics of patients with EGS diagnoses, including both disease severity and degree of physiologic derangement throughout the course of each patient care. This registry focused on patients with three common EGS diagnoses, acute appendicitis, acute cholecystitis, and small bowel obstruction, including those managed operatively and nonoperatively. The inclusion of patients managed nonoperatively marked the first time that the nonoperative management of surgical disease was included in an ACS NSQIP program.

The results of the ACS NSQIP EGS Pilot revealed the importance of assessing the quality of both operative and nonoperative EGS care. Discrepancies were identified in hospital performance on common surgical quality metrics when comparing operative and nonoperative management (Fig. 8.2) [17]. These findings demonstrate that providing high-quality operative care does not automatically translate into providing the same quality of nonoperative care. With nearly one-third of patient with common EGS diagnoses being managed nonoperatively, this highlights the importance of incorporating the nonoperative care of acute surgical disease into EGS quality initiatives [18].

Creating an EGS Quality Program

EGS care involves management of a highly heterogeneous group of patients being cared for at a highly heterogeneous group of hospitals [19]. This heterogeneity complicates QI efforts in EGS using Donabedian's structure, process, and outcome model for quality assessment. Currently,

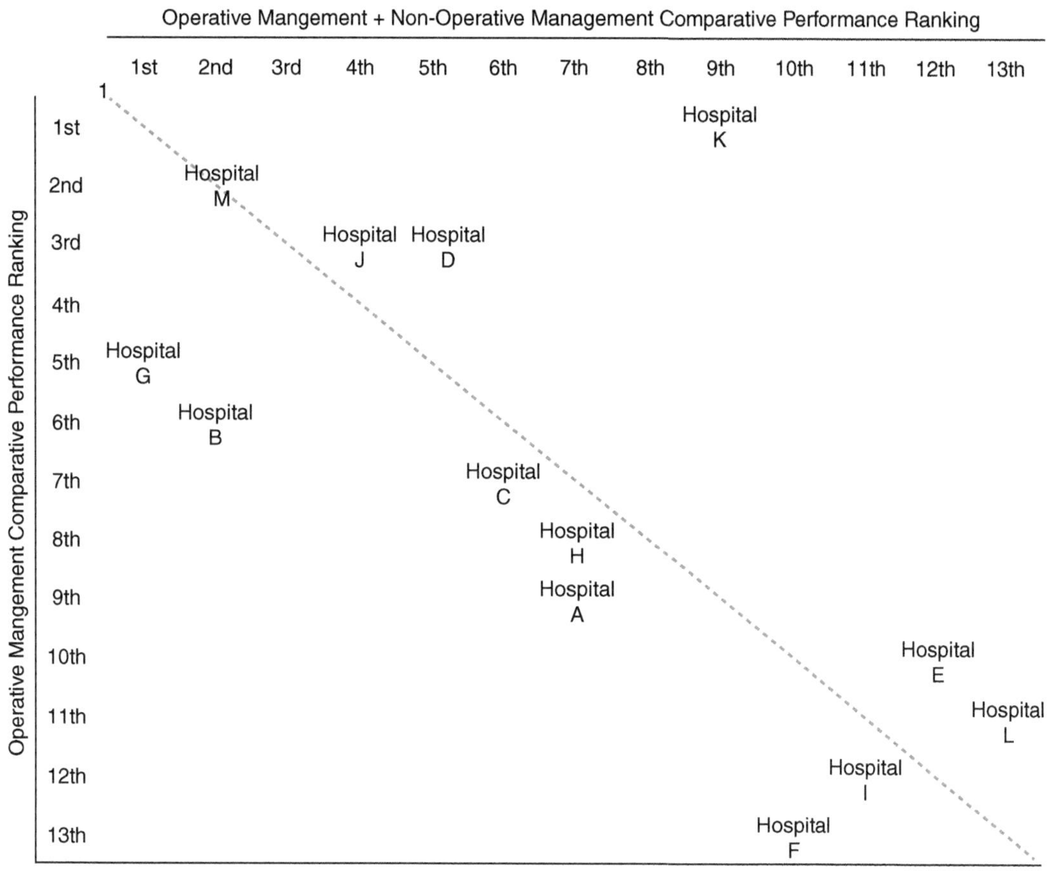

Fig. 8.2 Concordance of risk-adjusted hospital performance rankings for 30-day death or serious morbidity with and without the inclusion of patients managed nonoperatively in the ACS NSQIP EGS Pilot [17]

well-established structures and processes central to the delivery of high-quality EGS care are lacking, highlighting the need for development of an EGS quality program [20–23]. A successful quality program for EGS should be built upon four foundational principles: (1) strong surgical leadership and accountability, (2) structured tools for QI and organizational discipline, (3) change management and performance data, and (4) institutional commitment and resources.

Surgical Leadership and Accountability

Strong surgical leadership is vitally important to the success of any surgical quality program. The chief surgical quality officer should oversee the delivery of EGS care. This individual should be appointed by the department chair and have an adequate level of authority, credibility, and QI experience to effectively lead EGS QI efforts. The scope of oversight of the EGS program by the chief surgical quality officer must encompass the entire breadth of nonelective surgical care, both operative and nonoperative. While an EGS medical director is not always necessary, it is beneficial. A successful EGS quality program should have a clearly identified leader who oversees all aspects of EGS care provided at the hospital and is capable of addressing issues unique to EGS. To be successful, it is important that the leader of the EGS quality program has the support of institutional leadership and is granted sufficient authority to serve in their capacity as leader of the EGS program.

A hospital's credentialing process should delineate the required level of competency to provide EGS coverage at that institution and maintain accountability for the quality and safety of care that is provided. At most hospitals, EGS is considered a component of general surgery, and the credentialing process for EGS is the same as for general surgery. However, the leader of the EGS program should ensure that all surgeons providing EGS coverage for the hospital maintain the appropriate credentialing requirements and are capable of providing timely, high-quality emergency surgical care.

Multidisciplinary peer review is another important component of an effective EGS program. EGS program leaders should establish and lead periodic multidisciplinary EGS peer-review meetings, where selected cases, complications, delays in diagnosis or management, deaths, and sentinel events are examined in detail to identify areas for improvement in an effort to improve the quality of care provided. Representatives from all specialties involved in the care of EGS patients, including emergency medicine, radiology, surgery, anesthesia, critical care, and when appropriate internal medicine, should participate in multidisciplinary peer-review meetings. The focus of multidisciplinary peer review should not be punitive; rather, it should be to improve all aspects of EGS care in hopes of improving the quality of care delivered to patients.

Lastly, it is the responsibility of the chief surgical quality officer, in conjunction with the EGS quality program leader, to oversee the clinical data registry, review and interpret performance feedback, and disseminate performance feedback results to all EGS providers within the hospital. A quality program cannot be effective unless the data collected in the clinical registry is used to identify opportunities for improvement and stimulate frontline QI efforts.

Tools for Quality Improvement and Organizational Discipline

The foundation of a surgical quality program is a clinical data registry capable of systematically monitoring performance. Fundamental to any clinical registry is the systematic and accurate abstraction of well-defined clinical data points, process measures, and outcome measures by specially trained data abstractors. In the absence of a well-established, multicenter EGS-specific clinical data registry, a hospital looking to build an EGS quality program would have to rely on an institutional EGS registry. Reliable and clinically meaningful performance data are fundamentally important to any successful QI initiative. As discussed above, there are a number of unique aspects of assessing quality of EGS care. These nuances must be addressed for an EGS clinical data registry to be truly effective.

An effective EGS clinical data registry must incorporate several key factors unable to be addressed with existing registries. Patients with EGS diagnoses present to hospitals with tremendous variability in degree of physiologic derangement and disease severity. For example, consider two patients presenting to an emergency department with appendicitis. Both are young and otherwise healthy. Patient #1 has had 24 h of abdominal pain and is hemodynamically normal, and a mild leukocytosis is his only laboratory abnormality. Patient #2 has had pain for nearly a week and presented to the hospital in septic shock, with multisystem organ failure and rigid peritonitis. These patients would clearly not follow the same anticipated postoperative course.

Now, consider two hospitals, Hospital A and Hospital B, each of which performs 100 appendectomies in a given year. Hospital A performs appendectomies on 85 patients similar to Patient #1 and 15 on patients similar to Patient #2. Hospital B performs appendectomies on 15 patients similar to Patient #1 and 85 patients similar to Patient #2. Traditional clinical data registries are ill-equipped to account for severity of disease and physiologic derangement, complicating adequate risk adjustment. Consequently, comparative performance reports are likely to show that Hospital A has considerably worse outcomes following appendectomy than Hospital B.

To facilitate adequate risk adjustment for comparative performance assessment using EGS clinical data registries, it is necessary to include more granular data regarding severity of disease and physiologic derangement. Perhaps one of the most widely recognized and accepted tools for stratifying EGS disease severity is the American Association for the Surgery of Trauma's (AAST) EGS grading scale of 16 common emergency general surgery conditions, which grades the severity of each diagnosis from I to V based on clinical, imaging, operative, and pathologic criteria [24]. Incorporating a disease severity grading system such as this into an EGS clinical data registry is vital for adequate risk adjustment. Similarly, incorporating detailed physiologic data is imperative for an EGS registry. This includes data at the time of surgical consultation, perioperatively, and postoperatively. Emergency general surgeons encounter patients encounter patients at all time points in their course of disease and therefore face providing care under markedly variable physiologic conditions. To adequately account for this variability in disease, granular data points such as these are necessary to generate meaningful risk-adjusted comparative performance feedback to surgeons and hospitals.

Another important difference between an effective EGS clinical data registry and existing surgical registries is the inclusion of patients who are managed nonoperatively. As previously discussed, nonoperative management plays a significant role in many EGS diagnoses. The primary clinical data registries currently used for surgical QI assess the perioperative care provided to patients. As a result, patients who are primarily managed by surgeons for various diagnoses that do not require surgical intervention are left in a "blind spot" of surgical quality assessment.

Take, for example, two patients who present to an emergency department with perforated appendicitis. Patient #1 is taken to the operating room for a difficult appendectomy. She is started on deep vein thrombosis (DVT) prophylaxis postoperatively in accordance to the institutional clinical guidelines that were implemented in response to the hospital being a poor performer in postoperative VTE on their ACS NSQIP reports over the last several years. Patient #2 is managed nonoperatively. Interventional radiology is consulted for percutaneous abscess drainage, and DVT prophylaxis is held at their request. The procedure is delayed several times but ultimately is performed 36 h later. After the procedure, the surgical team forgets to order DVT prophylaxis, and she goes on to develop a pulmonary embolism. Most surgeons would consider both of these patients to be "surgical" patients, yet Patient #2 is not included in the existing clinical data registry that is used for surgical QI. Consequently, the adverse outcome she experienced under the care of her surgeon is not identified and an opportunity for QI is lost.

As highlighted by this example, an optimal EGS clinical data registry must include patients who are managed nonoperatively. While this may seem like a minor addition to existing registries, the incorporation of nonoperatively managed patients into current surgical registries introduces a number of significant challenges. Existing surgical registries classify patients by the operation that is performed and identify patients for inclusion from operating room lists. To include patients managed nonoperatively in an EGS registry, patients must instead be classified by their diagnosis and identified by an alternative methodology. Identifying patients for inclusion in an EGS registry by diagnosis can be complex. An effective EGS registry should include all or an unbiased sample of patients with EGS diagnoses. As an EGS clinical data registry is a tool for surgical QI, patients who are included should be managed or co-managed by a surgical team. The variability in how EGS services are structured and covered across hospitals precludes a uniform way to do this. Consequently, determining an optimal process for identifying patients by diagnosis requires significant foresight and planning by any hospital seeking to develop or participate in an EGS registry.

While there currently are no widely available EGS-specific tools for QI, hospitals seeking to evaluate performance in EGS can leverage existing data sources. Examples of data sources than can be used as tools for EGS QI include existing clinical data registries (i.e., ACS NSQIP), public databases (i.e., Hospital Consumer Assessment of Healthcare Providers and Systems (HCAHPS), Hospital Compare), proprietary databases (i.e., Press Ganey, United Healthcare), or existing clinical data registries (i.e., ACS NSQIP). Additionally, hospitals can evaluate performance on EGS-specific quality indicators that have been developed (Table 8.1).

Table 8.1 Quality indicators for emergency general surgery [25]

If a hospital provides EGS care, then the time from a computerized tomography scan or ultrasound being ordered STAT to the performance of the study should be ≤4 h
If a patient has undergone an EGS procedure and was found subsequently to have cancer, then postoperative care should include appropriate guideline directed oncologic follow-up and surveillance (as detailed by the National Comprehensive Cancer Network)
If a patient has undergone an EGS procedure, then the discharge or transfer summary should indicate: (a) Medical findings and diagnoses: a summary of the care, treatment, and services provided (b) A complete list of all medications and dosages to continue on discharge, including the purpose and side effects of new medications (c) Activity restrictions (d) Diet restrictions or recommendations (e) Wound/ostomy care instructions, if applicable (f) Home health services arranged, if applicable (g) Reasons to call the responsible provider or seek emergency medical attention (signs or symptoms of complications) (h) Follow-up appointment(s) (i) Contact information for the responsible provider
If an EGS patient is diagnosed with acute cholecystitis, then the patient should undergo a cholecystectomy within 72 h of symptom onset, or the reason for not doing so should be documented in the medical record
If an EGS patient is diagnosed with an uncontained perforated viscus, then surgery should begin within a timeframe consistent with the locally derived standard but ≤3 h from the decision to operate, or the reason for not doing so should be documented in the medical record
If an EGS patient has a small bowel obstruction and findings consistent with ischemia and/or impending perforation, then the patient should undergo surgical exploration within a timeframe consistent with the locally derived standard but ≤3 h from the decision to operate, or the reason for not doing so should be documented in the medical record
If a hospital provides EGS care, then the hospital should conduct, on at least a quarterly basis, a multidisciplinary review of patient morbidity and mortality involving all relevant EGS providers and include postmortem data when available
If a hospital provides EGS care, then the hospital should audit: (a) Unplanned readmissions to a critical care unit within 48 h of discharge to the ward (b) Unplanned postoperative readmissions within 30 days of discharge (c) Unplanned readmissions and operations within 30 days of discharge for patients previously managed nonoperatively (d) Unplanned returns to the operating room during the hospitalization or within 30 days of discharge
If a hospital provides EGS care, then a protocol should be in place for the preoperative hematologic preparation of patients taking common anticoagulants prior to emergency surgery
If a hospital provides EGS care, then a faculty- or attending-level radiologist should be available to read radiographic studies within 2 h
If a hospital provides EGS care, then the hospital should have a graded response strategy, such as a modified early warning score and an acute response team, in place to identify patients at risk of clinical deterioration as well as guidelines and defined responsibilities for escalation of care and involvement of senior staff
If a hospital provides EGS care, then the hospital should have a protocol in place regarding the availability of blood products
If a hospital provides EGS care, then the time from diagnosis of an intra-abdominal infection to source control (i.e., drainage, diversion, and/or resection of the pathology to control ongoing peritoneal contamination) should be monitored

Table 8.1 (continued)

If a hospital provides EGS care, then the hospital should ensure that EGS cases begin in a timely fashion based upon a locally defined tiering system through: (a) Monitoring the availability of the anesthesia and operating room staff (b) Monitoring the adequacy of access to the operating room (c) Having protocols in place to defer elective general surgery cases in order to give adequate priority to EGS patients (d) Having protocols in place for bypass or transfer of patients to a hospital with transfer agreements if timely access cannot be provided If a hospital provides EGS care, then the hospital should have a locally defined protocol to identify patients requiring admission to a critical care unit postoperatively based upon, at a minimum, the risk associated with the procedure, unresolved physiologic impairment or hemodynamic instability, the severity of the patient's comorbid conditions, and physician judgment
If a hospital provides EGS care, then the hospital should ensure timely access to surgical evaluation through: (a) Having a credentialed general surgeon on call at all times (b) Monitoring the time from general surgery consultation to the initial evaluation by a designated member of the general surgery team based upon a locally defined tiering system
If a hospital provides EGS care, then the hospital must ensure that the surgeon credentialed to perform the surgery is board eligible or certified by the American Board of Surgery or American Osteopathic Board of Surgery or fulfills the requirements of an alternative pathway as defined by the hospital
If a hospital provides EGS care, then the hospital should have a critical care specialist on call at all times or have protocols in place to provide critical care specialist on call at all times or have protocols in place to provide critical care services when needed through telemedicine or the transfer of patients to a hospital with transfer agreements

Lastly, hospitals can incorporate EGS clinical practice guidelines into the care of their EGS patients and monitor compliance. When incorporated into routine clinical practice, clinical practice guidelines can be a valuable tool for improving quality of care. The Cochrane Database of Systematic Reviews and the National Guideline Clearinghouse are both reliable sources of practice guidelines relevant to EGS. Additionally, specialty societies such as the Eastern Association for the Surgery of Trauma (EAST) and the Society of American Gastrointestinal and Endoscopic Surgeons (SAGES) have published guidelines to facilitate the delivery of high-quality EGS care. A list of EGS clinical practice guidelines is provided in Table 8.2.

Table 8.2 Examples of EGS clinical practice guidelines [26]

Clinical guidelines	Source
Antibiotics for uncomplicated diverticulitis	Cochrane Database
Early versus delayed laparoscopic cholecystectomy for people with acute cholecystitis	Cochrane Database
Laparoscopic repair for perforated peptic ulcer disease	Cochrane Database
Acute upper gastrointestinal bleeding: management	National Guideline Clearinghouse
Timing and type of surgical treatment of *Clostridium difficile*-associated disease	EAST Practice Management Guidelines
Evaluation and management of small bowel obstruction	EAST Practice Management Guidelines
Guidelines for diagnosis, treatment, and use of laparoscopy for surgical problems during pregnancy	Society of American Gastrointestinal and Endoscopic Surgeons

Change Management and Performance Data

The benefits of maintaining an EGS-specific registry are only assumed if the data collected are used to inform local QI initiatives. Data must be evaluated, interpreted, and disseminated to those participating in the care of EGS patients on a regular basis. Further, when opportunities for improvement are identified, they must be acted upon. An effective EGS quality program should include mechanisms that empower participating hospitals and caregivers to use their performance data to pursue QI within their institution. In order for durable changes in practice to occur, performance data must be used to demonstrate the efficacy of changes in practice using the performance data continuously being collected.

Institutional Commitment and Resources

For an EGS quality program to successfully stimulate QI, it is essential for the participating institution to commit to improving the quality of EGS care at their hospital and allocate the necessary resources to support QI efforts. Commitment of the institutional governing body and medical staff is key. The delivery of high-quality EGS care relies upon the support of hospital administrators and departmental leadership for those who participate in the care of patients with EGS diagnoses. Institutional leadership should encourage and support multidisciplinary collaboration in an EGS quality program that includes key stakeholders from emergency medicine, surgery, anesthesiology, critical care, interventional radiology, and nursing, among others.

An EGS quality leader, as previously discussed, should be granted sufficient authority by hospital and departmental leadership to oversee and uphold the standards of an EGS quality program. The institution must devote the necessary resources to support the timely delivery of emergent care, a quality program leader, a quality program manager, an EGS clinical data registrar, performance improvement specialist support, and administrative support. Providing high-quality EGS care is a time- and resource-intensive process that is not possible without the financial and infrastructural support of the participating institution. However, improving the quality of EGS care delivered can yield a substantial return on the institution's investment [7–9].

Conclusions

Quality improvement has become a major priority of contemporary healthcare. Surgery has become a proven leader in healthcare QI through the development of clinical data registries and the creation of a well-established infrastructure for conducting performance assessment. However, the unique characteristics of EGS have limited the ability to broadly incorporate these patients into existing surgical QI initiatives, leaving a large number of patients in a "blind spot" of surgical quality. This reality is becoming increasingly recognized and presents a tremendous opportunity for future QI efforts in acute care surgery. We hope that this chapter has provided an informative overview of surgical quality assessment, the resources that are currently available, and the opportunity that exists for building a durable QI infrastructure and program capable of improving the care of the acutely ill and injured for decades to come.

References

1. Kohn LT, Corrigan J, Donaldson MS, Institute of Medicine (U.S.). Committee on Quality of Health Care in America. To err is human : building a safer health system. Washington, D.C.: National Academy Press; 2000.
2. Donabedian A. Evaluating the quality of medical care. The Milbank Memorial Fund Quarterly. 1966;44(3):Suppl:166–206.
3. Institute of Medicine (U.S.). Committee on Quality of Health Care in America. Crossing the quality chasm : a new health system for the 21st century. Washington, D.C.: National Academy Press; 2001.
4. Cohen ME, Liu Y, Ko CY, Hall BL. Improved surgical outcomes for ACS NSQIP hospitals over time: evaluation of hospital cohorts with up to 8 years of participation. Ann Surg. 2016;263(2):267–73.
5. Guillamondegui OD, Gunter OL, Hines L, et al. Using the national surgical quality improvement program and the Tennessee surgical quality collaborative to improve surgical outcomes. J Am Coll Surg. 2012;214(4):709–14; discussion 714–706

6. Hall BL, Hamilton BH, Richards K, Bilimoria KY, Cohen ME, Ko CY. Does surgical quality improve in the American College of Surgeons National Surgical Quality Improvement Program: an evaluation of all participating hospitals. Ann Surg. 2009;250(3):363–76.
7. Birkmeyer JD, Gust C, Dimick JB, Birkmeyer NJ, Skinner JS. Hospital quality and the cost of inpatient surgery in the United States. Ann Surg. 2012;255(1):1–5.
8. Scally CP, Thumma JR, Birkmeyer JD, Dimick JB. Impact of surgical quality improvement on payments in medicare patients. Ann Surg. 2015;262(2):249–52.
9. Dimick JB, Weeks WB, Karia RJ, Das S, Campbell DA Jr. Who pays for poor surgical quality? Building a business case for quality improvement. J Am Coll Surg. 2006;202(6):933–7.
10. Science of improvement: establishing measures. Institute for Healthcare Improvement. How to improve web site. http://www.ihi.org/resources/Pages/HowtoImprove/ScienceofImprovementEstablishingMeasures.aspx. Accessed 5 Feb 2021.
11. Forum NQ. Patient Reported Outcomes (PROs) in performance measurement. Washington, DC: National Quality Forum; 2013.
12. Sakran JV, Ezzeddine H, Schwab CW, et al. Proceedings from the consensus conference on trauma patient-reported outcome measures. J Am Coll Surg. 2020;230(5):819–35.
13. Liu JB, Pusic AL, Matroniano A, et al. First report of a multiphase pilot to measure patient-reported outcomes in the American College of Surgeons National Surgical Quality Improvement Program. Joint Commission J Quality Patient Safety/Joint Commission Resources. 2019;45(5):319–28.
14. Ingraham AM, Haas B, Cohen ME, Ko CY, Nathens AB. Comparison of hospital performance in trauma vs emergency and elective general surgery: implications for acute care surgery quality improvement. Arch Surg. 2012;147(7):591–8.
15. Ingraham AM, Cohen ME, Raval MV, Ko CY, Nathens AB. Comparison of hospital performance in emergency versus elective general surgery operations at 198 hospitals. J Am Coll Surg. 2011;212(1):20–8.e21
16. Haider AH, Obirieze A, Velopulos CG, et al. Incremental cost of emergency versus elective surgery. Ann Surg. 2015;262(2):260–6.
17. Wandling M, Ko CY, Bankey PE, Cribari C, Cryer HG, Diaz JJ, Duane TM, Hameed SM, Hutter MM, Metzler III MH, Regner JL, Reilly PM, Reines HD, Sperry JL, Staudenmayer KL, Utter GH, Crandall ML, Bilimoria KY, Nathens AB. Expanding the scope of quality measurement in surgery to include non-operative care: results from the ACS NSQIP emergency general surgery pilot. J Trauma Cute Care Surg. 2017;83(5);837–45.
18. Wandling M, Nathens AB, Pavey ES, Chung JW, Yang AD, Shapiro MB, Ko CY, Bilimoria KY. Evaluating the blind spot of surgical quality: a national assessment of non-operative management. Jacksonville, FL: 2016 Association for Academic Surgery Academic Surgical Congress; 2016.
19. Stephens TJ, Peden CJ, Pearse RM, et al. Improving care at scale: process evaluation of a multi-component quality improvement intervention to reduce mortality after emergency abdominal surgery (EPOCH trial). Implementation Sci. 2018;13(1):142.
20. Tameron AM, Ricci KB, Oslock WM, et al. The association between self-declared acute care surgery services and critical care resources: results from a national survey. J Crit Care. 2020;60:84–90.
21. Santry HP, Strassels SA, Ingraham AM, et al. Identifying the fundamental structures and processes of care contributing to emergency general surgery quality using a mixed-methods Donabedian approach. BMC Med Res Methodol. 2020;20(1):247.
22. Ricci KB, Rushing AP, Ingraham AM, et al. The association between self-declared acute care surgery services and operating room access: results from a national survey. J Trauma Acute Care Surg. 2019;87(4):898–906.
23. Daniel VT, Rushing AP, Ingraham AM, et al. Association between operating room access and mortality for life-threatening general surgery emergencies. J Trauma Acute Care Surg. 2019;87(1):35–42.
24. Tominaga GT, Staudenmayer KL, Shafi S, et al. The American Association for the Surgery of Trauma grading scale for 16 emergency general surgery conditions: disease-specific criteria characterizing anatomic severity grading. J Trauma Acute Care Surg. 2016;81(3):593–602.
25. Ingraham A, Nathens A, Peitzman A, et al. Assessment of emergency general surgery care based on formally developed quality indicators. Surgery. 2017;162(2):397–407.
26. Wandling M, Nathens AB, Hoyt DB. Continual quality improvement in acute care surgery. In: Britt LD, Barie P, Jurkovich G, editors. Acute care surgery. 2nd ed. Philadelphia: Wolters Kluwer; 2019. p. 867–76.

Concepts in Emergency Research Exception from Informed Consent

9

Christine S. Cocanour and Isabelle A. Struve

Introduction

Informed consent is an ethical concept, codified in the law, and is in daily practice at every healthcare institution. It is the process of communication between patients and treating physicians that results in an agreement that allows the treating physician to perform a specific medical intervention. A valid informed consent requires disclosure, capacity, and voluntariness [1]. Disclosure requires that the physician must provide the patient the necessary information to make an autonomous decision. At a minimum, this must include the diagnosis, the procedure with its risks and benefits, as well as the alternatives with their risks and benefits. The information must be presented in language suited to the apprehension skills of the patient. Capacity is the ability of the patient to both understand and assess the information given, communicate their choices, and understand the consequences of their decision. Voluntariness requires that their decision be made without being subjected to external pressures such as coercion, manipulation, or undue influence.

Informed consent for clinical research requires more information and a different approach than informed consent for daily clinical practice. In the ideal situation, the consent process starts with a preliminary meeting at which the research team provides a clear description of the study's purpose and objectives, the procedures that the potential subject will undergo, the potential benefits (as an individual, to other patients, and to society), the potential harms, the probability of being assigned to any of the study arms, the implications of blinding, and the rights of the participant to receive updated information about the study and to agree or decline participation in the study at any point in time [2, 3]. A copy of the consent is given to the potential subject so that they can review the information with trusted family, friends, or advisors. The potential participant is allowed time to process the information before being asked to make a decision of whether they wish to participate. Referred to as the Experimental Subject's Bill of Rights, Table 9.1 lists information that must be given to a potential experimental subject [4, 5].

In the emergency setting, this consent process is not possible. Ethical concerns involving subjects who cannot provide consent was a barricade to emergency research. Standard, accepted medical therapy was not tested for either safety or efficacy in the emergency setting. In recognition of this potential harm, the government eventually permitted exception from informed consent in certain emergency research trials in order to (1) provide individuals in life-threatening situations

C. S. Cocanour (✉) · I. A. Struve
Department of Surgery, University of California Davis Health, Sacramento, CA, USA
e-mail: cscocanour@ucdavis.edu; istruve@ucdavis.edu

M. D. Zielinski, O. Guillamondegui (eds.), *The Acute Management of Surgical Disease*,
https://doi.org/10.1007/978-3-031-07881-1_9

Table 9.1 Experimental Subject's Bill of Rights

California law, under Health & Safety Code Section 24172 requires that any person asked to take part as a subject in a medical experiment, or any person asked to consent to such participation on behalf of another, is entitled to receive the following list of rights written in a language in which the person is fluent [4]. These are also found in the Basic HHS Policy for Protection of Human Research Subjects [5].
1. Be informed of the nature and purpose of the experiment.
2. Be given an explanation of the procedures to be followed in the medical experiment, and any drug or device to be utilized.
3. Be given a description of any attendant discomforts and risks reasonably to be expected from the experiment.
4. Be given an explanation of any benefits to the subject reasonably to be expected from the experiment, if applicable.
5. Be given a disclosure of any appropriate alternative procedures, drugs or devices that might be advantageous to the subject, and their relative risks and benefits.
6. Be informed of the avenues of medical treatment, if any, available to the subject after the experiment if complications should arise.
7. Be given an opportunity to ask any questions concerning the experiment or the procedures involved.
8. Be instructed that consent to participate in the medical experiment may be withdrawn at any time and the subject may discontinue participation in the medical experiment without prejudice.
9. Be given a copy of the signed and dated written consent form as provided for by Section 24173 or 24,178.
10. Be given the opportunity to decide to consent or not to consent to a medical experiment without the intervention of any element of force, fraud, deceit, duress, coercion, or undue influence on the subject's decision.

access to potentially life-saving therapies, (2) advance knowledge through collection of information about effectiveness and safety, and (3) improve therapies used in emergency medical situations that currently have poor clinical outcomes [6].

Informed consent for human subject research has not always been the standard, and as a consequence, patients have suffered. Because of this dark history, the evolution to include waiver or exception from informed consent in emergency research was momentous. This chapter will explore the history behind informed consent, informed consent for human subject research, and exception from informed consent (EFIC)/ waiver of informed consent (WIC). It will review the current guidelines for consent in emergency research as well as its applicability to specific research.

History of Informed Consent

Informed consent is a relatively new concept. Rooted in beneficence, the Hippocratic Oath pledges to do no harm, but the *Corpus Hippocraticum* bluntly advised keeping information away from the patient as the physician's primary task was to inspire confidence [7, 8]. In the medieval age, physicians continued to hold to Hippocratic traditions where authoritarianism and the obedience of patients were further influenced by Christian theology. Maintaining hope justified any deception on the part of the physician [9]. In the Age of Enlightenment, physicians began sharing more information with their patients, not to respect the patient's autonomy, but to allow the patient to better understand and be motivated to comply with the recommended treatment. In 1803, Percival published his treatise *Medical Ethics* which provided a modern foundation for medical ethics in North America [10]. Despite the influence of Reverend Thomas Gisborne who opposed lying to patients, Percival continued to emphasize the physicians' role of giving hope and comfort at the expense of truthfulness [8]. The AMA's first code of medical ethics was published in 1847 and borrowed heavily from Percival's treatise. However, truthfulness was only championed between physicians, not between physician and patient [8]. After its publication, Worthington Hooker, a Connecticut physician, made what is considered to be one of the most influential contributions to medical ethics by an American author in the nineteenth century when he denounced lying and deception in medicine [11].

The legal foundation of informed consent began in the early 1900s. Its roots are in early

English Common Law, which is a combination of customs, traditions, and case law that is distinct from legislative law. Informed consent is interpreted and grounded in the respect for autonomy and is derived from the legal theories of battery and negligence. Four cases that occurred from 1905 to 1914 are considered the early legal basis of informed consent [9]. In the *Mohr v. Williams* opinion, after entering into a contract, the physician can operate to the extent of the consent given but no further [12]. In *Pratt v. Davis*, there was no consent for hysterectomy, and the decision limited implied consent to emergencies or to when the patient understands the consequences of allowing a physician to exercise professional judgment [13]. In *Rolater v. Strain,* the opinion highlighted the patient's self-determination by stressing that a patient could give a carefully constrained consent, which would dictate precisely what the doctor could do [14]. *Schloendorff v. Society of New York Hospital* drew on the opinions of the previous three cases, and Judge Cardozo's landmark opinion is the first true description of a patient's right to self-determination [15]:

> In the case at hand, the wrong complained of is not merely negligence. It is trespass. Every human being of adult years and sound mind has a right to determine what shall be done with his own body; and a surgeon who performs an operation without his patient's consent commits an assault for which he is liable in damages. This is true, except in cases of emergency where the patient is unconscious, and where it is necessary to operate before consent can be obtained [15].

The next major development came in 1957 with the case of *Salgo v. Leland Stanford Jr. University Board of Trustees* [16]. This marked the first time that the term "informed consent" was used. The court determined that physicians have the duty to disclose any facts which are necessary to form the basis of an intelligent consent by the patient to the proposed treatment. It requires the disclosure of risks and alternatives, although it did give physicians discretion on what should be disclosed—a reasonable physician standard.

In 1973, the American Hospital Association adopted the first Patient's Bill of Rights which further led to the use of informed consent [17]. A marked increase in the numbers of malpractice awards and the increasing size of awards in the 1970s saw a skyrocketing of malpractice insurance premiums. Between 1975 and 1977, 25 states enacted informed consent laws in an attempt to decrease malpractice liability [8]. Statutory laws regarding informed consent now exist in all 50 states.

History of Informed Consent for Research

Cases that dealt with consent as it applied to medical research began in 1871 with *Carpenter v. Blake* in which the court ruled that a doctor who deviates from the usual, established method of treatment is liable for any resulting problems [18]. Because this rule accepted those treatments that had already been proven, experimentation put doctors at risk. In a 1934 case, *Brown v. Hughes*, the court determined that some experimentation had to be allowed or science would never advance [19]. A year later in *Fortner v. Koch*, the court recognized that "if the general practice of medicine and surgery is to progress, there must be a certain amount of experimentation carried on; but such experiments must be done with the knowledge and consent of the patient or those responsible for him, and must not vary too radically from the accepted method of procedure" [20]. Valid consent and an acceptable risk-benefit analysis would become important points in the debate on whether human subject research should be justified.

Human subject research did not become widespread in the United States until shortly before the beginning of World War II [9]. It was more common internationally. The atrocities committed by Nazi physicians in the name of research led to the 1946 trial before the Nuremberg military tribunal [21]. The judges established the certain basic principles that must be observed in order to satisfy moral, ethical, and legal concepts while conducting research on human subjects [21]. These ten principles became the Nuremberg Code which focused on protecting human subjects by requiring the subject's consent and setting boundaries within which the investigator may conduct research [22].

The Nuremberg Code was the first step in the regulation of research on humans. It was followed by the Declaration of Helsinki in 1964, which was drafted by the World Medical Association as a statement of ethical principles to provide guidance to physicians and other participants in medical research involving human subjects [23]. An influential document, American medical groups endorsed it, and eventually, it was used by the federal government as a basis for developing its own rules for human subject research.

Although courts and international organizations had recognized the importance of providing guidance and policies for human research subject protection, US government policies were slower to develop [24]. It was not until publicized cases where consent was lacking and through efforts of several influential scholars that the United States began to address this problem.

During the 1960s and 1970s, two particular cases attracted public attention to consent violations. A cancer study that took place in 1963 at the Jewish Chronic Disease Hospital in Brooklyn, New York, found that doctors had obtained permission from the hospital medical director to inject live cancer cells into chronically ill and debilitated patients, but they not only did not obtain the patient's consent, they told none of the patients that they were receiving live cancer cells [25, 26]. An even more egregious case came to light in 1972. Beginning in the early 1930s, the US Public Health Service conducted a study on the effects of untreated syphilis on black men in Alabama. It continued until *The New York Times* reported the study on its front page in 1972 [27].

In the 1960s, a Harvard physician, Henry K. Beecher, called for stricter protections for human research subjects [28, 29]. An Englishman, M.H. Pappworth, published *Human Guinea Pigs* in 1967, which chronicled his findings about more than 500 unethical experiments [30]. In 1972, psychiatrist Jay Katz and coauthors published a collection of writings from a variety of fields that related to the ethics of human research [26]. These publications, coupled with the publicized cases, stimulated discussion about the importance of conducting research while still protecting subjects' rights and led to the Federal Drug Administration (FDA) and the National Institutes of Health (NIH), both within the Department of Health, Education and Welfare, to propose their own solutions [24].

The first federal policy regarding human subject research developed at the Clinical Center of the NIH in 1953 [9, 24]. Despite the NIH championing informed consent, clinical researchers throughout the country did not adopt this approach but instead preferred to leave oversight directly to the investigators [9].

At the FDA, the Kefauver-Harris Bill emerged in the early 1960s due to concern about the use and control of drugs. The thalidomide debacle in Europe highlighted the necessity for more stringent drug testing and warning requirements and led to the inclusion of a consent requirement [31]. The consent provision was largely ignored until 1966 when the FDA, influenced by the public's anger surrounding the Jewish Chronic Disease Hospital Case, published the *Statement of Policy Concerning Consent for Use of Investigational New Drugs on Humans* [32]. This statement relied heavily on content from both the Nuremberg Code and the Declaration of Helsinki and brought the US policy into conformity with the international community. However, this statement did not apply to all human subject research but to only those under the jurisdiction of the FDA, that is, experimental drugs and devices.

In the early 1960s, the NIH was divided in its opinion regarding the need to regulate research on human subjects. A study commissioned to examine research protocols concluded that the NIH could not regulate research ethics without overstepping its bounds and intruding on investigators' authority. Despite this result, NIH Director James Shannon met with the National Advisory Health Council (NAHC) and convinced them to adopt a resolution to address the moral and ethical issues of clinical research. This led to the 1966 *Statement of Policy on Clinical Investigations Using Human Subjects* which required institutions receiving research grants to obtain prior committee review for proposed research [31, 33]. The review recommended consideration of three key elements: the rights and welfare of the subjects involved, the appropriateness of the methods used to obtain informed consent, and the risks and potential medical benefits of the investigation. Although it addressed the necessity of informed consent, it did not define informed consent.

In 1971, the Department of Health, Education, and Welfare (DHEW) expanded on the Surgeon General's policy with the Institutional Guide to DHEW Policy on Protection of Human Subjects also known as the DHEW Yellow Book. The Yellow Book defined informed consent as "the agreement obtained from a subject, or from his authorized representative, to the subject's participation in an activity" [34]. The Yellow Book also listed the elements of informed consent.

Piggybacking in part on the DHEW policy, Congress passed the National Research Act which established the National Commission for the Protection of Human Subjects of Biomedical and Behavioral Research (more commonly known as the National Commission) in 1974 [35]. The National Commission's mission was to provide ethical and policy analysis related to human research. In 1979, the National Commission passed the Belmont Report: Ethical Principles and Guidelines for the Protection of Human Subjects of Research. The Belmont report identified "three fundamental ethical principles applicable to research with humans—respect for persons, beneficence, and justice" [36]. In this report, the National Commission determined that in order to protect an individual's autonomy and dignity, consent was essential. Consent must include three conditions—information, comprehension, and voluntariness. At this same time, the National Commission also emphasized the Institutional Review Board (IRB) System [37]. In 1978, Congress established the President's Commission for the Study of Ethical Problems in Medicine and Biomedical and Behavioral Research. In response to the National Commission and the President's Commission, the Department of Health and Human Services (HHS) revised its human subjects regulations (CFR 45 §46, Subpart A).

In 1991, the CFR 45 §46 Subpart A was adopted by 16 government agencies and became known as the Common Rule. The Common Rule also includes a prolonged section detailing the general requirements for informed consent. CFR 45 §46.116 requires that the information be provided in language understandable to the subject; without such clear language, no consent will be considered informed. CFR 45 §46.116(a) details the eight elements that must be provided for an informed consent and are shown in Table 9.2.

The Common Rule set the framework for our current definition of informed consent. The next hurdle then became identifying when informed consent can be waived. In 1996, HHS identified three provisions in which an alteration or waiver of informed consent can occur. In the first provision under 45 CFR 46.116f, the IRB may approve the alteration or waiver of consent if all of the following conditions are met:

Table 9.2 The eight elements that must be provided for an informed consent as set forth in CFR 45 §46.116(a)

1. A statement that the study involves research, an explanation of the purposes of the research and the expected duration of the subject's participation, a description of the procedures to be followed, and an identification of any procedures which are experimental
2. A description of any reasonably foreseeable risks or discomforts to the subject
3. A description of any benefits to the subject or to others which may reasonably be expected from the research
4. A disclosure of appropriate alternative procedures or courses of treatment, if any, that might be advantageous to the subject
5. A statement describing the extent, if any, to which confidentiality of records identifying the subject will be maintained or research involving more than minimal risk
6. An explanation as to whether any compensation and an explanation as to whether any medical treatments are available if injury occurs and, if so, what they consist of or where further information may be obtained
7. An explanation of whom to contact for answers to pertinent questions about the research and research subjects' rights and whom to contact in the event of a research-related injury to the subject
8. A statement that participation is voluntary, refusal to participate will involve no penalty or loss of benefits to which the subject is otherwise entitled, and the subject may discontinue participation at any time without penalty or loss of benefits to which the subject is otherwise entitled [37, 39]

1. The research involves no more than minimal risk to the subjects.
2. The research could not practicably be carried out without the requested waiver or alteration.
3. If the research involves using identifiable private information or identifiable biospecimens, the research could not practicably be carried out without using such information or biospecimens in an identifiable format.
4. The waiver or alteration will not adversely affect the rights and welfare of the subjects.
5. Whenever appropriate, the subjects will be given additional information about the research after it is completed. The second provision found at CFR 46.116e pertains to research involving public benefit and service programs conducted by or subject to the approval of state or local officials. The third provision found in both CFR 21 §50.24 and CFR 45 §46.101 (i) pertains to emergency research.

Emergency Research

Emergency research involves the most vulnerable population of study subjects. They have no capacity to control what happens to them as they are unable to provide consent and the emergency circumstances require prompt action which does not allow time to locate and obtain consent from a legally authorized surrogate. Consent prior to entering a study prevented research in emergency settings and the ability to evaluate safety and efficacy of emergency treatments. It also prevented patients from accessing potential life-saving therapies.

Deferred consent was introduced in 1980 by Fost and Robertson to allow enrollment of subjects in a clinical trial in which consent was impossible because the subjects were comatose as a result of head trauma, permission was unlikely to be valid due to the emotional response of the next of kin, and it was necessary to enroll quickly to allow the therapies their intended effect [38]. They proposed three conditions: (1) there must be substantial reason for deferring consent, (2) consent should not be deferred any longer than is necessary to protect whatever interests deferral aims to protect, and (3) harm to the patients from deferring consent must be minimal. Beauchamp criticized these criteria as too vague to provide clear guidance [39]. From 1984 to 1987, the Brain Resuscitation Clinical Trial II (BRCT II) used deferred consent. They concluded that the use of deferred consent in resuscitation research is legally as well as ethically justified if the following conditions were met:

1. Study patients are comatose and therefore "incompetent."
2. Life-saving therapy must be administered immediately—and therefore an "emergency" exists.
3. The experimental therapy might be administered even if the patient were not in the research protocol.
4. The state of scientific knowledge is such that the clinician-investigator does not, and cannot, know whether standard or experimental therapy is best for his patient.
5. The possible risks of the experimental therapy do not expose the patient to meaningful additional risk [40].

In BRCT II, IRB approval was obtained in all but two participating hospitals with those two hospitals ultimately being dropped from the study because of inability to obtain the traditional prospective consent [41]. Opponents of deferred consent felt that a subject cannot consent meaningfully to something that has already happened and instead argued that there are conditions for the justifiability of resuscitation research without informed consent [42]. In 1993, a letter from the Director of the Office for Protection from Research Risks went out to Institutional Officials and Institutional Review Board Chairs throughout the country stating that deferred consent failed to constitute informed consent, and this mechanism should not be used after this time [43].

Informed consent in clinical research conducted in emergency circumstances came to a head in 1995 surrounding the execution of the National Acute Brain Injury Study: Hypothermia (NABISH) [44]. Arguments against the use of a waiver were that the research could be carried out practicably without a waiver, that the risks of experimental emergency treatments were too great, and that enrollment of minorities with waiver of consent particularly violated their rights. The IRBs that approved the trial believed that patients would incur no more than minimal additional risk by being entered into the trial. However, the Office of Protection from Research Risk differed and felt that minimal risk meant "risk to all persons and not just the persons who may become involved as subjects in the research" [44]. Therefore, for the first 9 months of this trial, it required prospective consent by the potential subject's surrogate. Because of low accrual, the NIH, the principal investigator, and the Patient Safety and Monitoring Board concluded that the trial should be stopped unless there was an ability to use waiver of consent. The DHHS then permitted the use of waiver of consent using "strictly limited circumstances" [45].

Later that year, the Secretary of Health and Human Services and the Commissioner of Food and Drugs proposed to amend the FDA's informed consent regulations to permit emergency care research. FDA proposed this action "in response to growing concerns that current rules are making high quality acute care research activities difficult or impossible to carry out at a time when the need for such research is increasingly recognized" [46]. It was opened for comments, and the vast majority of comments supported the proposal. In November 1996, the FDA amended its current informed consent regulations to permit harmonization of the DHHS policies on emergency research (CFR 21 §50.24 and CFR 45 §46.24) which is sometimes referred to as the final rule for waiver of informed consent in certain emergency research circumstances. The primary differences between the regulations before 1996 and after are the definition of the risks of research and the requirement for public disclosure and community consultation. Table 9.3 summarizes CFR 21 §50.24 requirements for exception from informed consent.

From 1996 to the present, there have been multiple studies looking at the implementation and application of informed consent in specific populations such as emergency surgery patients, trauma patients, etc. The next section will review a number of these studies and publications in more detail.

Dutton et al. explored the practical mechanics of obtaining patient consent for enrollment in resuscitation studies. Their goal was to identify how many patients had overt contraindications to

Table 9.3 Summary of the requirements for exception from informed consent. Adapted from CFR 21 §50.24(a)

1.	Human subjects are in a life-threatening situation, available treatments are unproven or unsatisfactory, and the collection of valid scientific evidence is necessary to determine the safety and effectiveness of interventions
2.	Obtaining consent is not feasible because:
(a)	The subject is unable to give consent as a result of their medical condition
(b)	The intervention must be administered before consent from the subject's legally authorized representative (LAR) is feasible
(a)	There is no way to prospectively identify subjects
3.	Participation in the research holds out the prospect of direct benefit to the subject because:
(a)	Subjects are facing a life-threatening situation that necessitates intervention
(b)	Appropriate preclinical studies have been conducted, and its evidence supports the potential for the intervention to provide direct benefit to the subjects
(c)	Risks associated with the investigation are reasonable in relation to what is known about the current standard therapy and the proposed intervention
4.	The clinical investigation could not practically be carried out without the waiver
5.	The investigator will attempt to contact a LAR and obtain consent within the potential therapeutic window. The efforts made to contact LARs will be summarized and made available to the IRB at the time of continuing review
6.	The IRB has approved the informed consent procedures and an informed consent document to be used when feasible
7.	Additional protections of the rights and welfare of the subjects will be provided, including, at least:
(a)	Consultation with representatives of the communities in which the clinical investigation will be conducted and from which the subjects will be drawn
(b)	Public disclosure to the communities about the study, its risks, and benefits prior to initiation of the study
(c)	Public disclosure of sufficient information following completion of the investigation to apprise the community and researchers of the study results

(continued)

Table 9.3 (continued)

(d)	Establishing an independent data monitoring committee to exercise oversight of the clinical investigation
(e)	If obtaining informed consent is not feasible from either the subject or their LAR, the investigator will attempt to contact within the therapeutic window a family member who is not the LAR and ask whether they object to the subject's participation in the investigation. The efforts made to contact family members will be summarized and made available to the IRB at the time of continuing review

consent, how many had occult contraindications, and how many had a legally authorized representative (LAR) available within 3 hours of hospital arrival [47]. The study performed in Baltimore analyzed 1734 patients. Only 20% were considered consentable, another 20% were potentially impaired, 37% were not consentable with 17% being objectively impaired (age <18 years, blood alcohol concentration above the legal limit, Glasgow Coma Scale <14, Abbreviated Injury Scale, brain >2, or methamphetamine or benzodiazepine screens positive), and 20% did not have a LAR. Twenty-three percent did have a LAR for consent. In their discussion, they note that from a patient's perspective, the informed consent process in emergency situations is inherently coercive. A need to find a LAR will further bias studies to less acute patients. Minors and females are likely to be overrepresented because they are more likely to have a LAR present, while adult male minorities will be underrepresented. Their study was limited in that they did not actually approach patients or family members for consent so they did not know how many would have consented to a research study.

Sims et al. looked at a community's attitudes and willingness to participate in emergency research. Their study was conducted in the context of community consultation for an upcoming trial investigating the use of vasopressin during hemorrhagic shock resuscitation [48]. The study took place at an urban level 1 trauma center in Philadelphia and the surrounding neighborhoods. Trauma patients ready for discharge and family members of patients with moderate to severe traumatic brain injuries were asked to participate in a structured interview. In addition, community-based organizations were contacted and invited to host a focus group that was led by a professional facilitator, observed by IRB members, and included a research team member to address any questions. Of 336 subjects invited to participate, 307 completed the survey. This included 172 trauma patients, 73 family members, and 64 community members. The three groups did not differ in respect to age, religion, or educational level, but patients were more likely to be male, white, and unemployed or disabled. The key concept of enrollment into a research study without consent was endorsed by the majority of participants. In contrast to previous reports, these subjects were more supportive of enrolling a community member without consent than they were to enrolling a family member or themselves. The authors suggested that this may be while the subjects perceived trauma research as important, they felt less strongly that they would personally benefit from the care associated with the emergency research. Patients and their families who were admitted following interpersonal violence were statistically less supportive of EFIC than those admitted following nonviolent mechanisms. The investigators suggested that the recent exposure to violence may have negatively impacted their sense of trust. The process of community consultation was considered valuable and confirms previous reports in which public disclosure and consultation activities that actively engage and educate participants positively influence their attitudes toward studies dependent upon exception from informed consent, essentially allowing them to be "partners" in the research process [48–51]. The study limitations may have reflected the positive views toward this particular research study rather than all emergency research studies. The face-to-face interaction may have been influenced the participants to respond in a way that they thought the researcher would approve. Because this was a convenience sample, this may not reflect the views of the community in general. Although the focus group format and the individual assessments allowed for in-depth dialogue and questions, it is very time-intensive.

Fox et al. reported their experience with waiver of consent in a multi-institutional, noninterventional observational emergency research study [52]. The PRospective Observational Multicenter Major Trauma Transfusion (PROMMTT) study enrolled trauma patients receiving at least one unit of red blood cells within 6 h of admission at ten US level 1 trauma centers. EFIC is primarily used in intervention studies in the emergency setting and requires that the research have potential for direct patient benefit and must require that the drug or device intervention be administered before a consent from the patient or their LAR can be obtained. Waiver of consent is usually used for any minimal risk study and by its definition does not involve an intervention. Although the information collected in this study was similar to that recorded in trauma registries, this study required that data collection be prospective to allow detail and accuracy. In developing this study, investigators expected a 30–60% refusal rate. Many patients would not be able to give consent because of severe injuries, no LAR would be available in a timely fashion, and even if a LAR was available, they may not be able to give an informed consent because of emotional distress. Another concern was consent bias. Enrolling only those patients who have the capacity to consent would limit the sample size, create selection bias, and reduce the validity and relevance of the research. All local IRBs approved the study, but one required that their investigators attempt consent, but they were allowed to retain data on patients that were unable to be consented. Of 121 subjects enrolled at this site, 46% of patients were able to be consented, and no patient or LAR refused to give consent. Thirty percent of patients died and 5% were discharged before consent could be attempted. Consent was attempted but not possible in 20% of patients. The 100% participation rate at the site requiring consent attempts was attributed to the very experienced staff at this site but also that this was a nonintervention study. Most studies that report refusal rates are intervention studies or randomized trials. In conclusion, the authors determined that waiver of consent can be a valuable tool for noninterventional observational emergency research. Deferred consent may be more appropriate for some studies, but in order to maximize study validity, investigators will need to work with their respective IRBs to create an appropriate consent process.

Rebers et al. reviewed 115 papers from 1997 to 2013 that discussed reasons not to ask for informed consent and/or conditions under which an exception to informed consent was considered acceptable [53]. Research on children or research that addressed the use of surrogate consent were excluded. Reasons for waiving the informed consent requirement fell into three main categories with ethical issues playing a role in all three: decrease of data validity and quality, distress or confusion of participants, and practical issues. Although not all papers included papers involving emergency research, each of the categories included examples from emergency research. In the area of decreased data validity and quality, participation bias was a key concern. Some patient groups may be less likely to give consent or may be physically unable to give consent due to their injuries. Requiring consent before an intervention in emergency situations may lead to an underestimation of the treatment effect if the intervention is delayed. Distress or confusion of participants may be magnified when confronted with the consent process during an emergency. Others have argued that patients may be negatively affected by the knowledge that it is not known which treatment is best. Practical problems are most often cited in emergency research as the reason why an informed consent should be waived. Patients are often incapacitated and unable to give consent; a LAR is not available, especially when the therapeutic window is short. A delay in treatment to obtain an informed consent may be ethically unacceptable if it has potential to adversely affect outcome. The authors stressed that informed consent should always remain the standard in research that requires an intervention. Compliance with guidelines applicable to their nation, institute and field of research are paramount when considering EFIC.

The establishment of EFIC and WIC more than 20 years ago has created a standard and ethical mechanism by which investigators can study questions and interventions in true emergent clinical states. The answers to these clinical questions are critical and ultimately can save many lives. The conditions and process by which EFIC and WIC are conducted should be routinely.

reported to the scientific community to not only educate but to also ensure that standards are met regarding the study of vulnerable populations not able to provide prospective informed consent [54].

Exception from informed consent has transformed the ability to perform emergency subject research, and as a result, management of acute traumatic injury and other time-dependent interventions have been able to be scientifically evaluated. However, the three ethical principles upon which informed consent is based—autonomy, beneficence, and justice—should always be considered when exception from informed consent is considered.

References

1. Cahana A, Hurst SA. Voluntary informed consent in research and clinical care: an update. Pain Pract. 2008;8:446–51.
2. Abaunza H, Romero K. Elements for adequate informed consent in the surgical context. World J Surg. 2014;38(7):1594–604.
3. Nijhawan LP, Janodia MD, Muddukrishna BS, et al. Informed consent: issues and challenges. J Adv Pharm Technol Res. 2013;4:134–40.
4. California Health and Safety Code 24172. http://leginfo.legislature.ca.gov/faces/codes_displaySection.xhtml?sectionNum=24172.&lawCode=HSC Accessed 29 Jan 2021.
5. Subpart A—basic HHS policy for protection of human research subjects; §46.116 general requirements for informed consent. https://www.ecfr.gov/cgi-bin/text-idx?SID=fb2d33c657de8fa6a803f044eb97356c&pitd=20210111&node=se45.1.46_1116&rgn=div8. Accessed 29 Jan 2021.
6. Guidance for institutional review boards, clinical investigators, and sponsors; exception from informed consent requirements for emergency research. https://www.fda.gov/files/about%20fda/published/Exception-from-Informed-Consent-Requirements-for-Emergency-Research.pdf. Accessed 7 Feb 2021.
7. Selections from the Hippocratic Corpus, Decorum XVI, in WHS Jones, trans., Hippocrates, 4 vols. (Cambridge, MA: Harvard University Press, 1923–31), 2:297, 299.
8. Cocanour CS. Informed consent-It's more than a signature on a piece of paper. Am J Surg. 2017;214(6):993–7.
9. Faden RR, Beauchamp TL. A history and theory of informed Consent. New York: Oxford University Press; 1986.
10. Percival T. Medical ethics: or a code of institutes and precepts adapted to the professional conduct of physicians and surgeons. 3rd ed. London: John Churchill; 1849.
11. Hooker W. Physician and patient or A practical view of the mutual duties, relations and interests of the medical profession and the community. New York: Baker and Scribner; 1849.
12. Mohr v. Williams, 95 Minn. 261, 104 N.W. 12, 108 N.W. 818; 1905.
13. Pratt v. Davis, 224 Ill. 300, 79 N.E. 562; 1906.
14. Rolator v. Strain, 39 OK 572, 137; 1913.
15. Schloendorff v. Society of New York Hospital, 104 N.E. 92, 211 N.Y. 125; 1914.
16. Salgo v. Leland Stanford Jr. Univ. Bd. Trustees. 154 Cal. App. 2d 560, 317 P.2d 170; 1957.
17. American Hospital Association. A patient's bill of rights. Chicago: American Hospital Association; 1992.
18. Carpenter v. Blake, 60 Barb. N.Y. 488; 1871.
19. Brown v. Hughes, 94 Colo. 295, 30 P.2d 259; 1934.
20. Fortner v. Koch, 272 Mich. 273, 261 N.W. 762 (Mich. 1935).
21. Trials of war criminals before Nuernberg, Nuremberg Military. https://www.loc.gov/rr/frd/Military_Law/pdf/NT_war-criminals_Vol-II.pdf. Accessed 7 Feb 2021.
22. Vaux KL, Schade SG. The search for universality in the ethics of human research: Andrew C. Ivy, Henry K. Beecher, and the Legacy of Nuremberg. In: Spicker SF, et al., editors. The use of human beings in research. Boston: Kluwer Academic; 1988. p. 3–16.
23. WMA Declaration of Helsinki—ethical principles for medical research involving human subjects. file:///C:/Users/Christine%20S%20Cocanour/Downloads/wma-declaration-of-helsinki-ethical-principles-for-medical-research-involving-human-subjects.pdf. Accessed 31 Jan 2021.
24. Wandler M. The history of the informed consent requirement in United States Federal Policy. http://nrs.harvard.edu/urn-3:HUL.InstRepos:8852197. Accessed 7 Feb 2021.
25. Hospital Accused on Cancer Study; Live Cells Given to Patients Without Their Consent, Director Tells Court; ALLEGATION IS DENIED; Chronic Disease Institution Defends Action—Value of Tests Is Praised—The New York Times (nytimes.com) https://timesmachine.nytimes.com/timesmachine/1964/01/21/97160985.html?pageNumber=31. Accessed 7 Feb 2021.
26. Katz J, Capron A, Glass E. Experimentation with human beings: the Authority of the investigator, subject, professions, and state in the human experimentation process. Russell Sage Foundation; 1972.

27. Heller, J. Syphilis victims in U.S. study went untreated for 40 years. New York Times July 25, 1972. https://timesmachine.nytimes.com/timesmachine/1972/07/26/80798097.pdf?pdf_redirect=true&ip=0. Accessed 31 Jan 2021.
28. Beecher HK. Experimentation in man. In: Ladimer I, Newman RW, editors. Clinical investigation in medicine 2–39; 1963.
29. Beecher HK. Consent in clinical experimentation: myth and reality. JAMA. 1966;195:34–5.
30. Pappworth MH. Human Guinea pigs: experimentation on man. Routledge & Kegan Paul PLC; 1967. p. 12–27.
31. The development of human subject research policy at DHEW. ACHRE Report, Part I, Chapter 3. https://ehss.energy.gov/ohre/roadmap/achre/chap3_2.html. Accessed 20 Feb 2021.
32. National Research Council (US) Committee on the use of third party toxicity research with human research participants. Intentional human dosing studies for Epa regulatory purposes: scientific and ethical issues. Washington (DC): National Academies Press (US); 2004. 2, The Regulatory Framework for Protecting Humans in Research. Available from: https://www.ncbi.nlm.nih.gov/books/NBK215883/
33. Stewart WH. Clinical research investigations using human subjects. In: Final report, Supplemental Vol. 1. Washington, D.C.: U.S. Government Printing Office; 1966. p. 473–4.
34. U.S. Department of Health, Education, and Welfare, The institutional guide to DHEW policy on protection of human subjects (Washington, D.C.: GPO, 1971) (ACHRE No. HHS-090794-A).
35. National Research Act of 1974. P.L. 348, 93d Cong., 2d Sess. (12 July 1974).
36. The National Commission. The Belmont report: ethical principles and guidelines for the protection of human subjects of research, pp. 4–20; 1979.
37. The National Commission, Report and Recommendations: institutional review boards; 1979. CFR 45 §46.116.
38. Fost N, Robertson JA. Deferring consent with incompetent patients in an intensive care unit. IRB. 1980;2(7):5–6.
39. Beauchamp TL. The ambiguities of "deferred consent". IRB: Rev Hum Subj Res. 1980;2:6–8.
40. Abramson NS, Meisel A, Safar P. Deferred consent: A new approach for resus- citation research. JAMA. 1986;255:2466.
41. Kelsey SF, Sutton-Tyrrell K, Abramson NS, et al. Randomized clinical trial of calcium entry blocker administration to comatose survivors of cardiac arrest: design, methods and patient characteristics. Control Clin Trials. 1991;1:525–45.
42. Miller BL. Philosophical, ethical, and legal aspects of resuscitation medicine. I. Deferred consent and justification of resuscitation research. Crit Care Med. 1988;16:1059–62.
43. Informed consent, legally effective and prospectively obtained (OPRR Letter, 1993) Number 93-3 Human Subject Protections. https://www.hhs.gov/ohrp/regulations-and-policy/guidance/legally-effective-and-prospectively-obtained/index.html. Accessed 20 Feb 2021
44. Clifton GL, Knudson P, McDonald M. Waiver of consent in studies of acute brain injury. J Neurotrauma. 2002;19(10):1121–6.
45. FEDERAL REGISTER. Action related to emergency research activity. 1995;60(143):38353.
46. FEDERAL REGISTER. Action related to emergency research activity. 1995;60(183):49086.
47. Dutton RP, Stansbury LG, Hemlock B, Hess JR, Scalea TM. Impediments to obtaining informed consent for clinical research in trauma patients. J Trauma. 2008;64(4):1106–12.
48. Sims CA, Isserman JA, Holena D, Sundaram LM, Tolstoy N, Greer S, Sonnad S, Pascual J, Reilly P. Exception from informed consent for emergency research: consulting the trauma community. J Trauma Acute Care Surg. 2013;74(1):157–65; discussion 165–6.
49. Biros M. Struggling with the rule: the exception form informed consent in resuscitation research. Acad Emerg Med. 2007;14:344–5.
50. Richardson LD, Wilets I, Ragin DF, et al. Research without consent: community perspectives from the community voices program. Acad Emerg Med. 2005;12:1082–90.
51. Triner W, Jacoby L, Shelton W, et al. Exception from informed consent enrollment in emergency medical research; attitudes and awareness. Acad Emerg Med. 2007;14:187–91.
52. Fox EE, Bulger EM, Dickerson AS, et al. Waiver of consent in noninterventional, observational emergency research: the PROMMTT experience. J Trauma Acute Care Surg. 2013;75(1 Suppl 1):S3–8.
53. Rebers S, Aaronson NK, van Leeuwen FE, Schmidt MK. Exceptions to the rule of informed consent for research with an intervention. BMC Med Ethics. 2016;17:9.
54. Klein L, Moore J, Biros M. A 20-year review: the use of exception from informed consent and waiver of informed consent in emergency research. Acad Emerg Med. 2018;25(10):1169–77.

Design and Impact of the American Association for the Surgery of Trauma Acute Care Surgery Fellowship

10

Erin L. Vanzant and Alicia M. Mohr

Introduction

Acute Care Surgery Fellowships were created to fill the need for expertise in emergency general surgery as well as trauma and surgical critical care. Acute care surgery is a subspecialty of general surgery, with its own curriculum, site-verified program requirements, and a certificate of completion. Since its inception, there have been both an increase in the number of accredited fellowship programs by the American Association for the Surgery of Trauma and a parallel increase in the number of interested applicants as well. The importance of recruitment and training of acute care surgeons is vital, as the acute care surgery model of practice continues to be implemented nationwide to address disparities in emergency general surgical care.

There are 4 million patients who visit the emergency department who require evaluation by emergency surgery physicians [1]. Of these, 3 million require admission. There are an additional 2–3 million trauma patients per year who also require evaluation and admission [1]. Delivery of care to this large number of patients is contingent on the ability to provide nonelective general surgical services. Traditionally, care of these patients has been dependent on general surgeons who take trauma and emergency general surgery call. The American College of Emergency Physicians conducted a survey of emergency physicians in 2005, and 75% felt that there was inadequate on-call surgeon-specialist coverage [1–3]. Subsequently in 2006, the Institute of Medicine reported that there was a national crisis in emergency care due to insufficient access to these providers [1].

As we entered the twentieth century, an increasing disparity between the need for delivery in medical care related to an ever-growing population was noted with a highly disproportionate number of general surgeons being trained. Between 1981 and 2006, only a 4% increase in the number of general surgeons was seen compared to a 31% increase in the population [3]. In addition, there are a decreasing number of physicians willing to participate in emergency call and an aging of the current workforce which further compounds the problem. The Association of American Medical Colleges predicted a 35% increase in surgeons would be required in order to meet demands of the growing population by 2025 [1, 3].

Surgical training has been evolving since its initiation. From the abandonment of pyramidal training programs to the current 80-hour work week limitations, surgical education has been molded into a specialty-specific, focused exposure, apprenticeship, with the adjunct of indepen-

E. L. Vanzant · A. M. Mohr (✉)
Department of Surgery, University of Florida College of Medicine, Gainesville, FL, USA
e-mail: rin.Vanzant@surgery.ufl.edu; alicia.mohr@surgery.ufl.edu

M. D. Zielinski, O. Guillamondegui (eds.), *The Acute Management of Surgical Disease*,
https://doi.org/10.1007/978-3-031-07881-1_10

dent learning [4]. These changes have affected every subspecialty in general surgery and have resulted in the development of increasingly subspecialized divisions. Concurrently, training in trauma, emergency general surgery, and surgical critical care has followed suit.

Trauma as a general surgery subspecialty training program has also evolved over the years. The "golden age of trauma" when injured patients underwent aggressive surgical exploration has since declined due to improvements in imaging, diagnostic techniques, and minimally invasive procedures. This has resulted in fewer surgical residents pursuing careers in trauma due to the thought of being a "nonoperative" discipline. This impression is also compounded by the need for high call burdens, 24-hour coverage, management of operative orthopedic and neurosurgical patients, and the perception of an undesired, stressful lifestyle compared to that of other surgical disciplines.

In 2003, the Committee to Develop the Reorganized Specialty of Trauma, Surgical Critical Care, and Emergency Surgery was formed through a joint meeting of the American College of Surgeons Committee on Trauma, the American Association for the Surgery of Trauma (AAST), the Western Trauma Association (WTA), and the Eastern Association for the Surgery of Trauma (EAST) [5, 6]. This committee formed a consortium to evaluate the problems facing the subspecialty of trauma and its future, in addition to developing a training paradigm to fit those needs. This Committee determined an increasing deficit in the operative training for traumatic exposure and hemorrhage control, in addition to an increasing need for a "surgical hospitalist" to address acute surgical patients without disrupting the scheduled elective daily operative procedures [5, 6].

Finally, with the resuscitation needs of traumatically injured patients, they determined that a need for surgical critical care training was also a necessity for residents pursuing a career in trauma. Therefore, the AAST formed an ad hoc Acute Care Surgery Committee to develop and reorganize the specialty of trauma, surgical critical care, and emergency surgery, redefining trauma surgery as acute care surgery (ACS), a model built to encompass trauma, critical care, as well as emergency surgery. In addition to this paradigm shift, they proposed the need for a 2-year fellowship to improve the quality of care and improve the shortage of trained physicians. Changes were made in the ACS model by incorporating training in emergency general surgery, surgical critical care, and surgical exposures necessary for the care of traumatically injured patients. They created the Acute Care Surgery Fellowship and training paradigm. The goal of the fellowship was to train a versatile surgeon, able to address the difficulties of caring for acutely ill patients in a variety of conditions, while facing the challenges of providing comprehensive care of patients every hour, day, and night.

History

The first piloted fellowship graduated Dr. John Cha from Denver Health Medical Center in 2007 having completed an SCC fellowship and second year in acute care surgical training which included rotations with thoracic, vascular, transplant, and interventional radiology services. In 2008, the first formal AAST ACS fellowship program began.

The initial curriculum was created based on defined operative expectations, as well as a focus on clinical experience. This was structured by dictating mandatory components, defining essential and desirable cases, while still allowing for some flexibility on rotations. Case selections were based on a wide range of trauma cases broken down into anatomical regions which included head and neck, thoracic, abdominal, vascular, ultrasound, as well as those defined in management of complex trauma and emergency general surgery. To increase operative experience in technically difficult areas, rotations in thoracic, transplant, hepatobiliary, and vascular surgery were encouraged however not mandated [7]. Since the establishment of the first fellowship, these requirements and the curriculum have continued to evolve.

In 2009, a written exam was instituted, followed by the institution of an additional midyear fellowship examination in 2015. The in-training exam was built to assess the baseline knowledge of the starting fellow allowing room for program directors to tailor education and experience to individual weaknesses, while the final exam allowed the opportunity to assess whether education metrics were being met. In addition to establishing examinations to track fellow progress, a case log system was established in 2010. A review of this log performed in 2014 revealed a high variability in individual fellow experience and case exposure [8]. In particular, there was noted to be a lack of exposure in several areas defined as essential by the curriculum particularly in the areas of head and neck, thoracic, and vascular surgery [8]. This led to revamped case log system in 2019 which will allow for future improved assessments of the surgical experiential training.

After assessing the need of accurate case numbers, the ACS fellowship curriculum was restructured from the rotation-based system in 2018. Thoracic and vascular surgery rotations were no longer optional and were made mandatory requirements of the fellowship with experiential goals. In addition to longitudinal requirements, there was also the establishment of a case minimum requirement to be performed in specific body regions. To further address potential gaps in exposure and training with regard to vascular and thoracic exposure in the trauma patient, a series of educational modules were developed and included detailed operative descriptions. With the explosion of virtual education in 2020, the AAST added weekly virtual Meet the Masters sessions to augment the ACS educational curriculum. Current fellows are required to keep a case log to evaluate proposed minimal essential case requirements, complete an in-service fellowship exam and final exam, as well as complete online educational modules/sessions. The AAST continues to evaluate the educational goals and needs of the fellows and refine the operative case requirements that were initially determined by consensus of the AAST ACS Committee.

Program Requirements

The AAST Board of Managers approved the original fellowship requirements in March of 2007. Since that time, two subsequent reviews have been performed which have led to restructuring of the fellowship [9]. The most recent requirements are available on the AAST website.[1] Programs seeking AAST fellowship approval should be robust academic centers with a commitment to education and must comply with the institutional guidelines for fellowship training. One of the most important aspects in establishing an ACS fellowship is the assurance that they will not detract from the existing general surgery residents' experience. Thus, support from the department chairman and the general surgery residency program director is mandatory. In an ACS fellowship, there must be core service support from the trauma and emergency general surgery division, in addition to the thoracic and vascular divisions. Additionally, while the acute care surgery year is not currently an ACGME verified fellowship, there must be an associated ACGME-approved SCC fellowship.

The goal of the second year is to allow fellows the opportunity to experience in depth the nuances of trauma and emergency general surgery, advance operative experience, and develop teaching skills and further research in ACS. Optional educational experiences during the ACS year include exposure to elective general surgery, international surgical rotations, focused ultrasound curricula, trauma system development, advanced endoscopy, orthopedics, neurosurgery, interventional radiology, pediatric trauma, and complex hepatobiliary/pancreatic, colorectal, and transplant surgery [9]. The essential and desirable case list includes operative experience in thoracic, vascular, and complex hepatobiliary/pancreatic procedures. These procedures are expected as a means of developing competency in the management of acute surgical emergencies in these anatomic regions. Fellowship programs should also provide

[1] https://www.aast.org/acute-care-surgery/current-acs-fellows/curriculum-and-case-numbers

opportunities to participate in research, injury prevention, intensive care unit administration, trauma systems, and quality improvement projects.

Step-by-Step Fellowship Establishment

The first step in establishing an ACS fellowship program is filling out the Program Information Form (PIF). The form requires information regarding the program director, all participating faculty, program caseload specifications, trauma information including a number of patients seen annually, operative trauma information, and acute care general surgery cases performed annually. Faculty will need to provide their caseload information, research accomplishments, publications, and participation in local or national committees. Some of the information can be obtained from the departmental billing office and/or the trauma registry. In addition to the facilities and resources available, the history of the surgical critical care fellowship must be provided. The PIF also requires an explanation of the structured curriculum, supervision policy, 360-degree evaluation process, and adjunctive educational offerings such as Advanced Trauma Operative Management and Advanced Surgical Skills Exposure in Trauma courses.

Once the PIF is complete and support is confirmed from all faculty including the chairman and the general residency program director, the fellowship is presented to the Graduate Medical Education (GME) office whereby the institution must support the fellowship. The goal of the designated institutional official and the GME Committee is to ensure no interference with resident education. They will also require proof that the institution can support the education requirements of the fellowship.

Finally, funding for the fellow salary needs to be approved. A proforma proposal will outline a mechanism for support. Some institutions may choose to provide the salary from the Acute Care Surgery Division or the Department of Surgery. There is a requirement by the AAST that fellows participate in a call schedule where they manage emergency general surgery patients and/or provide surgical critical care. If feasible, this may be an opportunity to support the funding, as the fellow should be general surgery board eligible or certified and may obtain privileges from the hospital to bill for patient care during these calls. During fellow calls, there is a requirement for full faculty backup in-house for operative trauma care and complex emergency general surgery. During the 1-year fellowship, there is graduated autonomy to independence for the fellows who are assessed by the core faculty.

Finally, upon PIF completion, the GME office approves the fellowship within the institution, and all support faculty are in agreement; the PIF is sent to the AAST. Once reviewed by at least two members of the ACS Committee, two representatives are then selected to visit the institution. A list of specific information to be reviewed during that visit will be provided. During the site visit, interviews are conducted of specific participating faculty, the general surgery program director, senior surgical residents, and other fellows as requested by the committee members. The program case numbers will be reviewed as well as the planned experiential training curriculum for the ACS fellow. Once the evaluation is complete, the committee members present the PIF and visit information to the entire committee who then vote whether or not to approve the program. Once approved, fellow interviews may ensue for the following year. The entire process generally requires 3–6 months to complete. Following approval and initiation of the program, a review by the AAST ACS Committee members will occur, and compliance with the AAST requirements will be assessed at defined intervals.

A Core Competence Committee should assess the fellow's progression through the fellowship and specifically evaluate the completion of milestones. There is also a requirement for a biannual review of the fellow's performance and case logs which should be discussed and provided to the fellow. Similarly, the ACS fellow should evaluate all participating faculty and educational experiences.

Impact

Since the inception of the acute care surgery practice model and fellowship, the number of hospitals employing both has steadily increased. Multiple studies have demonstrated the impact of instituting ACS practice models on patient care, as well as surgeon satisfaction [2, 7, 10]. A retrospective review looking at outcomes of emergency general surgery patients compared between level I trauma centers, non-trauma centers, and centers with ACS practices revealed that ACS groups have lower complication rates, lower hospital cost, time to the operating room, and shorter length of stays [10]. These findings have been validated by multiple studies, as well as other benefits of ACS practices including increased coverage with on-call staff, improved continuity of care, decreased time to surgical consultation, shorter time to the operative room, and improved patient throughput [3, 10]. The true impact of patient-centered outcomes and how it is impacted by the implementation of an ACS practice model still need to be studied on a national level. In addition to improved patient-centered outcomes, implementation of the ACS model has been shown to have positive surgeon-specific results. Surgeons have higher level of satisfaction with regard to call compared with the traditional call model; this also included non-acute care surgery surgeons. ACS surgeons report increased operative productivity with increased case numbers, improved billing, and increased work relative value units [3].

Surgeons who complete an Acute Care Surgery Fellowship are more likely to practice in hospital-based groups at level I trauma centers in urban communities, with the second largest number residing in level II centers and in suburban practices [3, 9]. These practitioners overall have expressed the added value of the ACS fellowship to their training with improvement in self-confidence, marketability, and preparedness for practice, and 93% would encourage others to complete an ACS fellowship [3, 7, 9]. In addition, ACS fellows have been seen to provide added value to residents, especially in the realm of being a surgical educator. A survey of general surgery residency programs with acute care surgery teams noted residents felt like they had improved operative experience, overall increased number of operations performed, enhanced perception of education, and improved patient outcomes [11].

As discussed previously, there is an increased need for well-trained surgeons to address the increased healthcare needs associated with the growing population. Not only is there an increased need for the overall number of surgeons but specifically an increased need for general surgeons and those willing to provide emergency general surgery services. As medical student and residency training has changed over the past decade, a shift toward choosing specialty based on lifestyle has emerged. This has led to fewer medical students choosing a career in general surgery according to surveys. In addition, more residents are choosing to specialize, and currently 80% of general surgery residents go on to further subspecialize. Recruitment in the field of SCC in the previous years has generally been poor with 40% of fellowships going unfilled in 2005 [3]. Over the past several years with the increase number of ACS fellowships and medical centers adapting to the acute care surgery model, there has been an increased interest in SCC and ACS fellowship training [7]. Since the establishment of the first ACS fellowship in 2006, an additional of 27 programs has been developed and approved by the AAST for training of these fellows, and the number of programs has continued to grow with numerous programs in various stages of accreditation. There has also been a linear increase in the number of applicants over the past several years, and as of 2019, only 15% of SCC fellowships went unfilled [12]. This increase in the number of applicants is likely due to increased exposure and understanding of acute care surgery as a career choice, as well as the potential for positive impact of ACS fellows on general surgery residency training.

Future Directions

In an era where surgical training has been significantly affected by ever-increasing oversight, reduced duty hours, increased focus on patient quality, and increased struggle for autonomy during training, the importance and desire for post-residency training continue to increase. At least 80% of residents go on to complete subspecialty training at the end of residency [1]. Given the increasing shortage of surgeons compared to population size and the reduced number of general surgeons willing to take emergency surgery call, there is an increase in importance to attract more medical students and residents into general surgery. There has been increasing success seen over the past several years likely secondary to increased numbers of ACS fellowships and practice models. Previous ACS fellows note factors that influence the choice of fellowship program include and are not limited to case diversity and scope, heavy clinical experience, leadership teaching, exposure to penetrating trauma, the presence of strong role models and mentors, as well as an inherent desire to acquire more complex skills [2]. Continued review and adaptability of these fellowships are likely to be vital to continue this trend. In addition, the growth in the number of trauma centers and the potential for the reduction of case volume in previously high-volume centers may require close monitoring and the need for re-evaluation and creative approaches to attract and improve trainee experience [2].

Other potential options for the future are the consideration of offering additional training tracts or tailoring programs to further meet fellow needs and interest. An example of this is Vanderbilt University's adaptation of the AAST ACS fellowship to create a global Acute Care Surgery Fellowship or the ability to create international surgical training experiences [13]. Similar to the healthcare disparities in the United States, many countries face similar shortages of access to surgical care, as well as organized infrastructure for the acutely ill and injured patient [13]. The focus of the program includes strong mentorship, development of research skills, grant writing, clinical skills, and knowledge of global surgical literature. The program curriculum was adapted to provide a foundation that could be used to help develop and implement systems for trauma and acute care surgery in low-/middle-income countries [13]. In addition to this, the fellowship should have the ability to adapt to further shape their future career and include research, quality improvement, trauma systems, teaching, and simulation training [7]. Such adaptations of acute care fellowship may attract more trainees to consider fellowship and future careers in providing trauma and emergency general surgery care.

Conclusion

The evolution of surgical training has led to a compartmentalization of specialties and an increase in postgraduate, discipline-specific fellowship training. The field of trauma and emergency general surgery has followed suit with the initiation of the Trauma and Acute Care Fellowship which also incorporates training in surgical critical care. Since the initiation of the first program, the number of fellow applicants has greatly expanded and continues to do so. Twenty-eight programs have been approved by the AAST to date (Table 10.1), and currently 269 ACS fellows have graduated as of July 2020. The curricula have been reviewed by the AAST ACS fellowship committee since the inception of the fellowship which has led to several positive changes in the training requirements over the last several years. It is anticipated that the discipline of trauma and acute care surgery will progress to a requirement for board certification in the future. In order to continue to attract medical students and residents to a career in ACS, continued efforts need to be made in not only expanding understanding of the ACS model but in also continuing to adapt fellowships to provide exceptional fellow experience and education.

Table 10.1 List of AAST-approved ACS fellowships

2020 AAST-approved programs	Location	Program director
Baystate Medical Center	Springfield, Massachusetts	A. Taylor Putnam, MD
Carolinas Medical Center	Charlotte, North Carolina	Rita Brintzenhoff, MD
East Carolina University/Vidant Medical Center	Greenville, North Carolina	Eric A. Toschlog, MD
Emory University/Grady Memorial Hospital	Atlanta, Georgia	Jason Sciarretta, MD
Hartford Hospital/University of Connecticut	Hartford, Connecticut	Jonathan Gates, MD, MBA
Indiana University	Indianapolis, Indiana	Mark E. Falimirski, MD
Massachusetts General Hospital	Boston, Massachusetts	David R. King, MD
Medical College of Wisconsin	Milwaukee, Wisconsin	Thomas Carver, MD
San Antonio Military Medical Center	San Antonio, Texas	Christopher E. White, MD
University of Arizona	Tucson, Arizona	Terence O'Keefe, MB, ChB, MSPH
University of California San Diego	San Diego, California	Amy Liepert, MD
University of California San Francisco	San Francisco, California	Andre Campbell, MD
University of California San Francisco—Fresno	Fresno, California	Nancy Parks, MD
University of Colorado School of Medicine	Denver, Colorado	Clay Cothren Burlew, MD
University of Florida	Gainesville, Florida	Alicia Mohr, MD
University of Maryland/R. Adams Cowley Shock Trauma Center	Baltimore, Maryland	Jose J. Diaz, MD, CNS
University of Nevada School of Medicine	Las Vegas, Nevada	Douglas Fraser, MD
University of New Mexico	Albuquerque, New Mexico	Jasmeet S. Paul, MD
University of Pennsylvania	Philadelphia, Pennsylvania	Niels D. Martin, MD
University of Pittsburgh Medical Center	Pittsburgh, Pennsylvania	Matt Rosengart, MD
University of Southern California	Los Angeles, California	Kenji Inaba, MD
University of Tennessee Health Science Center	Memphis, Tennessee	Dina Filiberto, MD
University of Texas Health Science Center	Houston, Texas	Bryan Cotton, MD, MPH
University of Utah	Salt Lake City, Utah	Alexander Colonna, MD, MSCI
Vanderbilt University Medical Center	Nashville, Tennessee	Raeanna Adams, MD, MBA
Wake Forest Baptist Medical Center	Winston-Salem, North Carolina	Nathan Mowery, MD
Wright State University	Dayton, Ohio	Mbaga Walusimbi, MD, MPH
Yale University	New Haven, Connecticut	Linda L. Maerz, MD

Rutgers New Jersey Medical School Under location Newark, New Jersey Under Program Director Ziad C. Sifri, MD

References

1. Khubchandani JA, Ingraham AM, Daniel VT, Ayturk D, Kiefe CI, Santry HP. Geographic diffusion and implementation of acute care surgery: an uneven solution to the National Emergency General Surgery Crisis. JAMA Surg. 2018;153(2):150–9.
2. Staudenmayer K, Bernard A, Davis KA, Doucet J, Haider A, Tres Scherer LR 3rd, et al. The current and future economic state of acute care surgery. J Trauma Acute Care Surg. 2019;87(2):413–9.
3. Davis KA, Jurkovich GJ. Fellowship training in acute care surgery: from inception to current state. Trauma Surg Acute Care Open. 2016;1(1):e000004.
4. Ginwalla RF, Rustin RB. The "global surgeon": is it time for modifications in the American surgical training paradigm? J Surg Educ. 2015;72(4):e100–3.
5. Committee to Develop the Reorganized Specialty of Trauma SCC, Emergency S. Acute care surgery: trauma, critical care, and emergency surgery. J Trauma. 2005;58(3):614–6.
6. Napolitano LM, Fulda GJ, Davis KA, Ashley DW, Friese R, Van Way CW 3rd, et al. Challenging issues in surgical critical care, trauma, and acute care surgery: a report from the Critical Care Committee of the American Association for the Surgery of Trauma. J Trauma. 2010;69(6):1619–33.
7. Gayed BN, Zarzaur BL, Livingston DH, Chiu WC, Davis KA, Tisherman SA, et al. Mapping the

increasing interest in acute care surgery-who, why and which fellowship? J Trauma Acute Care Surg. 2020;88(5):629–35.
8. Dente CJ, Duane TM, Jurkovich GJ, Britt LD, Meredith JW, Fildes JJ. How much and what type: analysis of the first year of the acute care surgery operative case log. J Trauma Acute Care Surg. 2014;76(2):329–38.
9. Jurkovich GJ, Davis KA, Burlew CC, Dente CJ, Galante JM, Goodwin JS 2nd, et al. Acute care surgery: an evolving paradigm. Curr Probl Surg. 2017;54(7):364–95.
10. Khalil M, Pandit V, Rhee P, Kulvatunyou N, Orouji T, Tang A, et al. Certified acute care surgery programs improve outcomes in patients undergoing emergency surgery: a nationwide analysis. J Trauma Acute Care Surg. 2015;79(1):60–3.
11. Dinan KA, Davis JW, Wolfe MM, Sue LP, Cagle KM. An acute care surgery fellowship benefits a general surgical residency. J Trauma Acute Care Surg. 2014;77(2):209–12.
12. NRMP Match [Online]. Specialty match program results 2016–2020. Available at: https://www.nrmp.org/fellowship-match-data
13. Merchant AI, Walters CB, Valenzuela J, McQueen KA, May AK. Creating a global acute care surgery fellowship to meet international need. J Surg Educ. 2017;74(5):780–6.

Surgical Rescue and Failure to Rescue

11

Anupamaa Seshadri, Alexandra Briggs, and Andrew Peitzman

Case Presentation

A 76-year-old woman is transferred directly to the medical intensive care unit from a community hospital after developing respiratory failure requiring intubation. She is febrile with a rising leukocytosis despite receiving antibiotics and has developed an acute kidney injury with increasing creatinine and oliguria. She has also developed a new vasopressor requirement. General surgery is consulted due to recent history of left colectomy with primary anastomosis for a large bowel obstruction. She is intubated, sedated, and not currently responsive to stimuli. Her abdominal exam is notable for abdominal distension and a wound that is clean and intact without surrounding erythema.

A. Seshadri
Department of Surgery, University of Pittsburgh Medical Center, Pittsburgh, PA, USA

Department of Surgery, Beth Israel Deaconess Medical Center, Boston, MA, USA
e-mail: aseshadr@bidmc.harvard.edu

A. Briggs
Department of Surgery, Dartmouth-Hitchcock Medical Center, Lebanon, NH, USA
e-mail: Alexandra.Briggs@hitchcock.org

A. Peitzman (✉)
Department of Surgery, University of Pittsburgh Medical Center, Pittsburgh, PA, USA
e-mail: peitzmanab@upmc.edu

Introduction

While postoperative mortality has been commonly used as a metric for quality in surgical care, failure to rescue has been embraced as a measure of quality of care in elective surgery. Failure to rescue is defined as the proportion of patients who experience a postoperative or post-hospitalization complication who subsequently die from that complication [1, 2]. Hospitals with the highest incidence of complications do not necessarily have the highest mortality. The difference in frequency of complications between high mortality and low mortality hospitals is not as great as is the difference in failure to rescue after the complication; in other words, mortality seems to be determined more by FTR of the patient after a complication than the frequency of complications. With the expanded understanding of the importance of FTR and its impact on mortality, FTR was formally endorsed as a quality measure for surgical care in 2010 by the National Quality Forum [3, 4]. As we learn more about how failure to rescue affects our patients, it is important to identify both the medical and surgical entities that result in failure to rescue, as well as to investigate the underlying epidemiology, system factors, and patient factors that lead to failure to rescue.

Emergency general surgery (EGS) patients are at 5x higher risk of complications and death than elective surgical patients and, thus, are logically

M. D. Zielinski, O. Guillamondegui (eds.), *The Acute Management of Surgical Disease*,
https://doi.org/10.1007/978-3-031-07881-1_11

at higher risk for failure to rescue [5]. It is therefore critical that EGS surgeons are aware of this entity and understand how to mitigate its effects. Importantly, precedent rates (death preceded by a complication) in emergency general surgery patients were reported to be 84.1%, similar to those published for elective operations. Failure to rescue in this EGS population was 12.8%, again comparable to published rates for elective surgery. Thus, for both elective surgery and EGS, FTR appears to be a reasonable quality metric.

Failure to rescue depends on both the type and the number of postoperative complications. Sixty percent of patients have a single complication, the majority of whom recover [6]. However, those patients who have multiple complications have significantly higher mortality than those with only one [7] (Fig. 11.1). Multiple studies have attempted to better delineate the timing and the causal pathways that lead to a patient developing secondary complications with the goal of interrupting the chain of events leading to death [8, 9]. While work is ongoing to detect those critical junctures where further complications can be averted, identification and aggressive treatment of the sentinel complication is essential to reduce risk of subsequent complications and FTR (Fig. 11.2).

In this chapter, we will discuss the epidemiology of failure to rescue, including the hospital and patient-level characteristics that lead to higher rates of failure to rescue, and review the current literature specific to EGS. We will also discuss the rescue of patients who develop pathology that requires surgical intervention for management. By understanding the medical and surgical complications that require surgical rescue and acknowledging the patient, provider, and system-based factors that influence failure to rescue, EGS surgeons will be equipped to improve outcomes in this vulnerable patient population.

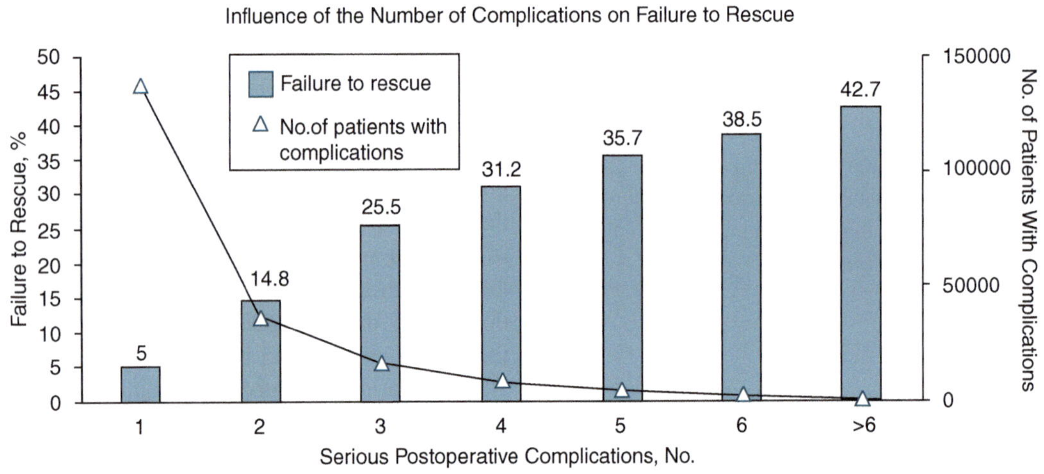

Fig. 11.1 Figure from Ferraris et al. demonstrating that failure to rescue increases with each serious postoperative complication that the patient suffers. (With permission from: Ferraris VA., et al. Identification of patients with postoperative complications who are at risk for failure to rescue. JAMA Surg. 2014;149 (11):1103–1108. doi:10.1001/jamasurg.2014.1338. Downloaded 4.3.16)

Odds ratios for secondary complications following the index complication

1° complication	Reintubation	Pneumonia	Dehiscence	Sepsis	Shock	Bleeding event	Cardiac arrest	Renal failure	Death
Pneumonia	17.1			7.3	13.0			11.8	6.2
Acute MI	11.7	5.1				4.3	12.0	8.7	7.7
Deep space infection			30.4	13.1	10.6			10.5	
Acute renal failure	11.3	6.0			11.2	11.3	25.3		
Bleeding-transfusion	(No odds ratio ≥ 3)								

Fig. 11.2 Results from Wakeam et al. demonstrating increased risk of secondary complications after index complication

Epidemiology and Causes of Failure to Rescue

When evaluating the causes of failure to rescue, it is important to look at the problem through multiple lenses. First, issues at the hospital and surgeon level can impact a wide swath of patients and are amenable to higher-level optimization. There are also patient-level issues that are often not modifiable, but recognition of these issues can lead to improved prognostication or identification of biases that can potentially be addressed. Finally, we will discuss methods by which surgeons and hospital systems can attempt to improve their safety culture to have a meaningful impact on their rates of failure to rescue.

Surgeon and Hospital Factors

The characteristics of hospitals that lead to increased or decreased rates of failure to rescue have been extensively studied both in surgery in general and in EGS specifically. Hospital macrosystem issues that impact FTR include number of intensive care unit beds, hospital patient volume, nurse staffing ratios, and extent of hospital technology/advanced specialties. It is estimated that 12–57% of observed variation in FTR is due to macrosystem issues [10]. Microsystem issues include culture of safety, communication, closed vs open ICUs, interpersonal and organizational dynamics, and rapid response teams [11]. Ghaferi et al. in 2009 found that in Medicare patients undergoing 6 major operations including pancreatectomy, esophagectomy, abdominal aortic aneurysm repair, coronary artery bypass grafting, aortic valve replacement, and mitral valve replacement, complication rates were similar between low-mortality and high-mortality hospitals, but failure to rescue rates correlated with mortality [12]. This implicated failure to rescue as the significant driver of mortality, as opposed to complication rates alone. The same group then studied Medicare patients undergoing high-risk cancer operations including esophagectomy, gastrectomy, and pancreatectomy and again reported that complication rates alone did not differ between low- and high-volume centers, but failure to rescue was significantly higher in low-volume centers [13]. This demonstrated that increased hospital volume for a particular case improved failure to rescue rates, which then improved mortality rates, in high-risk elective operations.

To better understand the hospital characteristics affecting failure to rescue rates, Sheetz et al. studied Medicare patients undergoing high-risk general or vascular surgery operations [10]. They found a decreased failure to rescue in hospitals that had teaching status, higher hospital technology (as defined by more operations that require high technology such as open heart surgery and solid organ transplantation), increasing nurse-to-patient ratio, and presence of more than 20 ICU beds. However, these factors did not account for all of the observed variation in failure to rescue rates across hospitals. Thus, while these factors are important and should be evaluated to better understand their impact on failure to rescue, other factors are also involved.

These factors were then studied specifically in the EGS population. Mehta et al. found no significant difference in complication rates between low mortality and high mortality hospitals in patients who underwent emergent bowel resection. However, they observed a 10.8× higher rate of FTR in the high mortality hospitals compared to the low mortality hospitals [14]. This demonstrated that the same signal is present within EGS patients as in the elective surgery population; failure to rescue drives mortality rates in post-surgical patients in the EGS population as well. The same group studied mortality rates in low-volume EGS surgeons as compared to high-volume surgeons and found that the low-volume surgeons had higher mortality rates despite similar complication rates [15]. This study did not specifically look at failure to rescue in low volume as compared to high-volume EGS surgeons.

Finally, as EGS pathology can occur on any day of the week and at any time of day, the "weekend effect" was studied to see whether differences in staffing and hospital resources caused by the weekend increased failure to rescue. Hatchimonji et al. found increased mortality on the weekend for those EGS patients who underwent emergent operations but found no increase in complications or failure to rescue [16]. Metcalfe et al. studied both operative and nonoperative patients admitted to an EGS service and found a slightly increased serious adverse event rate, failure to rescue, and in-hospital mortality in patients admitted on the weekend [17]. However, this effect was small. Taken together, these data seem to indicate that there is not a significant "weekend effect" on EGS patients, particularly those that require an emergent operation.

Targeting failure to rescue as a metric may significantly improve mortality, as was demonstrated by Fry et al. in a longitudinal retrospective study evaluating trends in mortality, complications, and failure to rescue over time [18]. The authors used Medicare data to compare trends in hospital mortality, serious complications, and failure to rescue in patients undergoing elective abdominal aortic aneurysm repair, colectomy, pancreatectomy, or lung resection, from a period of 2005–2006 and 2013–2014. They found that hospitals demonstrating a significant improvement in mortality had some improvement in rates of complications but a much more robust improvement in failure to rescue. More specifically, they found improvement in serious complications contributed 4–7% of the improvement in mortality, but improvement in FTR contributed 64–65%. This demonstrates, rather than solely targeting frequency of complications, focusing care to address failure to rescue once a complication has occurred can have significantly more impact on patient outcome.

Patient Factors

One patient population at significantly higher risk for failure to rescue is the geriatric population (see Chap. 39). Elderly patients have increased rates of mortality after surgery, with a higher rate of FTE [19, 20]. This is particularly evident in EGS patients, where preoperative optimization is typically impossible. Therefore, understanding the factors that predispose elderly patients to failure to rescue can potentially help mitigate this mortality increase and also allow improved prognostication for the patient and family.

It is clear that elderly patients are at increased risk for failure to rescue in EGS. Sheetz et al.

found a significantly higher rate of failure to rescue in the elderly as compared to younger patients who underwent emergent general or vascular surgery, with markedly higher failure to rescue rates in high mortality hospitals [21]. Interestingly, the same group studied different primary complications that lead to failure to rescue and found more failure to rescue after infectious or pulmonary complications in elderly patients, as opposed to cardiac complications [22]. This provides guidance that elderly patients require more vigilance to prevent infectious or pulmonary complications and may need more intensive therapy should those complications arise.

Patient volume also impacts outcome in elderly EGS patients. Mehta et al. found that individual surgeon volumes of geriatric EGS patients mattered; elderly patients who underwent an EGS operation had increased mortality and increased failure to rescue when their surgeon had a low geriatric EGS volume practice [23]. The same group also found a significantly increased failure to rescue in hospitals that had lower proportions of geriatric patients as compared to those that had higher proportions of geriatric patients; interestingly, this finding did not bear out with absolute number of geriatric patients [24]. These findings seem to demonstrate that elderly patients have better rescue rates and better outcomes when treated at centers that commonly care for high proportions of geriatric EGS patients, by surgeons with a high volume of geriatric EGS patients. This may indicate that geriatric EGS patients would be better served with centralized "centers of excellence" for specialized care, which is now being pursued by the American College of Surgeons through the Geriatric Surgery Verification program [25].

It is important to recognize that not all elderly patients are the same and there are patient-specific indicators that may predispose patients to worse failure to rescue rates. Khan et al. studied geriatric patients who underwent EGS and found that several factors increased the risk of failure to rescue in this population [26]. These included comorbidities such as chronic renal failure, COPD, and CHF, nutritional status as determined by albumin, and age >80. Using this information, they developed a scoring system to help prognosticate when encountering an elderly patient requiring emergent surgery. This group then evaluated the impact of frailty on the same population, using an EGS-specific frailty index [27]. They found that frailty was not only an independent contributor to failure to rescue, but it also increased the odds of failure to rescue threefold as compared with nonfrail status. While these identified risk factors are non-modifiable in the setting of EGS, recognizing that not all elderly patients pose the same risk for failure to rescue is important and can help with family discussions and prognostication in the perioperative setting and also warrant heightened vigilance in particularly vulnerable patients postoperatively.

Scarborough et al. studied the question of whether do-not-resuscitate (DNR) status in elderly EGS patients affects outcomes. They found that postoperative elderly patients who were DNR compared to propensity-matched full code patients had the same percentage of complications but a higher mortality rate and a higher FTR rate [28]. This is likely because of patient and provider reticence to pursue aggressive measures after the index complication in the setting of the patient's goals of care. Again, this is an important factor for counseling of patients in the perioperative setting and provides a chance for early palliative care and goals of care discussions in elderly EGS patients who are already DNR.

The elderly are not the only demographic group at risk for higher rates of failure to rescue. Previous work has shown racial and socioeconomic disparities in failure to rescue, and this is true of EGS patients as well. de Jager et al. found that low-income EGS patients in urban environments have higher odds of mortality, complications, and failure to rescue as compared to high-income EGS patients [29]. Furthermore, Metcalfe et al. found that uninsured EGS patients had higher odds of a major adverse event, mortality, and failure to rescue than privately insured patients [30]. These disparities need to be studied further, both to better understand the processes by which they lead to worse outcomes and to ameliorate these effects.

The Way Forward

While further research is ongoing to better delineate the specific factors leading to failure to rescue from an overall national hospital systems perspective, it is important for individual hospitals and surgeons to evaluate how to better manage complications to avoid failure to rescue. Root cause analysis (RCA) is a common method by which complications can be studied to better understand how they occur and what improvements can be implemented to prevent recurrent complications [31]. Johnston et al. studied the use of a Healthcare Failure Mode and Effects Analysis (HFMEA) on a surgical service to see how rapid responses and postoperative complications could be better managed [32]. This is a prospective systematic method where an interprofessional team including nursing assistants and nurses and physicians of varying levels in hierarchy, along with a patient, study the escalation of care events to see what process improvements could help prevent potential complications. In this study, the authors identified understaffing, communication failures including human factors and technological failure, and adherence to hierarchy as potential sources of failure to rescue. While these are interesting findings, this study also provides a structure for individual institutions to interrogate their own escalation processes. In response to this study, Ghaferi et al. stated that both HFMEA and RCA can be used as iterative processes to identify potential complications and prevent them, as well as study actual complications and learn from them [33]. Furthermore, the authors emphasize the importance of "safe culture," where all members of the care team are invested in improvement in safety and are willing to adapt.

As part of the effort to rapidly recognize complications and prevent secondary complications, multiple technological solutions have been trialed. These rely on the basic principle of track and trigger systems, which use parameters such as vital signs and urine output to create a score to risk stratify the patient for complications [34]. These systems, such as the Modified Early Warning System (MEWS) or the National Early Warning System (NEWS) employed by the National Health Service of the United Kingdom, have been used both in medical and surgical patients to attempt to improve the failure to rescue rate [35, 36]. Machine learning is now being adapted to take the electronically pulled data from electronic health records to continuously calculate risk scores to identify patients at risk of decompensation [37]. These systems still require refinement prior to widespread deployment for multiple reasons. First, while some clinical decompensations happen with predictable changes in vital signs or frequently checked labs, some pathologies may not be captured by these algorithms. Conversely, there is significant noise in the data as not all vital sign changes signal clinical decline, leading to alarm fatigue. Advancements in artificial intelligence will help improve these clinical models, but the involvement of a thoughtful clinician will always be required to avoid failure to rescue.

Rescue After Procedural Complications

While failure to rescue in surgical patients encompasses deaths after numerous postoperative complications, both medical and surgical in nature, here we will focus on some specific surgical complications that require rapid recognition and appropriate management to prevent catastrophic outcomes. These entities are summarized in Table 11.1.

Bile Duct Injury During Cholecystectomy

Laparoscopic cholecystectomy is one of the most commonly performed operations in the United States and globally [38], but complications from laparoscopic cholecystectomies can be devastating (see Chap. 16). The most common major complication from a laparoscopic cholecystectomy is an iatrogenic bile duct injury (BDI), with a reported incidence of 0.3–1.5% [38–40]. BDI occurs on a spectrum with multiple classification

Table 11.1 Postprocedural complications requiring rescue

Clinical Entity	Presenting Signs/Symptoms	Management Approach
Bile duct injury after cholecystectomy	fever, tachycardia, hypotension, hyperbilirubinemia	drainage for source control, OR for repair after sepsis control by expert HPB specialist
Gastrostomy tube complications		
Intestinal perforation	fever, tachycardia, peritonitis	OR for repair or resection of bowel
Buried bumper syndrome	peristomal leakage/irritation, resistance when using tube	removal of tube, replacement with looser fit
Inadvertent removal	known removal of tube, possible peritonitis	replacement at bedside if epithelialized tract; OR for gastrotomy closure and replacement of tube if no epithelialized tract
Central line complications		
Arterial placement	bleeding, thrombotic complications, CVA, AVF	Vascular Surgery consultation; removal with pressure vs OR for repair of vessel
Pneumothorax	hypoxia, hypotension	chest tube placement
Anastomotic leak	fever, abdominal pain, tachycardia	drainage for source control, OR for repair vs proximal diversion vs resection and reanastomosis
Enterocutaneous fistula	abdominal pain, visible drainage of succus	nutritional optimization (enteral vs TPN), excellent wound care, OR for repair vs resection if no spontaneous closure after optimization

schema including the Bismuth classification, the Stewart-Way classification, the Strasberg classification, and the Hannover classification, with the Bismuth and the Strasberg classifications used most commonly [41]. These classification systems all base their categories on the anatomic location of the injury, as higher injuries closer to or involving the right and left hepatic ducts become progressively more difficult to manage operatively.

The complications caused by iatrogenic BDI can be separated into short-term and long-term issues. In the short term, the typical main issue is bile leak and resultant sepsis, requiring source control. Long term, the complications can either be secondary to an unrepaired injury or an improperly repaired injury. These complications include recurrent cholangitis, anastomotic stricture, or secondary sclerosing cholangitis [42]. These complications have significant impact on the individual patient as well as the healthcare system as a whole.

O'Brien et al. studied the outcomes and cost of iatrogenic BDI after cholecystectomy in the United States and found that BDI was associated not only with increased hospital costs and length of stay but also with 30-day readmission and need for patients to be discharged to institutional post-acute care facilities [43]. They also found that the majority of BDI occurred during inpatient admissions as opposed to elective outpatient cases, which points to the increased difficulty of cholecystectomy in patients admitted for symptomatic biliary disease.

Prevention of BDI is the ideal strategy for mitigating the effects of this complication, which is most effectively done by achieving the critical view of safety [44]. There has been controversy as to whether intraoperative cholangiogram (IOC) should be done routinely or selectively in particularly difficult cases; intraoperative cholangiography does not seem to prevent BDI. However, IOC does seem to allow early diagnosis of bile duct injury when it occurs [45, 46]. Understand that bile duct injury occurs more commonly from misinterpretation of normal anatomy, rather than encountering aberrant anatomy.

Rystedt et al. [39] found that timing of biliary reconstruction with hepaticojejunostomy after BDI had no influence on long-term biliary patency, severe complications, or need for reintervention. This points to an important conclusion: as timing does not have a significant impact on long-term outcomes, resolution of sepsis and finding an appropriate expert to complete the hepaticojejunostomy should be performed prior to attempted repair.

This is echoed in a series of studies performed by Halle-Smith et al., who found significant cost improvement for major bile duct injuries with specialist repair, especially when performed immediately [42]. Specialist repair leads to fewer complications and should be performed whenever possible. Furthermore, with minor BDI, they found that not all injuries were managed surgically, as management with IR interventions including percutaneous drainage and percutaneous transhepatic cholangiographic (PTC) tube placement obviated the need for surgery [47]. Global consensus is moving toward these therapeutic strategies and was confirmed in a study by Khadra et al., where they found, over the past decades, mortality after BDI has not changed but there have been fewer long-term complications such as strictures [40]. In this study, this finding correlated to an increased use of PTC and an increased performance of the repair by hepatobiliary surgeons over time. Therefore, if a hepatobiliary specialist is available immediately, then immediate repair can be attempted. Otherwise, the patient should be managed in a multidisciplinary fashion to appropriately classify in the injury and determine the best modality and timing for repair.

Gastrostomy Tube Complications

Enteral access in patients for whom it is unsafe to swallow can be achieved in multiple ways, and the placement of a gastrostomy tube is a popular option for durable and convenient enteral access in these patients [48]. These tubes are placed by surgeons, gastroenterologists, and interventional radiologists, depending on local practice patterns. However, surgeons must be familiar with potential intraoperative and postoperative complications, especially as these patients often are managed outpatient or on a medical service after tube placement.

The most common immediate operative intervention requiring recognition and rescue is inadvertent intestinal perforation. While this complication is rare, occurring in 0.5%–1.3% of cases, it can have devastating consequences [49]. Ideally, performing all essential maneuvers during the initial placement of the tube will prevent the complication from occurring in the first place. These maneuvers include full insufflation of the stomach to maximize apposition against the abdominal wall, elevating the head of the bed to help displace the bowel inferiorly, and transillumination with demonstration of 1-to-1 movement of the operator's finger to the indented stomach wall endoscopically [48]. During the insertion of the needle through the tract that will be used for the tube, it is critical to continuously aspirate on the syringe while watching the screen closely. For a tract to be deemed "safe," the surgeon should only be able to aspirate air at the time he or she sees the needle entering the stomach endoscopically [49]. If air or bile is aspirated prior to that visualization, the tract is not safe, and the site cannot be used. Once the tube is placed, inadvertent bowel perforation may be suspected if the patient has fever, leukocytosis, and/or abdominal pain out of proportion to the procedure. If this is suspected, CT scan can help confirm the complication; the presence of a small amount of pneumoperitoneum on CT may be related to the procedure itself, but large-volume pneumoperitoneum should raise suspicion for perforation. In the case of bowel perforation, early antibiotics and surgical intervention are typically required for repair or resection of the involved bowel.

The two most common postoperative complications requiring surgical intervention are buried bumper syndrome and inadvertent tube removal. Buried bumper syndrome occurs when the inner bolster ("bumper") of the percutaneous endoscopic gastrostomy (PEG) tube erodes over time through the gastric mucosa into the abdominal wall. This occurs because of excessive traction from the external bolster being too tight against the skin and occurs in 0.3–2.4% of patients [49]. This typically presents as peristomal leakage and irritation, as well as potential resistance when the tube is used for feeds or medication. The treatment is removal of the tube and replacement with a more relaxed-fitting tube to prevent recurrence of the complication.

Inadvertent tube removal occurs in 1.6–4.4% of cases and can often be managed by immediate bedside replacement of a tube if the tract has matured. Correct placement of the new tube is confirmed with a contrasted plain film [49]. However, if the tube is newly placed within the previous 1–2 weeks, the tract created by the tube may not have yet epithelialized and matured and thus lead to a surgical emergency. Without a mature tract, the stomach can fall away from the abdominal wall, leading to free leakage of gastric contents into the peritoneum. Therefore, if a PEG is inadvertently removed, the patient must be immediately evaluated at the bedside with confirmation of the date of placement. If there is any evidence of peritonitis, broad-spectrum antibiotics and surgical exploration are required for source control and prevention of sepsis. Another feeding tube can be placed at the time of that operation to facilitate enteral access as well.

Line Complications

Central line placement, both temporary and tunneled, is a common procedure performed both by medical and surgical specialists. Numerous complications that require surgical intervention can result, and the emergency general surgeon should be prepared to recognize and manage these complications urgently. Prevention and management of line infections will not be addressed here but must be considered in all patients with central vascular access.

Arterial placement of central venous catheters results in 0.1–0.8% of patients but needs to be immediately recognized to prevent further problems [50]. Use of ultrasound to place central lines has decreased the incidence of arterial placement but has not eliminated this risk completely, and transduction of the line prior to dilation can help confirm placement if in question [51]. Arterial large bore line placement can lead to numerous downstream complications, including bleeding, hematoma, thrombus, stroke, pseudoaneurysm, or arteriovenous fistula formation [52]. Options for management of this complication include removing the catheter with prolonged manual pressure if the site is conducive to pressure, which may lead to thrombosis or incomplete control of bleeding, or removal of the catheter in the operating room with endovascular or surgical repair of the vessel. Involvement of a vascular surgeon in these cases can often be helpful with a large laceration, arteriovenous fistula, or pseudoaneurysm.

Pneumothorax is another common complication that can occur with upper torso central venous access, in up to 1% of line placements and most commonly with subclavian central line placement [52]. This can cause hemodynamic collapse early after placement and should be first in the differential when a patient is in distress after upper torso line placement. Pneumothoraces can be rapidly diagnosed based upon clinical presentation and immediate prior history of attempted line placement. When the diagnosis is less clear, bedside ultrasound or portable chest X-ray can also be used to evaluate for pneumothorax [53]. Typically, hemodynamically significant pneumothoraces or pneumothoraces with loss of >15% of the chest volume are managed with chest tube placement [52].

Anastomotic Leak

Anastomotic leak is a devastating postoperative complication, with an associated mortality rate as high as 35% [54]. While leaks overall occur in about 1–3% of small bowel anastomoses and 3–29% of colonic anastomoses, the creation of the anastomosis in an emergency surgery confers a significant increase in risk [54–57]. Unfortunately, there are numerous patient-specific risk factors that contribute to risk of anastomotic leak, including comorbidities, immunosuppressive medications, malnutrition, obesity, and tobacco use, but these factors cannot be optimized in the EGS patient [56–58]. However, knowledge of these risk factors allows the EGS surgeon to decide whether the patient is appropriate for an anastomosis during emergency surgery, which may lead to the decision to create a diverting stoma if an anastomosis is judged to be high-risk and higher suspicion postoperatively for development of leak. Intraoperative risk factors for leak include increased operative time and significant blood loss, including blood loss requiring transfusion [56–59]. For this reason, it is not recommended to perform an anastomosis during a damage control operation with its significant hypotension and blood loss. Of note, despite numerous studies, there is no clear evidence whether hand-sewn versus stapled anastomoses improve anastomotic leak risk in EGS patients [60].

Anastomotic leak can occur along a spectrum, ranging from a small leak that leads to a contained abscess to a large leak that leads to peritonitis; therefore, management of anastomotic leak depends on the location and severity of the leak. The first, most important step in management of an anastomotic leak is recognition of the leak. Anastomotic leaks can present as early as 1–2 days or as late as 30 days after the index operation, with common presenting symptoms including fever, tachycardia, and abdominal pain [61]. The second major step is source control. Once an anastomotic leak is suspected, CT scan with IV and oral contrast is typically performed for better delineation of the leak [61]. Small leaks may be managed with antibiotics alone or percutaneous drainage of intra-abdominal abscesses >3 cm in size [61]. Leaks leading to fistulae may respond to antibiotics and bowel rest, but if nonoperative management fails, surgery may be required. Large leaks generally require prompt operative intervention for source control, incorporating a range of intraoperative options: resection and reanastomosis, creation of a diverting ostomy proximal to the current anastomosis to facilitate healing, or takedown of the anastomosis and creation of an end ostomy. Resection and reanastomosis is the most common option for small bowel anastomotic leaks, particularly in more proximal anastomoses. For colonic leaks, typically the choice of operative repair depends on patient status, the site of the leak, and the quality of remaining tissue after debridement of the prior anastomosis [61].

Enterocutaneous Fistulae

Enterocutaneous fistulae (ECF) are an uncommon but serious complication from abdominal surgery, with a 10–30% mortality rate [62] (see Chap. 22). Hatchimonji et al. studied the rate of formation of enterocutaneous fistula in the EGS population and found it to be comparable to elective surgery at 1.1% [63]. The authors found that there was a significant increase in mortality in those EGS patients who developed an ECF as opposed to those who did not (10.1% versus 5.4%), as well as higher 30- and 90-day readmission rates.

The first principles of management of ECF include appropriate resuscitation and sepsis control. Patients with ECF will often present with malnutrition, dehydration, and electrolyte imbalance from fistula output, as well as potential sepsis if there is an intra-abdominal component of leak leading to undrained succus [62, 64]. Adequate IV access and IV fluid resuscitation and broad-spectrum antibiotics, along with electrolyte replacement, should be prioritized, with subsequent CT imaging of the abdomen to better delineate anatomy and to identify any undrained collections amenable to percutaneous drainage for source control. Should the patient be floridly septic despite minimally invasive methods for source control, early operation is required for rescue. If the patient remains stable with source control, subsequent management is directed toward nutritional optimization and management of the output, with a goal of either spontaneous closure or preoperative optimization for surgical management. As mortality from ECF is independently associated with serum albumin <3 g/dL, nutrition is critical both for closure of the fistula and overall health in these patients [65–68].

Opportunities for Surgical Rescue in Medical Patients

While failure to rescue can signify a missed postoperative complication, it can also describe a patient with a missed surgical problem who fails

Table 11.2 Medical entities requiring rescue

Clinical Entity	Presenting Signs/Symptoms	Management Approach
C. difficile colitis	diarrhea, abdominal pain, abdominal distention, tachycardia, hypotension	antibiotics, consideration for fecal transplantation, if worsening then OR for loop ileostomy and lavage vs total abdominal colectomy
Acute mesenteric ischemia	abdominal pain out of proportion, tachycardia, hypotension	heparinization if appropriate, OR for revascularization if needed and resection of necrotic bowel
Abdominal compartment syndrome	abdominal distention with bladder pressure > 20 mmHg, end organ dysfunction (renal failure, high airway peak pressures)	medical therapies including paracentesis and paralysis, OR for decompressive laparotomy if necessary

to survive because of delayed diagnosis and intervention. In this section, we will discuss pathologic entities commonly seen on medical services that, if not promptly recognized and managed (operatively if necessary), can lead to failure to rescue. These entities are summarized in Table 11.2.

Clostridium difficile Colitis

Clostridium difficile is a microorganism that causes infection when the host gut microbiome is disturbed, typically by antibiotics, allowing the organism to grow at a rate that overwhelms the normal flora [69]. The clinical manifestations of *C. difficile* infection range from mild diarrhea to fulminant infection with hypotension, organ failure, megacolon, and intestinal necrosis. Fulminant colitis occurs in 3–8% of patients with *C. difficile*, but as the patients often present initially with less severe colitis, recognition of progression of disease, prompt medical treatment, and early surgical intervention in these patients is critical for rescue [70].

The first step in rescue of patients with fulminant *C. difficile* is timely diagnosis. While often these patients have clear signs of diarrhea or previously diagnosed *C. difficile*, some patients have a variant of the disease without diarrhea [70]. Therefore, *C. difficile infection* should remain on the differential for patients with abdominal pain, leukocytosis, and recent antibiotic use, even in the absence of diarrhea. CT imaging of the abdomen in these patients may be a helpful diagnostic adjunct to evaluate inflammation of the colon.

Timing for surgical intervention in *C. difficile* infection remains controversial. It is agreed that uncomplicated mild *C. difficile* can often be managed with antibiotics alone and should not mandate surgical intervention. Patients who present with complicated disease, as defined by hypotension, ICU admission, ileus, mental status changes, WBC >35,000, lactate >2.2 mmol/L, or end organ failure, should undergo surgical management of their disease [71, 72]. However, when the disease progresses from an initial presentation of mild disease to more severe, it is difficult to determine when along the course of the disease one should operate. Should the disease progress to perforation or cause severe hypotension and critical illness, the subsequent mortality is high even when colectomy is performed, with a reported rate from 30 to 80% [70, 73]. Some retrospective studies have identified continuing elevation in white blood cell count or lactate as a signal that the disease is progressing and could benefit from surgical intervention [74, 75]. This remains an area of ongoing study, but these patients should be closely observed and surgical intervention should not be delayed until the patient is in extremis. This can be achieved by the development of institutional protocols for designating when surgical teams should be mandatorily involved in the care of *C. difficile* patients based on clinical, laboratory, or radiological findings, as well as a collaborative culture between medical and surgical teams.

There are multiple options for the surgical management of these patients. Over the past decades, the standard of care for these patients was to perform a total abdominal colectomy, as the external appearance of the colon often does not accurately convey the health of the mucosa and segmental colectomy often left disease behind [71]. However, an alternative strategy of a loop ileostomy and providing antegrade GoLytely intraoperatively and postoperative antegrade vancomycin flushes for 10 days has been described, with one group demonstrating a 100% resolution rate of *C. difficile*-associated disease symptoms and postoperative mortality of 19% [76]. The majority of these operations were performed laparoscopically, improving postoperative pain as well. (The uncommon patients who failed this approach did so because of abdominal compartment syndrome.) While this is not an appropriate management strategy in the patient with perforated *C. difficile* colitis, it remains a viable option even for patients with hypotension and critical illness.

Mesenteric Ischemia

Acute mesenteric ischemia is a surgical emergency that, while rare, carries high mortality of 50–80% [77] (see Chap. 19). Mesenteric ischemia is commonly misdiagnosed on presentation, with delay to diagnosis and treatment as a major determinant of outcome. Patients may present with tachycardia, hypotension, and abdominal pain, but particularly in the setting of patients that develop non-occlusive mesenteric ischemia, these patients may be intubated and unable to provide a clear exam. Therefore, vigilance for this clinical entity is critical to avoid missing this diagnosis.

Diagnosis starts with a clinical history and physical exam augmented by CT angiography of the abdomen with arterial and venous phases to evaluate for clot as well as to evaluate the integrity of the bowel [77, 78]. While fluid resuscitation and antibiotics are critical in the initial management of this entity, delay to surgical intervention directly impacts mortality in this patient population [79, 80]. Therefore, medical therapy for these critically ill patients should be concomitant with prompt surgical planning for definitive management. Surgical intervention must accomplish two goals: reestablishment of perfusion and resection of necrotic intestine. In the case of non-occlusive mesenteric ischemia, the vascular insult is secondary to low-flow, and typically an inflow procedure is not required. The principle of bowel resection is typically to resect the frankly necrotic bowel and, if any question of viability of other bowel, to perform the procedure as a damage-control operation.

Abdominal Compartment Syndrome

Intra-abdominal hypertension and abdominal compartment syndrome can occur both in medical and surgical patients and arising from numerous underlying etiologies. Intra-abdominal hypertension is defined by the World Society of the Abdominal Compartment Syndrome as intra-abdominal pressure >12 mmHg, with abdominal compartment syndrome defined as intra-abdominal pressure >20 mmHg with concomitant presence of organ failure related to this increased pressure [81]. This end-organ dysfunction may manifest as oliguria or as increased peak airway pressures if the patient is mechanically ventilated. While patients who develop abdominal compartment syndrome have a variety of presentations, the typical common denominator is an excessive fluid or blood product resuscitation that leads to third spacing of fluid and resultant increase in edema, ascites, and abdominal pressure. This leads to symptoms when the intra-abdominal pressure exceeds venous pressure, hampering venous return and causing end-organ dysfunction. While abdominal compartment syndrome is largely a clinical diagnosis, quantification of the abdominal pressure can be performed by obtaining a bladder pressure using an indwelling urinary catheter and a transducer [82].

While medical maneuvers such as paracentesis and pharmacologic paralysis can be used to temporize this condition, surgical laparotomy may be required for definitive management of abdominal compartment syndrome [83]. By simply opening the abdomen, this relieves the intra-abdominal pressure and allows ongoing medical management of the organ dysfunction caused by the compartment syndrome as well as the treatment of the underlying cause. The open abdomen is managed with a vacuum-assisted device until the acute episode abates, the patient is diuresed, and the edema resolves. Therefore, it is important to coordinate closely with medical services to determine which patients will benefit from laparotomy and perform this procedure promptly in those cases. It is sometimes necessary in these patients to perform complex abdominal wall closure once the patient has recovered sufficiently.

Case Resolution

Due to concern for intra-abdominal complications after her recent colectomy, a CT scan is obtained which demonstrates free air and fluid surrounding the site of her colonic anastomosis. She is taken to the operating room for exploration, during which feculent peritonitis is found, with visible dehiscence of the prior anastomosis. The prior anastomosis is resected, and an end colostomy is created due to the quality of the tissue and the extent of the contamination. Postoperatively, she improves and is subsequently able to be discharged to a skilled nursing facility.

References

1. Silver JH, Williams SV, Krakauer H, Schwartz JS. Hospital and patient characteristics associated with death after surgery: a study of adverse occurrence and failure to rescue. Med Care. 1992;30(7):615–29.
2. Hatchimonji JS, Kaufman EJ, Sharoky CE, Ma L, Garcia Whitlock AE, Holena DN. Failure to rescue in surgical patients: a review for acute care surgeons. J Trauma Acute Care Surg. 2019;87(3):699–706.
3. National Quality Forum. (2010). Safe practices for better healthcare—2010 update. Retrieved from: http://www.qualityforum.org/Publications/2010/04/Safe_Practices_10_Full.aspx
4. Needleman J, Buerhaus PI, Vanderboom C, Harris M. Using present-on-admission coding to improve exclusion rules for quality metrics: the case of failure-to-rescue. Med Care. 2013;51(8):722–30.
5. Havens JM, Peetz AB, Do WS, Cooper Z, Kelly E, Askari R, Reznor G, Salim A. The excess morbidity and mortality of emergency general surgery. J Trauma Acute Care Surg. 2015;78(2):306–11.
6. Tevis SE, Cobian AG, Truong HP, Craven MW, Kennedy GD. Implications of multiple complications on the postoperative recovery of general surgery patients. Ann Surg. 2016;263(6):1213–8.
7. Massarweh NN, Anaya DA, Kougias P, Bakaeen FG, Awad SS, Berger DH. Variation and impact of multiple complications on failure to rescue after inpatient surgery. Ann Surg. 2017;266(1):59–65.
8. Wakeam E, Hyder JA, Tsai TC, Lipsitz SR, Orgill DP, Finlayson SRG. Complication timing and association with mortality in the American College of Surgeons' National Surgical Quality Improvement Program database. J Surg Res. 2015;193(1):77–87.
9. Wakeam E, Hyder JA, Jiang W, Lipsitz SA, Finlayson S. Risk and patterns of secondary complications in surgical inpatients. JAMA Surg. 2015;150(1):65–73.
10. Sheetz KH, Dimick JB, Ghaferi AA. Impact of hospital characteristics on failure to rescue following major surgery. Ann Surg. 2016;263(4):692–7.
11. Smith ME, Wells EE, Friese CR, Krein SL, Ghaferi AA. Interpersonal and organizational dynamics are key drivers of failure to rescue. Health Aff (Millwood). 2018;37(11):1870–6.
12. Ghaferi AA, Birkmeyer JD, Dimick JB. Complications, failure to rescue, and mortality with major inpatient surgery in medicare patients. Ann Surg. 2009;250(6):1029–34.
13. Ghaferi AA, Birkmeyer JD, Dimick JB. Hospital volume and failure to rescue with high-risk surgery. Med Care. 2011;49(12):1076–81.
14. Mehta A, Efron DT, Stevens K, Manukyan MC, Joseph B, Sakran JV. Hospital variation in mortality after emergent bowel resections: the role of failure-to rescue. J Trauma Acute Care Surg. 2018;84(5):702–10.
15. Mehta A, Efron DT, Canner JK, Dultz L, Xu T, Jones C, Haut ER, Higgins RSD, Sakran JV. Effect of surgeon and hospital volume on emergency general surgery outcomes. J Am Coll Surg. 2017;225(5):666–75.
16. Hatchimonji JS, Kaufman EJ, Sharoky CE, Ma LW, Holena DN. A "weekend effect" in operative emergency general surgery. Am J Surg. 2019:S0002-9610(19)31157-2. https://doi.org/10.1016/j.amjsurg.2019.11.024.
17. Metcalfe D, Castillo-Angeles M, Rios-Diaz AJ, Havens JM, Haider A, Salim A. Is there a "weekend effect" in emergency general surgery? J Surg Res. 2018;222:219–24.
18. Fry BT, Smith ME, Thumma JR, Ghaferi AA, Dimick JB. Ten-year trends in surgical mortality, complications, and failure to rescue in Medicare beneficiaries. Ann Surg. 2020;271(5):855–61.
19. Finlayson EV, Birkmeyer JD. Operative mortality with elective surgery in older adults. Eff Clin Pract. 2001;4(4):172–7.
20. Ghaferi AA, Dimick JB. Importance of teamwork, communication, and culture on failure-to-rescue in the elderly. Br J Surg. 2016;103(2):e47–51.
21. Sheetz KH, Waits SA, Krell RW, Campbell DA Jr, Englesbe MJ, Ghaferi AA. Improving mortality following emergency surgery in older patients requires focus on complication rescue. Ann Surg. 2013;258(4):614–7.

22. Sheetz KH, Krell RW, Englesbe MJ, Birkmeyer JD, Campbell DA Jr, Ghaferi AA. The importance of the first complication: understanding failure to rescue after emergent surgery in the elderly. J Am Coll Surg. 2014;219(3):365–70.
23. Mehta A, Dultz LA, Joseph B, Canner JK, Stevens K, Jones C, Haut ER, Efron DT, Sakran JV. Emergency general surgery in geriatric patients: a statewide analysis of surgeon and hospital volume with outcomes. J Trauma Acute Care Surg. 2018;84(6):864–75.
24. Mehta A, Varma S, Efron DT, Joseph BA, Lunardi N, Haut ER, Cooper Z, Sakran JV. Emergency general surgery in geriatric patients: how should we evaluate hospital experience? J Trauma Acute Care Surg. 2019;86(2):189–95.
25. American College of Surgeons. Geriatric Surgery Verification Program. 2020; Available at: https://www.facs.org/Quality-Programs/geriatric-surgery.
26. Khan M, Azim A, O'Keeffe T, Jehan F, Kulvatunyou N, Santino C, Tang A, Vercruysse G, Gries L, Joseph B. Geriatric rescue after surgery (GRAS) score to predict failure-to-rescue in geriatric emergency general surgery patients. Am J Surg. 2018;215(1):53–7.
27. Khan M, Jehan F, Zeeshan M, Kulvatunyou N, Fain MJ, Saljuqi AT, O'Keeffe T, Joseph B. Failure to rescue after emergency general surgery in geriatric patients: does frailty matter? J Surg Res. 2019;233:397–402.
28. Scarborough JE, Pappas TN, Bennett KM, Lagoo-Deenadayalan S. Failure-to-pursue rescue: explaining excess mortality in elderly emergency general surgical patients with preexisting "do-not-resuscitate" orders. Ann Surg. 2012;256(3):453–61.
29. de Jager E, Chaudhary MA, Rahim F, Jarman MP, Uribe-Leitz T, Havens JM, Goralnick E, Schonfeld AJ, Haider AH. The impact of income on emergency general surgery outcomes in urban and rural areas. J Surg Res. 2020;245:629–35.
30. Metcalfe D, Castillo-Angeles M, Olufajo OA, Rios-Diaz A, Salim A, Haider AH, Havens JM. Failure to rescue and disparities in emergency general surgery. J Surg Res. 2018;231:62–8.
31. Charles R, Hood B, Derosier JM, Gosbee JW, Li Y, Caird MS, Biermann JS, Hake ME. How to perform a root cause analysis for workup and future prevention of medical errors: a review. Patient Saf Surg. 2016;10:20.
32. Johnston M, Arora S, Anderson O, King D, Behar N, Darzi A. Escalation of care in surgery: a systematic risk assessment to prevent avoidable harm in hospitalized patients. Ann Surg. 2015;261(5):831–8.
33. Ghaferi AA, Dimick JB. Understanding failure to rescue and improving safety culture. Ann Surg. 2015;261(5):839–40.
34. Ludikhuize J, Smorenburg SM, de Rooij SE, de Jonge E. Identification of deteriorating patients on general wards; measurement of vital parameters and potential effectiveness of the modified early warning score. J Crit Care. 2012;27(4):424.e7–13.
35. Heller AR, Mees ST, Lauterwald B, Reeps C, Koch T, Weitz J. Detection of deteriorating patients on surgical wards outside the ICU by an automated MEWS-based early warning system with paging functionality. Ann Surg. 2020;271(1):100–5.
36. Royal College of Physicians. National Early Warning Score (NEWS): Standardising the assessment of acute illness severity in the NHS; 2012. Available at: www.rcplondon.ac.uk/national-early-warning-score. Accessed July 2, 2020.
37. Loftus TJ, Tighe PJ, Filiberto AC, Balch J, Upchurch GR, Rashidi P, Bihorac A. Opportunities for machine learning to improve surgical ward safety. Am J Surg. 2020:S0002-9610(20)30091-X.
38. Pucher PH, Brunt LM, Davies N, Linsk A, Munshi A, Rodriguez HA, Fingerhut A, Fanelli RD, Asbun H, Aggarwal R, SAGES Safe Cholecystectomy Task Force. Outcome trends and safety measures after 30 years of laparoscopic cholecystectomy: a systematic review and pooled data analysis. Surg Endosc. 2018;32(5):2175–83.
39. Rystedt JM, Kleeff J, Salvia R, Besselink MG, Prasad R, Lesurtel M, Sturesson C, Abu Hilal M, Aljaiuossi A, Antonucci A, et al. Post cholecystectomy bile duct injury: early, intermediate or late repair with hepaticojejunostomy—an E-AHPBA multi-center study. HPB. 2019;21(12):1641–7.
40. Khadra H, Johnson H, Crowther J, McClaren P, Darden M, Parker G, Buell JF. Bile duct injury repairs: progressive outcomes in a tertiary referral center. Surgery. 2019;166(4):698–702.
41. Mercado MA, Doninguez I. Classification and management of bile duct injuries. World J Gastrointest Surg. 2011;3(4):43–8.
42. Halle-Smith JM, Hodson J, Stevens LG, Dassari B, Marudanayagam R, Perera T, Sutcliffe RP, Muiesan P, Isaac J, Mirza DF, Roberts KJ. A comprehensive evaluation of the long-term economic impact of major bile duct injury. HPB. 2019;21(10):1312–21.
43. O'Brien S, Wei D, Bhutiani N, Rao MK, Johnston SS, Patkar A, Vitale GC, Martin RCG. Adverse outcomes and short-term cost implications of bile duct injury during cholecystectomy. Surg Endosc. 2020;34(2):628–35.
44. Strasberg SM, Brunt LM. Rationale and use of the critical view of safety in laparoscopic cholecystectomy. J Am Coll Surg. 2010;211(1):132–8.
45. Flum DR, Dellinger EP, Cheadle A, Chan L, Koepsell T. Intraoperative cholangiography and risk of common bile duct injury during cholecystectomy. JAMA. 2003;289(13):1639–44.
46. Nickkholgh A, Soltaniyekta S, Kalbasi H. Routine versus selective intraoperative cholangiography during laparoscopic cholecystectomy: a survey of 2,130 patients undergoing laparoscopic cholecystectomy. Surg Endosc. 2006;20(6):868–74.
47. Halle-Smith JM, Hodson J, Stevens LG, Dasari B, Marudanayagam R, Perera T, Sutcliffe RP, Muiesan P, Isaac J, Mirza DF, Roberts KJ. A comprehen-

sive evaluation of the long-term clinical and economic impact of minor bile duct injury. Surgery. 2020;S0039-6060(20):30065–9.
48. Rahnemai-Azar AA, Rahnemaiazar AA, Naghshizadian R, Kurtz A, Farkas DT. Percutaneous endoscopic gastrostomy: indications, technique, complications and management. World J Gastroenterol. 2014;20(24):7739–51.
49. Stayner JL, Bhatnagar A, McGinn AN, Fang JC. Feeding tube placement: errors and complications. Nutr Clin Pract. 2012;27(6):738–48.
50. Guilbert M-C, Elkouri S, Bracco D, Corriveau MM, Beaudoin N, Dubois MJ, Bruneau L, Blair J-F. Arterial trauma during central venous catheter insertion: case series, review and proposed algorithm. J Vasc Surg. 2008;48(4):918–25.
51. Thompson C, Barrows T. Carotid arterial cannulation: removing the risk with ultrasound? Can J Anaesth. 2009;56(6):471–2.
52. Kornbau C, Lee KC, Hughes GD, Firstenberg MS. Central line complications. Int J Crit Illn Inj Sci. 2015;5(3):170–8.
53. Volpicelli G. Sonographic diagnosis of pneumothorax. Intensive Care Med. 2011;37(2):224–32.
54. Turrentine FE, Denlinger CE, Simpson VB, Garwood RA, Guerlain S, Agrawal A, Friel CM, LaPar DJ, Stukenborg GJ, Jones RS. Morbidity, mortality, cost, and survival estimates of gastrointestinal anastomotic leaks. J Am Coll Surg. 2015;220(2):195–206.
55. Guyton KL, Hyman NH, Alverdy JC. Prevention of perioperative anastomotic healing complications: anastomotic stricture and anastomotic leak. Adv Surg. 2016;50(1):129–41.
56. Sakr A, Emile SH, Abdallah E, Thabet W, Khafagy W. Predictive factors for small intestinal and colonic anastomotic leak: a multivariate analysis. Indian J Surg. 2017;79(6):555–62.
57. Nikolian VC, Kamdar NS, Regenbogen SE, Morris AM, Byrn JC, Suwanabol PA, Campbell DA, Hendren S. Anastomotic leak after colorectal resection: a population-based study of risk factors and hospital variation. Surgery. 2017;161(6):1619–27.
58. Telem DA, Chin EH, Nguyen SQ, Divino CM. Risk factors for anastomotic leak following colorectal surgery: a case-control study. Arch Surg. 2010;145(4):371–6.
59. Morse BC, Simpson JP, Jones YR, Joohnson BL, Knott BM, Kotrady JA. Determination of independent predictive factors for anastomotic leak: analysis of 682 intestinal anastomoses. Am J Surg. 2013;206(6):950–5.
60. Naumann DN, Bhangu A, Kelly M, Bowley DM. Stapled versus handsewn intestinal anastomosis in emergency laparotomy: a systematic review and meta-analysis. Surgery. 2015;157(4):609–18.
61. Chadi SA, Fingerhut A, Berho M, DeMeester SR, Fleshman JW, Hyman NH, Margolin DA, Martz JE, McLemore EC, Molena D, Newman MI, Rafferty J, Safar B, Senagore AJ, Zmore O, Wexner SD. Emerging trends in the etiology, prevention, and treatment of gastrointestinal anastomotic leakage. J Gastrointest Surg. 2016;20(12):2035–51.
62. Evenson AR, Fischer JE. Current management of enterocutaneous fistula. J Gastrointest Surg. 2006;10(3):455–64.
63. Hatchimonji JS, Passman J, Kaufman EJ, Sharoky CE, Ma LW, Scantling D, Xiong R, Holena DN. Enterocutaneous fistula after emergency general surgery: mortality, readmission, and financial burden. J Trauma Acute Care Surg. 2020; https://doi.org/10.1097/TA.0000000000002673.
64. Lloyd DAJ, Gabe SM, Windsor ACJ. Nutrition and management of enterocutaneous fistula. Br J Surg. 2006;93(9):1045–55.
65. Martinez JL, Luque-de-Leon E, Ballinas-Oseguera G, Mendez JD, Juarez-Oropoza MA, Roman-Ramos R. Factors predictive of recurrence and mortality after surgical repair of enterocutaneous fistula. J Gastrointest Surg. 2012;16(1):156–63.
66. de Vries FEE, Atema JJ, van Ruler O, Vaizey CJ, Serlie MJ, Boermeester MA. A systematic review and meta-analysis of timing and outcome of intestinal failure surgery in patients with enteric fistula. World J Surg. 2018;42(3):695–706.
67. Lynch CA, Delaney CP, Senagore AJ, Connor JT, Remzi FH, Fazio VW. Clinical outcome and factors predictive of recurrence after enterocutaneous fistula surgery. Ann Surg. 2004;240(5):825–31.
68. Owen RM, Love TP, Perez SD, Srinivasan JK, Sharma J, Pollock JD, Haack CI, Sweeney JF, Galloway JR. Definitive surgical treatment of enterocutaneous fistula: outcomes of a 23-year experience. JAMA Surg. 2013;148(2):118–26.
69. Bagdasarian N, Rao K, Malani PN. Diagnosis and treatment of Clostridium difficile in adults: a systematic review. JAMA. 2015;313(4):398–408.
70. Olivas AD, Umanskiy K, Zuckerbraun B, Alverdy JC. Avoiding colectomy during surgical management of fulminant Clostridium difficile colitis. Surg Infect. 2010;11(3):299–305.
71. Kautza B, Zuckerbrain BS. The surgical management of complicated Clostridium difficile infection: alternatives to colectomy. Surg Infect. 2016;17(3):337–42.
72. Surawicz CM, Brandt LJ, Binion DG, Ananthakrishnan AN, Curry SR, Gilligan PH, McFarland LV, Mellow M, Zuckerbrain BS. Guidelines for diagnosis, treatment, and prevention of Clostridium difficile infections. Am J Gastroenterol. 2013;108(4):478–98.
73. Briggs A, Peitzman AB. Surgical rescue in medical patients: the role of acute care surgeons as the surgical rapid response team. Crit Care Clin. 2018;34(2):209–19.
74. Pepin J, Vo TT, Boutros M, Marcotte E, Dial S, Dube S, Vasilevsky C-A, McFadden N, Patino C, Labbe A-C. Risk factors for mortality following emergency colectomy for fulminant Clostridium difficile infection. Dis Colon Rectum. 2009;52(3):400–5.
75. Lamontagne F, Labbe A-C, Haeck O, Lesur O, Lalancette M, Patino C, Leblalnc M, Laverdiere M, Pepin J. Impact of emergency colectomy on survival

of patients with fulminant Clostridium difficile colitis during an epidemic caused by a hypervirulent strain. Ann Surg. 2007;245(2):267–72.
76. Neal MD, Alverdy JC, Hall DE, Simmons RL, Zuckerbraun BS. Diverting loop ileostomy and colonic lavage: an alternative to total abdominal colectomy for the treatment of severe, complicated Clostridium difficile associated disease. Ann Surg. 2011;254(3):423–7.
77. Bala M, Kashuk J, Moore EE, Kluger Y, Biffl W, Gomes CA, Ben-Ishay O, Rubinstein C, Balogh ZJ, Civil I, Coccolini F, Leppaniemi A, Peitzman A, Ansaloni L, Sugrue M, Sartelli M, Di Saverio S, Fraga GP, Catena F. Acute mesenteric ischemia: guidelines on the World Society of Emergency Surgery. World J Emerg Surg. 2017;12:38.
78. Clair DG, Beach JM. Mesenteric ischemia. N Engl J Med. 2016;374(10):959–68.
79. Eltarawy IG, Etman YM, Zenati M, Simmons RL, Rosengart MR. Acute mesenteric ischemia: the importance of early surgical consultation. Am Surg. 2009;75(3):212–9.
80. Acosta-Merida MA, Marchena-Gomez J, Hemmersbach-Miller M, Roque-Castellano C, Hernandez-Romero JM. Identification of risk factors for perioperative mortality in acute mesenteric ischemia. World J Surg. 2006;30(8):1579–85.
81. Kirkpatrick AW, Roberts DJ, De Waele J, Jaeschke R, MLNG M, De Keulenaer B, Duchesne J, Bjorck M, Leppaniemi A, Ejike JC, Sugrue M, Cheatham M, Ivatury R, Ball CG, Blaser AR, Regli A, Balogh ZJ, D'Amours S, Debergh D, Kaplan M, Kimball E, Olvera C, Pediatric Guidelines Sub-Committee for the World Society of the Abdominal Compartment Syndrome. Intra-abdominal hypertension and the abdominal compartment syndrome: updated consensus definitions and clinical practice guidelines from the World Society of the Abdominal Compartment Syndrome. Intensive Care Med. 2013;39(7):1190–206.
82. Hunt L, Frost SA, Hillman K, Newton PJ, Davidson PM. Management of intra-abdominal hypertension and abdominal compartment syndrome: a review. J Trauma Manag Outcomes. 2014;8(1):2.
83. Luckianow GM, Ellis M, Governale D, Kaplan LJ. Abdominal compartment syndrome: risk factors, diagnosis, and current therapy. Crit Care Res Pract. 2012; https://doi.org/10.1155/2012/908169.

Small Bowel Obstruction

12

Andrew Medvecz and Oscar Guillamondegui

Case Report

A 72-year-old man with history of exploratory laparotomy for perforated diverticulitis approximately 3 years ago presents to the emergency department with a 24-hour history of nausea, vomiting, and bloating. He denies fevers and chills and has had no change in bladder function. He reports normally passing flatus regularly and having a bowel movement daily but has had neither of these today.

Overview

Small bowel obstruction (SBO) has been a source of significant morbidity and mortality among surgical patients for millennia. The disease's propensity for recurrence has led to many practice patterns and changes over the past century, and knowledge regarding appropriate management for this disease process continues to evolve. The management of SBO has significant economic and healthcare resource implications as it can account for 12–16% of surgical admissions annually and lead to over 300,000 annual operations [1]. For many patients, an admission for SBO will not be an isolated event, as this may be a harbinger for multiple recurrences and complications. This chapter will review the epidemiology and presentation of patients with SBO as well as current practice patterns and additional considerations when determining operative or nonoperative management of this vexing pathology.

Etiology

There is a diverse range of causes for small bowel obstruction; however, adhesive disease accounts for the most significant number of episodes and recurrences. Adhesive small bowel obstruction accounts for 75% of cases, with almost all a result of prior abdominal or pelvic operations. Postmortem studies from the 1970s showed that 51% of patients with minor, 72% with major, and 93% of patients with multiple intra-abdominal operations had developed adhesions [2]. Even 28% of patients without prior abdominal operation were found to have intra-abdominal adhesions. Open small bowel, colon, and gynecologic procedures account for the highest incidence of readmissions related to adhesive small bowel obstruction [3]. Time from prior abdominopelvic operation to obstruction varies widely, with some individuals demonstrating early obstruction 7–10 days following operation to initial episodes of adhesive SBO developing over 10 years following index abdominal operations.

A. Medvecz (✉) · O. Guillamondegui
Vanderbilt University Medical Center, Medical Arts Building, Nashville, TN, USA
e-mail: andrew.j.medvecz@vumc.org; oscar.guillamondegui@vumc.org

M. D. Zielinski, O. Guillamondegui (eds.), *The Acute Management of Surgical Disease*,
https://doi.org/10.1007/978-3-031-07881-1_12

Malignancy is the second-leading cause of small bowel obstruction. Primary small bowel tumors such as carcinoid, lymphoma, and small bowel carcinoma can account for the obstruction, and it may be caused by internal obstruction or external luminal compression. Metastatic malignancy to the small bowel can also account of small bowel obstruction. Tumors with known peritoneal spread such as colon, ovarian, pancreatic, and gastric neoplasms can lead to extraluminal compression or volvulus, leading to obstruction. Similarly, malignancy with hematogenous spread such as melanoma can also metastasize to the small bowel, leading to intraluminal or external compression [4].

Hernias are another cause of SBO. Ventral/incisional hernia from prior laparotomy are common lead points for SBO. Small hernias have greater likelihood of developing acute incarceration and obstruction. However, large ventral incisional hernias may also lead to SBO as there can be adhesions from chronic incarceration. Inguinal hernias are rarely associated small bowel obstruction; however, femoral and obturator hernias should be considered in the differential, more commonly in women.

Inflammatory bowel disease is another important etiology of small bowel obstruction because the management described below is more often medical and typically will not require operative management unless there is advanced disease. In particular, Crohn's disease can cause inflammatory perforations and interloop abscesses which can lead to partial or complete obstructions. The inflammatory process and subsequent adhesion formation associated with acute diverticulitis infectious etiologies such as tuberculosis are largely absent in economically advanced countries but should remain on the differential for patients exposed to populations endemic with tuberculosis.

Other causes of small bowel obstruction are less common but must also remain in the differential of a patient presenting with symptoms concerning for bowel obstruction. Intussusception of small bowel with small bowel or small bowel with cecum often associated with a lead point may present with obstruction. Accounting for less than 0.1% of mechanical small bowel obstructions, gallstone ileus remains a potential cause of obstruction. Accidental or psychiatric diagnosis-related consumption of non-digestible foreign bodies may also serve as a nidus for subsequent obstruction. Of note, other pathologies may mimic SBO, such as pneumonia, urinary tract infection, acute non-abdominal surgical intervention (e.g., joint replacement), and hypokalemia.

Diagnosis

The workup of patients presenting with concern for small bowel obstruction should undergo a thorough history and physical exam, imaging, and laboratory evaluation to assist in the diagnosis and management decisions. The AAST has created a grading system for intestinal obstruction due to adhesive disease which can be a useful tool in the diagnosis and management of bowel obstruction [5].

History and Physical Exam

Small bowel obstruction can most often be elucidated from the history of a patient presenting with diminished or absent flatus and abdominal distension. Many patients will experience nausea accompanied with bilious emesis [6]. Abdominal pain is variable, ranging from absent or mild abdominal pain to peritonitis suggesting ischemic bowel or perforation associated with the obstruction. Patients with prior obstructions may note similar clinical presentations as prior episodes. Past medical history includes known diagnoses of inflammatory bowel disease, malignancy, or diverticulitis. Prior surgical history should also be determined, not only to estimate an adhesive burden but also for operative planning (ex. presence of mesh, surgically-altered anatomy). Abdominal operations followed by pelvic operations have been associated with the highest risk of developing subsequent small bowel obstructions [7].

On physical exam, the first determination is the overall clinical status of the patient, whether they are "sick" or "not sick." Vital sign assessment including heart rate, blood pressure, respiratory rate, and oxygen status can suggest whether the patient is presenting with ischemia or associated aspiration from the obstruction. Bowel sounds are likely hypoactive or absent on abdominal exam. The abdomen will often be distended and tympanitic, and it may have tenderness associated with the distension. However, patients presenting with focal peritonitis should raise concern for bowel ischemia or generalized peritonitis with concern for perforation following the obstruction. The abdominal wall and groins should be examined for the presence of hernia. Rectal exam may be considered as well if differential includes distal obstructing lesion.

Laboratory Workup

A complete blood count (CBC) and basic metabolic panel (BMP) are routinely ordered for patients presenting with concern for obstruction. Of note is the white blood cell count, as leukocytosis may suggest the presence of ischemia or infectious etiology for the obstruction. Acute kidney injury manifested with elevated creatinine is a common finding in patients presenting with obstruction as many are dehydrated from inability to tolerate per os intake and persistent emesis. An elevated lactic acid level may portend ischemic changes or under-resuscitation.

Imaging

The goals of imaging studies in the setting of suspected small bowel obstruction are (a) identify the etiology for the obstruction, (b) assess ischemic bowel, and (c) aid in operative planning. Cross-sectional imaging with computed tomography (CT) scan of the abdomen and pelvis will most often be able to accomplish these goals. Intravenous iodinated contrast is used to aid with assessment of the bowel wall for ischemia. We do not routinely use enteral contrast given its poor tolerance by patients, often exacerbating nausea and emesis with the subsequent need for supine positioning for the CT scan although this may be considered in appropriately risk-stratified patients. CT scan can aid in characterizing the SBO, whether it is partial, complete, or a closed-loop obstruction. Partial obstructions may identify normal imaging or minimal intestinal distension with the presence of air distal to the small bowel. Higher-grade or complete obstructions will often have the hallmarks of small bowel distension. A transition point at which the dilated bowel becomes decompressed may suggest an anatomic location of the obstruction in settings of adhesive disease

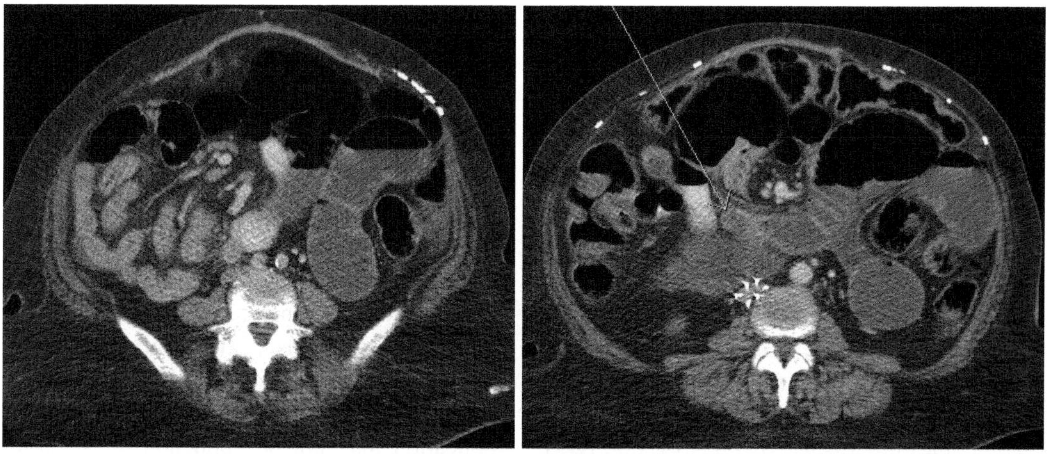

Fig. 12.1 Computed tomography images of patient with small bowel obstruction. The first image demonstrates dilated and decompressed loops of small bowel. The arrow in the second image demonstrates a transition point

(Fig. 12.1). Cross-sectional imaging also allows for assessment of ventral, obturator, and femoral herniae which may be difficult to assess on physical exam. Findings of mesenteric stranding or lack of bowel enhancement suggest ischemic changes to the bowel wall, and pneumoperitoneum or free fluid may suggest associated perforation, necessitating exploration.

Plain radiographs may be helpful in an initial evaluation of a patient presenting with nausea, vomiting, and distension; however, the specificity of dilated loops of small bowel on plain radiograph is low and typically results in CT scan. Plain radiographs do have a major role in the authors' subsequent management following the diagnosis of obstruction.

Management

The management of small bowel obstruction has often been described as having two arms: operative and nonoperative. However, to place a patient with obstruction into one of these two categories would be premature, as patients may cross from one algorithm to the other. Operative management should be considered the gold standard against which others are measured. Many patients, especially those presenting with suspected adhesive bowel disease, are candidates for nonoperative management. The decision of whether to pursue initial nonoperative management is complex and should utilize a shared decision-making model which involves the patient, surgeon, and consultants.

The principles of nonoperative management include bowel rest with nil per os status, nasogastric decompression typically with bilious and/or feculent output, and time. Serial abdominal exams are performed as well to confirm the obstruction does not progress to ischemia or perforation, thus requiring urgent operative management. Several studies have suggested the therapeutic benefit of water-soluble oral contrast which is given with a small bowel through radiographic study described earlier [8–10] (Fig. 12.2). The oral contrast, typically administered through the nasogastric tube, carries with it an osmotic load that can draw water into the lumen of the small bowel, thus allowing contrast and enteric content to pass through the point of obstruction. Progression of nonoperative management is followed with radiographic evidence of movement of contrast into the cecum. The patient will clinically begin to have flatus and ultimately have a bowel movement while concurrently having a decrease in the volume of nasogastric output as well as change to a non-bilious character. Successful resolution of small bowel obstruction with nonoperative management varies in studies, with ranges from 43 to 76% in several, large nonrandomized studies [7, 11–13]. Faster progression of contrast to the colon has been also associated with increased likelihood of successful nonoperative management [14].

Despite the success of nonoperative management in many patients with adhesive small bowel obstruction, operative management maintains a primary management for bowel obstruction. For those patients who fail nonoperative management, laparoscopy or laparotomy is indicated and has been found to have no difference in outcomes compared to those with operations in the first 24 h [6]. Indications for operative management, whether on initial presentation or during trial of nonoperative management, include evidence of generalized peritonitis suggesting perforation, lactic acidosis, leukocytosis, vital sign abnormalities (tachycardia), or radiographic signs of ischemia. Laparotomy for small bowel obstruction first involves exploration and identification of the transition point of obstruction. The etiology of the obstruction will dictate the operative proceedings. On entry to the abdomen, it should be explored for evidence of metastatic disease, especially in patients with reported history of malignancy. Intra-abdominal adhesions will require lysis, and ischemic or injured bowel should be resected. If an abdominal wall hernia is causing the obstruction, the hernia requires reduction and repair.

In recent years, laparoscopy has gained popularity in operative management of small bowel obstruction. There is evidence of shorter hospital stay and quicker return of bowel function, yet its application may not be applicable in all cases [15]. Great care must be taken entering the abdomen as the presence of adhesions and dilated small bowel increase the likelihood of enterot-

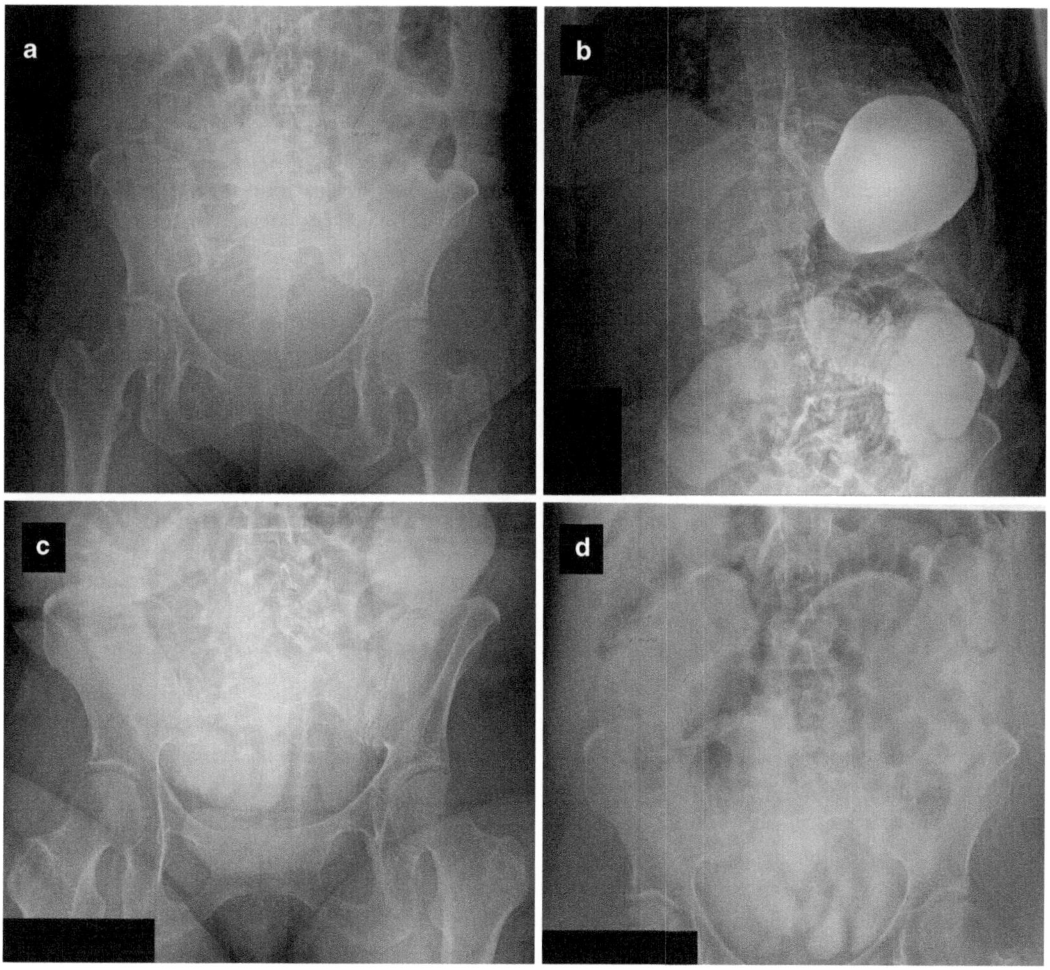

Fig. 12.2 Small bowel follow through in patient with adhesive small bowel obstruction. Images were taken at (**a**) time = 0, (**b**) time = 1 ½ h, (**c**) time = 3 ½ h, (**d**) time = 14 h. There is no progression of contrast to the colon

omy. After surveying the abdomen, the small bowel can be run backward from the ileocecal valve or forward from the ligament of Treitz. Dilated small bowel can be fragile and easily injured with laparoscopic graspers. Extensive lysis of adhesions may be undertaken laparoscopically given the comfort and laparoscopic skill of the surgeon. If not able to be completed laparoscopically, then conversion to a more targeted laparotomy may be possible. If bowel resection is ultimately required, exploration with laparoscopy may allow for more limited open exploration and thus smaller incision. While not the mainstay of surgical exploration for small bowel obstruction, laparoscopy remains a tool that can be used in select populations. The benefits of quicker return of bowel function, shorter hospital stay, and less morbidity can bring significant advantages to the management of these populations [15].

Small bowel obstruction in specific patient populations may require a different approached from the management decisions for adhesion-related issues. Patients with inflammatory bowel disease presenting with small bowel obstruction should be considered for medical management of the Crohn's stricture unless demonstrating bowel ischemia or closed loop obstruction as the disease process will make operative management challenging. For those patients who go on to require surgery, the American Society of Colon and Rectal Surgeons (ASCO) recommend resection of the affected bowel if causing the obstruction (Grade 1B) [16]. However, many patients should resolve their acute obstruction with bowel rest and a course of IV steroids. Consultation with gastroenterology should be considered, especially when determining appropriate course of action regarding inpatient and subsequent outpatient management with anti-inflammatory medication (Grade C, British Society of Gastroenterology) [17].

Outcomes

Successful management of a small bowel obstruction episode is characterized by return of bowel function and consumption of adequate oral nutrition. Retrospective studies have identified that the majority of small bowel obstructions are resolved without operative intervention [7, 14]. Yet the sinister aspect of small bowel obstruction that plagues surgeons is the potential for recurrence with both operative and nonoperative management. Nonoperative management does not eliminate the mechanical obstruction at the transition point, rather altering the bowel's absorption and physiology to alleviate the obstruction. Conversely, surgical management can eliminate the physical obstruction, whether most commonly from intra-abdominal adhesions or other causes such as hernia, malignancy, etc. With multiple operative interventions comes the risk of developing of new adhesive disease thus potentiating episodes of bowel obstruction. It further increases the risk for the development of incisional hernias.

Recent literature has focused on the likelihood of recurrence from small bowel obstruction. We evaluated the likelihood of recurrence of bowel obstruction in the setting of adhesive disease [13]. In the 10 years of follow-up, patients managed operatively during first episode of adhesive bowel disease were less likely to develop recurrence; however, patients undergoing operative management during subsequent admissions for adhesive disease had greater odds of developing recurrent obstruction. Behman similarly found a reduced risk of recurrence following operation for first episode of adhesive bowel disease [18]. With an increased emphasis on long-term patient-centered outcomes, recurrence should be discussed among providers and with patients during shared decision-making for treatment options. In some populations, earlier operative intervention be considered especially considering its impact on recurrence.

Recurrence of small bowel obstruction must be balanced with the morbidity and mortality of both operative and nonoperative management. We identified greater in-hospital mortality and complications in patients managed operatively our retrospective review of 10 years of follow up [13]. Other studies identified a mortality increase during readmission for small bowel obstruction following operative management [19]. There is also evidence that suggests that operative intervention during a first episode of adhesive small bowel obstruction is associated with lower long-term mortality risk [20]. The mixed results emphasize the importance of preoperative risk assessment for each patient, as the risk for morbidity and mortality vary widely among patients presenting with bowel obstruction.

Further study on the impact of operative and nonoperative management of small bowel obstruction is still needed. Given the potential for regional variability in practice patterns and the diversity in patient presentation, a large and standardized registry in emergency general surgery patients would aid in expanding research endeavors and improving patient care.

Our Practice

It is the authors practice to pursue nonoperative management including decompression, hydration, and bowel rest with a water-soluble contrast small-bowel follow through for most patients presenting with obstruction from adhesive disease, in line with guidelines from the Eastern Association for the Surgery of Trauma (EAST) [1]. Patients presenting with high-grade obstructions or those in whom water-soluble contrast does not lead to resolution will typically proceed toward operative exploration. Patients with signs or symptoms of acute peritonitis will undergo urgent/emergent exploration. If history or imaging suggest the source of the obstruction is malignancy, operative intervention will also be performed. In those patients with multiple comorbidities, we tend to manage with an extended effort at nonoperative treatment as long as the patient does not show signs of impending ischemia or perforation due to the operative and postoperative risks associated with this population. Patient education of the short- and long-term outcomes, specifically recurrence, are discussed when addressing treatment options and recommendations, all to optimize the outcome for every patient.

Case Report (Continued)

Computed tomography imaging demonstrated an obstruction of the mid-small bowel with a transition point in the left lower quadrant. A nasogastric tube was placed, and small bowel follow-through with water-soluble contrast was initiated. At 24 hours, the contrast had not progressed to the colon, and the patient had high nasogastric tube output and no bowel function. The patient was taken for laparotomy where significant intra-abdominal adhesions were encountered. A transition point was identified at an area of tethered small bowel to the abdominal sidewall, and small bowel resection and primary anastomosis were performed. The patient recovered well with return of bowel function on postoperative day 4 and discharged on postoperative day 6.

References

1. Maung AA, Johnson DC, Piper GL, et al. Evaluation and management of small-bowel obstruction: an Eastern Association for the Surgery of Trauma practice management guideline. J Trauma Acute Care Surg. 2012;73(5 SUPPL.4):362–9.
2. Weibel M, Manjo G. Peritoneal adhesions and their relation to abdominal surgery. Am J Surg. 1973;126(3):345–53.
3. Barmparas G, Branco BC, Schnüriger B, Lam L, Inaba K, Demetriades D. The incidence and risk factors of post-laparotomy adhesive small bowel obstruction. J Gastrointest Surg. 2010;14(10):1619–28.
4. Liang KV, Sanderson SO, Nowakowski GS, Arora AS. Metastatic malignant melanoma of the gastrointestinal tract. Mayo Clin Proc. 2006;81(4):511–6. https://doi.org/10.4065/81.4.5115.
5. Tominaga GT, Staudenmayer KL, Shafi S, et al. The American Association for the Surgery of Trauma grading scale for 16 emergency general surgery conditions: disease-specific criteria characterizing anatomic severity grading. J Trauma Acute Care Surg. 2016;81(3):593–602.
6. Bauer J, Keeley B, Krieger B, et al. Adhesive small bowel obstruction: early operative versus observational management. Am Surg. 2015;81(6):614–20.
7. Foster NM, McGory ML, Zingmond DS, Ko CY. Small bowel obstruction: a population-based appraisal. J Am Coll Surg. 2006;203(2):170–6.
8. Ceresoli M, Coccolini F, Catena F, et al. Water-soluble contrast agent in adhesive small bowel obstruction: a systematic review and meta-analysis of diagnostic and therapeutic value. Am J Surg. 2016;211(6):1114–25.
9. Choi H-K, Chu K-W, Law W-L. Therapeutic value of gastrografin in adhesive small bowel obstruction after unsuccessful conservative treatment a prospective randomized trial. Ann Surg. 2002;236(1):1–6.
10. Burge J, Abbas SM, Roadley G, et al. Randomized controlled trial of gastrografin in adhesive small bowel obstruction. ANZ J Surg. 2005;75(8):672–4.
11. Williams SB, Greenspon J, Young HA, Orkin BA. Small bowel obstruction: conservative vs. surgical management. Dis Colon Rectum. 2005;48(6):1140–6.
12. Miller G, Boman J, Shrier I, Gordon P. Natural history of patients with adhesive small bowel obstruction. Br J Surg. 2000;87:1240.
13. Medvecz AJ, Dennis BM, Wang L, Lindsell CJ, Guillamondegui OD. Impact of operative management on recurrence of adhesive small bowel obstruction: a longitudinal analysis of a statewide database. J Am Coll Surg. 2020;230(4):544–50.
14. Loftus T, Moore F, VanZant E, et al. A protocol for the management of adhesive small bowel obstruction. J Trauma Acute Care Surg. 2015;78(1):13–9.
15. Khaikin M, Schneidereit N, Cera S, et al. Laparoscopic vs. open surgery for acute adhesive small-bowel obstruction: patients' outcome and cost-effectiveness. Surg Endosc Other Interv Tech. 2007;21(5):742–6.
16. Strong S, Steele SR, Boutrous M, et al. Clinical practice guidelines for the surgical management of Crohn's disease. Dis Colon Rectum. 2015;58:1021–35.
17. Carter MJ, Lobo AJ, Travis SPL. Guidelines for the management of inflammatory bowel disease in adults. Gut. 2004;53(SUPPL. 5)
18. Behman R, Nathens AB, Mason S, et al. Association of surgical intervention for adhesive small-bowel obstruction with the risk of recurrence. JAMA Surg. 2019:1–8. Published online.

19. Wessels LE, Sise CB, Dunne CE, et al. Outcomes in adhesive small bowel obstruction from a large statewide database. J Trauma Acute Care Surg. 2019;86(4):1.
20. Behman R, Nathens AB, Haas B, Look Hong N, Pechlivanoglou P, Karanicolas P. Surgery for adhesive small-bowel obstruction is associated with improved long-term survival mediated through recurrence prevention: a population-based, propensity-matched analysis. J Trauma Acute Care Surg. 2019;87(3):636–44.

Large Bowel Obstruction

13

Nathan T. Mowery and Audrey L. Spencer

"The sun never sets on a bowel obstruction" has been considered as historical dogma in surgical training. Due to the high risk of complications, namely, intestinal ischemia and perforation, it has been a tenant of general surgery that these patients need aggressive intervention. In contrast to treatment for small bowel obstruction, which has largely moved to longer acceptable periods of observation, large bowel obstruction is still thought to be a time-sensitive diagnosis regardless of the underlying etiology.

While not as common as small bowel obstruction, colonic obstruction still represents 25% of all intestinal obstructions [1]. Furthermore, complication of large bowel diseases account for 47% of gastrointestinal emergencies [2]. The obstruction can come in many forms including, but not limited to, mechanical problems as in volvulus and cancer or physiologic in nature such as in Ogilvie's syndrome. Many clinicians differentiate between partial and complete obstruction to determine the time period available for intervention.

In this chapter, we will review the evidence for the management of large bowel obstruction, identify areas of controversy, and highlight future directions for refinement of current practices.

N. T. Mowery (✉) · A. L. Spencer
Department of Surgery, Wake Forest Baptist Medical Center, Winston Salem, NC, USA
e-mail: nmowery@wakehealth.edu; auspence@wakehealth.edu

Etiology/Pathology

The pathology that accounts for colonic obstructions is diverse. They range from benign and malignant tumors and strictures and volvulus-type pictures. Adhesive obstructions are possible in colonic obstruction but not seen with near the frequency seen in small bowel obstruction. The fact that the etiology is different from small bowel obstruction plays a key role in the more operative-based treatment of large bowel pathology.

Malignancy is the most common cause of colonic obstruction leading to emergent surgery accounting for approximately 70% of cases. This incidence is the largest driver of operative intervention over observation. This is not limited to colon cancer as distal tumors represent a significant portion of the cases. Overall 10% of the patients presenting with colonic obstruction have rectal cancer, while an additional 5% have anal cancer as the etiology [3].

The most common cause of benign colonic obstruction is volvulus which represents 5–15% of large bowel obstructions [4]. The mechanism of volvulus is when a mobile portion of the colon twists on a single point of attachment. Some patients have a longer mesentery genetically, while others develop redundancy over time due to issues with colonic motility as seen in severe constipation. The acquired mobility is more common and that explains why these patients present

M. D. Zielinski, O. Guillamondegui (eds.), *The Acute Management of Surgical Disease*,
https://doi.org/10.1007/978-3-031-07881-1_13

after their fourth decade of life [5]. Typical portions of the colon involved are the sigmoid colon (~60%), cecum (~40%), and transverse colon (~2%) [6]. Fig. 13.1 shows the typical types of volvulus.

A variety of other etiologies account for the remaining 15–25% of cases, including benign strictures from recurrent inflammation (most commonly diverticular disease), intussusception, adhesive disease, and hernias with incarceration. There are also exceptionally rare causes such as bezoar and retroperitoneal fibrosis that are clinically important to the individual but beyond the scope of this chapter. Despite the seemingly endless list of possible etiologies, the evaluation of colonic obstruction is repetitive in nature, and the management is comparable utilizing both endoscopic and surgical interventions.

Diagnosis/Pathology

The varied definition of large bowel obstruction in the scientific literature makes comparisons between treatment options and timing difficult. The most basic definition is obstipation with imaging demonstrating distended colon. In order to minimize morbidity, many authors have included "impending obstructions" such as tight strictures which are typically only found after intervention. The impending obstruction population needs to be studied, but the inclusion of such patients makes drawing conclusions about the time-sensitive nature of this disease process difficult. If we recognize that colon cancer is the most common cause of large bowel obstruction and is typically slow growing, a patient can tolerate "impending obstruction" for several days or weeks before they would develop complications.

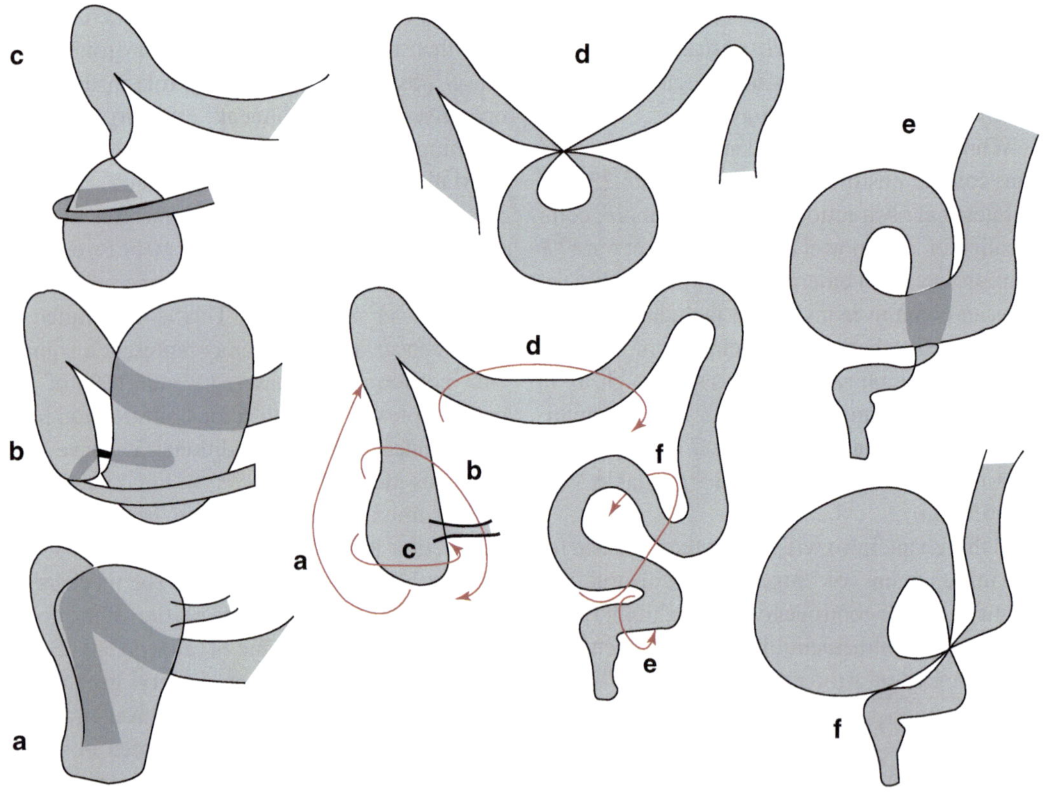

Fig. 13.1 Depiction of the three main types of colonic volvulus. Arrows represent the direction of volvulus accounting for the six presentations: (**a**) cecal bascule, (**b**) loop cecal volvulus, (**c**) axial cecal volvulus, (**d**) transverse colon volvulus, (**e**) organo-axial sigmoid volvulus, (**f**) classic sigmoid volvulus [7]

The clinical presentation of a large bowel obstruction is most commonly pain and bloating. Due to the distal nature of the obstruction, it does not have the classic nausea and vomiting seen in its small bowel counterpart. This can mean later presentation which is a key factor in its urgency and treatment as symptoms may not develop until just before abdominal catastrophe. Also due to the colonic flora and the potential for bacterial translocation, large bowel obstructions are more likely to present with systemic inflammatory response (SIRS) and electrolyte imbalances [8].

The presentation of colonic obstruction can be either acute or chronic. The presentation can point toward the etiology with a history of change in stool caliber or unintentional weight loss being more common in slow-evolving cancer. Acute pain is typically infraumbilical and crampy in nature. In the setting of large bowel volvulus, the nature of the pain can lead to the diagnosis. It has been shown that patients with sigmoid volvulus typically present with distention (79%), while cecal volvulus presents with pain (89%) [6].

While symptoms can help localize the source, imaging is required to further evaluate regardless of the etiology. Authors have suggested that plain x-ray should be utilized initially due to its lower cost and accessibility but has largely been replaced. Computed tomography (CT) is the standard diagnostic tool that would lead to most significant intervention. The global picture is essential for planning of treatment. Many consultants will not even proceed with adjuvants to non-operative therapy without a CT. While many surgeons learn the classic plain film appearance of colonic volvulus, they are not reliable and will miss up to 1/3 of the cases [9, 10]. Plain films may play a role in the patients at the extremes of physiology or in surveillance, but are otherwise relegated to irrelevant or a screening test for the evaluation of colonic obstruction. Another screening option is the ultrasound. Bedside ultrasound has higher sensitivity and the same specificity of plain x-ray but avoid moving the patient [11]. The later point could be of benefit in an ill unstable patient. The downside is that fact that some expertise is required with ultrasound limiting its widespread use.

Abdominal Computed Tomography

Virtually any hemodynamically stable patient suspected of colonic obstruction should get a CT scan secondary to its high sensitivity and specificity (both >90%) [12, 13]. CT can locate the obstructing lesions in 96% of cases and make correct diagnoses in 89% of cases. The use of triple contrast (intravenous, oral, and rectal) or the use of a computed tomographic enema allows an even more precise localization of the level of obstruction. It can also distinguish between an intraluminal cause of obstruction and an extraluminal compression. For patients diagnosed with a mass, a CT scan can also evaluate for the presence of distant metastasis which are present in 10% of cases of obstruction cancer [14].

Guidelines [15] would still recommend the use of CT even when free air is identified on screening imaging in the stable patient. As mentioned, this allows for identification of the scope of the disease and facilitates operative planning. Routine inclusion of the chest to look for distant spread in the case of colon cancer is not indicated.

Another essential trait of CT is the ability to differential true obstruction from the pseudo-obstructions such as toxic megacolon, paralytic ileus, and Ogilvie's syndrome [16]. In these diagnoses you will see the distended colon, but there will be a failure to identify a transition point.

Hydrosoluble Contrast Enema

Hydrosoluble contrast enema has historically been used to further evaluate colonic obstructions with regard to the nature of and degree of patency. The observed sensitivity of a contrast enema in the diagnosis of colonic obstruction is 80%, with specificity of 100% [12, 17, 18]. With the continued evolution of CT, this study has also been relegated as obsolete. CT scans, specifically with the addition of rectal contrast, gives equivalent information on the location of the tumor but also gives a wider picture of the local and regional spread.

Colonoscopy

Colonoscopy has two benefits which are as follows: it allows a direct visualization and potential biopsy of the cause of obstruction. It has limited roles in acute processes but is essential in evaluating chronic obstructions where malignancy becomes the dominant etiology. It also has the ability to evaluate for synchronous lesions which are seen in 10% of cases. The drawback is the availability. Many centers require consultation to gastroenterology for assistance which can add time to the evaluation process in an acute situation. Having a tissue diagnosis is attractive, but often delays in those results require practitioners to intervene before they return. Endoscopic evaluation still has some potential preoperative roles. One situation that would alter this would be in near obstructing colon cancer where endoluminal stents can be placed and markedly changes the therapeutic options available. A second role would be for the decompression of sigmoid volvulus to allow for transition to a semi-elective case.

Table 13.1 AAST grading for large and small bowel obstruction

Grade	AAST disease grade description	Intestinal obstruction–small and large bowel
I	Local disease	Partial obstruction
	Confined to the organ	
	Minimal abnormality	
II	Local disease	Complete obstruction, without bowel ischemia
	Confined to the organ	
	Severe abnormality	
III	Beyond the organ	Complete obstruction, bowel ischemic but viable
	Locally extension	
IV	Beyond the organ	Complete obstruction with gangrenous bowel OR perforation with local spillage
	Regional extension	
V	Beyond the organ	Perforation with diffuse peritoneal contamination
	Widespread extension	

Staging

Staging for bowel obstruction historically fell into two buckets—high grade and low grade. The distinction between the two categories was thought to be important given that high-grade obstructions (i.e., complete obstruction) classically required surgery and low-grade obstructions (i.e., partial obstruction) were thought to mostly resolve without surgical intervention. As practices have evolved and treatments have become less operative in nature, that distinction has become less important.

In 2014, the AAST set out to establish a uniform grading system (Table 13.1) for bowel obstruction with the intent to standardize both diagnosis and disease severity [19]. We previously lacked a method to characterize obstructions across differing institutions and geographic locations. The hope was to provide a framework to assist in measuring risk-adjusted outcomes and improve management protocols within the emergency general surgery realm as a whole.

This grading system has been applied to clinical cases involving both small and large bowel obstruction as the principles in management remain incredibly similar [20]. While formal recommendations for treatment based on severity of disease were not included in the AAST grading scale, the construction would favor more operative intervention as the grade increased.

Specific Pathologic Considerations

Obstructing Colon Cancer

Acute large bowel obstruction is the initial presentation in 7–29% of patients with colorectal cancer and represents one of the more common causes of surgical emergency. The most common location for the obstructing colorectal cancer is the sigmoid colon, and >75% of tumors are located distal to the splenic flexure. Emergency presentation of colorectal cancer is more common in advanced stages of the disease and frequently occurs in elderly patients with significant comorbidities.

Although resection of the tumor is the "gold standard" for the treatment of malignant colonic obstruction, in the past two decades, self-expanding endoluminal colonic stents have been introduced in the therapeutic armamentarium as the initial maneuver in the management of distal colonic obstruction, aiming to relieve the obstruction and avoid emergency surgery. Surgery is proposed as a second-stage definitive treatment once the acute obstruction has been resolved. Several studies have shown the feasibility of managing acute malignant obstruction by colonic stenting. However, there is ongoing debate on the advantages of this strategy compared with emergency surgery in this scenario.

Treatment

Intervention falls into two large categories: operative and nonoperative. The operative intervention required is guided by the location and presentation of the obstruction. Nonoperative therapy which can include endoscopically based intervention is limited by the patient's physiology, the resources available to the surgeon, and the degree of obstruction.

Nonoperative Observation

A key component of nonoperative management is how long the obstruction can safely be observed without intervention. While the "hard deadline of sunset" has softened over time, there is little support for the 5–7-day period often seen in small bowel obstructions.

Initial management of the patient with mechanical colorectal obstruction consists of supportive care that includes gastric decompression for patients with nausea or vomiting and intravenous fluid therapy with correction of electrolyte abnormalities. Subsequent treatment depends upon the etiology and location of the obstruction, medical comorbidities of the patient, as well as local resources and expertise of the available clinicians. Unlike the majority of small bowel obstructions which can be successfully managed nonoperatively, approximately 75 percent of large bowel obstructions ultimately require surgical intervention, whether emergently, urgently, or electively during the same hospital admission.

Endoscopic Intervention: Benign Disease

For patients with imaging signs of sigmoid volvulus, gastroenterology/colorectal surgery consultation should be obtained. Flexible sigmoidoscopy is generally suggested to initially decompress the colon to allow for semi-elective surgery (rather than as an emergency) and may be the only treatment necessary in high-risk patients. However, for patients able to tolerate an operation, elective resection during the same hospital stay is recommended for sigmoid volvulus because of the high rate of recurrence (up to 50 percent) with endoscopic decompression alone.

Endoscopic Intervention: Malignant Disease

The primary therapeutic use of endoscopy in the acute setting, much like in benign disease, is to convert emergent surgery to semi-elective surgery. The hope is that this would decrease the morbidity and mortality as emergent surgery almost universally carries an increased risk regardless of pathology. Colonic stents can be placed for two indications: palliation and as a bridge to semi-elective surgery. In the acute setting, which indication is being followed is unclear as some patients are not determined to be palliative until after the intervention. The concept of using stents as a "bridge to surgery" has become popular and is well-studied. The numerous case series have been combined into two systemic reviews, one with 598 patients [21] and one with 1198 patients [22]. These studies establish stenting as highly successful (>92%) and with low associated complications (perforation 3.7%). In a retrospective analysis of 5868 colostomies compared with 778 stents, the authors concluded that stent placement is less costly and associated with shorter length of hospital stay and fewer complications [23]. There are at least six existing randomized studies [24–29] on the topic. The variation in who received a stent coupled with the high rate of the studies being stopped early (three of six) makes a definitive statement difficult. When compared stent to emergent resection, most of the studies show equivalence. The attractive part of the stent is the association in the studies with an increased rate or primary anastomosis in the stent groups. Cheung et al. [25] showed that stenting leads to 67% of those patient being able to undergo successful laparoscopic single-stage surgery. The effect of stenting on anastomotic leak has had the opposite effect in two of the studies. Van Hooft et al. [29] showed leak rates 5 times greater in the stent group while Alcantara et al. [24] lower leak rates in the stent group (30.7% vs 0%).

In terms of oncologic outcomes, it would seem the outcomes are equivalent. There have been some noted differences in lymphatic invasion but that has not resulted in differences in long-term outcomes when used alone [30] or compared with emergency surgery [31–34].

Operative Intervention

Once the decision to proceed with surgical intervention has been made, the key point that must be determined is if an anastomosis will be done at the index operation or if a multistage plan is adopted. Regardless of the underling etiology, there is risk involved in creating a primary anastomosis. Two decades ago the default in unprepped colon resections was an ostomy. Historically, the leak rates of primary anastomoses were up to 50% and drove the decision to do multistage inventions. Modern leak rates are around 5% or slightly higher in the EGS population. The trauma literature was some of the first to describe how one-stage interventions in unprepped bowel could be performed. Also, the very utility of a preoperative bowel prep has been questioned with various colorectal studies reporting that they may not be helpful and could potentially be harmful. Finally, a greater understanding of the morbidity in ostomy takedowns which were usually thought as "risk free" now has been shown to have significant complications. All the above have moved toward a greater willingness to perform one-stage operations. Regardless of malignant or benign, there are some common surgical considerations.

Preoperative Bowel Preparation

Current recommendations do not advocate for the any type of bowel preparation (preoperative or intraoperative) prior to proceeding with emergency colon surgery for mechanical colorectal obstruction. The absence of mechanical bowel preparation is **not** a contraindication to primary anastomosis [35].

Bowel preparation can be considered but is not supported by evidence-based medicine. Numerous small studies show that successful bowel preparation with combined oral and mechanical bowel preparation prior to elective colorectal resections decreases rates of complications [36, 37]. This must be balanced against a large Cochrane analysis [38] of 18 trials with 5805 patients comparing preoperative bowel preparation in elective colon resection (2906 mechanical bowel preparation and 2899 without preperation) showing that mechanical bowel preparation has no effect on the rates of deep and superficial surgical site infections or, most importantly, anastomotic leaks. Currently bowel preparation would only be indicated when the surgeon plans of doing a simultaneous colonoscopy.

Benign Disease

In general, the surgical principles that apply to the malignant obstructions are true in benign disease as well. Whenever possible, a one-stage curative procedure is the preferred treatment for right- or left-sided colon obstruction, whether benign or malignant [39, 40]. There are some specific considerations such as mega-rectum in sigmoid volvulus cases where continuity will not improve the patient's quality of life, but for the most part one- or two-stage procedures are the norm in benign disease. The DIVERTI trial addressed the resection in perforated diverticulitis where a two-stage (proximal diversion) intervention was performed. They showed that two-stage was the safest choice. While not the exact population as the large bowel obstruction described in this chapter, it does outline the baseline in modern times. It is difficult to imagine a patient in current times that resection, anastomosis, and loop ileostomy for diversion would not be considered the default operation performed. Future literature should consider which patients can have the loop ileostomy omitted as studies with an arm that includes three-stage procedures or Hartman's procedures would be antiquated. Those procedures would be reserved for special anatomic situations.

Malignant Obstruction

Two groups of patients can be defined according to the location of the tumor with respect to the splenic flexure: those with proximal and distal obstructions. The choice of surgery will depend on the location of the obstruction, the general condition of the patient, the surgical findings, and the experience or resources of the hospital team.

Proximal Colonic Obstruction

Right hemicolectomy has been accepted as the treatment of choice for tumors proximal to the splenic flexure. A primary anastomosis between the small bowel and the colon has been considered safe in the emergency setting, with published anastomotic leak rates of 2.8–4.6% [18].

While a primary anastomosis is still the operation of choice, literature does bring into question who and how these operations should be done. Frago and colleagues examined a cohort of patient undergoing emergent colectomy (defined as occurring in the first 24 h) and found a leak rate of 16.4% on the 173 patients who underwent resection and primary anastomosis for proximal colonic cancer obstruction [41]. These authors highlighted the difference in leak rates between colorectal surgeons (those that had done an additional year of training) and general surgeons (colorectal 5.8% and general surgery 21%, $p < 0.05$). Interestingly the distal resection, which would be considered the more technically challenging operations that would benefit from colorectal training, did not show a difference in leak rates (6.3% colorectal and 8.9% in general surgery). These and other similar data have been used to suggest that these operations should be done by colorectal surgeons. These manuscripts do often not include data about the physiology in the patient groups and even less about the availability of the colorectal surgeons on nights and weekends. It is clear from emerging data that emergency general surgery patients have unique physiology and comorbidities and that these differences lead to markedly different outcomes [42]. In order to mitigate these poor outcomes, the acute care surgeon will need to adapt their techniques. In a single institution experience, Farrah et al. [43] showed leak rates could be decreased by performing a handsewn anastomosis rather than a stapled one (15.1% in the stapled vs 6.1% in the handsewn, $p = 0.003$). In the small bowel to colon anastomoses, the overall leak rate was similar to that presented in the colorectal literature of 14.7%, but when comparing stapled vs handsewn anastomoses, the leak could be decreased (18% stapled vs 10% handsewn, $p = 0.4$). Similar data was seen in a subsequent multi-institutional trial where the leak rates were not different despite the handsewn cohort having significantly lower albumin and higher lactate and were more likely to be on vasopressors [44] (Fig. 13.2).

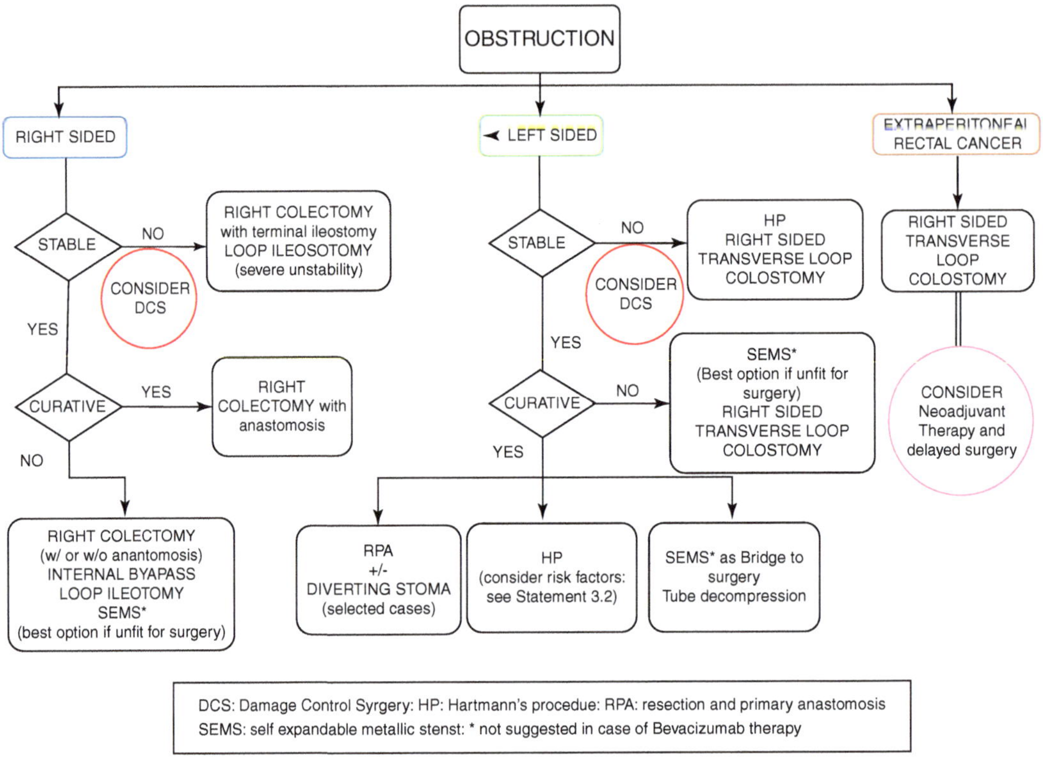

Fig. 13.2 Flowchart for the management of colonic obstruction due to colorectal cancer [15]

Distal Colonic Obstruction

The traditional surgical intervention was a three-stage procedure (proximal colostomy, second-stage tumor resection, and third-stage stoma closure) which has largely been relegated to being obsolete outside of extremely rare anatomic or physiologic situations. The issue is whether three low-risk interventions are better than one higher-risk operation. The literature has shown that staged resection does not improve survival and is instead associated with high morbidity and mortality rates [12, 17, 18, 39, 41, 45]. While many surgeons would still favor a two-stage procedure for high-risk patients, the literature has focused on what factors impart this increased risk and how they can be minimized. Most current research efforts examine which patients can safely undergo a one-stage procedure.

Prognostic factors for mortality in colonic obstruction have been identified: preoperative renal failure, American Society of Anesthesiologists class 3 or 4, and proximal colon lesions. The presence of all these factors could influence the choice of surgical technique.

There remain unique clinical situations where one-, two-, and three-stage procedures could be employed and where minimally invasive techniques could be utilized to improve outcomes. The surgical options available and the situations where they would be employed are the following.

The Three-Stage Management

While thought of as a "safe" surgery or a conservative intervention, this pathway has actually been proven to harm patients. Due to the morbidity of multiple interventions, increased complications have been shown in a comprehensive

Cochrane review [17] and in a prospective randomized trial. Kronberg and colleagues [46] showed similar oncologic outcomes and perioperative outcomes but shorter hospital days which is similar to the Cochrane results.

Currently, the role for three-stage intervention is limited to patient whose low rectal cancer advanced tumor characteristics would benefit from neoadjuvant treatment. It is also used for unresectable tumors or patients who are prohibitive operative risks. It could potentially be done under local anesthesia minimizing operative stress. The patient then can be evaluated to see if they can be made into an operative candidate to undergo definitive therapy.

Hartmann's Procedure (Two-Stage Procedure)

A Hartmann's procedure or two-stage procedure is still the preferred operation in emergent settings of distal obstructing tumors [47–49]. It allows cancer removal but avoids an anastomosis.

The comparison of two-stage procedures to others is complicated by the number of ostomies that are reversed and the wide range of reported complications with ostomy takedown. After a Hartmann's procedure is performed, only about 60% of ostomies are reversed due to age or comorbidities [17]. The morbidity (5–57%) and mortality (0–34%) varies greatly making determinations about the total complications difficult to determine [50].

Resection and Primary Anastomosis

The most attractive intervention is the one-stage procedure which minimizes hospital stays and all of the complications of subsequent operations. Surgical dogma has prevented progress in this area for many years, but recent studies have supported one-stage as a safe alternative [49, 51].

Efforts have focused on risk factors that would make one-stage intervention unsafe. There is data that supports primary anastomosis is feasible in both proximal and distal lesions [52, 53]. The factors that have been associated with anastomotic complications and may preclude one-stage intervention are malnutrition, chronic renal failure, and immunosuppression.

Mortality and anastomotic leak cannot be separated, and the risk of mortality has reproducibly been shown to be increased with age, ASA classification, operative urgency, and Duke's classification [47, 54, 55]. The decision to do a primary anastomosis or a stoma is often determined by real-time surgeon assessment. The main technical factors are a tension-free anastomosis and preservation of the blood supply to the anastomosis. If these two cannot be accomplished, then the surgeon should consider a stoma. The rate of leaks on the right side varies from 0.5 to 4.6% in perforated emergency cases and should be compared with 0.5–1.4% reported for elective surgery. Distal resection rates range from 3.5 to 30% in emergency versus 5–10% in elective cases [41, 56].

Subtotal Colectomy with Ileosigmoid or Ileorectal Anastomosis

One option to increase the safety of one-stage operation is to do a subtotal colectomy [14]. This avoids the colocolic anastomosis and eliminates the chance of missing a synchronous right side lesion in an unevaluated colon. Studies have shown that in patients with colonic obstruction, the leak rate is lower in ileocolic anastomosis than a colocolic anastomosis (<10% vs 18–20%) [14, 57].

The main drawback would be the incidence of diarrhea after surgery. There is evidence that 6 months out the functional difference between subtotal and segmental resection is minimal, 2 versus 3 bowel movements a day, but erratic follow-up and self-reported data may limit the validity of those outcomes [14]. In case of cecal perforation or ischemia and if synchronous neoplasms are present in the colon, this management is recommended [57]. There is data that leaving 10 cm of colon above the peritoneal reflection and resecting less than 10 cm of terminal ileum can result in less diarrhea [58].

Resection and Primary Anastomosis with Intraoperative "on Table" Irrigation

Surgeons have feared that the stool in the colon being anastomosed would lead to increased leak rates. There has been animal studies that have shown that intraluminal content is a larger predictor of anastomotic complications than peritonitis [59]. In patients who could not undergo preoperative bowel preparation, the surgeons would irrigate burden in patients undergoing colonic resection. While it makes some practical sense, the literature would not support it having any effect on complications [49, 51]. One potential use is if the surgeon intends to do a colonoscopy to look for synchronous lesions. The use of a lavage would allow for better visualization of the colon [60]. Much like preoperative bowel prep which has faded in terms of importance over the years, the importance of intraluminal stool burden has not been an important predictor of anastomotic complications. Many of the complications can be explained based on patient comorbidities and physiology rather than the presence or lack of stool.

Resection and Primary Anastomosis with Intraluminal Device

There is a variety of intraluminal devices that have been proposed to decrease the complication rates in high-risk anastomoses. Devices fell into a few categories such as decompression devices, intracolonic devices, and biodegradable devices. They were intended either to decompress the colon by stenting the sphincter open or to protect the anastomosis from being bathed in stool. In principle they may have value, but unfortunately they have not been shown to work, and their use is reserved to a few non evidence-based uses [61].

Resection and Primary Anastomosis with Proximal Diverting Stoma

The use of a loop ileostomy or colostomy to protect a distal anastomosis has been considered an alternative to Hartmann's procedure. There has been data in the perforated diverticulitis literature that proximal diversion is associated with a greater number of ostomies being reversed [62]. Data supporting proximal diversion in the malignant obstruction group has not been as supportive. In an American College of Surgeons' National Surgical Quality Improvement Program Procedure Targeted Colectomy databases study, 2323 patients with no diversion were compared to 204 patients with diversion. They found the diversion group was more likely to have complications (sepsis, blood transfusions, readmission within 30 days). It could be assumed that there was a large selection bias that not be accounted for in such a large retrospective database study but should give pause to the routine use of diverting ileostomy [63].

Laparoscopic Versus Open Resection

The concept of laparoscopic surgery for acute large bowel obstruction is relatively new. The literature in non-acute situations suggests shorter hospital stays and faster return to daily activities with equivalent if not superior oncologic outcomes [64, 65]. The adoption of laparoscopic surgery in the emergent setting has been slower. There have been case reports that suggest it is safe but without comparisons to open resection [66, 67].

Perforation

One situation to consider is colon cancers presenting perforated. Typically, these patients were associated with poor outcomes due to the fact they were often both septic and had advanced tumor characteristics. It is true that perioperative mortality is tied to the presence of perforation with free perforation having the highest mortality (19%) which is significantly higher than contained perforations and no perforation (0% and 5%, p.038) [2]. Despite worse oncologic resection characteristics, the 5-year survival is not predicted by the presence of perforation but, like

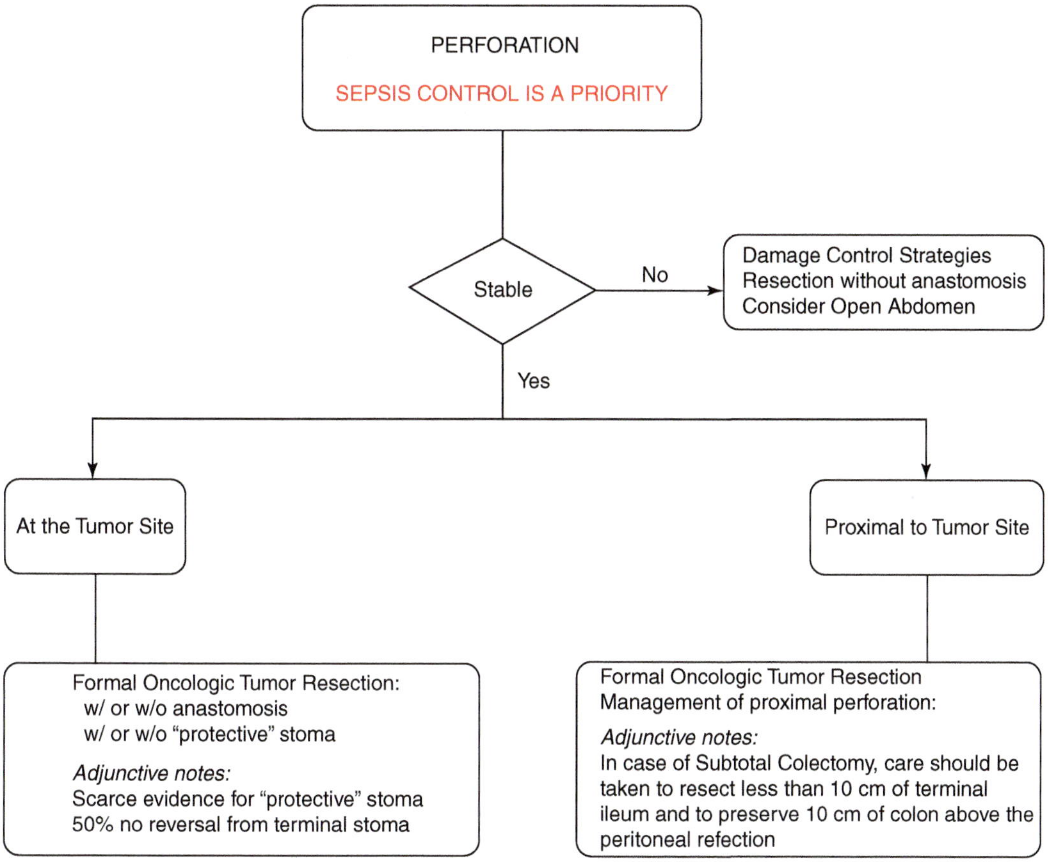

Fig. 13.3 Flowchart for the management of colonic perforation die to colorectal cancer [15]

most pathologies, is a by-product of the comorbidities and physiology [2]. The first priority must be control of the perforation with the completeness of the oncologic surgery taking a back seat. Sepsis is the most immediate threat to a perforated patients' life and is certainly time dependent (Fig. 13.3) [15].

Specific Surgical Considerations for Benign Disease

Sigmoid Volvulus

Any patient with volvulus presenting with signs of impaired intestinal blood flow or perforation should be taken to the operating room in an expeditious fashion following initiation of resuscitation and broad-spectrum IV antibiotics. Resection should ideally be performed without detorsion of the affected bowel segment to avoid unnecessary return of toxic waste products and bacterial load into the venous circulation [68]. When considering which operation to perform, whether it be a Hartmann's procedure or a segmental resection with colorectal anastomosis, one must take into consideration the physiologic status of the patient. In patients with hemodynamic instability or gross contamination secondary to perforation, a Hartmann's procedure is the preferred operation [69].

In stable patients with little to no enteric spillage, resection of the redundant colon with colorectal anastomosis is a reasonable option and has been shown to be a viable choice in large patient series [70].

The decision to create a protective ostomy should be based on comfort level of the surgeon while taking into consideration patient factors such as nutrition status, overall health, and level of the anastomosis.

The initial treatment of sigmoid volvulus, in the absence of ischemia or perforation, has largely been endoscopic. Detorsion is the necessary first step, either by sigmoidoscopy or colonoscopy, and has been reported to be successful in up to 95% of cases [69]. Long-term recurrence rates of volvulus have been quoted as high as 75% in some patient populations, necessitating definitive surgical management in appropriate surgical candidates. Following successful endoscopic detorsion, a rectal tube is often placed to allow for ongoing colonic decompression and to prevent retorsion prior to sigmoidectomy. Without overt signs of intestinal ischemia, it is acceptable to allow for a period of several days in order to completely resuscitate the patient and optimize from a medical standpoint prior to surgery.

Once the patient has been adequately prepared for surgery, a segmental sigmoid resection with colorectal anastomosis is the most appropriate procedure for definitive therapy. A protective ostomy is rarely utilized; however it may be necessary based on patient-specific factors such as age, level of contamination, and nutritional and hemodynamic status. Complete resection of all redundant colon is paramount to minimize risk of recurrent volvulus. Both laparoscopic and open methods have been utilized; however, there is no definitive evidence to suggest outcomes are improved when minimally invasive techniques are used. The theoretical benefit of reduced postoperative pain and decreased hospital length of stay have not borne out in the literature; however, the ultimate choice of technique should be based on surgeon experience and level of comfort [71, 72].

For those patients with high or unacceptable surgical risk, nonresectional techniques and nonsurgical management have both been described. Several small series have described low recurrence rates following both intraperitoneal and extraperitoneal sigmoidopexy; however this has not been validated through larger studies. In patients felt to be at high risk for anastomotic leak or who would not otherwise tolerate a formal resection, sigmoidopexy does remain an option but is generally not considered first-line therapy. For patients with comorbidities that are prohibitive to surgery, a consistent bowel regimen and dietary modifications have become the mainstay of therapy [69].

Cecal Volvulus

As in the case of sigmoid volvulus, immediate surgical intervention is necessary for any patient diagnosed with cecal volvulus and presenting with signs of intestinal ischemia or perforation. In contrast to sigmoid volvulus, endoscopic decompression is typically not recommended given that endoscopic intervention tends to be ineffective for this anatomic location and conveys a higher risk of bowel perforation. In any case involving nonviable bowel, the entirety of the involved segment should be removed, and the operative surgeon may [73, 74] elect to perform an ileocolic anastomosis plus or minus a diverting ileostomy or bring up an ileostomy with a long mucous fistula. The large majority of the data supporting these statements comes from studies published 20 years ago and are somewhat outdated. However, morbidity rates following cecectomy for volvulus are not insignificant, and in cases involving perforation or contamination, expert consensus continues to rely on the judgment of the independent surgeon in such circumstances.

Patients who present with cecal volvulus without signs of intestinal ischemia may be better suited for segmental resection. Unfortunately, the published data on this subset of patients is even less substantial. Several small case series report zero recurrence of cecal volvulus when segmental resection is performed, however carrying with it higher rates of associated morbidity and mortality compared to patients undergoing cecopexy alone. In otherwise healthy patients, segmental resection is the preferred method of treatment for cecal volvulus, while cecopexy may be reserved for patients with extensive medical comorbidities or comparatively higher operative risk.

Pseudo-Obstruction

Acute pseudo-obstruction is an entity most commonly described in older patients, residents of nursing homes, or hospitalized individuals following surgery and traumatic injury. It is crucial to rule out sources of mechanical obstruction, ischemia, and perforation prior to initiating therapy. While a diagnosis is typically made before bowel becomes compromised, those patients presenting in extremis, with perforation or with a cecal diameter >12 cm, will likely require immediate surgical intervention.

For stable patients, the treatment algorithm lies largely in reversing the underlying etiology. Initial steps involve hydration, correction of underlying electrolyte abnormalities, and avoidance of narcotic pain medications. Nasogastric and rectal tube decompression often provide moderate relief, and in some instances, anticholinergic agents may prove beneficial. Avoidance of osmotic agents and stimulant laxatives is generally encouraged as these can lead to worsening of symptoms. Up to 90% of cases will see complete resolution utilizing medical therapies and without requiring surgical intervention.

When conservative measures prove ineffectual or are otherwise contraindicated, endoscopic decompression is recommended as part of a step-up management scheme in the treatment of colonic pseudo-obstruction. The goal of endoscopic therapy is to access the right colon with minimal to no insufflation, placement of a decompression tube, and evacuation of gas. Most patients will resolve their pseudo-obstruction without further need for intervention and, once they begin to show signs of bowel recovery, will likely need dietary modifications and an appropriate bowel regimen. Additional endoscopic management includes percutaneous cecostomy tube placement. While the use of this technique has been controversial in the surgical community, there are no currently available studies which look at outcomes related to percutaneously placed cecostomy tubes specifically for colonic pseudo-obstruction. What we do know is that they are associated with a relatively high morbidity rate, nearly 40%, and are fraught with complications including dislodged tube, peritonitis, bleeding, infection, and buried bumper syndrome.

In general, percutaneous cecostomy tubes are to be avoided if possible. Surgical intervention remains the last line of defense in cecal pseudo-obstruction [73, 74].

Approximately 10% of patients with pseudo-obstruction will fail conservative measures and progress to need for surgery. Both mortality and morbidity rates increase substantially for those patients requiring surgical intervention; thus all efforts to relieve the pseudo-obstruction by non-surgical means is advised. Cecal dilation >14 cm and symptom duration >4 days are all associated with worse outcomes; however in certain instances, surgery cannot be avoided [75, 76].

Both surgical cecostomy and resection have been demonstrated in small case series to be of benefit, although there is no data directly comparing one method to the other. The choice of which procedure to perform will undoubtedly remain preference of the surgeon based on independent patient factors and the quality of the involved bowel at the time of the procedure.

Benign Stricture

There is a significant lack of published literature related to efficacy of treatment for benign colonic stricture. Given the wide variability in etiology of benign stricture, the exact cause of obstruction secondary to narrowing of the colonic lumen must be investigated thoroughly to rule out an acute process. Strictures related to an acute episode of inflammatory bowel disease such as Crohn's or ulcerative colitis can usually be addressed with immunomodulators and steroids. Other causes of stricture may not be as clinically obvious and warrant a more extensive workup.

The preferred method for treatment of benign stricture, similar to pseudo-obstruction, is a step-up approach where surgical intervention is reserved for those with complete obstruction, evidence of perforation, and peritonitis or those who fail conservative therapies. Several advanced endoscopy techniques now exist, allowing for a multidisciplinary approach to benign colonic stricture. Balloon dilation has been shown to be effective over the long term in >60% of patients and, although it carries a small risk of perforation, can generally be performed under light sedation [77].

It is considered a reasonable first step in patients presenting with both anastomotic and inflammatory strictures. Endoscopic administration of corticosteroid injections also serves as an adjunct to enhance the effectiveness of balloon dilation in Crohn's strictures. While the true efficacy has yet to be borne out in the literature, its theoretical benefit lies in avoiding repeat need for dilation.

Savary dilation is an alternative technique to endoscopy utilizing serial bougies over a fluoroscopically guided wire. Small series have suggested this is a cheaper technique when compared to balloon dilation, and while repeated intervention is occasionally necessary, most patients have excellent outcomes with very low-risk profiles [77].

Endoscopic stent placement has been a successful approach to strictures involving the proximal gastrointestinal tract. Its effectiveness in treating colonic strictures is less convincing. Often used to temporize obstructive symptoms related to malignancy, endoscopic stent placement for benign disease has not been as effective [77].

The risk of stent occlusion, migration, and perforation seem to outweigh any potential benefit, and larger prospective trials have not been pursued as a result.

Colonic Anastomosis in Open Abdomen

For many years, the principles of damage control surgery have been incorporated into treatment algorithms for the emergency general surgery population [78]. Despite their underlying fundamental differences, patients presenting with severe physiologic derangement secondary to late complications of intra-abdominal sepsis and hemorrhage often require laparotomy with immediate source control and temporary abdominal closure similar to their trauma counterparts [79]. The utility of damage control principles and the ultimate outcome is not nearly as well studied in the EGS population as it has been in the trauma cohort. This includes abdominal closure rates and when is the optimal timing to restore intestinal continuity. The decision between colostomy creation and a colonic anastomosis has yet to be definitely proven in the scientific literature and remains largely a practice based upon surgeon-specific experience and judgment.

Given the paucity of data relating to these scenarios specifically in the emergency general surgery population, evidence-based decisions must be extrapolated from more heterogeneous studies. In patients undergoing laparotomy for intra-abdominal sepsis or hemorrhage, all reasonable attempts should be made to avoid leaving the abdomen open as it is associated with significant morbidity and mortality. Mortality rates associated with open abdomen have been quoted as high as 35% in the non-trauma population with notable rates of severe complications such as enteroatmospheric fistula, intra-abdominal abscess, hernia, and delayed fascial closure [80]. While there has been concern regarding historical overuse of the open abdomen, there are certainly instances in which such a management scheme is necessary. Once a decision has been made to leave an abdomen open following intestinal resection, the dilemma becomes one of either performing an anastomosis or creating an ostomy to restore continuity.

Several patient-specific factors should help guide the decision to create a colostomy or to perform a colonic anastomosis. In patients with significant medical comorbidities, short life expectancy or intra-abdominal pathology such as significant intra-abdominal contamination, near-frozen abdomen, or destructive perforations with significant tissue loss, colostomy creation may be unavoidable. Patients with persistent physiologic derangements such as shock state, ongoing large volume crystalloid or blood product resuscitation, and ongoing intestinal ischemia may also necessitate colostomy creation given that ultimate closure of the abdominal wall should be a priority and occur in as timely a fashion as possible to reduce rates of complication. Abdominal compartments that are left open for second look surgery and in patients where physiologic stability has been established, the decision to restore intestinal continuity is multifactorial.

In 2010, Ordonez et al. [81] retrospectively analyzed a series of 112 patients undergoing laparotomy for intra-abdominal sepsis. All patients had bowel resection performed and were managed with an open abdomen with temporary abdominal closure. A total of 34 patients underwent primary anastomosis, while the remaining 78 patients had a diverting ostomy created. There was no significant difference demonstrated in hospital mortality, anastomotic leak rate, or development of fistula. A subsequent prospective analysis of 51 patients treated with open abdomen for perforated diverticulitis, 38 patients underwent primary anastomosis with the remainder treated with a diverting stoma [82]. The overall mortality rate for the study was 10% which is consistent across patients treated with open abdomen, and >75% of the surviving patients were discharged from the hospital with intestinal continuity restored.

Both of these studies, along with several others, have demonstrated the relative safety of performing a primary colonic anastomosis in an open abdomen with the condition that adequate source control has been obtained and the patient has been appropriately resuscitated without ongoing physiologic derangement prior to restoring continuity.

For the patients who do ultimately require ostomy creation, surgeons must decide the optimal placement within the abdominal wall. Given that the majority of patients undergoing laparotomy in a damage control scenarios are by definition an emergent procedure, very little preoperative planning is likely to take place. Hernia rates in patients requiring emergent laparotomy often exceed 20% 1 year after their initial surgery [83]. Many of these patients go on to require additional surgery, especially in those with colostomy creation and subsequent takedown. These same patients are at higher risk for repeat laparotomy for adhesive bowel obstructions and incarcerated hernias. Complex abdominal wall reconstruction has become the mainstay in treatment of patients who have undergone multiple prior abdominal wall surgeries. The approach to these procedures is further complicated by the various tissue planes that have been disrupted during prior surgery.

To the extent possible, all patients who are to undergo laparotomy should ideally be marked for ideal stoma placement preoperatively. With increasing preponderance of obesity in the general population, and the difficulty in managing an ostomy in the outpatient setting, it is generally recommended that ostomies be sited above the belt line where abdominal wall thickness is minimized and should avoid natural skin creases [84]. Function takes precedence over appearance and aesthetics. Placement through the rectus muscle itself assists in prevention in stoma retraction and development of parastomal hernias. However, despite best intentions, many patients with ostomy creation and/or takedown will go on to develop large, complex ventral hernias and may require abdominal wall reconstruction.

Thankfully, in the last decade, techniques in abdominal wall reconstruction and hernia repair have made significant advancements including laparoscopic and robotic approaches. While the presence of a prior ostomy may add a certain level of complexity to an abdominal wall reconstruction, a retrospective study of 169 patients over 8 years showed that outcomes in abdominal wall reconstruction specifically utilizing a component separation technique were no different between those with rectus complex violation and those without [85]. Being mindful and intentional with ostomy siting is essential in the surgical process, but the site does not preclude patients from reconstruction at a later point in time.

Palliative Patients

Three randomized prospective trials [86–88] have compared the use of stents versus diverting ostomies in palliative patients with obstruction from unresectable colorectal cancer. In general all three favor stents with positive effect being shorter hospital stays, earlier return to a diet, and improved quality of life. There were concerns in one of the studies [87] about the rate of perforations with stents, but this has not been viewed as prohibitive reason to avoid stents.

Overall survival in palliative patients who have stents placed compared to surgery has had mixed results. While stents have been associated with shorter hospital stays, lower rates of stoma creation, [45, 89] and an earlier start of chemotherapy, they have been unable to show increased survival. To the contrary, studies have shown resection of the primary tumor was associated with a better prognosis compared with the stent group [45, 90]. A mean survival rate of 15.9–23.7 months was observed in the resection group compared with 4.4–7.6 months in the stent group.

Conclusions

Colonic obstruction still remains a time-sensitive diagnosis that requires timely intervention to optimize patient outcomes. Endoscopic interventions such as stents have increased the options on hand, but the evidence is not convincing enough to exclude the need for surgical intervention. In general, surgery has move toward a one-stage procedure with two-stage procedure being the exception. Adjuvants such as bowel preparation and diverting proximal ostomies have limited use and have not been associated with improved outcomes. To the contrary primary anastomosis even in unprepped bowel has been shown to be safe. Benign disease continues to follow classic teaching. Most surgeons would treat adhesive disease and benign strictures the same as their malignant counterparts. If physiology permits, left-sided volvulus should be decompressed to allow for a semi-elective surgical intervention. Given that right hemicolectomy with primary anastomosis is the treatment of right-sided volvulus, surgery should proceed based on patient physiology.

References

1. Arezzo A, et al. Stent as bridge to surgery for left-sided malignant colonic obstruction reduces adverse events and stoma rate compared with emergency surgery: results of a systematic review and meta-analysis of randomized controlled trials. Gastrointest Endosc. 2017;86(3):416–26.
2. Zielinski MD, et al. Emergency management of perforated colon cancers: how aggressive should we be? J Gastrointest Surg. 2011;15(12):2232–8.
3. Deans GT, Krukowski ZH, Irwin ST. Malignant obstruction of the left colon. Br J Surg. 1994;81(9):1270–6.
4. Halabi WJ, et al. Colonic volvulus in the United States: trends, outcomes, and predictors of mortality. Ann Surg. 2014;259(2):293–301.
5. Jones DJ. ABC of colorectal diseases. Large bowel volvulus. BMJ. 1992;305(6849):358–60.
6. Lau KC, et al. A study of large-bowel volvulus in urban Australia. Can J Surg. 2006;49(3):203–7.
7. Vandendries C, et al. Diagnosis of colonic volvulus: findings on multidetector CT with three-dimensional reconstructions. Br J Radiol. 2010;83(995):983–90.
8. Kahi CJ, Rex DK. Bowel obstruction and pseudo-obstruction. Gastroenterol Clin N Am. 2003;32(4):1229–47.
9. Atamanalp SS. Sigmoid volvulus: Diagnosis in 938 patients over 45.5 years. Tech Coloproctol. 2013;17(4):419–24.
10. Taourel P, et al. Helical CT of large bowel obstruction. Abdom Imaging. 2003;28(2):267–75.
11. Chen SC, et al. Ultrasonography is superior to plain radiography in the diagnosis of pneumoperitoneum. Br J Surg. 2002;89(3):351–4.
12. Frager D, et al. Prospective evaluation of colonic obstruction with computed tomography. Abdom Imaging. 1998;23(2):141–6.
13. Gerhardt RT, et al. Derivation of a clinical guideline for the assessment of nonspecific abdominal pain: the guideline for abdominal pain in the ED setting (GAPEDS) phase 1 study. Am J Emerg Med. 2005;23(6):709–17.
14. Hennekinne-Mucci S, et al. Emergency subtotal/total colectomy in the management of obstructed left colon carcinoma. Int J Color Dis. 2006;21(6):538–41.
15. Pisano M, et al. 2017 WSES guidelines on colon and rectal cancer emergencies: obstruction and perforation. World J Emerg Surg. 2018;13:36.
16. Hayakawa K, et al. Radiological diagnosis of large-bowel obstruction: nonneoplastic etiology. Jpn J Radiol. 2012;30(7):541–52.
17. De Salvo GL, et al. Curative surgery for obstruction from primary left colorectal carcinoma: primary or staged resection? Cochrane Database Syst Rev. 2004;2:CD002101.

18. Gainant A. Emergency management of acute colonic cancer obstruction. J Visc Surg. 2012;149(1):e3–e10.
19. Shafi S, et al. Measuring anatomic severity of disease in emergency general surgery. J Trauma Acute Care Surg. 2014;76(3):884–7.
20. Hernandez MC, et al. The American Association for the Surgery of Trauma Severity Grade is valid and generalizable in adhesive small bowel obstruction. J Trauma Acute Care Surg. 2018;84(2):372–8.
21. Khot UP, et al. Systematic review of the efficacy and safety of colorectal stents. Br J Surg. 2002;89(9):1096–102.
22. Sebastian S, et al. Pooled analysis of the efficacy and safety of self-expanding metal stenting in malignant colorectal obstruction. Am J Gastroenterol. 2004;99(10):2051–7.
23. Varadarajulu S, et al. Endoscopic stenting versus surgical colostomy for the management of malignant colonic obstruction: comparison of hospital costs and clinical outcomes. Surg Endosc. 2011;25(7):2203–9.
24. Alcantara M, et al. Prospective, controlled, randomized study of intraoperative colonic lavage versus stent placement in obstructive left-sided colonic cancer. World J Surg. 2011;35(8):1904–10.
25. Cheung HY, et al. Endolaparoscopic approach vs conventional open surgery in the treatment of obstructing left-sided colon cancer: a randomized controlled trial. Arch Surg. 2009;144(12):1127–32.
26. Ghazal AH, et al. Colonic endolumenal stenting devices and elective surgery versus emergency subtotal/total colectomy in the management of malignant obstructed left colon carcinoma. J Gastrointest Surg. 2013;17(6):1123–9.
27. Ho KS, et al. Endoscopic stenting and elective surgery versus emergency surgery for left-sided malignant colonic obstruction: a prospective randomized trial. Int J Color Dis. 2012;27(3):355–62.
28. Pirlet IA, et al. Emergency preoperative stenting versus surgery for acute left-sided malignant colonic obstruction: a multicenter randomized controlled trial. Surg Endosc. 2011;25(6):1814–21.
29. van Hooft JE, et al. Colonic stenting versus emergency surgery for acute left-sided malignant colonic obstruction: a multicentre randomised trial. Lancet Oncol. 2011;12(4):344–52.
30. Iversen LH, et al. Self-expanding metallic stents as bridge to surgery in obstructing colorectal cancer. Br J Surg. 2011;98(2):275–81.
31. Dastur JK, et al. Comparison of short-and long-term outcomes following either insertion of self-expanding metallic stents or emergency surgery in malignant large bowel obstruction. Tech Coloproctol. 2008;12(1):51–5.
32. Kavanagh DO, et al. A comparative study of short- and medium-term outcomes comparing emergent surgery and stenting as a bridge to surgery in patients with acute malignant colonic obstruction. Dis Colon Rectum. 2013;56(4):433–40.
33. Saida Y, et al. Long-term prognosis of preoperative "bridge to surgery" expandable metallic stent insertion for obstructive colorectal cancer: comparison with emergency operation. Dis Colon Rectum. 2003;46(10 Suppl):S44–9.
34. Tilney HS, et al. Comparison of colonic stenting and open surgery for malignant large bowel obstruction. Surg Endosc. 2007;21(2):225–33.
35. Jimenez Fuertes M, Costa Navarro D. Resection and primary anastomosis without diverting ileostomy for left colon emergencies: is it a safe procedure? World J Surg. 2012;36(5):1148–53.
36. Kiran RP, et al. Combined preoperative mechanical bowel preparation with oral antibiotics significantly reduces surgical site infection, anastomotic leak, and ileus after colorectal surgery. Ann Surg. 2015;262(3):416–25; discussion 423–5.
37. Scarborough JE, et al. Combined mechanical and oral antibiotic bowel preparation reduces incisional surgical site infection and anastomotic leak rates after elective colorectal resection: an analysis of colectomy-targeted ACS NSQIP. Ann Surg. 2015;262(2):331–7.
38. Guenaga KF, Matos D, Wille-Jorgensen P. Mechanical bowel preparation for elective colorectal surgery. Cochrane Database Syst Rev. 2011;9:CD001544.
39. Breitenstein S, et al. Systematic evaluation of surgical strategies for acute malignant left-sided colonic obstruction. Br J Surg. 2007;94(12):1451–60.
40. Deen KI, et al. Surgical management of left colon obstruction: the University of Minnesota experience. J Am Coll Surg. 1998;187(6):573–6.
41. Frago R, et al. Differences between proximal and distal obstructing colonic cancer after curative surgery. Color Dis. 2011;13(6):e116–22.
42. Becher RD, et al. A critical assessment of outcomes in emergency versus nonemergency general surgery using the American College of Surgeons National Surgical Quality Improvement Program database. Am Surg. 2011;77(7):951–9.
43. Farrah JP, et al. Stapled versus hand-sewn anastomoses in emergency general surgery: a retrospective review of outcomes in a unique patient population. J Trauma Acute Care Surg. 2013;74(5):1187–92; discussion 1192-4.
44. Bruns BR, et al. Stapled versus hand-sewn: a prospective emergency surgery study. An American Association for the Surgery of Trauma multi-institutional study. J Trauma Acute Care Surg. 2017;82(3):435–43.
45. Lee WS, et al. The outcome after stent placement or surgery as the initial treatment for obstructive primary tumor in patients with stage IV colon cancer. Am J Surg. 2012;203(6):715–9.
46. Kronborg O. Acute obstruction from tumour in the left colon without spread. Int J Color Dis. 1995;10(1):1–5.
47. Biondo S, et al. Large bowel obstruction: predictive factors for postoperative mortality. Dis Colon Rectum. 2004;47(11):1889–97.
48. Meyer F, et al. Emergency operation in carcinomas of the left colon: value of Hartmann's procedure. Tech Coloproctol. 2004;8(Suppl 1):s226–9.

49. Trompetas V. Emergency management of malignant acute left-sided colonic obstruction. Ann R Coll Surg Engl. 2008;90(3):181–6.
50. Frago R, et al. Current management of acute malignant large bowel obstruction: a systematic review. Am J Surg. 2014;207(1):127–38.
51. Ortiz H, et al. Comparative study to determine the need for intraoperative colonic irrigation for primary anastomosis in left-sided colonic emergencies. Color Dis. 2009;11(6):648–52.
52. Hsu TC. Comparison of one-stage resection and anastomosis of acute complete obstruction of left and right colon. Am J Surg. 2005;189(4):384–7.
53. Chiappa A, et al. One-stage resection and primary anastomosis following acute obstruction of the left colon for cancer. Am Surg. 2000;66(7):619–22.
54. Tekkis PP, et al. The Association of Coloproctology of Great Britain and Ireland study of large bowel obstruction caused by colorectal cancer. Ann Surg. 2004;240(1):76–81.
55. Zorcolo L, et al. Toward lowering morbidity, mortality, and stoma formation in emergency colorectal surgery: the role of specialization. Dis Colon Rectum. 2003;46(11):1461–7; discussion 1467-8.
56. Veyrie N, et al. Anastomotic leakage after elective right versus left colectomy for cancer: prevalence and independent risk factors. J Am Coll Surg. 2007;205(6):785–93.
57. Single-stage treatment for malignant left-sided colonic obstruction: a prospective randomized clinical trial comparing subtotal colectomy with segmental resection following intraoperative irrigation. The SCOTIA Study Group. Subtotal colectomy versus on-table irrigation and anastomosis. Br J Surg. 1995;82(12):1622–7.
58. Papa MZ, et al. Avoiding diarrhea after subtotal colectomy with primary anastomosis in the treatment of colon cancer. J Am Coll Surg. 1997;184(3):269–72.
59. Ravo B, et al. The importance of intraluminal anastomotic fecal contact and peritonitis in colonic anastomotic leakages. An experimental study. Dis Colon Rectum. 1988;31(11):868–71.
60. Sasaki K, et al. One-stage segmental colectomy and primary anastomosis after intraoperative colonic irrigation and total colonoscopy for patients with obstruction due to left-sided colorectal cancer. Dis Colon Rectum. 2012;55(1):72–8.
61. Morks AN, Havenga K, Ploeg RJ. Can intraluminal devices prevent or reduce colorectal anastomotic leakage: a review. World J Gastroenterol. 2011;17(40):4461–9.
62. Bridoux V, et al. Hartmann's procedure or primary anastomosis for generalized peritonitis due to perforated diverticulitis: a prospective multicenter randomized trial (DIVERTI). J Am Coll Surg. 2017;225(6):798–805.
63. Shwaartz C, et al. Should patients with obstructing colorectal cancer have proximal diversion? Am J Surg. 2017;213(4):742–7.
64. Guillou PJ, et al. Short-term endpoints of conventional versus laparoscopic-assisted surgery in patients with colorectal cancer (MRC CLASICC trial): multicentre, randomised controlled trial. Lancet. 2005;365(9472):1718–26.
65. McLeod RS, Stern H, C.E.B.R.i.S. Group. Canadian Association of General Surgeons Evidence Based Reviews in surgery. 10. Laparoscopy-assisted colectomy versus open colectomy for treatment of non-metastatic colon cancer: a randomized trial. Can J Surg. 2004;47(3):209–11.
66. Dudley HA, Racliffe AG, McGeehan D. Intraoperative irrigation of the colon to permit primary anastomosis. Br J Surg. 1980;67(2):80–1.
67. Gash K, et al. The role of laparoscopic surgery for the management of acute large bowel obstruction. Color Dis. 2011;13(3):263–6.
68. Madiba TE, Thomson SR. The management of cecal volvulus. Dis Colon Rectum. 2002;45(2):264–7.
69. Vogel JD, et al. Clinical practice guidelines for colon volvulus and acute colonic pseudo-obstruction. Dis Colon Rectum. 2016;59(7):589–600.
70. Atamanalp SS. Treatment of sigmoid volvulus: a single-center experience of 952 patients over 46.5 years. Tech Coloproctol. 2013;17(5):561–9.
71. Basato S, et al. Comparison of two surgical techniques for resection of uncomplicated sigmoid volvulus: laparoscopy or open surgical approach? J Visc Surg. 2014;151(6):431–4.
72. Cartwright-Terry T, et al. Laparoscopy in the management of closed loop sigmoid volvulus. Color Dis. 2008;10(4):370–2.
73. Benacci JC, Wolff BG, Cecostomy. Therapeutic indications and results. Dis Colon Rectum. 1995;38(5):530–4.
74. Bertolini D, et al. Severe delayed complication after percutaneous endoscopic colostomy for chronic intestinal pseudo-obstruction: a case report and review of the literature. World J Gastroenterol. 2007;13(15):2255–7.
75. Vanek VW, Al-Salti M. Acute pseudo-obstruction of the colon (Ogilvie's syndrome). An analysis of 400 cases. Dis Colon Rectum. 1986;29(3):203–10.
76. Jain A, Vargas HD. Advances and challenges in the management of acute colonic pseudo-obstruction (Ogilvie syndrome). Clin Colon Rectal Surg. 2012;25(1):37–45.
77. Kwon YH, Jeon SW, Lee YK. Endoscopic management of refractory benign colorectal strictures. Clin Endosc. 2013;46(5):472–5.
78. Stawicki SP, et al. The concept of damage control: extending the paradigm to emergency general surgery. Injury. 2008;39(1):93–101.
79. Coccolini F, et al. The open abdomen in trauma and non-trauma patients: WSES guidelines. World J Emerg Surg. 2018;13:7.
80. Sartelli M, et al. The role of the open abdomen procedure in managing severe abdominal sepsis: WSES position paper. World J Emerg Surg. 2015;10:35.

81. Ordonez CA, et al. Deferred primary anastomosis versus diversion in patients with severe secondary peritonitis managed with staged laparotomies. World J Surg. 2010;34(1):169–76.
82. Kafka-Ritsch R, et al. Damage control surgery with abdominal vacuum and delayed bowel reconstruction in patients with perforated diverticulitis Hinchey III/IV. J Gastrointest Surg. 2012;16(10):1915–22.
83. Fink C, et al. Incisional hernia rate 3 years after midline laparotomy. Br J Surg. 2014;101(2):51–4.
84. Whitehead A, Cataldo PA. Technical considerations in stoma creation. Clin Colon Rectal Surg. 2017;30(3):162–71.
85. Garvey PB, et al. Violation of the rectus complex is not a contraindication to component separation for abdominal wall reconstruction. J Am Coll Surg. 2012;214(2):131–9.
86. Fiori E, et al. Palliative management of malignant rectosigmoidal obstruction. Colostomy vs. endoscopic stenting. A randomized prospective trial. Anticancer Res. 2004;24(1):265–8.
87. van Hooft JE, et al. Early closure of a multicenter randomized clinical trial of endoscopic stenting versus surgery for stage IV left-sided colorectal cancer. Endoscopy. 2008;40(3):184–91.
88. Xinopoulos D, et al. Stenting or stoma creation for patients with inoperable malignant colonic obstructions? Results of a study and cost-effectiveness analysis. Surg Endosc. 2004;18(3):421–6.
89. Watt AM, et al. Self-expanding metallic stents for relieving malignant colorectal obstruction: a systematic review. Ann Surg. 2007;246(1):24–30.
90. Frago R, et al. Outcomes in the management of obstructive unresectable stage IV colorectal cancer. Eur J Surg Oncol. 2010;36(12):1187–94.

14 Abdominal Wall Hernias

Jacob A. Quick, Lucas R. A. Beffa,
and Stephen L. Barnes

Case Presentation

A 45-year-old male presents to the emergency room with 3 days of worsening abdominal pain, nausea, and vomiting. He has a past medical history of hypertension, diabetes mellitus, and atrial fibrillation for which he takes aspirin. He has a previous surgical history of exploratory laparotomy 5 years ago for perforated diverticulitis resulting in a Hartmann's procedure. He then had colostomy reversal 6 months following that operation without incident. He developed an incisional hernia in the midline and underwent laparoscopic repair with an intraperitoneal mesh 3 years ago.

He is tachycardic, tachypneic, and hypotensive. His BMI is 42, and he has a non-reducible recurrent midline incisional hernia with surrounding skin erythema. He is exquisitely tender over the hernia which is unable to be manually reduced. He has a leukocytosis of 26,000/L, hemoglobin of 16 g/dL, and a high anion gap metabolic acidosis. CT imaging shows free fluid in an incarcerated incisional hernia with bowel obstruction. There is concern for possible bowel pneumatosis. There is a clear transition point in the hernia sac. No other acute abnormalities.

The patient is taken emergently to the operating room after appropriate fluid resuscitation where an exploratory laparotomy is performed. Strangulated small bowel is resected and primary anastomosis performed. The previous intraperitoneal mesh has been contaminated with succus. The decision was made not to remove the previous intraperitoneal mesh at the time of surgery. The hernia defect was assessed and found to be 15 cm wide and 26 cm in length. The remaining fascial defect was able to be closed, however, under tension.

Postoperative day 5, the patient develops redness and cellulitis of the incision. The wound is opened, and purulent material is drained. The following day, there continues to be significant drainage from the wound which now appears bilious in nature consistent with an enteroatmospheric fistula. CT imaging reveals fascial dehiscence with air and fluid surrounding

J. A. Quick (✉) · S. L. Barnes
University of Missouri, Columbia, MO, USA
e-mail: barnesste@health.missouri.edu

L. R. A. Beffa
Department of Surgery, University of Colorado School of Medicine, Denver, CO, USA
e-mail: Beffal@ccf.org

M. D. Zielinski, O. Guillamondegui (eds.), *The Acute Management of Surgical Disease*,
https://doi.org/10.1007/978-3-031-07881-1_14

the intraperitoneal mesh. The patient is taken back to the operating room where the anastomosis is resected, and healthy bowel is anastomosed in a two-layered hand-sewn fashion. The previous mesh was also removed. The fascia was able to be closed with absorbable suture primarily.

The patient improves and returns 1 month later with bulging under the incision. CT confirms recurrent hernia. The patient then undergoes abdominal wall reconstruction with permanent synthetic mesh in the retromuscular position after weight loss and improved control of his diabetes 6 months after the last operation.

Introduction

An abdominal hernia is defined as any defect in the abdominal wall. Hernias are common across the world, especially in the United States where an estimated 1 in 4 people will have a hernia during their lifetime [1]. Defects vary in both the cause and location of the hernia. There were an estimated 2.3 million inpatient abdominal hernias repaired in the United States from 2001 to 2010 [1]. The rate of acute hernia emergency varies depending on age, sex, and location of the hernia. In the United States, rates of emergent incisional hernia repair averaged 10 per 100,000 person-years from 2001 to 2010 [1]. Incisional hernias comprise the largest number of emergent repairs when compared to inguinal, femoral, or umbilical hernias. When performed emergently, hernia repairs are associated with a high recurrence, worse outcomes, and an increase in postoperative complications when compared to elective hernia surgery [2]. Emergent hernia repair remains a challenging problem faced by general surgeons. Seemingly simple, yet surprising complex, hernia surgery remains one of the most debated topics in the general surgery literature. Effective repair of hernias demand expert knowledge of anatomy and identification of the correct surgical planes.

When faced with a hernia emergency, there are multiple decisions to consider. The foremost priority is to deal with the acute problem, whether that be obstruction, strangulation, perforation, or peritonitis. Emergent hernia repairs are unique in that there are two issues to address: the first is to address the immediate threat to the patient's life and second to repair the hernia defect. This may result in a suture-only repair of the defect in the acute setting. Based on the size and complexity of the hernia, primary repair may not always be possible nor advisable. This begs the question, if a defect cannot be primarily closed, is a prosthetic repair favored? Patients with previous prosthetic hernia repairs become more complex and raise questions regarding management of the existing mesh prosthesis. These remain challenging questions for even the most experienced surgeons and have few straightforward answers.

Careful intraoperative decision-making is paramount to achieve optimal patient outcomes. The choice of repair becomes the focal point after addressing any threats to the patient's life. Mesh implantation may increase infection risk-contaminated fields. Conversely, if no mesh is used, the patient's risk of recurrent hernia and associated sequelae such as dehiscence may also be high. Further, definitive hernia repair may need to be delayed if a patient's physiology dictates resuscitation in the ICU. In select scenarios, it is in the patient's best interest to temporarily manage the defect and return to the operating suite at a later date for definitive repair.

The aim of this chapter is to provide evidence-based guidance for general surgeons to address acute hernia emergencies safely. The chapter will focus on presentation and diagnostic approach to acute hernias, as well as describe the intraoperative decision-making for different types of hernia. Finally, we'll discuss the role of prosthetic mesh in repairing acute hernias.

Hernia Presentation and Diagnostic Approach

Many patients with abdominal wall hernias are unaware of their existence until pain, obstruction, or disfigurement prompt investigation. Some will cite a single physical event, following which they noted a bulge or sharp pain, while others may describe a long-standing discomfort noticeable at the end of each day, which resolves with rest. Aside from pain, nonurgent hernias cause a wide array of nonspecific symptoms.

Incarceration occurs when a hernia cannot be reduced despite attempts to return the contents to peritoneal cavity. Incarceration is not always a surgical emergency, however. Many hernias are chronically incarcerated as scarring and adhesions develop within the hernia sac. These types of hernia, however, can progress acutely and require emergent operative intervention. Strangulation occurs when mesenteric blood flow is compromised. Mesenteric vessels, typically at the neck of a hernia, become compressed and/or twisted, leading to ischemia requiring emergency surgical intervention. It should be noted that venous outflow is obstructed first, leading to progressive venous engorgement and hastening the ischemic process.

Diagnosis of an acutely incarcerated or strangulated hernia begins with an accurate history and physical examination. Like most acute processes, the initial presenting symptom of acute hernia is typically pain. Pain may be sharp or dull and is regularly described as a "deep" pain that worsens with movement, coughing, or straining. Associated symptoms may include nausea, obstructive symptoms, or fever. Clinical signs in addition to a nonreducible bulge may include overlying skin changes, which often suggest strangulation. While a hernia may simply be defined as an abdominal wall defect, there are over 50 named hernias throughout the abdominal cavity, and each may present with their characteristic symptoms and have unique anatomy, approach, repair, and complications. Groin hernias may produce radiating pain to the scrotum, labia, or the thigh if a femoral or obturator hernia is present. Parastomal hernias will frequently be associated with ostomy prolapse and obstruction. Conversely, Richter's hernias commonly result in strangulation, but without obstruction, as they involve herniation of the antimesenteric border only. Spigelian hernias present below the umbilicus, lateral to the right rectus muscle. Occurring within the layers of the semilunar line, Spigelian hernias may not be associated with a mass as the hernia is contained beneath the external oblique fascia and frequently as acute intestinal obstruction. Diagnosis may be obscured by elements of the physical examination such as obesity, chronic scarring, and skin changes or other causes. In approximately one-quarter of patients, physical examination will fail to elucidate the presence of a hernia, and in these cases, additional diagnostic modalities may be beneficial in the acute setting [3].

Ultrasonography

Ultrasound is a viable diagnostic option for many patients. Inexpensive, and readily available, ultrasonography is widely utilized at the bedside by emergency department providers and surgeons alike. Advances in ultrasound training and expertise have led to an increasing number of centers favoring ultrasound as an initial diagnostic imaging technique for acute hernias. The sensitivity and specificity of ultrasound to identify hernias has been reported to be up to 100% and remains the only dynamic imaging modality readily available for emergent diagnosis. In some series, it has shown to be superior to computed tomography imaging with regard to rates of detection, cost, time, and interobserver reliability across those interpreting images [4, 5].

When not immediately visualized, the ability of ultrasound to identify a hernia can be improved with the use of the Valsalva maneuver, which will aid in enlarging the sac contents. However, this is not likely necessary with acutely incarcerated hernias and may produce worsening pain when the probe is positioned over the hernia. When a hernia is present, ultrasound findings include identification of bowel within the hernia sac, characterized by hypoechoic fluid within the lumen. Peristalsis may be seen as well and is suggestive of viability. Herniated fat will appear hyperechoic, and pain typically will be elicited upon compression with the ultrasound probe. When a hernia can be palpated, and manual reduction has not been confirmed, ultrasound may also be utilized. Using ultrasound guidance, directed reduction may be attempted. This technique may aid in reduction of difficult to palpate hernias, such as in obese patients, or with femoral or obturator hernias [6].

While ultrasound has a number of distinct advantages, including perfusion analysis with Doppler modes, it is adversely affected by obesity. Obesity is one of the biggest challenges of using ultrasound to identify herniation. Pannus adipose tissue, edema, and related anatomical distortion make it difficult to identify landmarks and fascial borders. This becomes even more difficult when scanning for a suspected inguinal hernia [5].

Computed Tomography (CT)

The use of CT imaging for the evaluation of abdominal or inguinal pain has become ubiquitous. For the diagnosis of hernia, CT has shown to have sensitivities and specificities above 80% in most series [7]. Despite these numbers, CT can both over- and underdiagnose hernias and has relatively low interobserver reliability [8]. This presents concerns with accurate diagnosis in occult hernias. Acutely incarcerated hernias, however, will be readily apparent on CT imaging, with a near 100% sensitivity and specificity.

A key advantage to CT imaging is the ability to identify other abnormalities that may not be imaged with localized ultrasound, as well as provide additional information, such as the presence of occult contralateral hernias, hollow viscus anatomy, and free intraperitoneal air that may change the operative approach to an acute hernia event. Acutely incarcerated or strangulated midline incisional hernias may present as a solitary mass and point of pain, while the underlying anatomy will reveal a "swiss-cheese" defect, with multiple hernias that may not be clinically palpable during initial evaluation.

In the case of a suspected but unconfirmed hernia, CT imaging can be utilized to characterize the defect and contents of the sac. This is especially true in the obese population. Excess adipose tissue may obscure not only the fascial defect, but edema stemming from panniculus morbidus may preclude palpation of the hernia sac and contents. Similarly, Spigelian and Richter's hernias may require CT to correctly identify their presence.

Just as the sensitivity and specificity of physical examination can be increased by asking a patient to stand or Valsalva, the sensitivity of CT scan can be increased via prone positioning. Although not likely an issue in the urgent or emergent arena, this may prove helpful in identifying occult defects, including those in the femoral or obturator spaces [9].

CT findings suggestive of bowel strangulation, such as thickened or hypoenhanced intestinal walls, should prompt emergent surgical intervention. Additional findings, such as free intraperitoneal air, pneumatosis intestinalis, or free fluid are all suggestive of strangulation as well [10].

Additional Diagnostic Adjuncts

While no laboratory studies exist to diagnose a hernia, several markers may hasten surgical intervention when a clear need for emergency repair is not readily apparent. Acidosis, specifically lactic acidosis, has been shown to be predictive of strangulation and is commonly ordered upon arrival to the emergency department. Other laboratory results, such as leukocytosis, elevated CPK, and D-dimer, have also been shown to be predictive of strangulation and may assist in the decision for emergent surgical intervention [11].

Indications for Emergent Repair

Most literature regarding hernia repair stems from the elective surgical patient. Patients presenting to the emergency department with easily reducible hernias are unlikely to require emergent operation. If concern for reduction in masse exists, then admission with serial examination may be warranted. This rare instance occurs when the external hernia sac and contents are reduced from their initial position, into the preperitoneal space. The hernia appears reduced externally; however the incarcerating scar/orifice remains and can still lead to strangulation and thus warrants repeat examinations. Otherwise, patients should undergo risk factor modulation, such as glucose and nutrition optimization, smoking cessation, weight loss, and cardiovascular optimization in preparation for elective repair. Hernia patients who present with acute incarceration or strangulation require urgent or emergent operative intervention.

Obvious indicators of strangulation, such as hemodynamic instability, acidosis, peritonitis, or skin necrosis, warrant emergent surgical intervention. Fortunately, most patients do not present in extremis. Classically, the quartet of fever, continuous pain, tachycardia, and leukocytosis have been used to determine if strangulation is present. While predictive, this specific constellation of symptoms rarely present together. The decision to operate is often complicated by distractors, such as patient age and comorbidities. It is crucial for the acute care surgeon to acknowledge that delay to surgical intervention in the setting of a possible strangulated hernia is linearly associated with worse outcomes. Early surgical intervention is warranted whenever there is a concern for strangulation [12, 13].

Barring overt signs pointing to the need for emergent operation, surgeons must distinguish between incarceration, strangulation, and obstruction. This may not be abundantly clear and highlights the importance of holding a high index of suspicion. When in doubt, patients should proceed to the operating room as soon as feasible. In select settings, a brief resuscitation period may be employed. This allows for a safer approach in the operating room and limits dire events during anesthetic induction. It should be noted, however, that resuscitation should not preclude nor delay operative intervention when strangulation is suspected or confirmed.

Groin Hernia

Most acute groin hernias are direct and indirect inguinal hernias and are most commonly identified in either young or elderly men. Often accompanied by a history with recent straining or heavy lifting, inguinal hernias are typically easier to diagnose than other groin hernias. Classically, obturator and femoral hernias occur in thin, elderly, multiparous women and are associated with vague thigh or pelvic pain. Physical examination may demonstrate a bulge below the inguinal ligament in femoral hernias. Due to nonspecific symptoms, obturator and femoral hernias frequently present with delayed diagnosis and strangulation. As such, both of these relatively rare groin hernias have disproportionately high-mortality and morbidity [14, 15]. Acutely incarcerated or strangulated groin hernias require surgical intervention emergently. No viable non-operative treatment options exist. Unfortunately, surgical intervention is not always a simple answer. Entire texts exist describing the various methods of surgical management of groin hernias. Here we'll focus on several widely utilized techniques.

Surgical Approach

In the case of bowel strangulation, a bowel resection must be performed with viable margins. This can prove challenging with inguinal hernias because of incisional limitations and relatively narrow hernial orifices found in many inguinal, femoral, and obturator hernias. Via a standard inguinal incision, whether that be suprainguinal or infrainguinal, it is at times possible to deliver viable bowel through the existing hernia defect and perform adequate resection and anastomosis. In many instances, the hernia orifice must be enlarged to perform resection. It is important to delineate the anatomical structures when performing this maneuver to avoid potential complications. This is especially important with femoral hernias, as division of the iliopubic tract or the inguinal ligament may be required. In this region, it is also critical to avoid injuring the femoral vein, which can be difficult to identify secondary to scarring and acute inflammation.

After freeing viscera from the hernia defect, viability must be assessed and resection performed as necessary. Multiple variables determine the ability to perform anastomosis via the inguinal incision, including defect size, bowel mobility, concomitant intra-abdominal adhesions, and surgeon skill. When anastomosis cannot be performed through the groin, it can be accomplished via a transabdominal approach with standard anastomotic techniques. Some published series show up to a 20% need for laparotomy with strangulated inguinal hernias requiring resection [16, 17]. Laparoscopy is an option for stable patients, and success is largely dependent upon individual surgeon skill and experience.

In the case of peritonitis or severe abdominal pain, perforation may have already occurred. Abdominal pain is associated with perforation and necrosis within the abdominal cavity. This presents surgical approach dilemma. The hernia must be addressed, as well as the intra-abdominal contents. For stable patients, a laparoscopic or robotic approach to the abdomen is an excellent option to evaluate bowel viability. This may be combined with a minimally invasive groin hernia repair when viable bowel is identified and therefore should be considered as the first approach in the operating room. If non-viable bowel is identified, resection can either be performed via a transabdominal approach laparoscopically or open.

Following bowel and resection repair, the next step is to complete repair of the hernia defect. Bassini's hernia repair technique continues to stand the test of time. In 1866, Eduardo Bassini suffered a serious groin wound and subsequently developed a fistula. His personal interest in hernia repair became his legacy, as he studied with Billroth and pioneered the tissue repair that now bears his name. The Bassini repair involves thorough dissection of the inguinal region and begins by opening the inguinal canal. Dividing the cremaster fully exposes the deep ring and allows for dissection in the preperitoneal space. Bassini's classic repair involves suturing the internal oblique, transversus abdominis, and transversalis fascia to the shelving edge of the inguinal ligament.

The Shouldice method of inguinal hernia repair has proven to have low recurrence rates and low rates of complication. Developed in the 1940s, it has been refined and modified several times, and is often referred to as the "modernized Bassini repair," despite distinct differences. Namely, the Shouldice method involves a four-layered reconstruction with two running sutures that imbricate the tissue. The layers are sutured medial-to-lateral and back again, imbricating four layers within the two suture lines [18].

While these operations have been a mainstay of surgical training for decades, the techniques are rarely employed electively and often performed incorrectly. Many surgeons simply approximate tissue bundles located cranially, to tissue bundles located caudally. This not only results in an anatomically incorrect repair, but one which has high rates of recurrence and complication. It is therefore critical to meticulously dissect and identify the layers of the abdominal wall and inguinal canal. Commonly dubbed the "complete dissection," exposure of these individual elements (internal oblique, transversus muscle, and transversalis fascia) will result in approximation of the correct tissue layers. Another common misstep is identifying the shelving edge of the inguinal ligament too superficially. This can result in a sheet-fold configuration and will result in a closed but potential space for hernia recurrence. Again, full dissection precludes this common pitfall. With the external oblique retracted caudally, the deepest portion of the inguinal ligament is exposed with the femoral sheath. The iliopubic tract, lacunar, and Cooper's ligaments can then not only palpated, but visualized. This will prevent suture placement in the incorrect and superficial fold of the inguinal ligament.

For femoral hernias, McVay's repair is typically performed [19]. Another variation on Bassini's repair, McVay, sutured the internal oblique, transversus muscle, and transversalis fascia to Cooper's ligament. This maneuver closes the space medial to the femoral vessels, preventing recurrent femoral herniation. However, to accomplish this, the medial portion of the iliopubic tract must be excised lateral to the vessels toward the lacunar ligament, thus exposing Cooper's ligament and proper suture placement. This move should be made with trepidation to avoid dividing the inguinal ligament or lacerating the femoral vein. While recoverable, both technical complications can result in significant morbidity if not properly addressed. McVay's repair is often more difficult to perform secondary to untoward tension and may require a relaxing incision on the rectus muscle. In fact, many surgeons routinely do a relaxing incision for all but the smallest hernia defects.

Developed in the 1980s, the Lichtenstein repair involves anterior placement of and recreation of the deep inguinal ring with nonabsorbable prosthetic mesh. This technique is the most common method of elective open inguinal hernia repair today. Lichtenstein tension-free hernioplasty is considered by many surgeons and hernia societies to be the criterion standard for elective open inguinal hernia repair due to its low recurrence and complication rate [20, 21]. The technique may be modified for femoral herniorrhaphy by suturing the inferior edge of mesh to Cooper's ligament instead of the inguinal ligament. Additional modifications must also be made to accomplish femoral herniorrhaphy, such as excising a portion of the iliopubic tract. The decision to use prosthetic mesh is complex and is discussed later in this chapter.

Minimally invasive approaches to acute groin hernias should be considered for stable patients. A common fear of laparoscopy with acutely incarcerated hernias is the inability to reduce the hernia contents. In one series of over 300 patients operated on for acute incarceration and strangulation, only 6 required conversion to an open procedure to complete the operation [22]. This suggests most hernias can be reduced and resections performed laparoscopically or robotically. Another common issue is the hernia repair itself. Laparoscopic and robotic techniques sans mesh are not viable options in the adult patient, and therefore fear of mesh infection often precludes surgeons to employ minimally invasive techniques. However, as discussed later in this chapter, mesh infection is a relatively rare occurrence [23].

Ventral Hernia

Ventral hernias may occur spontaneously, as the result of congenital defects, or following surgery, and include all anterior abdominal wall hernias. When ventral hernias result in an acute surgical issue, such as acute obstruction, incarceration, and strangulation, a thorough history is paramount. Very often, patients may have had previous hernia repairs, prosthetics, and multiple surgical procedures that have the potential to change the surgical approach. Additionally, preoperative imaging can be helpful in planning. Symptoms of acute incarceration and obstruction are similar to those seen with other hernias and include pain, a palpable mass, and obstructive symptoms. Likewise, patients with compromised vascular flow may present in extremis and unstable and represent a true surgical emergency.

Surgical Approach

Both minimally invasive and open techniques are commonly employed for acutely incarcerated and strangulated ventral hernias. As the dominant approach for many decades, open approaches offer more familiar tissue reconstruction techniques and thus remain a popular option for many surgeons.

Large ventral hernias rarely present with strangulation, but are frequently chronically incarcerated. Despite their chronic nature, surgical emergencies occur and are often obstructive in nature. Acute incarceration with obstruction typically requires operation on an urgent basis, but without clear signs for operation, it may be prudent to pursue nonoperative means initially. These include nasogastric decompression, nothing per mouth, intravenous resuscitation, and frequent ambulation. Worsening pain, acidosis, tachycardia, leukocytosis, or skin changes should prompt timely surgical intervention.

Incisional hernia approaches should begin just superior or inferior to the border of the existing scar, in order to gain peritoneal entry with minimal adhesions. Many surgeons will start superficially and excise the entirety of the existing scar just under the dermis and then begin deeper dissection in an untouched tissue plane. This is a safe method to gain open access to the abdomen and limits iatrogenic visceral injury. Care should be taken with electrocautery, and a combination of sharp and controlled blunt techniques are recommended for the subcutaneous dissection and exposure of the hernia sac. Electrocautery visceral injuries can be occult and the extent of injury difficult to ascertain, increasing the risk for delayed complications to arise in the days following operation. Transverse or incisional hernias located off-midline present unique entry and repair challenges. It is generally best to utilize the existing scar as a guide. There are instances, however, where a hernia located at a previous stoma site, for example, is best approached via a midline laparotomy given its proximity to the midline.

Once the hernia sac is exposed circumferentially, the dissection is carried down to the intact fascia. The hernia sac is then opened and contents examined. Adhesiolysis should be done sharply, with limited use of blunt techniques or electrocautery. Blunt adhesiolysis, while effective for loose adhesions, can lead to unnecessary visceral injury when dense scar tissue is encountered. If resection is required, standard techniques of resection and anastomosis are applied.

Regarding minimally invasive approaches, abdominal entry should be gained in an untouched plane. There is no evidence favoring one entry technique over another and should be based upon surgeon preference and experience [24]. One of the main issues limiting minimally invasive surgery in the acute setting is surgeon skill with a potentially difficult lysis of adhesions associated with acutely incarcerated, obstructed, or strangulated hernias. Bowel distension frequently limits visualization and is commonly cited as a reason for conversion to an open operation. Moreover, laparoscopic lysis of adhesions has a significantly higher rate of enterotomy creation than do open techniques. A missed enterotomy can be a devastating complication. Therefore, minimally invasive approaches should be considered carefully. One study found that laparoscopic adhesiolysis was safest in patients with less than three laparotomies and whose small bowel diameter was less than 4 cm [25].

Repair of the acute ventral hernia can similarly be approached via open or with minimally invasive techniques. Like groin hernias, the inability to reduce the hernia, perform a resection when necessary, and complete a prosthetic repair laparoscopically or robotically causes much consternation among surgeons. It is important for surgeons to address both their own limitations and the limitations arising from patient factors (obesity, bowel dilatation, gross contamination) when choosing surgical approach.

Tissue repair of elective ventral hernia repair has largely been replaced by prosthetic repair due to decreased recurrence and relatively low complication rates with mesh prosthetics [26]. Details regarding mesh are included later in this chapter. For patients with gross contamination or established peritonitis, mesh is ill-advised, as the infection rates are higher than most would be willing to accept. For those patients, a tissue repair should be completed, with or without absorbable mesh. Small defects (<3 cm) may not require additional flap creation or absorbable prosthetic and can likely be repaired via a simple suture technique [11]. There is no clear superiority of interrupted over running suture nor a specific suture material used in these techniques [27].

For larger defects requiring repair in contaminated and dirty surgical fields, absorbable mesh may be considered to aid in bridging the gap. There is some debate regarding the utility and long-term outcomes of these meshes and is covered in more detail later in this chapter. Tissue-only methods have been well-described for many years. Timing of reconstruction is often debated. Some surgeons claim advanced repairs should be done early, prior to development of a larger defect, while others initially repair with absorbable mesh or temporary closure and then return to place synthetic nonabsorbable mesh as part of the delayed definitive repair months later [28].

Larger defects and hernia sacs typically require large dissections. This may result in creation of potential spaces within the abdominal wall during closure, putting patients at risk for seroma formation and surgical site events. Many surgeons utilize drains in the subcutaneous space or above mesh when the fascia is unable to be reapproximated. Despite the widespread use of drains, there is sparse evidence supporting the practice, and in some series, infection rates are higher in patients with drains in place [29–31]. Suture approximation of skin and subcutaneous flaps is also frequently done, but with similar results [32]. Additional component separation techniques (either posterior or anterior based) in the acute setting for large hernia defects (> 10 cm wide) are not well studied. In our experience, these surgical approaches are not advisable given the significant additional operative time, increase risk for wound complications, and reducing options for recurrent hernia repairs in the future should the acute hernia repair fail.

In select instances, such as hemodynamic instability, it may be prudent to leave the incision open [11]. Patients in shock with hemodynamic compromise secondary to sepsis are at high risk to develop compartment syndrome and may not be able to be closed at the first operation. In this rare occurrence, surgeons should strive to achieve closure at the earliest possible time to avoid the sequelae of the open abdomen, such as enteroatmospheric fistulae [33]. When leaving the wound open, several options exist for temporary coverage. Commercial varieties, including hook-and-loop closures (Wittmann Patch, Starsurgical Inc., Burlington, WI) and negative pressure dressings (Abthera™, KCI USA, Inc., San Antonio, TX), may assist in temporary closure. Great care should take place to avoid enteroatmospheric fistula development. Negative pressure wound therapy, while effective, can result in dressing erosion and fistula formation. Specially designed dressings are available, but do not eliminate the risk of fistula. Surgeon-created devices typically involve placing a plastic barrier (X-ray cassette drape, slush drape, or IV fluid bag) placed over the viscera, with a towel or dressing as the next layer. A complex vacuum-sealed external dressing to manage ascites and fluid may then be utilized [34]. Negative pressure wound dressings have shown improved closure rates, as well as lessened times to closure, and are the preferred method to address open abdominal wounds [35, 36].

Large defects or defects unable to be closed at the initial operation will require abdominal wall reconstruction in the elective setting. Posterior-based component separation techniques are preferred over anterior approaches due to favorable closure rates with low risk of recurrence. The transversus abdominis release (TAR) technique has gained popularity in recent years due to its ability to reestablish domain with tissue reconstruction. The TAR is indicated for large hernia defects that cannot be closed with traditional approaches, in patients with noncompliant abdominal walls or in those with multiply recurrent hernias leading to large aggregate defects. Also referred to as a posterior component separation, it is associated with low recurrence rates and morbidity [37, 38]. Evolving from the work of Rives and Stoppa, the TAR involves creation of the retrorectus space by dissecting the posterior sheath away from the overlying rectus muscle. As the dissection extends laterally, the neurovascular bundles are identified and preserved, while the posterior sheath is incised medial to the semilunaris. The transversus abdominis is then divided, and the transversalis fascia advanced en bloc with the posterior rectus sheath. After completing this bilaterally, the medial cut edges of the rectus sheath leaflets are approximated. Mesh may be placed in the retromuscular space, further strengthening the repair. The TAR technique is capable of gaining 8–12 cm of distance toward the midline bilaterally. This equates to native tissue coverage of up to a 24 cm defect and is thus our method of choice when addressing large defects.

Anterior component separations continue to have a role for the modern acute care surgeon. Several variations exist: the two most common being external oblique only and the posterior rectus sheath and external oblique release [39]. Ramirez popularized anterior component separation in 1990 by releasing both the posterior rectus sheath from the rectus muscle dividing the external oblique muscle which allow myofascial advancement of the abdominal wall for a tension-free closure for large midline hernia defects [38]. There are several advantages and disadvantages to anterior component releases. Major advantages include extraperitoneal mesh placement and can be an alternative approach for large recurrent hernias that have previously undergone a posterior component separation now with recurrence. Disadvantages include raising lipocutaneous skin flaps, which are prone to seroma formation and skin necrosis, and have higher rates of SSI compared to posterior component separation techniques [40]. These wound issues were mitigated by the advent of endoscopic release of the external oblique fascia which saved the creation of large lipocutaneous flaps. While this approach has been shown to be successful, however, the growing popularity of the TAR approach, these have been utilized less. Both of these complex reconstructive techniques have little utility in the acute setting. While in ideal conditions, it may be feasible to perform a complex repair, often the physiology of the acute setting prevents complex tissue reconstruction.

Parastomal Hernia

It is not surprising that stoma creation has a high likelihood of resulting in hernia formation, with reported incidence of more than 50% in some series [41]. The very nature of stoma maturation deliberately creates a hernia. Multiple methods have been proposed to avoid herniation of other bowel loops or organs, including circumferential fascial suture placement and prophylactic mesh. One of the most important points regarding parastomal hernias is location of the ostomy site and occurs long before hernia development. Most, if not all, ostomies created through the semilunaris will result in a hernia. When violated, this key anatomical landmark will almost always result in hernia formation. Only in rare instances should an ostomy be placed lateral to the rectus muscle.

In patients with parastomal hernias who present acutely, obstructive symptoms are common. Additionally, patients may present with prolapse, leaking/poorly fitting appliances and/or pain. Initial evaluation should be to evaluate the viability and patency of the stoma. In cases of acute incarceration without the ability to perform adequate taxis, operative repair should follow.

Classically, patients underwent ostomy transplantation to a new location within the abdominal wall. In the setting of perforation, established peritonitis, and gross contamination, this is still the most viable option, as simple suture repair has an unacceptable recurrence rate. When viable bowel is identified, and the hernia can be reduced, one of two prosthetic repairs should commence. The keyhole technique has been utilized for many years and involves splitting the mesh around the stoma and suturing it to the fascia. While a popular method, recurrence remains relatively high. First described in 1980, Dr. Sugarbaker's technique involves placement of intraperitoneal mesh, from which the proximal aspect of the ostomy protrudes from the side. This technique is widely utilized both for hernia repair and prophylactically at the time of ostomy creation.

Hernia in Cirrhotic Patients

Increased intra-abdominal pressure and malnutrition contribute to the high incidence of hernias in patients with cirrhosis. Ideally, these hernias would be approached electively, with optimization of hepatic function and ascites prior to a surgical emergency [42, 43]. Hernias in cirrhotic patients tend to enlarge rapidly and frequently lead to complications and worsened outcomes [44] (Fig. 14.1). Even with emergent surgical

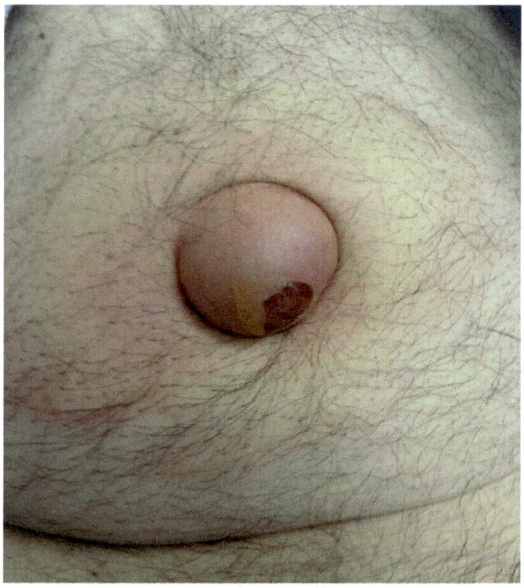

Fig. 14.1 Acutely strangulated umbilical hernia in a patient with cirrhosis

intervention, a ruptured umbilical hernia in a patient with cirrhosis can have up to a 20% mortality. Without surgery, mortality approaches 80% [45, 46].

Following initial resuscitation of a patient with cirrhosis with concomitant complicated hernia, surgeons should consider preoperative management of ascites as it will influence early and late complications. Transjugular intrahepatic portosystemic shunt (TIPS) is an effective method to decrease portal hypertension. There is evidence showing improved wound complications and long-term outcomes with urgent repair of complicated hernias in cirrhotic patients when preoperative TIPS is employed [47]. Selected patients who meet criteria with ruptured umbilical hernias and cirrhosis should undergo urgent evaluation for liver transplant [48].

Most surgeons prefer an open approach to acute hernias in patients with cirrhosis. Large-volume ascites generally preclude adequate visualization via minimally invasive techniques. In the presence of skin necrosis or leaking ascites requiring wound management, the benefit of minimally invasive approaches is less likely. Similar to other acute hernias, the initial management should be directed at addressing potential life threats and performing resection as necessary. Ascites present at the time of operation should be drained intraoperatively while being cognizant of expected fluid shifts in the setting of large-volume ascites evacuation. Traditionally, acute hernias were repaired with nonabsorbable suture; however there is evidence that mesh is safe and decreases recurrence in the presence of cirrhotic ascites [44, 49]. We recommend utilizing mesh, except in the instance of bacterial peritonitis or gross contamination as outlined later in the chapter. No evidence exists as to the ideal position of mesh placement, but as in other hernias, we recommend placing mesh in the extraperitoneal sublay position.

Intra-abdominal drains are a simple and effective means to accomplish decreased abdominal pressure postoperatively. We routinely place a closed suction drain into the peritoneum and leave it in place until the drainage decreases or enough time has lapsed to allow for adequate wound healing [50]. Drains should be placed through the abdominal wall in a “Z” fashion, penetrating the fascial layers at angles to one another, with a long subcutaneous component to reduce leakage following drain removal.

Flank Hernia

Lateral abdominal wall defects remain a challenging problem due to the complex anatomy and proximity of the hernia defect to bony structures. Lateral abdominal wall hernias are classified into four main locations as defined by the European Hernia Society Classification Guidelines: subcostal (L1), flank (L2), iliac (L3), and lumbar (L4) [51]. The true risk of incarceration is unknown due to the rarity of lateral abdominal hernias. Only case reports exist with strangulation, incarceration, or obstruction [52]. Flank hernias with a wide neck may have a low risk of incarceration or obstruction [53].

Surgical approach can be performed open or utilizing a minimally invasive approach depending on the comfort and skill set of the surgeon. There are very few medical trials focusing on lateral abdominal wall defects; however, mesh should be used for a definitive repair when appropriate. Mesh can be placed preperitoneal or intraperitoneal using open, laparoscopic, or robotics approaches. Closure of the defect is preferable; otherwise eventration of the mesh and abdominal wall bulging is common. Patient expectations should be managed preoperatively. It is uncommon to regain a truly symmetric result following repair of these hernias. Often, the lateral abdominal musculature does not engage or contract in a similar fashion as the unaffected side due to some degree of muscular denervation, which creates an asymmetric abdominal figure.

Due to the paucity of literature, outcomes for flank hernias vary widely. Recurrence rates following open repair range from 0 to 15% [54, 55]. Laparoscopic approaches tend to have a lower recurrence rates, lower wound complications, and shorter lengths of stay [56]. Currently, there are no studies evaluating the efficacy of robotic surgery in the setting of flank hernia repairs.

In the emergent setting, similar goals as described previously for other hernia repairs remain true for the flank hernias. The first priority is to correct the emergent life-threatening issue. Primary closure of the hernia defect should follow. If defect closure is not possible, then a bridging absorbable or biologic mesh would be the next preferred option. Traumatic flank hernias do not necessitate immediate repair in and of themselves unless presenting with a life-threatening problem such as evisceration. Traumatic flank hernias can typically be managed nonoperatively in the acute setting and addressed later after the patient recovers from their injuries. Bender et al. describe their experience with traumatic flank hernias resulting from high-speed blunt trauma. Although rare, the few hernias that were repaired at time of laparotomy had a high recurrence and complication rate [57]. A recent metanalysis of traumatic flank hernias show no significant difference between early and late repair, although recommendations were weak due to the low quality of the studies [58]. Elective repair of flank hernias have been shown to have high success rate with low postoperative complications [59]. Traumatic flank hernia repair should be delayed in lieu of elective repair once patient is recovered from their injuries when possible.

Fixation of mesh, if used, can be challenging given the confinements and anatomy of the lateral abdominal wall. Retroperitoneal structures including ureter, nerves, and major vasculature need to be considered when performing mesh fixation. One unique fixation method in lateral abdominal defects remains bone anchor fixation particularly to the iliac crest or the pubic bone. This can be a very useful and strong point for mesh fixation, especially if your ability for adequate mesh overlap at the time of surgery is limited [60]. Bone anchors are made by several various third-party vendors; Fig. 14.2 depicts a Mitek bone anchor system by Johnson and Johnson.

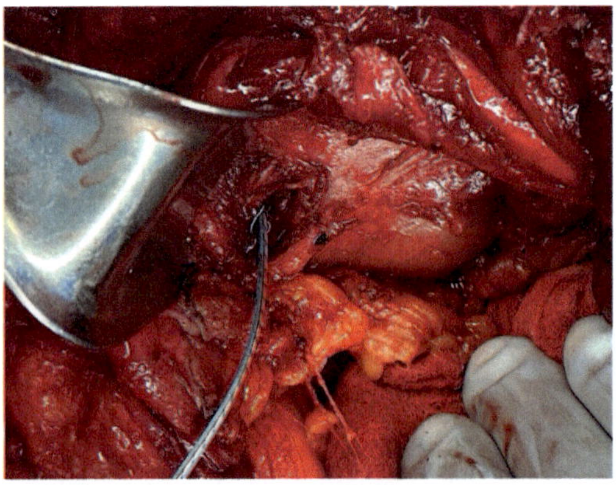

Fig. 14.2 Bone anchor fixation for flank hernia repair

Mesh Characteristics

The ideal hernia repair is one that is durable with minimal morbidity to the patient. Unplanned and emergent hernia repairs carry a significant increase in both perioperative morbidity and mortality when compared to elective hernia repairs [61, 62]. Mesh implantation is associated with the highest rates of both short-term and long-term complications, including infection, chronic pain, and abnormal wound healing [63]. When operating in an emergent setting, the choice to use mesh or a tissue-based repair is a frequent dilemma that is not easily reconciled. The risks and benefits to the patient need to be carefully weighed and several clinical factors contemplated prior to making that decision. However, if the surgeon proceeds with a mesh-based hernia repair, there are several key mesh characteristics that warrant consideration.

Hernia mesh is described using four main descriptors: mesh material, pore size, weight, and barrier coating. Mesh materials fall into several broad categories: synthetic permanent, biologic, and synthetic absorbable. Synthetic permanent mesh is comprised of three main polymers: polypropylene (PP), polyester (PE), or expanded polytetrafluoroethylene (ePTFE). Polypropylene is a monofilament material that is inert and undergoes little oxidation [64]. Polyester can be either monofilament or multifilament. Biologic meshes are collagen-rich materials derived from either human, porcine, or bovine sources [65]. ePTFE is a permanent synthetic laminar mesh that carries an excellent anti-adhesion profile, yet due to its lack of pores, it makes it unacceptably susceptible to infection. Its use in emergent or acute hernia repairs has no role and should be avoided [66]. Synthetic absorbable meshes are typically porous and designed to completely absorb over time. These include poly-4-hydroxybutyrate (Phasix™, Davol Inc., Warwick, RI) [67] and polyglactin-910 (Vicryl®, Ethicon, New Brunswick, NJ).

Pore size describes the amount of space not comprised by mesh material. These are grossly categorized into three groups: macroporous, microporous, and laminar. Macroporous mesh is usually considered >75 μm, while <75 μm is considered microporous. Laminar meshes have no pores and are rather a flat sheet. An example of laminar mesh is ePTFE. The importance of this characteristic comes with the ability for macrophages to clear bacteria from mesh. Microporous meshes have increased foreign material density and make it more difficult for macrophages to clear bacteria from the mesh itself. Whereas, macroporous meshes by definition have greater space between the material thus reducing foreign material burden and allowing macrophages better access to any bacterial contamination and thus perform better in contaminated settings. Laminar-based meshes, such as ePTFE, are the most susceptible to infection with the lowest ability to clear bacteria due to its laminar construct.

The location of mesh placement within the abdominal will determine if a coated or non-coated mesh is warranted. If a mesh is placed outside the peritoneal cavity, then an uncoated mesh is preferable, whether this be a preperitoneal, retromuscular, or onlay based repair. Alternatively, any synthetic mesh placed against the visceral contents would benefit from an anti-adhesion barrier coating in order to separate the mesh material from the abdominal organs. The barrier coating is a main reason why intraperitoneal mesh has a very low salvage rate if a mesh infection were to occur [68]. This addition of a barrier coating material alters mesh composition and interferes with the ability to clear mesh from bacterial contamination, thus limiting its ability to be used in contaminated settings [69]. Additionally, the barrier coating can consist of a separate mesh material itself, such as ePTFE. These "composite" meshes can have excellent anti-adhesive profiles [70].

There are multiple characteristics to consider when choosing a mesh for hernia repair. The choice of mesh product should be dictated by the clinical scenario and goals of the operation. Each mesh construct has advantages and disadvantages, and it is vital to have a basic understanding of the mesh material so that a suitable mesh can be placed in the appropriate clinical setting.

Permanent Synthetic Mesh

The choice to use permanent synthetic mesh in the acute setting continues to evolve with growing support in the medical literature. Macroporous mesh withstands contaminated settings well due to the large pores being able to be cleared by macrophages of any potential bacterial contamination. Similarly, a multifilament mesh has more difficulty with bacterial clearance due to the microstructure of the strands being woven together. Thus macroporous, monofilament synthetics may be the best choice for contaminated fields.

Mesh location is important as well. Inlay mesh, sewn to the edges of the defect, should be avoided when possible due to the extremely high recurrence rates. Onlay mesh placed on the anterior surface of the fascia, outside the abdominal cavity has also been associated with high recurrence rates. Sublay mesh can be broken down into three sub-positions, retromuscular, preperitoneal, and intraperitoneal, and is the most desired location.

When a hernia emergency is encountered, there is often ischemia, perforation, or contaminated fluid within the hernia sac or abdominal cavity due to translocation of intestinal flora. Traditionally, these contaminated settings have been a contraindication to use permanent synthetic mesh for hernia repair. Recent studies have shown there to be at least safe use of synthetic permanent macroporous monofilament mesh in an extraperitoneal position, either retromuscular or preperitoneal sublay, with outcomes similar to elective hernia repairs [71–75]. Even laparoscopic intraperitoneal onlay mesh (IPOM) can be used in the clean-contaminated settings in select clinical scenarios such as laparoscopic cholecystectomy and hysterectomy without increased risk to the patient [76]. However, given the altered properties of intraperitoneal mesh constructs and their limited salvageability, their use in grossly contaminated fields should be avoided [77].

Uncoated, macroporous, midweight, monofilament permanent mesh placed in an extraperitoneal sublay position remains a safe choice for the management of the acute hernia emergency, even in contaminated settings. Permanent synthetic mesh produces lower recurrence rates and similar postoperative morbidity to absorbable or biologic mesh in a contaminated field [65]. Table 14.1 summarizes several studies that highlight the use of permanent synthetic mesh in the contaminated setting with reported outcomes.

Absorbable Synthetic Mesh

Similar to biologic mesh, absorbable mesh is an attractive adjunct because it eventually absorbs and leaves no permanent foreign material in situ. These mesh constructs are most commonly made from one of two materials: poly-4-hydroxybutyrate (Phasix™, Davol Inc., Warwick, RI) [67] and polyglactin-910 (Vicryl®, Ethicon, New Brunswick, NJ). Both these materials provide temporary scaffolding to allow collagen deposition within the abdominal wall. Polyglactin 910 mesh has been available for decades; however, it should not be considered a viable option for definitive hernia repair. A newer absorbable biosynthetic mesh has recently gained popularity which is constructed of poly-4-hydroxybutyrate [78]. This can be formed into woven polymers that are similar in feel to a plastic material.

Poly-4-hydroxybutyrate (PHB) has recently been advocated for use in contaminated complex abdominal wall reconstruction. While there is a paucity of evidence to support its use in these settings, however, there are some reports. Roth et al. found a similar hernia recurrence rate and wound complication rates when using poly-4-hydroxybutyrate in the retromuscular position to permanent synthetic mesh at 18 months [79]. Mess et al. also found a similar rate of hernia recurrence and wound complications when compared to synthetic mesh using poly-4-hydroxybutyrate in abdominal wall reconstruction on long-term follow-up [80]. Given the similar outcomes between permanent synthetic mesh and PHB, the additional and significant cost of PHB would not seem to be clinically justified even in contaminated settings. Furthermore, there are no long-term studies supporting its use, which may show a significant increase in hernia recurrence rate after 5 years since the complete absorption of PHB is 18 months [81].

Absorbable synthetic mesh remains controversial, but does have several attractive qualities, namely, biodegradation over time. There is a significant increase in cost with these products when compared to permanent synthetic mesh. Further studies are clearly warranted on these products; however, poly-4-hydroxybutyrate does appear to have at least comparable outcomes after hernia surgery to permanent synthetic mesh.

Biologic Mesh

Biologic mesh was seen initially as an excellent option for hernia repair. It has several attractive qualities. It is made from an acellular collagen matrix that promotes tissue ingrowth and provides scaffolding for collagen deposition [82]. Additionally, there is no synthetic material that is implanted, and therefore its use in contaminated settings was thought to be ideal [82]. These traits propagated an explosion of biologic mesh into the general and acute care surgery armamentarium.

As biologics were implanted with little long-term clinical evidence of performance, several downsides began to emerge. There was no evidence of reduction in seromas or surgical site events with biologic mesh compared to those used with synthetic mesh, even in the contaminated setting [74, 83]. There is evidence to the contrary with increased persistent bacterial biofilms and increased difficulty in clearing infected biologic mesh when compared to contaminated

Table 14.1 Studies examining the use of permanent synthetic mesh in the contaminated setting with reported outcomes

Author	*n*	Material	Position	CDC Class	SSO (%)	SSI (%)	Recurrence (%)
Carbonell [23]	100	Polypropylene	Retrorectus	III/IV	26/34	7.1/19	7
Majumder [26]	57	Polypropylene/polyester	Retromuscular	II/III	22.8	12.3	8.9
Warren [42]	402	Polypropylene	Retromuscular/onlay/IPOM	II/III/IV	42.5	14.2	10.5
Ion [43]	56	Polypropylene/composite	Retrorectus/ inlay	II	7	N/A	N/A
Brahmahatt [44]	27	Polypropylene/polyethylene/PTFE	IPOM	N/A	44	22	19

CDC Class Centers for Disease Control and Prevention Wound Classification, I, clean; II, clean contaminated; III, contaminated; IV, dirty. *SSO* Surgical site occurrence. *SSI* Surgical site infection. *IPOM* intraperitoneal onlay mesh synthetic mesh [84, 85]. Biologic mesh, at best, has a similar recurrence rate compared to synthetic mesh when used in retromuscular based repairs [86]. Multiple other studies have shown higher recurrence rates of biologic mesh when used as definitive hernia repair when compared to permanent synthetic mesh [74, 85, 87].

Significant economic burden is associated with the use of biologics. There have been multiple studies demonstrating a significantly higher cost associated with biologic mesh repairs when compared to synthetic mesh repairs [88, 89]. While cost should not be the primary driver for clinical decisions, fiscal responsibility should play a role for the modern surgeon when considering all aspects of the case.

Biologic mesh has little, if any role, for implantation in the elective setting, but there are some rare instances that it may be beneficial in the acute setting. Biologic mesh can be viewed as a safe option for severely contaminated and high-risk hernias. However, it should not be viewed as a durable hernia repair. When compared to synthetic mesh place in the appropriate sublay position, there is little benefit [65]. Biologic grafts have higher hernia recurrence rates, less bacterial clearance, and higher rates of wound complications and are less cost-effective than synthetic mesh. In the acute setting, biologic mesh has a limited role as a temporizing hernia solution when synthetic mesh is contraindicated or to promote tissue coverage over exposed viscera.

Conclusion

Diagnosis of the acute hernia emergency is usually straightforward. In some instances, however, imaging may be beneficial when the diagnosis is in question, such as with femoral or Spigelian hernias. Emergent operative intervention is warranted for patients with indicators of strangulation, such as hemodynamic instability, acidosis, peritonitis, or skin necrosis. Most patients undergoing an emergent operation are approached via open techniques, but minimally invasive techniques should be considered in patients not in extremis. Immediate threats to life must be addressed swiftly and definitively. Only after these have been remedied can hernia repair commence. Each hernia location has specific nuances that should be considered in the acute setting. Lightweight, macroporous meshes should be utilized in most circumstances, barring gross contamination. Biologic and laminar prosthetics should be avoided. Complex abdominal wall reconstruction, such as component separation techniques, should be reserved for the elective setting. In cases where the defect may not be initially closed, use of negative pressure therapy is the preferred method to address open abdominal wounds.

References

1. Beadles CA, Meagher AD, Charles AG. Trends in emergent hernia repair in the United States. JAMA Surg. 2015;150(3):194–200.
2. Helgstrand F, Rosenberg J, Kehlet H, Bisgaard T. Outcomes after emergency versus elective ventral hernia repair: a prospective nationwide study. World J Surg. 2013;37(10):2273–9.
3. Baucom RB, Beck WC, Holzman MD, Sharp KW, Nealon WH, Poulose BK. Prospective evaluation of surgeon physical examination for detection of incisional hernias. J Am Coll Surg. 2014;218(3):363–6. https://doi.org/10.1016/j.jamcollsurg.2013.12.007.
4. Beck WC, Holzman MD, Sharp KW, Nealon WH, Dupon WD, Poulose BK. Comparitive effectiveness of dynamic abdominal sonography for hernia vs computed tomography in the diagnosis of incisional hernia. J Am Coll Surg. 2013;216(3):447–53.; quiz 510-1. https://doi.org/10.1016/j.jamcollsurg.2012.11.012.
5. Jamadar DA, Jacboson JA, Morag Y, Girish G, Ebrahim F, Gest T, Franz M. Sonography of inguinal region hernias. AJR. 2006;187:185–90.
6. De Kok BM, Puylaert JBCM, Zijta FM. Ultrasound-guided reduction of an incarcerated obturator hernia in an elderly patient. J Clin Ultrasound. 2018;46(6):415–8. https://doi.org/10.1002/jcu.22562.
7. Robinson A, Light D, Kasim A, Nice C. A systematic review and meta-analysis of the role of radiology in the diagnosis of occult inguinal hernia. Surg Endosc. 2013;27(1):11–8. https://doi.org/10.1007/s00464-012-2412-3. Epub 2012 Jun 26
8. Holihan JL, Cherla D, Blair KJ, Chua SS, Hasapes JP, Matta EJ, Shiralkar KG, Surabhi VR, Tammisetti VS, Ko TC, Liang MK. Computed tomography in ventral hernia diagnosis: have we improved? A quality improvement initiative. J Surg Res. 2018;224:97–101. https://doi.org/10.1016/j.jss.2017.11.055.
9. Miyaki A, Yamaguchi K, Kishibe S, Ida A, Miyauchi T, Naritaka Y. Diagnosis of inguinal hernia by prone-

vs. supine-position computed tomography. Hernia. 2017;21(5):705–13. https://doi.org/10.1007/s10029-017-1640-9. Epub 2017 Aug 10.
10. Cox VL, Tahvildari AM, Johnson B, Wei W, Jeffrey RB. Bowel obstruction complicated by ischemia: analysis of CT findings. Abdom Radiol (NY). 2018;43(12):3227–32. https://doi.org/10.1007/s00261-018-1651-8.
11. Birindelli A, Sartelli M, Di Saverio S, et al. 2017 update of the WSES guidelines for emergency repair of complicated abdominal wall hernias. World J Emerg Surg. 2017;12:37. https://doi.org/10.1186/s13017-017-0149-y.
12. Martínez-Serrano MA, Pereira JA, Sancho J, Argudo N, López-Cano M, Grande L. Specific improvement measures to reduce complications and mortality after urgent surgery in complicated abdominal wall hernia. Hernia. 2012;16(2):171–7. https://doi.org/10.1007/s10029-011-0875-0.
13. Koizumi M, Sata N, Kaneda Y, Endo K, Sasanuma H, Sakuma Y, Ota M, Lefor AT, Yasuda Y. Optimal timeline for emergency surgery in patients with strangulated groin hernias. Hernia. 2014;18(6):845–8.
14. Hachisuka T. Femoral hernia repair. Surg Clin North Am. 2003;83(5):1189–205. https://doi.org/10.1016/S0039-6109(03)00120-8.
15. Kulkarni SR, Punamiya AR, Naniwadekar RG, Janugade HB, Chotai TD, Singh TV, Natchair A. Obturator hernia: a diagnostic challenge. Int J Surg Case Rep. 2013;4(7):606–8. https://doi.org/10.1016/j.ijscr.2013.02.023.
16. Ram BR, Goud VS, Kumar DR, Reddy BK, Boda KS, Madipeddi V. Strangulated groin hernia repair: a new approach for all. J Clin Diagn Res. 2016;10(4):PC04–6. https://doi.org/10.7860/JCDR/2016/18037.7613.
17. Romain B, Chemaly R, Meyer N, Brigand C, Steinmetz JP, Rohr S. Prognostic factors of postoperative morbidity and mortality in strangulated groin hernia. Hernia. 2012;16(4):405–10. https://doi.org/10.1007/s10029-012-0937-y.
18. Chan CK, Chan G. The Shouldice technique for the treatment of inguinal hernia. J Minim Access Surg. 2006;2(3):124–8. https://doi.org/10.4103/0972-9941.27723.
19. Rutledge RH. McVay herniorrhaphy. Op Tech Gen Surgery. 1999;1(2):116–31.
20. HerniaSurge Group. International guidelines for groin hernia management. Hernia. 2018;22(1):1–165. https://doi.org/10.1007/s10029-017-1668-x.
21. Sakorafas GH, Halikias I, Nissotakis C, Kotsifopoulos N, Stavrou A, Atonopoulos C, Kassaras GA. Open tension free repair of inguinal hernias; the Lichtenstein technique. BMC Surg. 2001;1:3. https://doi.org/10.1186/1471-2482-1-3.
22. Deeba S, Purkayastha S, Paraskevas P, et al. Laparoscopic approach to incarcerated and strangulated inguinal hernia. JSLS. 2009;13:327–31.
23. Lin YT, Weng TY, Tam KW. Effectiveness and safety of mesh repair for incarcerated or strangulated hernias: a systematic review and meta-analysis. World J Surg. 2020;44(7):2176–84. https://doi.org/10.1007/s00268-020-05430-4.
24. Recknagel JD, Goodman LR. Clinical perspective concerning abdominal entry techniques. J Minim Invasive Gynecol. 2020:S1553-4650(20)30341-1. https://doi.org/10.1016/j.jmig.2020.07.010.
25. Farinella E, Cirocchi R, La Mura F, et al. Feasibility of laparoscopy for small bowel obstruction. World J Emerg Surg. 2009;4:3. https://doi.org/10.1186/1749-7922-4-3.
26. Luijendijk RW, Hop WC, van den Tol MP, de Lange DC, Braaksma MM, Ijzermans JN, Boelhouwer RU, de Vries BC, Salu MK, Wereldsma JC, Bruijninckx CM, Jeekel J. A comparison of suture repair with mesh repair for incisional hernia. N Engl J Med. 2000;343(6):392–8. https://doi.org/10.1056/NEJM200008103430603.
27. Muysoms FE, Antoniou SA, Bury K, Campanelli G, Conze J, Cuccurullo D, de Beaux AC, Deerenberg EB, East B, Fortelny RH, Gillion JF, Henriksen NA, Israelsson L, Jairam A, Jänes A, Jeekel J, López-Cano M, Miserez M, Morales-Conde S, Sanders DL, Simons MP, Śmietański M, Venclauskas L, Berrevoet F, European Hernia Society. European Hernia Society guidelines on the closure of abdominal wall incisions. Hernia. 2015;19(1):1–24. https://doi.org/10.1007/s10029-014-1342-5. Epub 2015 Jan 25.
28. Rawstorne E, Smart CJ, Fallis SA, Suggett N. Component separation in abdominal trauma. J Surg Case Rep. 2014;2014(1):rjt133. https://doi.org/10.1093/jscr/rjt133.
29. Shermak MA, Rotellini-Coltvet LA, Chang D. Seroma development following body contouring surgery for massive weight loss: patient risk factors and treatment strategies. Plast Reconstr Surg. 2008;122(1):280–8.
30. Luo Y, Masood DE, Mohammed Jinnaah S, Tacey M, Hodgson R. Do drain tubes help reduce risks of postoperative complications in complex incisional hernia repair (as defined by a recent court ruling)? ANZ J Surg. 2020;90(6):1080–5. https://doi.org/10.1111/ans.15875.
31. Luo Y, Mohammed Jinnaah S, Masood D, Hodgson R. Drain tube use in incisional hernia repair: a national survey. Hernia. 2020; [published online ahead of print, 2020 Jan 8]; https://doi.org/10.1007/s10029-019-02115-3.
32. Alhussini MA, Awad AT, Kholosy HM. Using quilting sutures in decreasing seroma formation after managing large ventral hernias: a comparative study. Hernia. 2019;23:717–22. https://doi.org/10.1007/s10029-018-1850-9.
33. Gross DJ, Smith MC, Zangbar-Sabegh B, Chao K, Chang E, Boudourakis L, Muthusamy M, Roudnitsky V, Schwartz T. Challenge of uncontrolled enteroatmospheric fistulas. Trauma Surg Acute Care Open. 2019;4(1):e000381. https://doi.org/10.1136/tsaco-2019-000381.
34. Turza KC, Campbell CA, Rosenberger LH, Politano AD, Davies SW, Riccio LM, Sawyer RG. Options for closure of the infected abdomen. Surg Infect

(Larchmt). 2012;13(6):343–51. https://doi.org/10.1089/sur.2012.014. Epub 2012 Dec 10.
35. Miller PR, Meredith W, Johnson JC, et al. Prospective evaluation of vacuum-assisted fascial closure after open abdomen: planned ventral hernia rate is substantially reduced. Ann Surg. 2004;239:608–16.
36. van Hensbroek PB. Wind J. Dijkgraaf MGW, et al. Temporary closure of the open abdomen: a systematic review of delayed primary fascial closure in patients with an open abdomen. World J Surg. 2009;33:199–207.
37. Petro CC, Como JJ, Yee S, Prabhu AS, Novitsky YW, Rosen MJ. Posterior component separation and transversus abdominis muscle release for complex incisional hernia repair in patients with a history of an open abdomen. J Trauma Acute Care Surg. 2015;78(2):422–9. https://doi.org/10.1097/TA.0000000000000495.
38. Novitsky YW, Elliott HL, Orenstein SB, Rosen MJ. Transversus abdominis muscle release: a novel approach to posterior component separation during complex abdominal wall reconstruction. Am J Surg. 2012;204(5):709–16.
39. Ramirez OM, Ruas E, Dellon AL. "Components separation" method for closure of abdominal-wall defects: an anatomic and clinical study. Plast Reconstr Surg. 1990;86(3):519–26.
40. Maloney SR, Schlosser KA, Prasad T, et al. Twelve years of component separation technique in abdominal wall reconstruction. Surgery. 2019;166(4):435–44.
41. Kann BR. Early stomal complications. Clin Colon Rectal Surg. 2008;21:23–30. https://doi.org/10.1055/s-2008-1055318.
42. Gray SH, Vick CC, Graham LA, et al. Umbilical herniorrhaphy in cirrhosis: improved outcomes with elective repair. J Gastrointest Surg. 2008;12:675–81. https://doi.org/10.1007/s11605-008-0496-9.
43. Eker HH, van Ramshorst GH, de Goede B, Tilanus HW, Metselaar HJ, de Man RA, Lange JF, Kazemier G. A prospective study on elective umbilical hernia repair in patients with liver cirrhosis and ascites. Surgery. 2011;150:542–6.
44. Ammar SA. Management of complicated umbilical hernias in cirrhotic patients using permanent mesh: randomized clinical trial. Hernia. 2010;14:35–8.
45. Chatzizacharias NA, Bradley JA, Harper S, Butler A, Jah A, Huguet E, Praseedom RK, Allison M, Gibbs P. Successful surgical management of ruptured umbilical hernias in cirrhotic patients. World J Gastroenterol. 2015;21:3109–13.
46. McKay A, Dixon E, Bathe O, Sutherland F. Umbilical hernia repair in the presence of cirrhosis and ascites: results of a survey and review of the literature. Hernia. 2009;13:461–8.
47. Telem DA, Schiano T, Divino CM. Complicated hernia presentation in patients with advanced cirrhosis and refractory ascites: management and outcome. Surgery. 2010;148(3):538–43. https://doi.org/10.1016/j.surg.2010.01.002.
48. Malespin M, Moore CM, Fialho A, de Melo SW, Benyashvili T, Kothari AN, di Sabato D, Kallwitz ER, Cotler SJ, Lu AD. Case series of 10 patients with cirrhosis undergoing emergent repair of ruptured umbilical hernias: natural history and predictors of outcomes. Exp Clin Transplant. 2019;17(2):210–3. https://doi.org/10.6002/ect.2017.0086.
49. Hew S, Yu W, Robson S, Starkey G, Testro A, Fink M, Angus P, Gow P. Safety and effectiveness of umbilical hernia repair in patients with cirrhosis. Hernia. 2018;22:759–65. https://doi.org/10.1007/s10029-018-1761-9.
50. Triantos CK, Kehagias I, Nikolopoulou V, Burroughs AK. Surgical repair of umbilical hernias in cirrhosis with ascites. Am J Med Sci. 2011;341(3):222–6. https://doi.org/10.1097/MAJ.0b013e3181f31932.
51. Muysoms FE, Miserez M, Berrevoet F, et al. Classification of primary and incisional abdominal wall hernias. Hernia. 2009;13(4):407–14.
52. Henriksen NA, Kaufmann R, Simons MP, et al. EHS and AHS guidelines for treatment of primary ventral hernias in rare locations or special circumstances. BJS Open. 2020;4(2):342–53.
53. Katkhouda N, Alicuben ET, Pham V, et al. Management of lateral abdominal hernias. Hernia. 2020;24(2):353–8.
54. Carbonell AM, Kercher KW, Sigmon L, et al. A novel technique of lumbar hernia repair using bone anchor fixation. Hernia. 2005;9(1):22–5.
55. Moreno-Egea A, Alcaraz AC, Cuervo MC. Surgical options in lumbar hernia: laparoscopic versus open repair. A long-term prospective study. Surg Innov. 2013;20(4):331–44.
56. Yavuz N, Ersoy YE, Demirkesen O, Tortum OB, Erguney S. Laparoscopic incisional lumbar hernia repair. Hernia. 2009;13(3):281–6.
57. Bender JS, Dennis RW, Albrecht RM. Traumatic flank hernias: acute and chronic management. Am J Surg. 2008;195(3):414–7; discussion 417.
58. Karhof S, Boot R, Simmermacher RKJ, van Wessem KJP, Leenen LPH, Hietbrink F. Timing of repair and mesh use in traumatic abdominal wall defects: a systematic review and meta-analysis of current literature. World J Emerg Surg. 2019;14:59.
59. Zhou DJ, Carlson MA. Incidence, etiology, management, and outcomes of flank hernia: review of published data. Hernia. 2018;22(2):353–61.
60. Mukherjee K, Miller RS. Flank hernia repair with suture anchor mesh fixation to the iliac crest. Am Surg. 2017;83(3):284–9.
61. Simon KL, Frelich MJ, Gould JC, Zhao HS, Szabo A, Goldblatt MI. Inpatient outcomes after elective versus nonelective ventral hernia repair. J Surg Res. 2015;198(2):305–10.
62. Kurt N, Oncel M, Ozkan Z, Bingul S. Risk and outcome of bowel resection in patients with incarcerated groin hernias: retrospective study. World J Surg. 2003;27(6):741–3.
63. Borab ZM, Shakir S, Lanni MA, et al. Does prophylactic mesh placement in elective, midline lapa-

rotomy reduce the incidence of incisional hernia? A systematic review and meta-analysis. Surgery. 2017;161(4):1149–63.
64. Rastegarpour A, Cheung M, Vardhan M, Ibrahim MM, Butler CE, Levinson H. Surgical mesh for ventral incisional hernia repairs: understanding mesh design. Plast Surg (Oakv). 2016;24(1):41–50.
65. Köckerling F, Alam NN, Antoniou SA, et al. What is the evidence for the use of biologic or biosynthetic meshes in abdominal wall reconstruction? Hernia. 2018;22(2):249–69.
66. Stremitzer S, Bachleitner-Hofmann T, Gradl B, et al. Mesh graft infection following abdominal hernia repair: risk factor evaluation and strategies of mesh graft preservation. A retrospective analysis of 476 operations. World J Surg. 2010;34(7):1702–9.
67. Deeken CR, Matthews BD. Characterization of the mechanical strength, resorption properties, and histologic characteristics of a fully absorbable material (Poly-4-hydroxybutyrate-PHASIX mesh) in a porcine model of hernia repair. ISRN Surg. 2013;2013:238067.
68. Warren JA, Love M, Cobb WS, et al. Factors affecting salvage rate of infected prosthetic mesh. Am J Surg. 2020;
69. Sanchez VM, Abi-Haidar YE, Itani KM. Mesh infection in ventral incisional hernia repair: incidence, contributing factors, and treatment. Surg Infect. 2011;12(3):205–10.
70. Liu H, van Steensel S, Gielen M, Vercoulen T, Melenhorst J, Winkens B, Bouvy ND. Comparison of coated meshes for intraperitoneal placement in animal studies: a systematic review and meta-analysis. Hernia. 2019; https://doi.org/10.1007/s10029-019-02071-ys.
71. Carbonell AM, Criss CN, Cobb WS, Novitsky YW, Rosen MJ. Outcomes of synthetic mesh in contaminated ventral hernia repairs. J Am Coll Surg. 2013;217(6):991–8.
72. Bondre IL, Holihan JL, Askenasy EP, et al. Suture, synthetic, or biologic in contaminated ventral hernia repair. J Surg Res. 2016;200(2):488–94.
73. Krpata DM, Blatnik JA, Novitsky YW, Rosen MJ. Evaluation of high-risk, comorbid patients undergoing open ventral hernia repair with synthetic mesh. Surgery. 2013;153(1):120–5.
74. Majumder A, Winder JS, Wen Y, Pauli EM, Belyansky I, Novitsky YW. Comparative analysis of biologic versus synthetic mesh outcomes in contaminated hernia repairs. Surgery. 2016;160(4):828–38.
75. Campanelli G, Nicolosi FM, Pettinari D, Avesani EC. Prosthetic repair, intestinal resection, and potentially contaminated areas: safe and feasible? Hernia. 2004;8(3):190–2.
76. Praveen Raj P, Ganesh MK, Senthilnathan P, Parthasarathi R, Rajapandian S, Palanivelu C. Concomitant laparoscopic intraperitoneal onlay mesh repair with other clean contaminated procedures-study of feasibility and safety. J Laparoendosc Adv Surg Tech A. 2015;25(1):33–6.
77. Cobb WS, Carbonell AM, Kalbaugh CL, Jones Y, Lokey JS. Infection risk of open placement of intraperitoneal composite mesh. Am Surg. 2009;75(9):762–7; discussion 767-768.
78. Utsunomia C, Ren Q, Zinn M. Poly(4-Hydroxybutyrate): current state and perspectives. Front Bioeng Biotechnol. 2020;8:257.
79. Roth JS, Anthone GJ, Selzer DJ, et al. Prospective evaluation of poly-4-hydroxybutyrate mesh in CDC class I/high-risk ventral and incisional hernia repair: 18-month follow-up. Surg Endosc. 2018;32(4):1929–36.
80. Messa CA, Kozak G, Broach RB, Fischer JP. When the mesh goes away: an analysis of Poly-4-Hydroxybutyrate mesh for complex hernia repair. Plast Reconstr Surg Glob Open. 2019;7(11):e2576.
81. Martin DP, Badhwar A, Shah DV, et al. Characterization of poly-4-hydroxybutyrate mesh for hernia repair applications. J Surg Res. 2013;184(2):766–73.
82. Novitsky YW. Biology of biological meshes used in hernia repair. Surg Clin North Am. 2013;93(5):1211–5.
83. Liang MK, Berger RL, Nguyen MT, Hicks SC, Li LT, Leong M. Outcomes with porcine acellular dermal matrix versus synthetic mesh and suture in complicated open ventral hernia repair. Surg Infect. 2014;15(5):506–12.
84. Kallick E, Nistico L, Longwell M, et al. Resistance of synthetic and biologic surgical meshes to methicillin-resistant Staphylococcus aureus biofilm: an in vitro investigation. Int J Biomater. 2019;2019:–1063643.
85. Sandvall BK, Suver DW, Said HK, et al. Comparison of synthetic and biologic mesh in ventral hernia repair using components separation technique. Ann Plast Surg. 2016;76(6):674–9.
86. Darehzereshki A, Goldfarb M, Zehetner J, et al. Biologic versus nonbiologic mesh in ventral hernia repair: a systematic review and meta-analysis. World J Surg. 2014;38(1):40–50.
87. Slater NJ, van der Kolk M, Hendriks T, van Goor H, Bleichrodt RP. Biologic grafts for ventral hernia repair: a systematic review. Am J Surg. 2013;205(2):220–30.
88. FitzGerald JF, Kumar AS. Biologic versus synthetic mesh reinforcement: what are the pros and cons? Clin Colon Rectal Surg. 2014;27(4):140–8.
89. Reynolds D, Davenport DL, Korosec RL, Roth JS. Financial implications of ventral hernia repair: a hospital cost analysis. J Gastrointest Surg. 2013;17(1):159–66; discussion p.166–157.

15 Acute Cholecystitis

Jarrett Santorelli and Todd Costantini

Case Presentation

A previously healthy 44-year-old female presents to the emergency department with severe constant pain located in the right upper quadrant. The patient reports her pain began 10 h ago, is slowly worsening with time, and is now associated with nausea and 1 episode of emesis. She reports prior pain in this region, often after eating fatty foods, but it has always been self-limited and she has never pursued further evaluation. On exam the patient is noted to be febrile to 38.7 °C, her heart rate is 107, and she has tenderness and guarding localized to the right upper quadrant.

Introduction

Acute calculous cholecystitis is a complication of cholelithiasis, a condition that afflicts more than 20 million Americans annually with approximately 120,000 cholecystectomies performed for acute cholecystitis every year in the United States [1–3]. Gallstones have been documented to account for 90–95% of cases of acute cholecystitis [4]. Gallstone formation is known to be a multifactorial process associated with body mass index (BMI), diet, family history, diabetes and hemolytic disease with a prevalence of gallstones approximately 10–15% of the population [4]. Because of the asymptomatic nature of cholelithiasis (81%), diagnosis is based upon a combination of physical exam findings, laboratory evaluation and imaging studies. Classic symptoms for presentation of acute cholecystitis include nausea, vomiting, fever, right upper quadrant or epigastric pain, right shoulder pain and a positive Murphy's sign (patient "catches" their breath during inspiration while right upper quadrant palpated). Laboratory evaluation typically demonstrates elevated white blood cell count but also may show an increase in C—reactive protein and liver function tests.

Imaging

Abdominal pain remains one of the most common presenting symptoms to the emergency department (ED) with right upper quadrant pain accounting for a significant number of visits. Following physical exam and laboratory evaluation, imaging studies are often performed for further patient evaluation. Recently, a meta-analysis was performed to analyze the accuracy of imag-

J. Santorelli · T. Costantini (✉)
Division of Trauma, Surgical Critical Care, Burns and Acute Care Surgery, Department of Surgery, UC San Diego School of Medicine, San Diego, CA, USA
e-mail: jsantorelli@health.ucsd.edu; tcostantini@health.ucsd.edu

M. D. Zielinski, O. Guillamondegui (eds.), *The Acute Management of Surgical Disease*,
https://doi.org/10.1007/978-3-031-07881-1_15

ing studies in the diagnosis of acute cholecystitis. They found that ultrasound was frequently used to detect cholecystitis but demonstrated a large margin of error [4, 5]. When using ultrasound for evaluation, a convex multifrequency probe is used to evaluate the right upper quadrant. Multiple sonographic signs have been developed, and when several of these signs are present together, sensitivity for acute cholecystitis rises. The major sonographic signs associated with acute cholecystitis include gallbladder wall thickening (>3 mm), a positive Murphy's sign, pericholecystic fluid, distended gallbladder, gallstones, and sludge. When combining the findings of clinical presentation with a positive sonographic Murphy's sign and gallbladder wall thickening (>3 mm), sonography has a positive predictive value of up to 94% [6, 7]. However, the sensitivity of ultrasound for acute cholecystitis in the literature has been reported from 40 to 91% [7–9].

Computed tomography (CT) imaging is being used increasingly in the ED for evaluation of patient's with abdominal pain. When evaluated for its diagnostic accuracy, however, there is a lack of definitive evidence for its accuracy in the diagnosis of acute cholecystitis [5, 10]. There are multiple reasons for the shortcoming of CT for the diagnosis of acute cholecystitis. First, in contrast to ultrasonography, CT has demonstrated limited ability to detect gallstones and is unable to evaluate for focal tenderness. Second, the risks of radiation must be considered as an abdominal CT exposes the patient to significantly more radiation that may not be worthwhile for a test demonstrating sensitivity of 65–75% [11].

Hepato-imino diacetic acid (HIDA) scan is a well-established scintigraphic imaging technique that is considered by many to be the gold standard imaging technique for the diagnosis of acute cholecystitis. It has been shown to have a higher sensitivity and specificity compared to other imaging techniques and seen to be as high as 97% in recent reviews [5]. A recent study compared histopathologic findings post cholecystectomy with HIDA results demonstrating a sensitivity of 91.7% for acute cholecystitis [7]. In 2012, Kiewiet et al. demonstrated in a large meta-analysis that the sensitivity of abdominal ultrasound was 81% compared to a sensitivity of 96% for HIDA. [5].

Tokyo Guidelines for Diagnosis of Acute Cholecystitis

Despite being one of the most common surgical diseases, diagnosis of acute cholecystitis remains problematic as clinical diagnosis can be incorrect in up to 23% of patients [7, 12]. In 2007 discussions by global experts at the Tokyo Consensus Meeting created guidelines for diagnosis and severity of acute cholecystitis. Following validation studies issues with ambiguity were identified, and the criteria were revised in 2013 [13]. With the new diagnostic criteria, the decision was made to designate the presence of local signs of inflammation and systemic signs of inflammation. These new diagnostic criteria, seen in Table 15.1, were validated by a multicenter study of 451 patients with acute cholecystitis, which found that their use improved sensitivity and specificity to 91.2% and 96.9%, respectively [13–15]. The guidelines were again revised in 2018, and after a large literature review including literature with 216 articles, little evidence was found concerning the diagnostic criteria, and thus they were unchanged in the publication of the 2018 guidelines (Table 15.1).

Table 15.1 Tokyo Guidelines 18 diagnostic criteria [14]

A. Local signs of inflammation.	1. Murphy's sign. 2. RUQ mass/pain/ tenderness.
B. Systemic signs of inflammation.	1. Fever. 2. Elevated CRP. 3. Elevated WBC.
C. Imaging findings.	1. Wall thickening. 2. Hypoechoic layer. 3. Debris. 4. Distended gallbladder.
Suspected diagnosis	One item in A + one item in B
Definite diagnosis	One item in A + one item in B + C

In summary, the diagnosis of pathologically confirmed acute cholecystitis may be difficult but can most reliably be made with a combination of physical exam findings, laboratory findings consistent with inflammation, and imaging findings. Ultrasound remains the initial imaging test of choice due to its low cost, widespread availability, and relatively high sensitivity and specificity [13–15].

Management of Acute Cholecystitis

Cholecystectomy remains one of the most common surgical procedures performed each year. Prior to the 1800s, patients diagnosed with biliary colic underwent cholecystostomy procedures where the gallbladder was opened and drained and stones were removed as surgeons feared death if the organ was removed. In 1882, Dr. Carl Langenbuch performed the first successful cholecystectomy at the Lazarus Hospital in Berlin, curing his patient who had suffered for 16 years, overnight. By the early 1900s, hundreds of cholecystectomies had been performed, and open cholecystectomy for biliary colic became the gold standard. It wasn't until 1985 this approach was changed when German surgeon Erich Mühe removed the first gallbladder after his construction of the "galloscope," after being inspired by the work of Kurt Semm a German gynecologists [16].

Severity Grading

The initial management of acute calculous cholecystitis is often dictated by the patient's current clinical status, disease severity, and underlying comorbidities. Despite being one of the most common surgical diseases, diagnosis of acute cholecystitis remains problematic as clinical diagnosis can be incorrect in up to 23% of patients [7, 12]. At this time there are multiple severity grading systems which are often used to dictate further care. The two most commonly used severity grading systems include the Tokyo Guidelines (Table 15.2) and the American Association for the Surgery of Trauma (AAST) severity grading (Table 15.3) [17]. In 2007 discussions by global experts at the Tokyo Consensus Meeting created guidelines for diagnosis and severity of acute cholecystitis. These new diagnostic criteria, referred to as the Tokyo Guidelines, were validated by a multicenter study of 451 patients with acute cholecystitis, finding that their use sensitivity and specificity for acute cholecystitis were 91.2% and 96.9%, respectively [7, 14, 18]. In these criteria, acute calculous cholecystitis is broken up into mild, moderate, and severe disease. In a case series published by Yokoe et al., the prognosis for grade 3 patients was found to be significantly worse than for grades 1 and 2 [14, 18]. Additional studies have found that the length of hospital stay is significantly increased in patients with higher TG18 severity grades [19–22]. More recently a multivariate analysis has demonstrated that the TG13 severity grade was an independent predictor of both length of hospital stay and conversion to

Table 15.2 Tokyo Guidelines 18 grading scale [14]

Grade	Classification	Criteria
Grade 1	Mild acute cholecystitis	Acute cholecystitis in a healthy individual without organ dysfunction
Grade 2	Moderate acute cholecystitis	Acute cholecystitis with any one of: 1. WBC >18,000. 2. Palpable tender mass in the RUQ. 3. Duration of symptoms >72 h. 4. Marked local inflammation.
Grade 3	Severe acute cholecystitis	Acute cholecystitis with dysfunction of any one system 1. Cardiovascular dysfunction (hypotension). 2. Confusion or AMS. 3. Respiratory dysfunction PaO_2/FiO_2 <300). 4. Renal dysfunction (oliguria, creatinine >1.5). 5. Hepatic dysfunction (PT/INR >1.5). 6. Hematologic dysfunction (platelets <100,000).

Table 15.3 AAST EGS grade descriptions of acute cholecystitis severity [17]

Grade	Description	Imaging	Operative
Grade 1	Localized GB inflammation	Wall thickening, pericholecystic fluid, non-visualization of GB	Localized inflammatory changes
Grade 2	Distended gallbladder with purulence or hydrops, necrosis/ gangrene	Above plus air in gallbladder lumen, wall, or biliary tree	Distended gallbladder with pus/ hydrops, non-perforated necrosis
Grade 3	Non iatrogenic perforation with bile in the RUQ	Extraluminal fluid collection limited to RUQ	Non-iatrogenic gallbladder wall perforation with bile limited to RUQ
Grade 4	Pericholecystic abscess, bilioenteric fistula, gallstone ileus	RUQ abscess, bilioenteric fistula, gallstone ileus	Pericholecystic abscess, bilioenteric fistula, gallstone ileus
Grade 5	Grade 4 + generalized peritonitis	Free intraperitoneal fluid	Above with peritonitis

open surgery [19]. Finally both conversion rates from laparoscopic to open cholecystectomy and intraoperative biliary complications are both significantly increased in patients with higher severity grade [14, 19, 20].

The AAST developed a clinical, radiologic, operative, and pathologic grading system for EGS diseases, including acute cholecystitis in an attempt to create a more universal anatomic severity grading system focusing on distinct anatomic changes. A study by Hernandez et al. found that increasing AAST severity score was associated with mortality, morbidity, complication severity, duration of stay, need for cholecystostomy tube, open procedure, and conversion from laparoscopic to open procedure [17]. This same study concluded that the AAST grading system is superior to the Tokyo Severity Grading scale with greater associations for key clinical outcomes. The ability to rapidly assign disease severity from degree of anatomic injury is (1) simple to calculate, (2) does not require multiple laboratory values, and (3) does not require development of organ failure to associate with outcome. A second study again confirmed that anatomic grade is independently associated with multiple patient outcomes; however, it appears to lack the ability to differentiate between lower grades. For example, perforated cholecystitis is represented by grade 3 disease; therefore the majority of disease presentation is classified as grade 1 or grade 2 with limited ability to differentiate and prognosticate differences between these levels [23–26]. While both severity grading scales have pros and cons, universal adoption of any grading system, whether it be the TG or AAST, has the potential to improve prognostication and risk stratification as well as create a common language across health care systems.

Role of Antibiotics for Acute Cholecystitis

Perioperative Antibiotic Therapy

The treatment of mild or low-grade acute cholecystitis with intravenous antibiotics with or without surgical intervention is currently widely accepted and practiced. While it appears there is little data to support this practice, it is currently the recommendation of many guidelines, including the Surgical Infection Society and the Infectious Diseases Society of America, to start empiric antibiotic therapy upon diagnosis of acute cholecystitis [27–30]. This recommendation is based upon consensus of the TG meeting as well as a comprehensive review of the management of acute cholecystitis by Strasberg et al. [1, 27, 30, 31] On close review, these recommendations appear to be based on few small studies that have shown the presence of bactobilia on pathologic specimen. However, the incidence of bactobilia in patients with acute cholecystitis is between 23 and 72%, and a recent retrospective study showed that the prevalence of positive bile cultures was not related to severity of acute cholecystitis or outcome [28, 32–36]. It is clear that early cholecystectomy for patients with mild or moderate cholecystitis is associated with decreased morbidity and shorter hospital length of stay [37]. In these patients, we recommend no need for empiric antibiotic therapy and that only perioperative pre-incision antibiotics necessary to cover skin flora be given.

Antibiotics for Use with Nonoperative Management

Multiple studies have challenged the need for antibiotics when attempting to perform conservative (nonoperative) management of acute calculous cholecystitis. A prospective randomized controlled trial performed by Mazeh et al. demonstrated little effect of antibiotics in patients managed conservatively, as well as their use being associated with increased LOS during the index admission. During these patients' elective interval cholecystectomy, there was a lower rate of positive cultures in the non-antibiotic group possibly suggesting that antibiotic usage results in bacterial overgrowth [27]. Additionally, we have limited evidence upon whether antibiotics commonly prescribed for acute cholecystitis are able to reach therapeutic levels in bile especially in the case of biliary obstruction. Coccolini and co-workers reported a rise in the prevalence of resistant bacteria in bile cultures from patients with acute cholecystitis. While the recommendations of this chapter are to undergo operative removal or drainage of the gallbladder for management of acute cholecystitis (and not undergo conservative management with interval elective treatment), this discrepancy strongly demonstrates the need for evidence-based guidelines on the use of antibiotics in clinical practice and in individual patients [28]. The most common clinically significant pathogens associated with advanced cholecystitis are *E. coli*, *Klebsiella*, and, in immunocompromised individuals, enterococcus [38]. Commonly prescribed antibiotic regimens, which may be appropriate in patients with moderate to severe cholecystitis who have sepsis or are unable to undergo early cholecystectomy or biliary drainage, targeting the above pathogens can be seen in Table 15.4.

Table 15.4 Antibiotic regimen for acute cholecystitis [17]

Community-acquired moderate acute cholecystitis	Cefuroxime, ceftriaxone
Community-acquired severe acute cholecystitis with physiologic dysfunction or immunocompromised state	Imipenem, meropenem, doripenem, piperacillin-tazobactam, ciprofloxacin, levofloxacin, or cefepime each in combination with metronidazole

Timing of Cholecystectomy

Cholecystectomy, whether open or laparoscopic, remains the gold standard for treatment of cholecystitis either at the time of the initial attack or 2–3 months after the initial attack has subsided. Since the introduction of laparoscopic cholecystectomy, the timing of cholecystectomy in acute disease has been debated as the laparoscopic approach has clear benefits. However, there has been concern for increased technical difficulty in patients with acute cholecystitis and need for conversion to an open procedure. It is difficult to compare outcomes of early vs late cholecystectomy as there remain variable definitions of early timing (24 h–7 days). In 2013, a review performed by Gurusamy et al. compared cholecystectomy at less than 7 days vs greater than 6 weeks demonstrating no significant difference in conversion rate, complication, or the incidence of ductal injuries [39, 40]. Menahem et al. performed a subsequent meta-analysis that included multiple randomized trials which supported these findings and also demonstrated a lower hospital stay in the early cholecystectomy group [41]. In a recent randomized controlled trial performed by Gutt et al., patients who underwent laparoscopic cholecystectomy within 24 h of admission had a lower morbidity, shorter length of stay, and lower hospital costs [37]. Another recent study by Cao et al. compared four groups of laparoscopic cholecystectomy timing, finding that cholecystectomy performed less than 72 h from admission was associated with significant reductions in mortality, complications, bile duct leaks, bile duct injuries, wound infections, conversion rates, length of hospital stay, and blood loss [42]. The findings from the above reports are echoed in the most recent TG18 management bundle which recommends operative intervention or biliary drainage within 72 h or more urgently for severe disease [43].

Operative Technique

Removal of the gallbladder currently remains the only definitive management of acute cholecystitis. Prior to wide use of the laparoscopic approach this was performed via open cholecystectomy. In the 1990s, performance of laparoscopic cholecystectomy became widespread; however, this was matched with a sharp increase in the number of major bile duct injuries as this new approach was being adopted widely [1]. The critical view of safety is a central tenet of performing safe laparoscopy cholecystectomy involving identification of the cystic duct and artery with their complete dissection off the cystic plate. Calot's triangle is cleared of fat and fibrous tissue, and only two structures, the cystic duct and cystic artery, should be connected to the lower end of the gallbladder (Fig. 15.1). During laparoscopic surgery complete removal from the cystic plate creates difficulty in completing clipping of the ducts, and thus this step was modified to mobilization of the lower 1/3. In terms of validation of this technique, there are several studies including thousands of patients in which the critical view was used for cystic duct identification without any biliary injury due to misidentification [44–46]. Critical view of safety is part of the culture of safety in cholecystectomy (COSIC) which has been taken up by the Society of American Gastrointestinal and Endoscopic Surgeons (SAGES) in an effort named "Safe Cholecystectomy." In 2014, the so-called SAGES Safe Cholecystectomy Task Force met and performed an expert Delphi consensus to encourage a culture focused on reducing biliary injury. At the conclusion, the top 5 factors for safe practice in laparoscopic cholecystectomy included (1) establishing the critical view of safety, (2) understanding relevant anatomy, (3) appropriate intraoperative retraction and exposure, (4) knowing when to call for help, and (5) recognizing the need for conversion to an alternate procedure [47]. Interestingly, only 2 of the top 5 factors included technical skills highlighting the importance of the need to continue to improve knowledge in these areas and prioritize future trainees' understanding of the anatomy, the critical view, and safe intraoperative decision-making. In 2016 the IRCAD Hepatobiliary and Pancreatic surgical experts also convened to develop a set of recommendations on safe laparoscopic cholecystectomy. These recommendations again emphasized the importance of the establishment of the critical view of safety while also highlighting use on intraoperative cholangiography and the important role that partial cholecystectomy can play during difficult cholecystectomy [48].

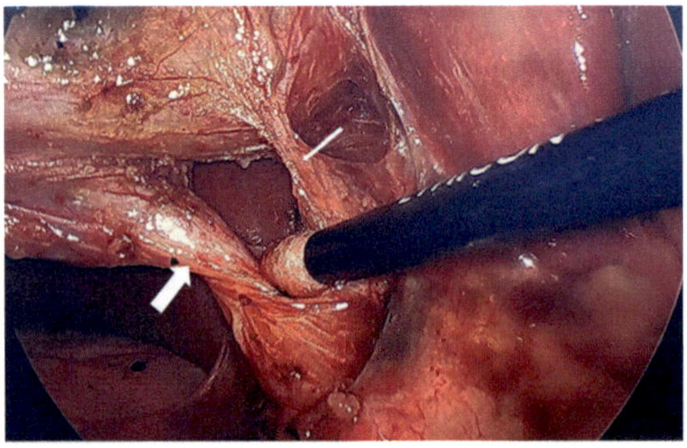

Fig. 15.1 Critical view of safety during laparoscopic cholecystectomy
Critical view of safety demonstrating the cystic duct (wide arrow) and cystic artery (thin arrow) entering the gallbladder with the liver clearly visualized behind the infundibulum

Robotic Cholecystectomy

As technology continues to develop and improve, the robotic surgical system has been introduced as another technique that may be used to perform minimally invasive surgery. Robotic surgery has touted significant benefits to the surgeon including reported lower heart rate and even reduced mental strain; however, in many cases it is associated with increased cost and increased operative time [49, 50]. In a recent review comparing laparoscopic cholecystectomy with robotic cholecystectomy, including five randomized controlled trials, there was no statistically significant differences in intraoperative complications, postoperative complications, readmission rate, hospital stay, estimated blood loss, or a difference in conversion rates. Significant findings demonstrated that robotic cholecystectomy was associated with longer operative time, a higher rate of incisional hernia, and increased hospital costs [49]. Additionally a systematic review performed by Huang et al. also demonstrated the previously seen increased operative time as well as the overall hospital costs being significantly greater when performed robotically [51, 52]. While robotic surgery has been shown to reduce complications, conversion rates, blood loss, and hospital stay compared to laparoscopic surgery in some procedures, it appears that robotic surgery fails to demonstrate any of these benefits when performing cholecystectomy [49, 53–55]. Until procedure length and hospital costs can be reduced, laparoscopic cholecystectomy should remain the approach of choice.

Subtotal Cholecystectomy

It has become clear that a deep understanding of the anatomy and clinical decision-making during the procedure are essential in the performance of safe laparoscopic cholecystectomy. In accordance with both the SAGES and IRCAD recommendations, it is essential to understand when it is time to call for help as well as when it is time to perform a "bail out" procedure [47, 48]. Biliary injuries are more common when operations are more difficult secondary to acute or chronic inflammation creating difficulty in establishing the critical view of safety [1, 44, 56]. The first description of a bail out procedure during cholecystectomy was performed in 1898 by Hans Kehr where the posterior wall of the gallbladder and infundibular cuff were left in place. However, throughout the history of cholecystectomy there have been many additional reports of both partial and subtotal cholecystectomy, but the extent of resection has never been defined leading to significant confusion when using these terms. In an attempt to clarify terminology moving forward, Strasberg et al. proposed no longer using the term partial cholecystectomy. Additionally designation whether or not a closed remnant gallbladder is produced by the procedure should determine the use of the modifying term fenestrating (an open gallbladder remnant remains) (Fig. 15.2a) and reconstituting (a closed functional gallbladder remnant remains, Fig. 15.2b) be introduced [57]. On review there is limited data comparing the short- and long-term outcomes of the two techniques, and likely each is associated with their own unique complications. When performing the reconstituting technique, a gallbladder remnant is created. In 1966, Bodvall and Overgaard first defined the term gallbladder remnant in 1966 which was defined as a wider part of

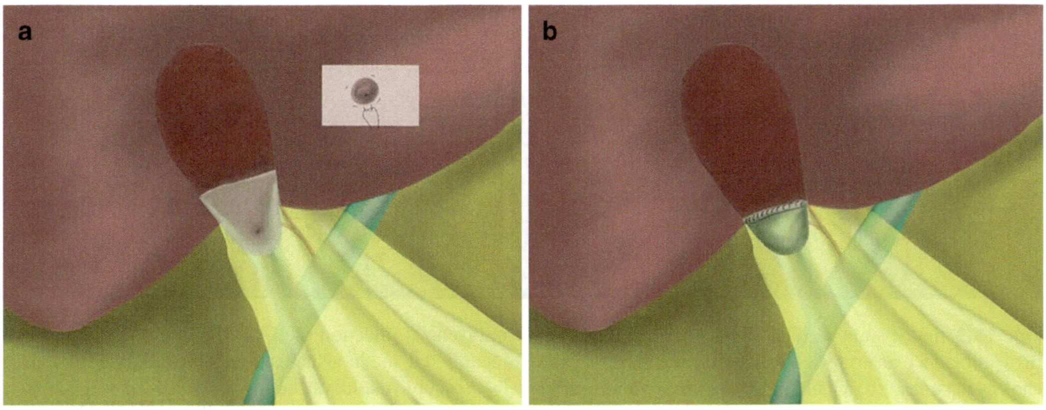

Fig. 15.2 Subtotal cholecystectomy. (**a**) Fenestrating subtotal cholecystectomy with open gallbladder remnant remaining with purse string suture of cystic duct orifice. (**b**) Reconstituting subtotal cholecystectomy with closed gallbladder remnant remaining

the free end of the cystic duct that gives the appearance of a diminutive gallbladder [57, 58]. This description was first applied to a previous case causing symptoms, and the subject was again approached in 2009 by Pernice and Andreoli [59]. On further review it appears gallbladder remnants may become symptomatic requiring a second operation. With regard to the fenestrating subtotal cholecystectomy, biliary leak remains a major concern. However, systematic review and meta-analysis performed by Elshaer et al. in 2015 demonstrated that while fistula was more common with the fenestrating technique, they seemed to resolve spontaneously in most cases when not complicated by a retained CBD stone [33]. More recently a study performed by Van Dijk et al. reviewed both the short-term and long-term complications and morbidity of the two techniques [60]. Fenestrating subtotal cholecystectomy was associated with a higher rate of postoperative bile leak, longer hospital stay, and higher rate of completion cholecystectomies, while reconstituting subtotal cholecystectomy was associated with an increased recurrence of biliary events. Patient-reported outcomes and quality of life were found to be equal between the two groups [60]. It seems both procedures represent viable and safe techniques when difficult anatomy prevents visualization of the critical view of safety, and which technique is used depends on surgeon preference and skill level as well as intraoperative findings.

Indocyanine Green Cholangiography

New and innovative operative techniques are being established to aid in the safe identification of the biliary tree. Intraoperative visualization of the bile ducts using near infrared light in coordination with the fluorescent dye indocyanine green (ICG) is becoming increasingly common. ICG is given as an intravenous agent prior to the start of the operation. The dye is water soluble and bound to plasma proteins which is metabolized by the hepatic parenchyma and subsequently secreted into bile. With the use of a near infrared laparoscope, the bile ducts are seen to be fluorescent allowing for identification of the cystic duct, common bile duct, and common hepatic duct (Fig. 15.3). There are multiple dosage schemes noted on literature review ranging from fixed dosage of 2.5 mg to a dosage of 0.5 mg/kg. Zarrinpar et al. showed a dose of 0.25 mg/kg administered at least 45 minutes prior to visualization facilitates intraoperative anatomical identification [61, 62]. In a systematic review performed by Vlek et al., visualization rates of the biliary structures with ICG appeared to be equally good for either 2.5 mg fixed dosage or 0.5 mg per kg dosage of ICG. In comparison to intraoperative cholangiography, no ducts need to be incised in patients undergoing ICG cholangiography [63]. Vlek et al. concluded that ICG pro-

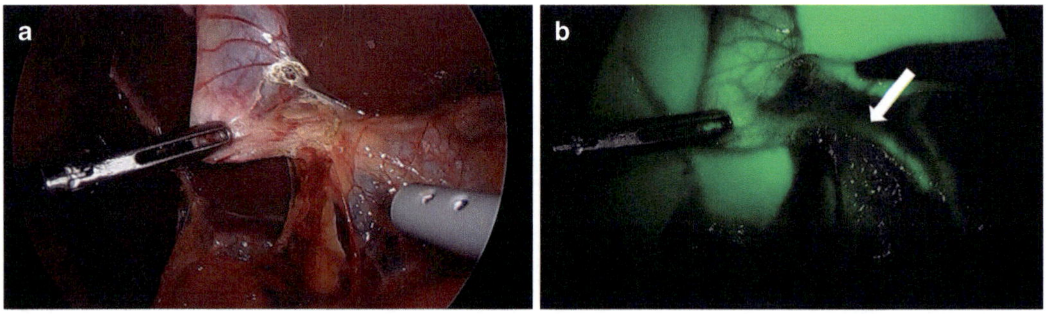

Fig. 15.3 Indocyanine green cholangiography (ICG). (**a**) Gallbladder anatomy visualized during laparoscopic cholecystectomy. (**b**) Gallbladder anatomy viewed after intravenous injection of ICG. The cystic duct (arrow) is identified to aid in visualization of the biliary ducts during laparoscopic cholecystectomy

vided equal visualization of the bile ducts; however no randomized trials have been performed to date. There are several limitations regarding the widespread use of ICG. First, in order to utilize the technology, the laparoscope must be equipped with the near infrared technology and have an accompanying tower. There is also concern that the amount of intra-abdominal adipose tissue can effect visualization. Osayi et al. have reported improved visualization of the cystic duct junction in patients with lower BMI, while other studies have reported no difference across BMI groups [63–65].

Cholecystostomy Tube

Percutaneous cholecystostomy (PC) is considered a treatment option under the TG13 practice guidelines for patients with grade 2 disease with symptoms longer than 96 h and/or patients at high risk for surgery and in grade 3 disease as a temporizing measure for all patients planned for delayed cholecystectomy [43]. A Cochrane review in 2012 included two randomized clinical trials to evaluate the benefits and risks of PC in high-risk surgical patients compared to conservative treatment or emergency laparoscopic cholecystectomy; however, the authors were unable to draw conclusions and create any guidelines given the poor quality of evidence that was available [66, 67]. Chou et al. found that when cholecystostomy was performed within 1 day of admission, there was a lower bleeding rate and shorter hospital stay [68]. In a study by Bala et al., 37% of high-risk patients required permanent cholecystostomy with tube-related complications occurring in 31% of patients, most commonly tube dislodgement [69]. Additionally, while patients undergoing PC were seen to have a significantly elevated mortality rate when compared to those who are not, it is clear that this rate is likely related to selection bias with inability to create an adequate cohort of matched patients to truly analyze the effects of PC. The rate of recurrence of symptoms within 1 year of PC in patients who survive the first episode and did not undergo cholecystectomy varies from 6 to 20% across various studies [66]. A systematic review by Macchini et al. demonstrates a recurrence rate of approximately 12.1% [70]. Up to this point, it seemed that while PC has been generally been accepted as a bridging technique to laparoscopic cholecystectomy, it seems more recent studies have outlined its potential use as definitive treatment with rates of patients not undergoing cholecystectomy after PC ranging from 43 to 94%. The recently performed multicenter, randomized CHOCOLATE trial demonstrated that laparoscopic cholecystectomy is superior to percutaneous catheter drainage in the treatment of high-risk patients (defined as APACHE II score of 7–14) with acute calculous cholecystitis and reduced the rate of major complications as well as reducing healthcare costs questioning the utility of PC [71].

Endoscopic Ultrasound

While laparoscopic cholecystectomy remains the ideal management for patients with acute cholecystitis, some patients presenting with severe disease or severe comorbidity are not candidates for an operative intervention nor candidates for conservative management. While percutaneous cholecystostomy is the most well-established technique, evolving technology endoscopic transpapillary gallbladder drainage (ETGBD) and endoscopic ultrasound-guided-transmural gallbladder drainage (EUS-TGBD), using a transgastric or trans duodenal puncture and drain or stent placement, have been suggested as novel techniques. Inoue et al. evaluated long-term outcomes in high-risk surgical patients, who underwent ET-GBD vs percutaneous drainage [72]. The study demonstrated success rates up to 94% with recurrence rates of 0% compared to 17% in the percutaneous group demonstrating the technique feasibility. EUS-TGBD was initially performed using self-expanding metal stents (SEMS); however, it has now moved toward the use of lumen approximating metal stents (LAMS) (Fig. 15.4). While most of the literature consists

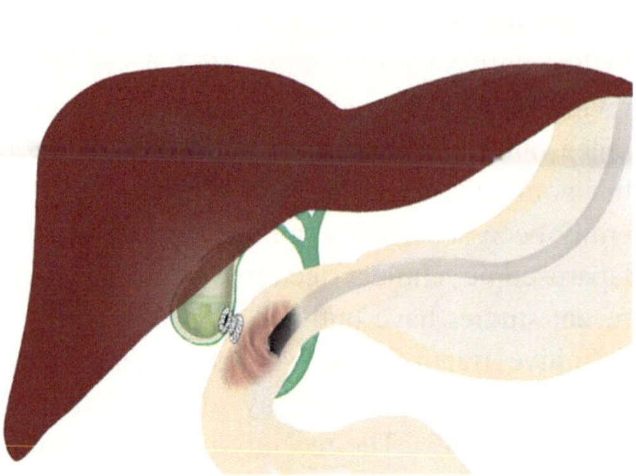

Fig. 15.4 Endoscopic transduodenal lumen apposing metal stent for biliary drainage

of case reports and case series, a recent meta-analysis was performed by Manta et al. that included 62 studies with 226 patients. Overall LAMS were successfully placed in 95% of patients with clinical success in 91% while acting as a definitive treatment with an incidence of adverse events noted to be approximately 10%. In comparison, percutaneous cholecystostomy is associated with biliary peritonitis, bleeding, pneumothorax in up to 12%, and other potential complications from premature tube removal in up to an additional 12% of patients [73, 74]. A study by Kedia et al. found that hospital length of stay, time to clinical resolution, adverse event rate, number of interventions, and post procedure pain scores were significantly higher for the percutaneous compared to endoscopic procedures [75, 76]. Overall while endoscopic biliary drainage may not be widely available, it represents a safe and effective approach in patients that are high risk for operative intervention.

Outcomes

While cholecystectomy is a commonly performed, safe operation, overall complication rates range from 5 to 15% in the literature. The most serious complication is bile duct injury with an incidence 0.3–1.5% [63, 77, 78].There has been many classification systems used to define these injuries; however they are often defined by the classification system created by Strasberg et al. and are also commonly associated with vascular injuries, especially arterial injuries [56, 79, 80]. As previously mentioned, technical skill, operative decision-making, and thorough understanding of the anatomy are all imperative in preventing iatrogenic injury. Complete and early diagnosis of the extent of the injury and possible associated vascular injuries are extremely important for operative planning and better outcomes. While the technical aspects of management of these injuries is complex and outside the scope of this chapter, it is important to understand reconstruction requires expert multidisciplinary teams, and it is best to refer patients to tertiary care centers equipped with advanced endoscopy, advanced interventional radiology, and hepatobiliary surgical techniques.

References

1. S S. Acute calculous CHolecystitis. N Engl J Med. 2008;358(26):2804–11.
2. Everhart JEKM, Hill M, Maurer KR. Prevalence and ethnic differences in gallbladder disease in the United States. Gastroenterol. 1999;117:632–9.
3. Urbach DR, Stukel TA. Rate of elective cholecystectomy and the incidence of severe gallstone disease. CMAJ. 2005;172:1015–9.
4. Zenobi MAE, Domanico A, Arienti V. Update on bedside ultrasound (US) diagnosis of acute cholecystitis (AC). Intern Emerg Med. 2016;11:261–4.
5. Kiewiet JJLM, Bipat S, et al. A systematic review and meta-analysis of diagnostic performance of imaging in acute cholecystitis. Radiology. 2012;264(3):708–20.
6. Smith EADJ, Elsayes KM, Menias CO, Bude RO. Cross-sectional imaging of acute and chronic gallbladder inflammatory disease. Am J Roentgenol. 2009;192:188–96.
7. Kaoutzanis C, Davies E, Leichtle S, Welch K, Winter S, Lampman R, Arneson W. Abdominal ultrasound versus hepato-imino diacetic acid scan in diagnosing acute cholecystitis-what is the real benefit? J Surg Res. 2014;188:44–52.
8. Chatziioannou SNMW, Ford PV, Dhekne RD. Hepatobiliary scintigraphy is superior to abdominal ultrasonography in suspected acute cholecystitis. Surgery. 2000;127:609.
9. Kalimi RGG, Caplin D, et al. Diagnosis of acute cholecystitis: sensitivity of sonography, cholescintigraphy, and combined sonography-cholescintigraphy. J Am Coll Surg. 2001;193:609.
10. Trowbridge RLRN, Shojania. Does this patient have acute cholecystitis? JAMA. 2003;289(1):80–6.

11. Shaespear JA, Rzvani M. CT findings of acute cholecystitis and its coplications. Gastrointestinal imaging. 2009;194:1523–9.
12. Freitas JEMS, Fink-Bennett DM, Bree RL. Suspected acute cholecystitis. Comparison of hepatobiliary scintigraphy versus ultrasonography. Clin Nucl Med. 1982;7:364.
13. Yokoe MTT, Strasber S, Slomkin J, Mayumi T, Gomi H, Pitt H, Garden J, Kiriyama S, et al. TG13 diagnostic criteria and severity grading of acute cholecystitis (with videos). J Hepatobiliary Pancreat Sci. 2013;20:35–46.
14. Yokoe MHJ, Takada T, Strasber S, Slomkin J, Mayumi T, Gomi H, Pitt H, Garden J, Kiriyama S, et al. Tokyo guidelines 2018: diagnostic criteria and severity grading of acute cholecystitis (with videos). J Hepatobiliary Pancreat Sci. 2018;25:41–54.
15. Naidu KBE, Gananadha S, Mosse CT. The yield of fever, inflammatory markers and ultrasound in the diagnosis of acute cholecystitis: a validation of the 2013 Tokyo guidelines. World J Surg. 2016;40:2892–7.
16. W R. The first laparoscopic cholecystectomy. J Soc Laparosc Robotic Surg. 2001;5:89–94.
17. Hernandez MMB, Aho J, Haddad N, Saleem H, Zeb M, Morris D, Jenkins D, Zielinski M. Validation of the AAST EGS acute cholecystitis grade and comparison with the Tokyo guidelines. Surgery. 2018;163: 739–46.
18. Yokoe MTT, Hwang TL, Endo I, Akazawa K, Miura F, et al. Validation of TG13 severity grading in acute cholecystitis: Japan-Taiwan collaborative study for acute cholecystitis. J Hepatobiliary Pancreat Sci. 2017;24:338–45.
19. Paul Wright GSK, Johnson J, Hefty MT, Chung MH. Predicting length of stay and conversion to open cholecystectomy for acute cholecystitis using the 2013 Tokyo guidelines in a US population. J Hepatobiliary Pancreat Sci. 2015;22:795–801.
20. Kamalapurkar DPT, Siriwardhane M, Hollands M, Johnston E, Pleass H, et al. Index cholecystectomy in grade II and III acute calculous cholecystitis is feasible and safe. ANZ J Surg. 2015;85:854–9.
21. Amirthalingam V LJ, Woon W, Shelat V. Tokyo Guidelines 2013 may be too restrictive and patients with moderate and severe acute cholecystitis can be managed by early cholecystectomy too. Surg Endosc 2017;31:2892–2900.
22. Ambe PC, Christ H, Wassenberg D. Does the Tokyo guidelines predict the extent of gallbladder inflammation in patients with acute cholecystitis? A single center retrospective analysis. BMC Gastroenterol. 2015;20:142.
23. Vera KPK, Schuster K, Davis K. Validation of a new American Association for the Surgery of Trauma (AAST) anatomic severity grading system for acute cholecystitis. J Trauma Acute Care Surg. 2018;84(4):650–4.
24. Savage SAKC, Priest EL, Crandall ML, Rodriguez BC, Shafi S. Validating a new grading scale for emergency general surgery diseases. Surg Res. 2015;196(2):264–9.
25. Shafi SPE, Crandall ML, Klekar CS, Nazim A, Aboutanos M, Agarwal S, Bhattacharya B, Byrge N, Dhillon TS, et al. Multicenter validation of American Association for the Surgery of Trauma grading system for acute colonic diverticulitis and its use for emergency general surgery quality improvement program. J Trauma Acute Care Surg. 2016;80(3):405–10.
26. Hernandez MCAJ, Habermann EB, Choudhry AJ, Morris DS, Zielinski MD. Increased anatomic severity predicts outcomes: validation of the American Association for the Surgery of Trauma's emergency general surgery score in appendicitis. J Trauma Acute Care Surg. 2017;82(1):73–9.
27. Mazeh HMI, Dior U, Simanovsky N, Shapiro M, Freund H, Eid A. Role of antibiotic therapy in mild acute calculus cholecystitis: a prospective randomized controlled trial. World J Surg. 2012;36:1750–9.
28. van Dijk ARP, Tasma T, van Dieren S, Hugh T, Boermeester M. Systematic review of antibiotic treatment for acute calculous cholecystitis. BJS. 2016;103:797–811.
29. Solomkin JSMJ, Bradley JS, Rodvold KA, Goldstein EJC, Baron EJ, et al. Diagnosis and management of complicated intra-abdominal infection in adults and children: guidelines by the Surgical Infection Society and the Infectious Diseases Society of America. Clin Infect Dis. 2010;50:133–64.
30. Yoshida MTT, Kawarada Y, Tanaka A, Nimura Y, Gomi H, et al. Antimicrobial therapy for acute cholecystitis: Tokyo guidelines. J Hepatobiliary Pancreat Sci. 2007;14:83–90.
31. Mayumi T, Kawarada Y, et al. Results of the Tokyo consensus meeting Tokyo guidelines. J Hepatobiliary Pancreat Sci. 2007;14:114–21.
32. Galili OES, Matter I, Madi H, Brodsky A, Galis I. The effect of bactibilia on the course and outcome of laparoscopic cholecystectomy. Eur J Clin Microbiol Infect. 2008;27:797–803.
33. Elshaer MGG, Thomas K, Sorge R, Al-Hamali S, Ebdewi H. Subtotal cholecystectomy for "difficult gallbladders" systematic review and meta-analysis. JAMA. 2015;150(2):159–68.
34. Bang CS, Yoon JH, Kim YJ, Kim JB, Baik GH, Suk KT, et al. Clinical impact of body mass index on bactibilia and bacteremia. BMC Gastroenterol. 2014;14:104.
35. Darkahi BSG, Liljeholm H, Videhult P, Melhus Å, Rasmussen IC. Biliary microflora in patients undergoing cholecystectomy. Surg Infect. 2014;15:262.
36. Lykkegaard Nielsen MMF, Justesen T, Scheibel JH, Lindenberg S. Wound sepsis after elective cholecystectomy. Restriction of prophylactic antibiotics to risk groups. Scand J Gastroenterol. 1981;16:937–40.
37. Gutt CN, Encke J, Koninger J, et al. Acute cholecystitis: early versus delayed cholecystectomy, a multicenter randomized trial. Ann Surg. 2013;258:385–93.
38. Solomkin JSMJ, Bradley JS, et al. Diagnosis and management of complicated intra-abdominal infec-

tion in adults and children: guidelines by the surgical infection society and the infectious diseases society of America. Surg Infect. 2010;11:79–109.
39. Bagla PSJ, Riall T. Management of acute cholecystitis. Curr Opin Infect Dis. 2016;29(5):508–13.
40. Gurusamy KSNM, Davidson BR. Early versus delayed laparoscopic cholecystectomy for acute gallstone pancreatitis. Cochrane Database Syst Rev. 2013; https://doi.org/10.1002/14651858.CD010326.pub2.
41. Menahem BMA, Fohlen A, et al. Delayed laparoscopic cholecystectomy increases the total hospital stay compared to an early laparoscopic cholecystectomy after acute cholecystitis: an updated meta-analysis of randomized controlled trials. HPB (Oxford). 2015;17:857–62.
42. Cao AMEG, Cox MR. Early laparoscopic cholecystectomy is superior to delayed acute cholecystitis: a meta-analysis of case-control studies. Surg Endosc. 2016;30:1172–82.
43. Mayumi TOK, Takada T, Strasberg S, Slomkin J, Schlossberd D, Pitt H, et al. Tokyo guidelines 2018: management bundles for acute cholangitis and cholecystitis. J Hepatobiliary Pancreat Sci. 2018;25:96–100.
44. Strasberg SBM. The critical view of safety. Annals of Surgery. 2017;265(3):464–5.
45. Yegiyants SCJ. Operative strategy can reduce the incidence of major bile duct injury in laparoscopic cholecystectomy. Am Surg. 2008;74:985–7.
46. Avgerinos CKD, Touloumis Z, et al. One thousand laparoscopic cholecystectomies in a single surgical unit using the "critical view of safety" technique. J Gastrointest Surg. 2009;13:498–503.
47. Pucher PBM, Fanelli R, Asbun H, Aggarwal R. SAGES expert Delphi consensus: critical factors for safe surgical practice in laparoscopic cholecystectomy. Surg Endosc. 2015;29:3074–85.
48. Conrad CWG, Asbun H, Dallemagne B, et al. IRCAD recommendation on safe laparoscopic cholecystectomy. J Hepatobiliary Pancreat Sci. 2017;24:603–15.
49. Han CSX, Yao L, Yan P, Li M, Hu L, Tian H, Jing W, Du B, Wang L, Yang K, Guo T. Robotic-assisted versus laparoscopic cholecystectomy for benign gallbladder diseases: a systematic review and meta-analysis. Surg Endosc. 2018;32:4377–92.
50. Heemskerk J, et al. Relax, it's just laparoscopy! A prospective randomized trial on heart rate variability of the surgeon in robot-assisted versus conventional laparoscopic cholecystectomy. Dig Surg. 2014;31:225–32.
51. Huang YCT, Maddern G, Samra J. Robotic cholecystectomy versus convensiontal laparoscopic cholecystectomy: a meta-analysis. Surgery. 2016;161(3):628–36.
52. Breitenstein SNA, Puhan M, Held U, Weber M, Clavien PA. Robotic-assisted versus laparoscopic cholecystectomy: outcome and cost analyses of a case-matched control study. Ann Surg. 2008;247:987–93.
53. Zhou J, et al. Robotic versus laparoscopic distal pancreatectomy: a meta-analysis of short-term outcomes. PLoS One. 2016;11(3)
54. Chang S-J, et al. Comparing the efficacy and safety between robotic-assisted versus open pyeloplasty in children: a systemic review and meta-analysis. World J Urol. 2015;33(11):1855–65.
55. Zhagn X, et al. Robot-assisted versus laparoscopic-assisted surgery for colorectal cancer: a meta-analysis. Surg Endosc. 2016;30(12):5601–14.
56. Strasberg SHS. An analytical review of vasculobiliary injury in laparoscopic and open cholecystectomy. HPB. 2011;13:1–14.
57. Strasberg SPM, Brunt M. Subtotal cholecystectomy—"Fenestrating" vs "Reconstituting" subtypes and the prevention of bile duct injury: definition of the optimal procedure in difficult operative conditions. J AM Coll Surg. 2016;222(1):89–96.
58. Bodvall BOB. Cystic duct remnant after cholecystectomy: incidence studied by cholegraphy in 500 cases, and significance in 103 reoperations. Ann Surg. 1966;163:382.
59. Pernice LMAF. Laparoscopic treatment of stone recurrence in a gallbladder remnant: report of an additional case and literature review. J Gastrointest Surg. 2009;13:208.
60. van Dijk ADS, Lameris W, Vries E, et al. Short- and Long-Term outcomes after a reconstituting and fenestrating subtotal cholecystectomy. J AM Coll Surg. 2017;225(3):371–9.
61. Hiwastashi KOH, Setoyama T, Ando K, Ogura Y, Aridome K, Maenohara S, Natsugoe S. Evaluation of laparoscopic cholecystectomy using indocyanine green cholangiography including cholecystitis. Medicine. 2018;97(30)
62. Zarrinpar ADE, Mobley C, et al. Intraoperative laparoscopic near-infrared fluorescence cholangiography to facilitate anatomical identification: when to give indocyanine green and how much. Surg Innov. 2016;23:360–5.
63. Vlek S, van Dam D, Rubinstein S, Lange-de Klerk E, Schoonmade L, Tuynman J, Meijerink W, Ankersmit M. Biliary tract visualization using near infrared imaging with indocyanine green during laparoscopic cholecystectomyL results of a systematic review. Surg Endosc. 2017;31:2731–42.
64. Osayi SNWM, Chaudhry UI, Drosdeck JM, Perry KA, Noria SF, Hazey JW, Muscarella P, Melvin WS, Narula VK. Near infrared fluorescent cholangiography facilitates identification of biliary anatomy during laparoscopic cholecystectomy. Surg Endosc Other Interv Tech. 2014;28(267)
65. Pen˜as-Herrero I dlS-HC, Perez-Miranda M. Endoscopic ultrasound-guided gallbladder drainage for the management of acute cholecystitis. J Hepatobiliary Pancreat Sci. 2015;22:35–43.
66. Stanek A, Dohan A, Barkun J, Barkun A, Reinhold C, Valenti D, Cassinotto C, Gallix B. Percutaneous cholecystostomy: a simple bridge to surgery or an alterna-

tive option for the management of acute cholecystitis? Am J Surg. 2018;216:595–603.
67. Gurusamy KSRM, Davidson BR. Percutaneous cholecystostomy for highrisk surgical patients with acute calculous cholecystitis. Cochrane Database Syst Rev. 2013;(8) https://doi.org/10.1002/14651858.CD007088.pub2.
68. Chou CKLK, Chan CC, et al. Early percutaneous cholecystostomy in severe acute cholecystitis reduces the complication rate and duration of hospital stay. Medicine. 2015;94(27):e1096.
69. Bala MMI, Mazeh H, Yuval J, Eid A, Almogy G. Percutaneous cholcystostomy is safe and effective option for acute calculous cholecystitis in select group of high-risk patients. Eur J Trauma Emerg Surg. 2015;42:761–6.
70. Macchini DDL, Oldani M, et al. Timing of percutaneous cholecystostomy tube removal: a systematic review. Minverva Chir. 2016;71(6)
71. Loozen CSH, Duijvendijk P, Bessel M, Gouma D, Nieuwenhuijzen G, Kelder J, Donkervoort S, Boerma D, et al. Laparoscopic cholecystectomy versus percutaneous catheter drainage for acute cholecystitis in high risk patients (CHOCOLATE): multicentre randomised clinical trial. BMJ. 2018:363.
72. Inoue T OF, Kachi K, et al. Long-term outcomes of endoscopic gallbladder stenting in high-risk surgical patients with calculous cholecystitis (with videos). Gastrointest Endosc. 2016;83:905–13.
73. Manta RMM, Galloro G, Conigliaro R, Zullo A. Endoscopic ultrasound-guided gallbladder drainage for acute cholecystitis with a lumen apposing metal stent: a systematic review of case series. Eur J Gastroenterol Hepatol. 2018;30(7):695–8.
74. Bakkaloglu HYH, Guloglu R, Taviloglu K, Tunca F, Aksoy M, et al. Ultrasound guided percutaneous cholecystostomy in high-risk patients for surgical intervention. World J Gastroenterol. 2006;12:7179–82.
75. Kedia PSR, Kumta NA, Widmer J, Jamal-Kabani A, Weaver K, et al. Endoscopic gallbladder drainage compared with percutaneous drainage. Gastrointest Endosc. 2015;82:1031–6.
76. Anderloni ABA, Vieceli F, Khashab M, Hassan C, Repici A. Endoscopic ultrasound-guided transmural stenting for gallbladder drainage in high-risk patients with acute cholecystitis: a systematic review and pooled analysis. Surg Endosc. 2016;30:5200–8.
77. Deziel DJMK, Economou SG, Doolas A, Ko ST, Airan. Complications of laparoscopic cholecystectomy: a national survey of 4,292 hospitals and an analysis of 77,604 cases. Am J Surg. 1993;165:9–14.
78. Flum DRDE, Cheadle A, Chan L. Koepsell T intraoperative cholangiography and risk of common bile duct injury during cholecystectomy. JAMA. 2003;289:1639–44.
79. Davidoff AMPT, Murray EA, Hillern DJ, Johnson RD, Baker ME. Mechanisms of major biliary injury during laparoscopic cholecystectomy. Ann Surg. 1992;215:196–202.
80. Strasberg SHM, Soper N. An analysis of the problem of biliary injury during laparoscopic cholecystectomy. J Am Coll Surg. 1995;1:101–25.

Appendicitis

16

David H. Kim and Lillian S. Kao

Case Report

A 27-year-old previously healthy male presented to the emergency room with a 36-h history of periumbilical pain that migrated to his right lower quadrant. He denied nausea or vomiting but had no appetite. He denied fever or chills. Positive clinical findings included right lower quadrant tenderness and right lower quadrant referred pain when palpating his left lower quadrant. Laboratory values were notable for a leukocytosis of 16,000 cells/L and an elevated C-reactive protein of 12 mg/L. An abdominal ultrasound was non-diagnostic, but the computed tomography (CT) scan showed a dilated appendix with periappendiceal fat stranding.

Surgical consultation was obtained. After a discussion of the risks, benefits, and alternatives to surgery, the patient decided to proceed with surgery. Laparoscopic appendectomy was uneventful, and non-perforated acute appendicitis was confirmed.

The patient progressed well postoperatively and was discharged home the next morning.

Introduction

Appendicitis is one of the most common diagnoses the general surgeon will encounter. The individual lifetime risk of appendicitis is 8.6% for males and 6.7% for females [1]. The lifetime risk of appendectomy is 12% for males and 23.1% for females [1]. The workup and treatment strategies are constantly evolving as the results of new trials become available. An understanding of the literature is necessary to be able to counsel patients regarding the alternative strategies and their associated risks and benefits.

Workup

The initial evaluation starts with a complete history and physical exam. Classically described symptoms include anorexia, nausea, vomiting, and periumbilical pain which migrates to the right lower quadrant. Migratory tenderness is present in 5–60% of patients [2]. The physical examination may be notable for fever and tachycardia in addition to tenderness to palpation at McBurney's point which is located approximately one-third of the way from an imaginary

D. H. Kim (✉) · L. S. Kao
Department of Surgery, McGovern Medical School at the University of Texas Health Science Center, Houston, TX, USA
e-mail: David.H.Kim@uth.tmc.edu; Lillian.S.Kao@uth.tmc.edu

M. D. Zielinski, O. Guillamondegui (eds.), *The Acute Management of Surgical Disease*,
https://doi.org/10.1007/978-3-031-07881-1_16

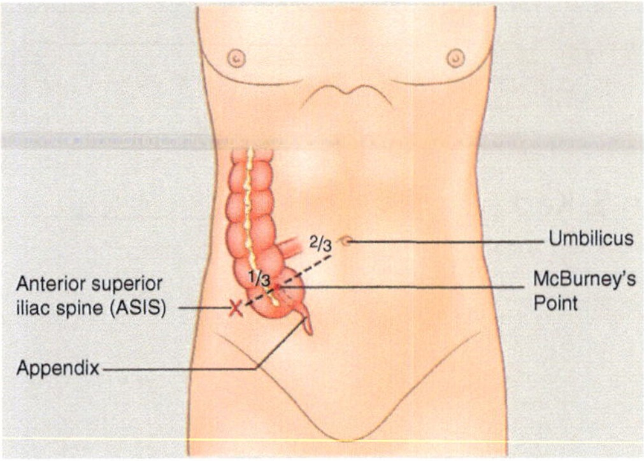

Fig. 16.1 McBurney's point. [With permissions from Sellars H, Boorman P. Surgery, 2017-08-01, Vol 35 (8), 432–438]

line running from the right anterior superior iliac spine to the umbilicus. (Fig. 16.1) Other signs associated with acute appendicitis include the Rovsing's sign where palpation of the left lower quadrant causes pain in the right lower quadrant, the psoas sign where extension of the right hip against resistance causes pain suggesting a retrocecal appendix, and the obturator sign where internal rotation of the right hip causes pain suggesting the appendix lies in the pelvis. Although these and other signs are historically taught, each has a relatively low sensitivity for the diagnosis of acute appendicitis.

Laboratory tests that are obtained during the workup include a complete blood count; leukocytosis is usually present in patients with acute appendicitis. A C-reactive protein may also be ordered to help rule the diagnosis out. In adults with a normal white blood cell count and C-reactive protein, the likelihood of acute appendicitis is low, and imaging may not be required to rule out the diagnosis. One study of 98 patients found a 100% negative predictive value when the white cell count and C-reactive protein levels are both normal (white cell count $<11 \times 10^9$ cells/L and C-reactive protein <10 mg/L) [3]. Chemistries may also be ordered if the patient has been vomiting to ensure normal electrolytes and renal function.

Diagnosis Prediction Models

Several different risk prediction models and scoring systems have been described to assist in the diagnosis of acute appendicitis and in decision-making around obtaining imaging. Most of these models are based on single institution retrospective analyses [4].

The most widely known scoring system is the Alvarado score. Originally described by Alvarado in 1986, the score is a 10-point clinical scoring system for the diagnosis of acute appendicitis based on the patient's symptoms, exam, and laboratory values [5]. Higher scores increase the likelihood of the diagnosis.

The appendicitis inflammatory response score (AIRS) is another scoring system described in 2012. The authors used prospectively collected data to stratify the risk of appendicitis [6]. This score also utilizes various elements of the history, physical exam findings, and labs.

The adult appendicitis score (AAS) was described in 2014 and is similarly comprised of physical exam findings and laboratory values [7]. Patients are stratified into low, intermediate, and high probability of having acute appendicitis. A 2020 review of 5345 adult patients in the United Kingdom examined 15 risk prediction models to determine which model best identifies patients with right lower quadrant pain who were at low risk of appendicitis. In this study, 28% of women and 12% of men underwent a negative appendectomy; 73% of women and 36% of men received preoperative imaging. In this patient population, the authors found that the AAS performed best for women (failure rate of 3.7%) and the appendicitis inflammatory response score (AIRS) performed best for men (failure rate of 2.4%) [8]. However, there have not been any studies comparing outcomes based on routine use of a prediction score.

Imaging

Historically, the use of diagnostic imaging was viewed as extraneous in the context of classic symptoms and an acceptable negative appendectomy rate of 10–20%. However, imaging of patients with suspected appendicitis has increased over time. Among patients diagnosed with appendicitis, over 70% of children and over 80% of adults underwent CT imaging [9].

Table 16.1 Sensitivity and specificity of imaging techniques [12, 13]

	Sensitivity	Specificity
Ultrasound (children)	88%	94%
Ultrasound (adults)	83%	93%
CT (children)	94%	95%
CT (adults)	94%	94%
MRI	97%	95%

CT, ultrasound, and MRI are the imaging modalities of choice for suspected appendicitis. CT is most commonly used in adults as it is typically rapidly available and has a higher sensitivity than ultrasound (Table 16.1). Despite the lower sensitivity, ultrasound is typically first-line imaging modality in children and pregnant patients to limit exposure to ionizing radiation. When ultrasound is non-diagnostic in this population, MRI is recommended [10, 11].

Currently, controversy exists around the optimal use of CT scans and imaging. The debate is centered on the trade-off between use of routine CT imaging to reduce the risk of an unnecessary operation and avoidance of CT scans to minimize exposure to and risks of ionizing radiation, particularly in children.

As the accuracy of imaging improved over time, prospective observational studies reported increased use of both ultrasound and CT with a concurrent decreased in negative appendectomy rates [14, 15]. Lack of imaging in adult patients has been associated with a three times greater odds of negative appendectomy [15]. A small 2007 randomized controlled trial also supported routine imaging in adults. In the trial, patients with right lower quadrant pain were randomized to receive mandatory versus selective CT imaging. The selective cohort underwent roughly one-third less CT scans. Although the trial was underpowered, the mandatory cohort had a trend toward decreased negative appendectomy and perforation rates [16].

With the increasing use of imaging, concern has grown for the risks of increased exposure to ionizing radiation. In response, the Image Gently and Image Wisely campaigns were started to advocate for safe and effective imaging for children and adults, respectively. Strategies to reduce ionizing radiation include using radiation doses as low as reasonably achievable (ALARA) and promoting an ultrasound-first strategy. In a single-center study, an ultrasound-first strategy resulted in a near-zero CT rate without any delay in treatment or increase in negative appendectomy rates [17]. However, the strategy also resulted in an increased use of MRI which corresponded with increased costs. Despite data to suggest that dose reduction programs and ultrasound-first strategies can decrease radiation exposure, these tactics have not been widely adopted across centers, particularly non-children's hospitals [14, 15].

An additional strategy for reducing ionizing radiation exposure that has been evaluated in adolescents and young adults (15–44 years) is the use of low-dose CT. In 2012, a single institution randomized trial showed that the negative appendectomy rate for low-dose CT (3.5%) was non-inferior to standard-dose CT (3.2%) [18]. This led to a much larger multi-institutional randomized controlled trial in 2017 which confirmed the findings of the prior trial; low-dose CT was non-inferior to standard CT with negative appendectomy rates of 3.9% and 2.7%, respectively [19]. Based on these trials, CT can be utilized with lower radiation doses without significant clinical detriment.

Pathology

The general belief is that appendiceal obstruction is the inciting insult of appendicitis. This leads to edema and distention of the appendiceal wall resulting in ischemia and perforation. Fecaliths, enlarged lymphoid follicles, and tumors are potential etiologies of luminal obstruction. Bacterial overgrowth and luminal distention occur due to ongoing mucus secretion. This increases the transmural pressure of the appendix which leads to occlusion of blood and lymphatic vessels. Over time, this causes overt ischemia of the appendix.

Enteric flora are the typical bacterial organisms associated with appendicitis. *Bacteroides* and *Escherichia coli* are virtually ubiquitous with *Peptostreptococcus*, *Pseudomonas*, and *Lactobacillus* being very common as well [20].

Rarely, a specimen will have serosal appendicitis on histopathologic examination. This describes a serosal inflammatory reaction due to a non-appendiceal source. This occurs in approximately 0.01% of patients [21]. The cause of this inflammation may be obvious at the time of surgery though often no primary source can be found. If the serositis can adequately be explained by another intra-abdominal source seen at surgery, no additional investigation is required. When unexplained, the surgeon must be vigilant to any new clinical signs the patient may present with that require additional workup.

Unexpected neoplasms are found in around 1% of appendectomy specimens [22, 23]. Carcinoid tumors, adenocarcinoma, and mucinous neoplasms are the most commonly encountered tumors. If significant concern for malignancy exists during the index operation, then it is prudent to perform a formal right hemicolectomy. This can be performed using a laparoscopic or open approach depending on the surgeon's expertise. If a mucinous neoplasm is suspected, then care should be taken not to rupture the neoplasm which could lead to pseudomyxoma peritonei.

If the malignancy is discovered after histopathologic examination of the appendix, then a staging workup should be performed. Further treatment will be dictated by the tumor biology and the tumor stage. If no metastatic disease, carcinoid tumors that invade the lamina propria/submucosa and are ≤1 cm in size (T1) do not require further resection beyond appendectomy [24]. Patients with high T stages, incomplete resection, or positive nodes should undergo a staging workup. The management of higher T stages and larger tumors is controversial with a wide range of recommendations. Ideally, further management of the patient would involve a multidisciplinary team to determine the best individual treatment course. If the patient is found to have an adenocarcinoma after appendectomy and no metastases, then a formal right hemicolectomy should be performed. Low-grade mucinous neoplasms with negative margins and without perforation or peritoneal involvement do not require additional resection beyond appendectomy [25]. High-grade mucinous neoplasms with the same criteria can usually be treated with appendectomy alone but should be considered on a case by case basis [25]. Mucinous adenocarcinomas should undergo formal right hemicolectomy [25].

Management Based on Disease Severity

The treatment of acute appendicitis has traditionally been operative, with nonoperative management considered for factors such as severity of disease and patient comorbidities. Traditionally, acute appendicitis has been stratified by (1) uncomplicated or simple appendicitis and (2) complicated appendicitis which includes appendicitis associated with gangrene, perforation, phlegmon, or abscess. Alternatively, various individual and single institution grading scales have been previously reported [26]. More recently, the American Association for the Surgery of Trauma (AAST) developed a grading scale for 16 emergency general surgery conditions which include acute appendicitis. The scale provides a uniform reliable scoring system to predict risk and outcomes and to aid quality improvement and resource management. The grading scale increases with severity ranging from Grade I (minimal) to V (severe). The grades are defined based on four categories: clinical, imaging, operative, and pathologic findings (Table 16.2) [27].

A large retrospective study evaluated the AAST grading system as a predictor of disease severity. The authors examined 1099 patients and found that increasing duration of symptoms correlated with increasing severity of appendicitis. Higher AAST grades had longer symptom dura-

Table 16.2 AAST grading scale. [With permissions from Tominaga GT, Staudenmayer KL, Shafi S, et al. The American Association for the Surgery of Trauma grading scale for 16 emergency general surgery conditions: Disease-specific criteria characterizing anatomic severity grading. *J Trauma Acute Care Surg.* 2016;81 (3):593–60)]

AAST grade	Description	Clinical criteria	Imaging criteria (CT findings)	Operative criteria	Pathologic criteria
A. Acute Appendicitis					
I	Acutely inflamed appendix, intact	Pain, leukocytosis and right lower quadrant (RLQ) tenderness	Inflammatory changes localized to appendix +/− appendiceal dilation +/− contrast nonfilling	Acutely inflamed appendix, intact	Presence of neutrophils at the base of crypts, submucosa +/− in muscular wall
II	Gangrenous appendix, intact	Pain, leukocytosis, and RLQ tenderness	Appendiceal wall necrosis with contrast nonenhancement +/− air in appendiceal wall	Gangrenous appendix, intact	Mucosa and muscular wall digestion; not identifiable on hematoxylin-eosin stain
III	Perforated appendix with local contamination	Pain, leukocytosis, and RLQ tenderness	Above with local periappendiceal fluid +/− contrast extravasation	Above, with evidence of local contamination	Gross perforation or focal dissolution of muscular wall
IV	Perforated appendix with periappendiceal phlegmon or abscess	Pain, leukocytosis, and RLQ tenderness; may have palpable mass	Regional soft tissue inflammatory changes, phlegmon or abscess	Above, with abscess or phlegmon in region of appendix	Gross perforation
V	Perforated appendix with generalized peritonitis	Generalized peritonitis	Diffuse abdominal or pelvic inflammatory changes +/− free intraperitoneal fluid or air	Above, with addition of generalized purulent contamination away from appendix	Gross perforation

tion, longer operative times, and increased costs [28]. Another single institutional retrospective study of 334 patients had similar findings. Grade of appendicitis based on preoperative CT imaging was strongly correlated to operative findings. Also, increasing AAST grade was associated with open procedures, complications, and increased length of stay [29]. Subsequently, a large prospective multicenter study of 2909 patients aimed to validate the AAST grading system as a predictor of 30-day outcomes. The authors found a significant correlation between increasing grade and length of stay, infectious complications, Clavien-Dindo complications, and secondary interventions. They also showed a significant correlation with 30-day complications in addition to readmission rates [30].

In 2019 the AAST published a summary guideline for treatment of acute appendicitis based on grade [31]. Laparoscopic appendectomy is recommended as an option for all AAST grades of appendicitis (Table 16.3). Nonoperative management is provided as an alternative for simple appendicitis (AAST Grade I) and for appendicitis with an associated phlegmon or abscess (AAST Grade IV) . However, these guidelines may be modified once updated with the results of all new randomized trials comparing operative to nonoperative management [32].

Table 16.3 AAST management guidelines [31]. [Modified from Schuster KM, Holena DN, Salim A, Savage S, Crandall M. American Association for the Surgery of Trauma emergency general surgery guideline summaries 2018: acute appendicitis, acute cholecystitis, acute diverticulitis, acute pancreatitis, and small bowel obstruction. *Trauma Surg Acute Care Open.* 2019;4 (1):e000281]

AAST Grade	Clinical criteria	Recommended management
I	Acutely inflamed appendix (non-perforated)	Laparoscopic appendectomy; nonoperative treatment with antibiotics may be reasonable
II	Gangrenous appendix (non-perforated)	Laparoscopic appendectomy
III	Perforated appendix with minimal RLQ contamination	Laparoscopic appendectomy
IV	Perforated appendix with periappendiceal phlegmon/ abscess	Laparoscopic appendectomy; nonoperative treatment with antibiotics +/– drain may be reasonable in select patients
V	Perforated appendix with generalized peritonitis	Laparoscopic appendectomy if patient stable

Nonoperative Management

Acute Appendicitis: AAST Grades I–III

Several trials have challenged the dogma that laparoscopic appendectomy is the gold standard for treatment of acute appendicitis. The first randomized controlled trial comparing antibiotics alone to appendectomy was published in 1995. The trial enrolled 40 patients with 1 patient failing initial antibiotic alone therapy and 7 patients having a recurrence within the 1-year follow-up [33]. Since that time, several additional randomized controlled trials in the adult population have shown similar results. These trials focused mainly on patients with uncomplicated appendicitis (AAST Grade I). Systematic reviews and meta-analyses of these trials have demonstrated that initial nonoperative therapy has a lower complication rate but a fairly high failure and recurrence rate, ranging from 10 to 26% [34–41]. Longer-term, 5-year outcomes have been reported for the 2015 APPAC (Antibiotic Therapy vs Appendectomy for Treatment of Uncomplicated Acute Appendicitis) trial [42]. The rates of recurrence for nonoperative management of simple appendicitis based on CT were 27.3% at 1 year, 34% at 2 years, 35.2% at 3 years, 37.1% at 4 years, and 39.1% at 5 years [43].

A multicenter pragmatic trial, Comparison of Outcomes of antibiotic Drugs and Appendectomy (CODA), has recently been completed and will provide further information regarding short- and long-term clinical and patient-reported outcomes [32]. CODA, unlike prior trials, did not exclude patients with gangrenous appendicitis or a localized perforation (AAST Grades II and III).

Based on the current available evidence, nonoperative therapy with antibiotics alone is an option to operative management for acute AAST Grade I appendicitis. The risks and benefits should be discussed with patients to encourage shared decision-making based on patients' preferences and values.

Appendicitis with Phlegmon or Abscess: AAST Grade IV Appendicitis

Patients with acute appendicitis will present with a phlegmon or abscess 3.8% of the time [44]. Traditionally, adult patients who are hemodynamically stable with a phlegmon or abscess have been treated with antibiotics with or without drain placement. A recent systematic review and meta-analysis suggests that the management paradigm is shifting. Gavriilidis et al. reviewed 18 observational studies and 3 randomized trials comparing nonoperative management to appendectomy in patients with complicated appendicitis defined as a phlegmon or abscess. When both observational studies and randomized trials were included in the analysis, nonoperative management was associated with a lower incidence of overall complications, abdominal and pelvic abscesses, and wound infections as compared to a surgical approach. When only randomized trials were included, there were no significant differences in these outcomes, although the confidence interval was not precise enough to rule out a clinically significant difference (OR 0.46, 95% CI 0.17–1.29) [45].

The pediatric population with complicated appendicitis may benefit from early surgical intervention. A 2011 randomized trial investigating early vs interval appendectomy in children showed a benefit with early intervention. Appendectomy during the initial hospital stay led to a statistically significant decrease in time away from normal activities (13.8 vs 19.4 days) and lower adverse event rate (30% vs 55%) when compared to interval appendectomy 6–8 weeks after initial nonoperative treatment [46]. A more recent 2018 study of pediatric patients with complicated appendicitis showed less complications with early appendectomy than late (26.7% vs 34.6, $p < 0.01$) [47]. Current guidelines recommend early appendectomy for complicated appendicitis [11].

In summary, based on the best available evidence, both the World Society of Emergency Surgery and AAST guidelines recommend laparoscopic appendectomy as first-line therapy in patients with perforated appendicitis with a phlegmon or abscess (AAST Grade IV) with the caveat that select patients may be treated with antibiotics and/or percutaneous drain placement [11, 48]. The subset of patients in whom initial nonoperative management is the preferred treatment strategy needs to be further defined. Furthermore, given that both these guidelines have been published recently, their impact on changing practice has yet to be assessed.

Interval Appendectomy

After initial nonoperative management either with antibiotics alone or in conjunction with percutaneous drains, the question remains as to perform routine interval appendectomy to do with the appendix. Traditionally, interval appendectomy was performed after initial nonoperative treatment 6–8 weeks after resolution. This was done to prevent the risk of recurrent appendicitis over the patient's lifetime. The risk of recurrent appendicitis is up to 20% in children [49]. Risk of recurrent appendicitis after initial nonoperative management in adults varies in the literature but is between 5 and 14% [50, 51]. These recurrences usually occurred within 1 year of the initial diagnosis of appendicitis.

Currently, most would recommend against routine interval appendectomy in asymptomatic patients to prevent recurrence [52]. A more compelling argument for interval appendectomy is to rule out neoplasm as the inciting cause of appendicitis. A 2019 study of patients who were successfully treated nonoperatively compared interval appendectomy to follow-up MRI. This study was terminated early after accruing 60 patients due to the high incidence of neoplasms. They found an underlying neoplasm in 20% of the study participants with 29% of patients >40 years old having a neoplasm [53]. Physicians should engage patients in shared decision-making regarding personal risk factors for a neoplasm along with risks and benefits of interval appendectomy after successful initial nonoperative management.

Operative Management

The AAST guideline recommends laparoscopic appendectomy for all grades of appendicitis. Historically, surgical dogma was to perform the appendectomy as soon as possible due to the perceived increased risk of perforation. However, studies suggest that a delay in performing an appendectomy in less than 24 hours may not increase the rate of perforation, gangrene, or abscess [54].

General principles for operative management include prompt resuscitation if the patient is hemodynamically unstable and administration of appropriate preoperative antibiotics prior to incision, with re-dosing as indicated during the case.

There are multiple approaches for appendectomy including open and laparoscopic. An alternative approach includes natural orifice transluminal endoscopic surgery (NOTES).

Open Appendectomy

Although the AAST guideline recommends laparoscopic appendectomy when feasible, an open appendectomy may be necessary. Several incisions can be utilized for the open procedure. The choice of incision should be made based on the surgeon's comfort level and patient factors such as scars from previous abdominal incisions. The McBurney incision is centered over McBurney's point which is 1/3 the distance from the anterior superior iliac spine (ASIS) to the umbilicus. The skin incision is made perpendicular to the line from the ASIS to the umbilicus. The paramedian, pararectus, and midline incision are also reasonable alternatives to the McBurney incision.

When utilizing the McBurney incision, subcutaneous tissues are dissected until the external oblique aponeurosis is encountered. This is split along the direction of its fibers, and the external oblique, internal oblique, and transversus abdominis muscles are bluntly split using a clamp until the transversalis fascia and peritoneum are exposed (Fig. 16.2). These are elevated and incised sharply to gain access to the peritoneum. A finger sweep is utilized to identify the inflamed appendix and deliver it to the wound. Alternatively, the ascending colon is identified and the taenia followed caudad until the appendix is identified. Once the appendix is delivered into the wound, the mesoappendix is transected between clamps prior to suture ligating it to control the appendiceal artery. Once the appendiceal base is exposed after transection of the mesoappendix, the base is doubly ligated using a suture of choice prior to transecting the appendix and passing off the field. Some surgeons prefer to dunk the appendiceal stump using a purse string suture though this is not mandatory.

The peritoneum is then closed using a running absorbable suture prior to reapproximating the split muscle layers in a similar fashion. The subcutaneous tissues are closed in layers as well. The skin may be left open when a class 4 wound is encountered to present surgical site infection.

Laparoscopic Appendectomy

Based on the AAST guidelines, laparoscopic appendectomy is the preferred surgical approach when feasible. Patients who undergo laparoscopic appendectomy have less superficial surgical site infections, shorter length of stays, and less pain with equivalent outcomes when compared to open appendectomy [55]. It has been shown in multiple studies to be safe in children, pregnant patients, obese patients, and the elderly [48].

After induction of anesthesia, the patient is positioned supine with the left arm tucked allowing both the surgeon and assistant to stand on the patient's left. If the patient did not void preoperatively, a urinary catheter may be placed which may reduce the risk of bladder injury [56].

There are multiple different options for entry into the abdomen, initiation of pneumoperitoneum and trocar placement. Options for placement of the initial trocar include an open or Hasson technique, insufflation with a Veress needle followed by use of an optical trocar, or direct entry into the abdomen with an optical trocar. Although single incision laparoscopic surgery is an option, the traditional approach is to use three trocars. When using an open technique, a peri- or transumbilical 10–12 mm trocar is placed, and the abdomen is insufflated. Two additional 5 mm trocars are inserted under direct visualization so as to allow for triangulation (Fig. 16.3). For example, the additional trocars may be placed above the pubis symphysis and in the left lower quadrant. The patient is placed in the Trendelenburg position with the right side elevated.

The small bowel is swept out of the pelvis cephalad. The ascending colon is identified and the taeniae coli followed caudad to their confluence at the base of the cecum. The appendix is elevated with an atraumatic laparoscopic grasper. Gentle blunt dissection may be required to expose the appendix due to the local inflammatory reaction. When encountering a retrocecal appendix, the white line of Toldt must be incised to enter the retroperitoneum for exposure.

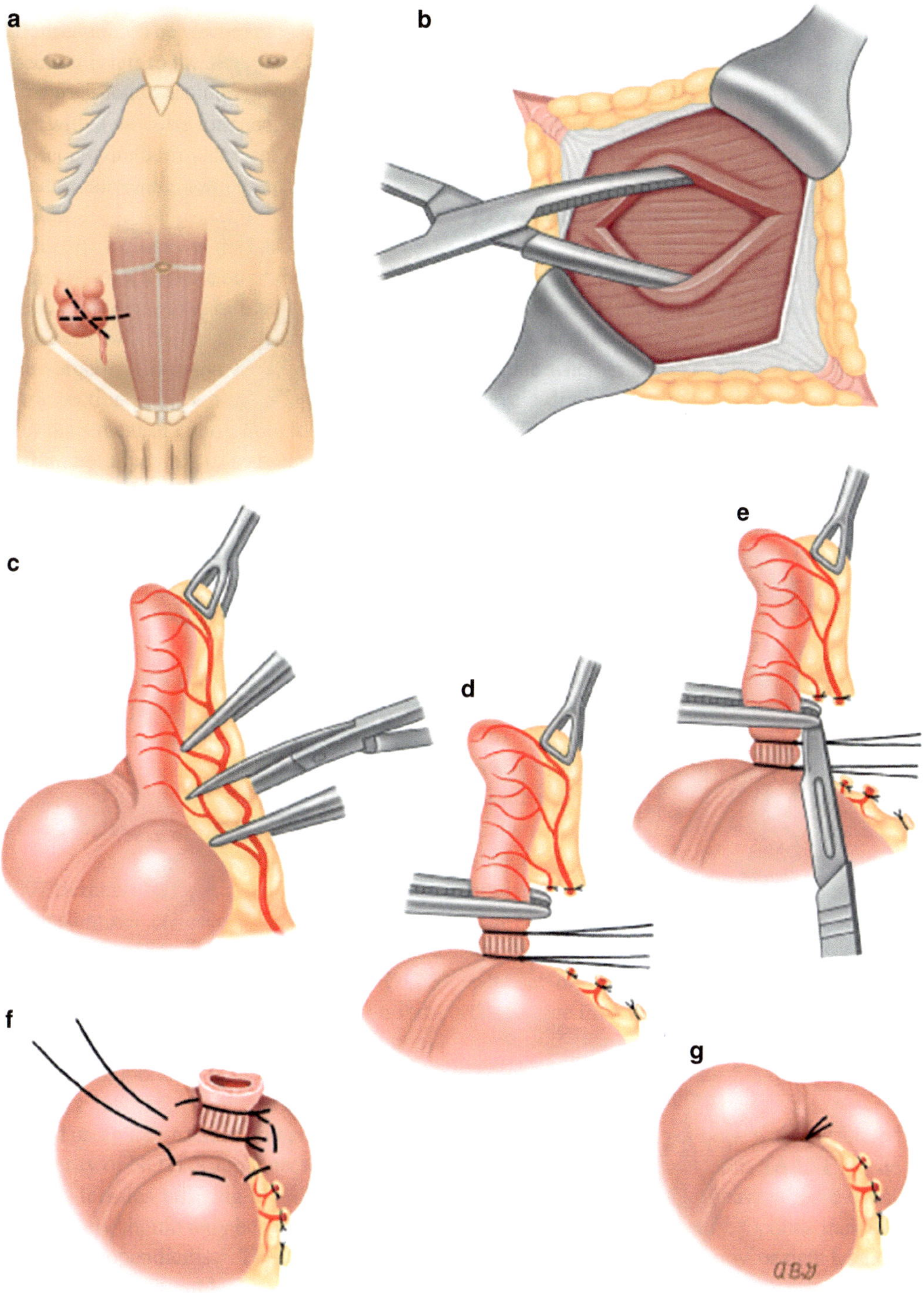

Fig. 16.2 Open appendectomy. (**a**) Incision centered over McBurney's point. B) Splitting the muscle along its fibers bluntly. (**c**) Transection of the mesoappendix. (**d**, **e**) Ligation and transection of the appendix. (**f**) Purse-string suture to "dunk" the stump (optional). (**g**) Completed appendectomy with "dunked" stump. [With permissions from: Smink D, Soybel DI. Management of acute appendicitis in adults. In: UpToDate, Post TW (Ed), UpToDate, Waltham, MA. (Accessed on [9/1/20].) Copyright © 2020 UpToDate, Inc. For more information visit www.uptodate.com]

cion for neoplasm is high, a formal right hemicolectomy should be performed adhering to sound oncologic principles. When considering ileocecectomy, if there is any concern for the vascular status of the proposed anastomosis, then a right hemicolectomy should be performed. Laparoscopic ileocecectomy or right hemicolectomy can be performed if the surgeon is comfortable with these techniques; otherwise, they may be performed after converting to an open procedure.

Special Populations

Pregnancy

Appendicitis occurs less frequently in pregnant patients when compared to age-matched non-pregnant patients and presents most frequently during the second trimester [68]. Pregnant patients frequently have atypical presentations of appendicitis. Non-specific abdominal complaints are most common. However, patients who have a classic presentation should lead to a high index of suspicion for appendicitis. Leukocytosis is also non-specific and common in pregnancy.

Ultrasound is the imaging modality of choice in the pregnant patient. If the diagnosis is unclear after ultrasound, MRI should follow. If MRI is unavailable, then low-dose CT should be considered [10].

Once the diagnosis of acute appendicitis is established, prompt surgical resection should occur. Nonoperative management should not be considered in pregnant patient with uncomplicated appendicitis due to the increased rate of complications compared with operative intervention [69]. Outcomes from surgery are similar to those in non-pregnant patients except when perforation is present. Perforated appendicitis leads to a significantly higher rate of fetal loss than non-perforated appendicitis [70]. Though some literature suggests laparoscopic compared to open appendectomy increases the risk of fetal loss, a 2019 systematic review and meta-analysis found no difference in fetal loss between the two approaches [71, 72]. Further, the authors found that patients who underwent laparoscopic appendectomy had shorter hospital stays and less wound infections [72]. Laparoscopy is safe in all trimesters and should not be delayed due to pregnancy if an indication for surgery is present [69]. During the second and third trimesters, initial port placement may require adjustment due to fundal height [69]. Typical insufflation pressures of 15 mmHg have been shown to be safe though some recommend lower continuous pressure and to adjust pressures based on the patient's intraoperative hemodynamics [69].

Obesity

Laparoscopy is preferred over open appendectomy in obese patients. Laparoscopic surgery is associated with less wound infections, lower hospital length of stay, operative time, and cost [73].

Normal-Appearing Appendix

On occasion, the surgeon may encounter a grossly normal appearing appendix. It is prudent to examine the abdomen for another source of the patient's symptoms. Some conditions to consider include Crohn's disease, Meckel's diverticulitis, pelvic inflammatory disease, right-sided diverticulitis, and ectopic pregnancy. It is still recommended that the appendix be resected as up to 30% of normal-appearing appendices have appendicitis after histologic examination [74]. Appendectomy with a grossly normal appendix also aids future evaluation by removing appendicitis in the differential.

Chronic Appendicitis

Patients suffering from chronic appendicitis are typically described as having persistent (usually more than 1 week) right lower quadrant pain which resolves after appendectomy. The pain may be constant or intermittent and patients often have a no leukocytosis. Histopathologic examination reveals chronic inflammation or fibrosis of the appendix [75].

Postoperative Management

Postoperative management after uncomplicated appendicitis includes pain control with a multimodal approach and early ambulation. No further antibiotic therapy is indicated. A regular diet may be started immediately, and the patient is usually discharged on the first postoperative day although same-day discharge is becoming more frequent. Studies have not demonstrated any difference in short-term readmission rates or wound complications [76, 77].

Antibiotic therapy beyond the perioperative period (24 h) is not indicated for AAST Grade I-II appendicitis. Typical postoperative management for complicated appendicitis (Grades III-V) includes broad-spectrum postoperative antibiotics. Recent evidence suggests that the duration of postoperative antibiotics for complicated appendicitis should not exceed 4 postoperative days after source control. The 2015 multicenter STOP-IT trial showed that there is no benefit to extended antibiotic therapy (8 days) versus fixed duration (4 ± 1 days) when adequate source control is obtained from an intra-abdominal infection [78].

Fast-track pathways for various surgical procedures have been implemented with great success. These aim to decrease hospital length of stay without increasing complication rates. Generally, these have been described for elective procedures but have started to be used for emergent cases as well. Fast-track appendectomy pathways for uncomplicated appendicitis outline appropriate patient selection for participation, antibiotic administration, laparoscopy as the initial approach, local anesthesia, and postoperative pain medications given in the operating room and post-anesthesia care unit (PACU). Extensive counseling on postoperative care and restrictions are provided. The patient typically must meet several PACU criteria before discharge home. This has increased the number of patients who received same-day discharge after uncomplicated appendicitis without increasing morbidity or mortality [79, 80].

Similarly, fast-track pathways for complicated appendicitis have decreased hospital length of stay without significantly increasing complication or readmission rates [81]. Fast-track pathways typically pertain to patients without a discrete abscess or who require a percutaneous drain (i.e., AAST Grades I–III). Although the specifics may vary between institutions, such protocols include early resumption of a diet postoperatively, transition to oral antibiotics if extended administration is indicated, and minimization of unnecessary labs. Patients are discharged home when their pain is controlled on oral medications and they are tolerating oral intake.

Outcomes

Overall, the outcomes associated with appendicitis are good. Developed health systems have a mortality rate ranging from 0.09% to 0.24% [82, 83]. Less developed countries have a higher mortality rate of 1–4% [84, 85].

Surgical site infections (SSI) are the most common complication. Superficial SSIs have an incidence of 2.5%–5.4%, while organ space infections have an incidence of 1.3%–3% [55, 86–89]. Laparoscopic appendectomies have a lower risk of superficial SSI (OR 0.37, 95% CI 0.32–0.43) but higher risk of organ space infections (OR 1.44, 95% CI 1.21–1.73) [55].

Other less common complications include bleeding, usually from the mesentery, and appendiceal stump leak at the cecal staple line. Stump appendicitis is a rare clinical entity that can occur when an inappropriately long appendiceal stump is left after appendectomy. The true incidence of stump appendicitis is unknown, but it should be considered in the differential diagnosis in patients with abdominal pain after appendectomy [90].

Summary

As our understanding of appendicitis evolves, so have the diagnostic and treatment strategies. Clinical suspicion for appendicitis is typically accompanied with an imaging study to decrease the number of negative appendectomies and the costs associated with them. Although CT remains widely used for the diagnosis of appendicitis, there are strong advocates for use of non-ionizing techniques, particularly in children. Laparoscopic appendectomy is the standard of care for uncomplicated and complicated appendicitis though select patients may benefit from nonoperative treatment. Antibiotic therapy alone is an increasingly offered alternative for uncomplicated appendicitis, and results from recent and ongoing trials can be used to inform shared decision-making. Finally, fast-track pathways are becoming increasingly popular in facilitating early discharge and cost savings.

References

1. Addiss DG, Shaffer N, Fowler BS, Tauxe RV. The epidemiology of appendicitis and appendectomy in the United States. Am J Epidemiol. 1990;132(5):910–25.
2. Birnbaum BA, Wilson SR. Appendicitis at the millennium. Radiology. 2000;215(2):337–48.
3. Sengupta A, Bax G, Paterson-Brown S. White cell count and C-reactive protein measurement in patients with possible appendicitis. Ann R Coll Surg Engl. 2009;91(2):113–5.
4. Kularatna M, Lauti M, Haran C, et al. Clinical prediction rules for appendicitis in adults: which is best? World J Surg. 2017;41(7):1769–81.
5. Alvarado A. A practical score for the early diagnosis of acute appendicitis. Ann Emerg Med. 1986;15(5):557–64.
6. Andersson M, Andersson RE. The appendicitis inflammatory response score: a tool for the diagnosis of acute appendicitis that outperforms the Alvarado score. World J Surg. 2008;32(8):1843–9.
7. Sammalkorpi HE, Mentula P, Leppaniemi A. A new adult appendicitis score improves diagnostic accuracy of acute appendicitis--a prospective study. BMC Gastroenterol 2014;14:114.
8. Bhangu A, Collaborative RSGobotWMR. Evaluation of appendicitis risk prediction models in adults with suspected appendicitis. Br J Surg. 2020;107(1):73–86.
9. Wang RC, Kornblith AE, Grupp-Phelan J, Smith-Bindman R, Kao LS, Fahimi J. Trends in Use of Diagnostic Imaging for Abdominal Pain in U.S. Emergency Departments. AJR Am J Roentgenol. 2021;216(1):200–8.
10. Kave M, Parooie F, Salarzaei M. Pregnancy and appendicitis: a systematic review and meta-analysis on the clinical use of MRI in diagnosis of appendicitis in pregnant women. World J Emerg Surg. 2019;14:37.
11. Di Saverio S, Podda M, De Simone B, et al. Diagnosis and treatment of acute appendicitis: 2020 update of the WSES Jerusalem guidelines. World J Emerg Surg. 2020;15(1):27.
12. Doria AS, Moineddin R, Kellenberger CJ, et al. US or CT for diagnosis of appendicitis in children and adults? A meta-analysis. Radiology. 2006;241(1):83–94.
13. Barger RL Jr, Nandalur KR. Diagnostic performance of magnetic resonance imaging in the detection of appendicitis in adults: a meta-analysis. Acad Radiol. 2010;17(10):1211–6.
14. Cuschieri J, Florence M, Flum DR, et al. Negative appendectomy and imaging accuracy in the Washington state surgical care and outcomes assessment program. Ann Surg. 2008;248(4):557–63.
15. Drake FT, Florence MG, Johnson MG, et al. Progress in the diagnosis of appendicitis: a report from Washington State's surgical care and outcomes assessment program. Ann Surg. 2012;256(4):586–94.
16. Lee CC, Golub R, Singer AJ, Cantu R Jr, Levinson H. Routine versus selective abdominal computed tomography scan in the evaluation of right lower quadrant pain: a randomized controlled trial. Acad Emerg Med. 2007;14(2):117–22.
17. Anderson KT, Bartz-Kurycki M, Austin MT, et al. Approaching zero: implications of a computed tomography reduction program for pediatric appendicitis evaluation. J Pediatr Surg. 2017;52(12):1909–15.
18. Kim K, Kim YH, Kim SY, et al. Low-dose abdominal CT for evaluating suspected appendicitis. N Engl J Med. 2012;366(17):1596–605.
19. Group L. Low-dose CT for the diagnosis of appendicitis in adolescents and young adults (LOCAT): a pragmatic, multicentre, randomised controlled non-inferiority trial. Lancet Gastroenterol Hepatol. 2017;2(11):793–804.
20. Bennion RS, Baron EJ, Thompson JE, Jr., et al. The bacteriology of gangrenous and perforated appendicitis--revisited. Ann Surg 1990;211(2):165–171.
21. Pranesh N, Sathya V, Mainprize KS. Serosal appendicitis: incidence, causes and clinical significance. Postgrad Med J. 2006;82(974):830–2.
22. Charfi S, Sellami A, Affes A, Yaich K, Mzali R, Boudawara TS. Histopathological findings in appendectomy specimens: a study of 24,697 cases. Int J Color Dis. 2014;29(8):1009–12.
23. Teixeira FJR Jr, Couto Netto SDD, Akaishi EH, Utiyama EM, Menegozzo CAM, Rocha MC. Acute appendicitis, inflammatory appendiceal mass and the risk of a hidden malignant tumor: a systematic review of the literature. World J Emerg Surg. 2017;12:12.
24. Network NCC. Neuroendocrine and adrenal tumors (Version 2.2020). https://www.nccn.org/professionals/physician_gls/f_guidelines.asp#site. Accessed 12 Dec 2020.
25. Glasgow SC, Gaertner W, Stewart D, et al. The American Society of Colon and Rectal Surgeons, clinical practice guidelines for the management of appendiceal neoplasms. Dis Colon Rectum. 2019;62(12):1425–38.

26. Garst GC, Moore EE, Banerjee MN, et al. Acute appendicitis: a disease severity score for the acute care surgeon. J Trauma Acute Care Surg. 2013;74(1):32–6.
27. Tominaga GT, Staudenmayer KL, Shafi S, et al. The American Association for the Surgery of Trauma grading scale for 16 emergency general surgery conditions: disease-specific criteria characterizing anatomic severity grading. J Trauma Acute Care Surg. 2016;81(3):593–602.
28. Collins CM, Davenport DL, Talley CL, Bernard AC. Appendicitis grade, operative duration, and hospital cost. J Am Coll Surg. 2018;226(4):578–83.
29. Hernandez MC, Aho JM, Habermann EB, Choudhry AJ, Morris DS, Zielinski MD. Increased anatomic severity predicts outcomes: validation of the American Association for the Surgery of Trauma's emergency general surgery score in appendicitis. J Trauma Acute Care Surg. 2017;82(1):73–9.
30. Vasileiou G, Ray-Zack M, Zielinski M, Qian S, Yeh DD, Crandall M. Validation of the American Association for the Surgery of Trauma emergency general surgery score for acute appendicitis-an EAST multicenter study. J Trauma Acute Care Surg. 2019;87(1):134–9.
31. Schuster KM, Holena DN, Salim A, Savage S, Crandall M. American Association for the Surgery of Trauma emergency general surgery guideline summaries 2018: acute appendicitis, acute cholecystitis, acute diverticulitis, acute pancreatitis, and small bowel obstruction. Trauma Surg Acute Care Open. 2019;4(1):e000281.
32. Davidson GH, Flum DR, Talan DA, et al. Comparison of outcomes of antibiotic drugs and appendectomy (CODA) trial: a protocol for the pragmatic randomised study of appendicitis treatment. BMJ Open. 2017;7(11):e016117.
33. Eriksson S, Granström L. Randomized controlled trial of appendicectomy versus antibiotic therapy for acute appendicitis. Br J Surg. 1995;82(2):166–9.
34. Varadhan KK, Humes DJ, Neal KR, Lobo DN. Antibiotic therapy versus appendectomy for acute appendicitis: a meta-analysis. World J Surg. 2010;34(2):199–209.
35. Wilms IM, de Hoog DE, de Visser DC, Janzing HM. Appendectomy versus antibiotic treatment for acute appendicitis. Cochrane Database Syst Rev. 2011;(11):Cd008359.
36. Liu K, Fogg L. Use of antibiotics alone for treatment of uncomplicated acute appendicitis: a systematic review and meta-analysis. Surgery. 2011;150(4):673–83.
37. Ansaloni L, Catena F, Coccolini F, et al. Surgery versus conservative antibiotic treatment in acute appendicitis: a systematic review and meta-analysis of randomized controlled trials. Dig Surg. 2011;28(3):210–21.
38. Mason RJ, Moazzez A, Sohn H, Katkhouda N. Meta-analysis of randomized trials comparing antibiotic therapy with appendectomy for acute uncomplicated (no abscess or phlegmon) appendicitis. Surg Infect. 2012;13(2):74–84.
39. Varadhan KK, Neal KR, Lobo DN. Safety and efficacy of antibiotics compared with appendicectomy for treatment of uncomplicated acute appendicitis: meta-analysis of randomised controlled trials. BMJ. 2012;344:e2156.
40. Sallinen V, Akl EA, You JJ, et al. Meta-analysis of antibiotics versus appendicectomy for non-perforated acute appendicitis. Br J Surg. 2016;103(6):656–67.
41. Harnoss JC, Zelienka I, Probst P, et al. Antibiotics versus surgical therapy for uncomplicated appendicitis: systematic review and meta-analysis of controlled trials (PROSPERO 2015: CRD42015016882). Ann Surg. 2017;265(5):889–900.
42. Salminen P, Paajanen H, Rautio T, et al. Antibiotic therapy vs appendectomy for treatment of uncomplicated acute appendicitis: the APPAC randomized clinical trial. JAMA. 2015;313(23):2340–8.
43. Salminen P, Tuominen R, Paajanen H, et al. Five-year follow-up of antibiotic therapy for uncomplicated acute appendicitis in the APPAC randomized clinical trial. JAMA. 2018;320(12):1259–65.
44. Andersson RE, Petzold MG. Nonsurgical treatment of appendiceal abscess or phlegmon: a systematic review and meta-analysis. Ann Surg. 2007;246(5):741–8.
45. Gavriilidis P, de'Angelis N, Katsanos K, Di Saverio S. Acute Appendicectomy or conservative treatment for complicated appendicitis (phlegmon or abscess)? A systematic review by updated traditional and cumulative meta-analysis. J Clin Med Res. 2019;11(1):56–64.
46. Blakely ML, Williams R, Dassinger MS, et al. Early vs interval appendectomy for children with perforated appendicitis. Arch Surg. 2011;146(6):660–5.
47. Saluja S, Sun T, Mao J, et al. Early versus late surgical management of complicated appendicitis in children: a statewide database analysis with one-year follow-up. J Pediatr Surg. 2018;53(7):1339–44.
48. Gorter RR, Eker HH, Gorter-Stam MA, et al. Diagnosis and management of acute appendicitis. EAES consensus development conference 2015. Surg Endosc. 2016;30(11):4668–90.
49. Hall NJ, Jones CE, Eaton S, Stanton MP, Burge DM. Is interval appendicectomy justified after successful nonoperative treatment of an appendix mass in children? A systematic review. J Pediatr Surg. 2011;46(4):767–71.
50. Nitecki S, Assalia A, Schein M. Contemporary management of the appendiceal mass. Br J Surg. 1993;80(1):18–20.
51. Kaminski A, Liu IL, Applebaum H, Lee SL, Haigh PI. Routine interval appendectomy is not justified after initial nonoperative treatment of acute appendicitis. Arch Surg. 2005;140(9):897–901.
52. Deakin DE, Ahmed I. Interval appendicectomy after resolution of adult inflammatory appendix mass—is it necessary? Surgeon 2007;5(1):45–50.
53. Mällinen J, Rautio T, Grönroos J, et al. Risk of appendiceal neoplasm in periappendicular abscess in patients treated with interval appendectomy vs

follow-up with magnetic resonance imaging: 1-year outcomes of the peri-appendicitis Acuta randomized clinical trial. JAMA Surg. 2019;154(3):200–7.
54. Bhangu A. Safety of short, in-hospital delays before surgery for acute appendicitis: multicentre cohort study, systematic review, and meta-analysis. Ann Surg. 2014;259(5):894–903.
55. Sauerland S, Lefering R, Neugebauer EA. Laparoscopic versus open surgery for suspected appendicitis. Cochrane Database Syst Rev. 2004;(4):Cd001546.
56. Nason GJ, Baig SN, Burke MJ, et al. On-table urethral catheterisation during laparoscopic appendicectomy: is it necessary? Can Urol Assoc J. 2015;9(1–2):55–8.
57. Bernhardt J, Gerber B, Schober HC, Kähler G, Ludwig K. NOTES—case report of a unidirectional flexible appendectomy. Int J Color Dis. 2008;23(5):547–50.
58. Yagci MA, Kayaalp C. Transvaginal appendectomy: a systematic review. Minim Invasive Surg. 2014;2014:384706.
59. Yang E, Nie D, Li Z. Comparison of major clinical outcomes between transvaginal NOTES and traditional laparoscopic surgery: a systematic review and meta-analysis. J Surg Res. 2019;244:278–90.
60. Moore CB, Smith RS, Herbertson R, Toevs C. Does use of intraoperative irrigation with open or laparoscopic appendectomy reduce post-operative intra-abdominal abscess? Am Surg. 2011;77(1):78–80.
61. Bi LW, Yan BL, Yang QY, Cui HL. Peritoneal irrigation vs suction alone during pediatric appendectomy for perforated appendicitis: a meta-analysis. Medicine (Baltimore). 2019;98(50):e18047.
62. Hajibandeh S, Hajibandeh S, Kelly A, et al. Irrigation versus suction alone in laparoscopic appendectomy: is dilution the solution to pollution? A systematic review and meta-analysis. Surg Innov. 2018;25(2):174–82.
63. St Peter SD, Adibe OO, Iqbal CW, et al. Irrigation versus suction alone during laparoscopic appendectomy for perforated appendicitis: a prospective randomized trial. Ann Surg. 2012;256(4):581–5.
64. Anderson KT, Putnam LR, Bartz-Kurycki MA, et al. Povidone-iodine irrigation for pediatric perforated appendicitis may be protective: a Bayesian pilot randomized controlled trial. Ann Surg. 2020;271(5):827–33.
65. Cheng Y, Zhou S, Zhou R, et al. Abdominal drainage to prevent intra-peritoneal abscess after open appendectomy for complicated appendicitis. Cochrane Database Syst Rev. 2015;(2):Cd010168.
66. Li Z, Zhao L, Cheng Y, Cheng N, Deng Y. Abdominal drainage to prevent intra-peritoneal abscess after open appendectomy for complicated appendicitis. Cochrane Database Syst Rev. 2018;5(5):Cd010168.
67. Abdulhamid AK, Sarker SJ. Is abdominal drainage after open emergency appendectomy for complicated appendicitis beneficial or waste of money? A single Centre retrospective cohort study. Ann Med Surg (Lond). 2018;36:168–72.
68. Andersson RE, Lambe M. Incidence of appendicitis during pregnancy. Int J Epidemiol. 2001;30(6):1281–5.
69. Pearl JP, Price RR, Tonkin AE, Richardson WS, Stefanidis D. SAGES guidelines for the use of laparoscopy during pregnancy. Surg Endosc. 2017;31(10):3767–82.
70. Babaknia A, Parsa H, Woodruff JD. Appendicitis during pregnancy. Obstet Gynecol. 1977;50(1):40–4.
71. Prodromidou A, Machairas N, Kostakis ID, et al. Outcomes after open and laparoscopic appendectomy during pregnancy: a meta-analysis. Eur J Obstet Gynecol Reprod Biol. 2018;225:40–50.
72. Lee SH, Lee JY, Choi YY, Lee JG. Laparoscopic appendectomy versus open appendectomy for suspected appendicitis during pregnancy: a systematic review and updated meta-analysis. BMC Surg. 2019;19(1):41.
73. Ciarrocchi A, Amicucci G. Laparoscopic versus open appendectomy in obese patients: a meta-analysis of prospective and retrospective studies. J Minim Access Surg. 2014;10(1):4–9.
74. Phillips AW, Jones AE, Sargen K. Should the macroscopically normal appendix be removed during laparoscopy for acute right iliac fossa pain when no other explanatory pathology is found? Surg Laparosc Endosc Percutan Tech. 2009;19(5):392–4.
75. Mussack T, Schmidbauer S, Nerlich A, Schmidt W, Hallfeldt KK. Chronic appendicitis as an independent clinical entity. Chirurg. 2002;73(7):710–5.
76. Cairo SB, Raval MV, Browne M, Meyers H, Rothstein DH. Association of same-day discharge with hospital readmission after appendectomy in pediatric patients. JAMA Surg. 2017;152(12):1106–12.
77. Grigorian A, Kuza CM, Schubl SD, et al. Same-day discharge after non-perforated laparoscopic appendectomy is safe. J Investig Surg. 2019;34:270–5.
78. Sawyer RG, Claridge JA, Nathens AB, et al. Trial of short-course antimicrobial therapy for intraabdominal infection. N Engl J Med. 2015;372(21):1996–2005.
79. Cash CL, Frazee RC, Abernathy SW, et al. A prospective treatment protocol for outpatient laparoscopic appendectomy for acute appendicitis. J Am Coll Surg. 2012;215(1):101–5; discussion 105–106.
80. Frazee RC, Abernathy SW, Davis M, et al. Outpatient laparoscopic appendectomy should be the standard of care for uncomplicated appendicitis. J Trauma Acute Care Surg. 2014;76(1):79–82; discussion 82–73.
81. Frazee R, Abernathy S, Davis M, Isbell T, Regner J, Smith R. Fast track pathway for perforated appendicitis. Am J Surg. 2017;213(4):739–41.
82. Bliss LA, Yang CJ, Kent TS, Ng SC, Critchlow JF, Tseng JF. Appendicitis in the modern era: universal problem and variable treatment. Surg Endosc. 2015;29(7):1897–902.
83. Faiz O, Clark J, Brown T, et al. Traditional and laparoscopic appendectomy in adults: outcomes in English NHS hospitals between 1996 and 2006. Ann Surg. 2008;248(5):800–6.

84. Ali N, Aliyu S. Appendicitis and its surgical management experience at the University of Maiduguri Teaching Hospital Nigeria. Niger J Med. 2012;21(2):223–6.
85. Ohene-Yeboah M, Togbe B. An audit of appendicitis and appendicectomy in Kumasi, Ghana. West Afr J Med. 2006;25(2):138–43.
86. Cueto J, D'Allemagne B, Vazquez-Frias JA, et al. Morbidity of laparoscopic surgery for complicated appendicitis: an international study. Surg Endosc. 2006;20(5):717–20.
87. Bennett J, Boddy A, Rhodes M. Choice of approach for appendicectomy: a meta-analysis of open versus laparoscopic appendicectomy. Surg Laparosc Endosc Percutan Tech. 2007;17(4):245–55.
88. van Rossem CC, Schreinemacher MH, Treskes K, van Hogezand RM, van Geloven AA. Duration of antibiotic treatment after appendicectomy for acute complicated appendicitis. Br J Surg. 2014;101(6):715–9.
89. Fleming FJ, Kim MJ, Messing S, Gunzler D, Salloum R, Monson JR. Balancing the risk of postoperative surgical infections: a multivariate analysis of factors associated with laparoscopic appendectomy from the NSQIP database. Ann Surg. 2010;252(6):895–900.
90. Liang MK, Lo HG, Marks JL. Stump appendicitis: a comprehensive review of literature. Am Surg. 2006;72(2):162–6.

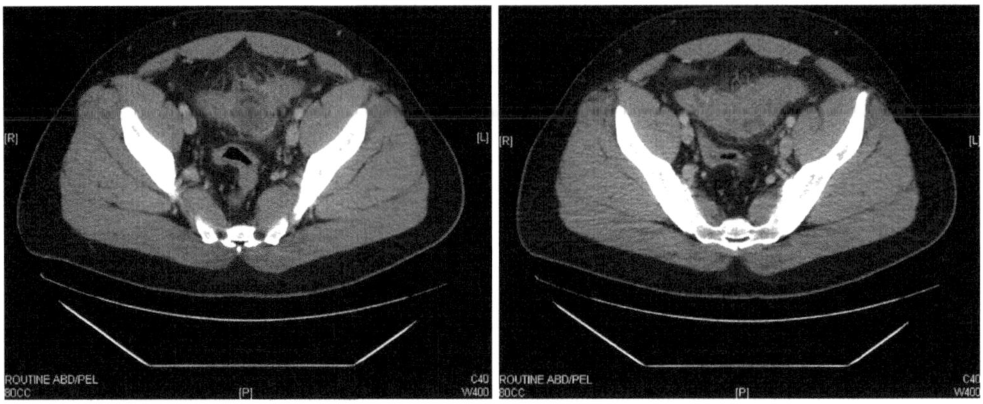

Figs. 17.1 and 17.2 Contrasted CT of the abdomen and pelvis showing pericolonic fat stranding and formation of pericolic phlegmon consistent with acute sigmoid diverticulitis. No organized or drainable fluid collections are present

Introduction

Acute colonic diverticulitis has continued to increase in frequency over the last two decades [1, 2]. As a fundamental emergency surgical disease, 75 per 100,000 people will require inpatient stays annually, though true prevalence is poorly understood as outpatient cases of acute colonic diverticulitis are rarely studied. Incidence of acute colonic diverticulitis is exacerbated by common problems of modern society including obesity, smoking, diet (especially low-fiber diets), a sedentary lifestyle, and the use of aspirin and NSAIDs [1, 2]. Annually, diverticulitis costs the US healthcare system $2.6 billion dollars [2].

Acute colonic diverticulitis occurs when colonic diverticuli become inflamed. Diverticuli become more common with age and with exposure to a Western diet and lifestyle. Uncoordinated contractions of the colon raise intraluminal pressure, which is exacerbated by low-fiber diets [1]. This results in formation of colonic diverticuli, most common in the sigmoid colon. The exact mechanism of subsequent inflammation is unclear but may result from occlusion of the diverticular lumen, leading to bacterial overgrowth and perforation, much like with appendicitis. An alternative theory postulates that an acute perforation of the diverticular fundus results in inflammation that progresses to diverticulitis [1].

Though incidence of diverticulosis increases with age, diverticulitis is most rapidly increasing in populations less than 50 years of age—the diagnosis of which is undoubtedly facilitated by improvements and availability of computed tomography. Despite increasing occurrence in younger populations, older age groups are more likely to have complicated diverticulitis, characterized by abscess formation, peritonitis, fistula formation, and the need for surgical intervention. Approximately 1 in 5 patients will require surgical intervention during their index hospitalization [1, 2]. The Hartmann's procedure remains the most common surgical intervention, and, indeed, 1/3 of all colonic resections and colostomies are attributable to diverticular disease [2]. Mortality remains low with this disease process, however, with a 1% mortality rate in patients managed without surgery and a 4% mortality in those requiring surgical intervention [1].

In this chapter, we will discuss factors predisposing patients to acute colonic diverticulitis, including high-risk populations. Special attention will be paid to modern grading scales for emergency general surgery (EGS) diseases. Advances in medical and surgical management will be discussed, as well as surgical controversies and the management of complicated forms of acute colonic diverticulitis.

Grading Scales for Acute Colonic Diverticulitis

The classic grading scale for acute colonic diverticulitis was proposed by Hinchey et al. in 1978 and modified by Kaiser et al. in 2005 [3, 4]. This grading scale encompassed the progression from uncomplicated diverticulitis to complicated diverticulitis with peritonitis, initially based upon operative findings but updated to incorporate imaging. Despite the widespread adoption of this grading system, it remains specific only to diverticulitis, and the general construct is not applicable to other inflammatory processes in the EGS spectrum. The Hinchey classification also failed to account for different aspects of complicated disease.

In 2014, the American Association for the Surgery of Trauma (AAST) developed and published grading scales for the classification of EGS conditions. Included in this series of disease processes was the grading scale for acute colonic diverticulitis [5]. Though many individual EGS diseases have individual grading systems, such as the Hinchey classification, they did not translate well from one pathophysiology to another. Many diseases have no grading systems at all. In an effort to design a uniform grading system, learned once and applied across the spectrum of EGS diseases, the new grading scale created categories of progressively worsening disease classified in a variety of manners.

Table 17.1 demonstrates the grading scale for acute colonic diverticulitis. Disease processes are graded on a severity scale of 1 (mild) to 5 (the most severe). Increasing grades represent the progression from uncomplicated inflammatory processes to regional inflammation/abscess to systemic inflammatory pathology. As not every EGS disease is treated surgically, scores may be based on clinical criteria, such as physical exam and laboratory studies, imaging criteria, operative findings, or pathologic specimens. If a patient's disease process is scored in more than one category, such as clinical and imaging, the highest grade is used as the overall score.

After creation of the grading scales, multiple studies were performed to validate whether the grading scales were indeed easy to use and predictive of worsening outcomes with increasing grades. An initial validation study showed mod-

Table 17.1 AAST EGS grading scale for acute colonic diverticulitis. The goal of uniform grading systems is to apply a single scale to a spectrum of disease processes. Disease process is graded on a severity scale of 1 (mild) to 5 (the most severe)

AAST grade	Description	Clinical criteria	Imaging criteria (CT findings)	Operative criteria	Pathologic criteria
I	Colonic inflammation	Pain; leukocytosis; minimal or no tenderness	Mesenteric stranding; colon wall thickening	N/A	N/A
II	Colon micro-perforation or pericolic phlegmon without abscess	Local tenderness (single or multiple areas) without peritonitis	Pericolic phlegmon; foci of air (single or multiple); no abscess	Pericolic phlegmon with no abscess	Inflamed colon with microscopic perforation
III	Localized pericolic abscess	Localized peritonitis	Pericolic abscess	Pericolic abscess	Inflamed colon with perforation
IV	Distant and/or multiple abscesses	Localized peritonitis at multiple locations	Abscess or phlegmon away from the colon	Abscess or phlegmon away from the colon	Inflamed colon with perforation
V	Free colonic perforation with generalized peritonitis	Generalized peritonitis	Free air and free fluid	Perforation with generalized fecal and purulent contamination	Inflamed colon with perforation

erate inter-rater reliability and a significant association between higher grades and complications, as well as longer length of stay [6]. A follow-up multi-center validation also demonstrated significant associations between higher EGS grades in acute colonic diverticulitis and clinical outcomes [7]. Inter-rater reliability was rated as high in the multi-center validation. An additional study published in 2020 compared the AAST grading scale for acute colonic diverticulitis to the modified Hinchey classification. This study demonstrated equivalent ability to predict the need for intervention and likelihood of complications, demonstrating non-inferiority with the existing standard [8].

As Ebersole et al. noted in their 2020 comparative study, the AAST EGS classification may be preferable to the modified Hinchey classification, in that it is applicable preoperatively, or even if no intervention is required. Overall, the AAST grading scales have provided a common language for EGS surgeons to use in order to facilitate clinical management, to ensure effective communication in hand-offs and transfers and to facilitate research on EGS diseases. Additionally, the structure of the scales remains standardized regardless of the disease process, meaning a clinician who learns the grading scale for acute colonic diverticulitis will understand the grading framework for appendicitis, perforated ulcers, breast infections, and a diversity of other EGS pathology. The use of the AAST EGS grading scale for acute colonic diverticulitis is encouraged for EGS providers, to facilitate care and promote research.

Risk Factors

The prevalence of diverticular disease has increased over the past century from reports around 2–10% in the early 1900s to up to 50% in patients 60 years and above [9]. Hospitalizations and need for surgical intervention is also increasing.

The so-called Western diet comprising refined carbohydrates, red meats, and low-fiber foods has long been associated with a higher risk of diverticular disease. Other risk factors include smoking, chronic use of opioids, nonsteroidal inflammatory drugs, obesity with high visceral to skeletal fat ratios, and sedentary lifestyle.

It is surmised that these risk factors result in alteration of gastrointestinal motility and lead to increased intraluminal pressure which causes herniation of mucosa through a weekend colonic wall near perforating blood vessels. The exact mechanism by which a diverticulum becomes inflamed, converting diverticulosis to diverticulitis, is not clear though several hypotheses exist. Some have postulated that a narrow-necked diverticulum may lead to bacterial overgrowth within the outpouching resulting in infection, while others hypothesize that inspissated stool can cause erosion through the diverticulum leading to peritonitis [10].

Presentation and Diagnosis

Patients with acute diverticulitis may present in the outpatient setting or via the emergency department. Focused history taking and physical examination are important in the initial evaluation of patients presenting with acute abdominal pain. Inflammatory diverticular disease typically presents with a constellation of symptoms that usually include left lower quadrant abdominal pain and fevers [11, 12]. Pain may radiate to the suprapubic region, groin, or back. Changes in bowel movements, diarrhea, nausea, vomiting, and anorexia may also be present. Symptoms are often recurrent but are not usually provoked by an inciting event.

Initial Assessment

The abdominal examination of a patient with acute diverticulitis will vary depending on the degree of inflammation, stage of disease, and segment of colon involved. Mild symptoms are associated with low-grade disease. Commonly, patients present with left lower quadrant tenderness to palpation. In moderate disease, evidence of localized left lower quadrant peritonitis may be seen on examination as evidenced by rebound tenderness or voluntary guarding. Generalized peritonitis is concerning and is associated with the high-grade diverticulitis and systemic illness. Digital rectal examination, if performed, is usually nonspecific but may be helpful in the presence of stricture and large bowel obstruction or to evaluate for rectal pathology.

Presence of systemic symptoms should raise concern for high-grade disease, and hemodynamic derangement prompts early assessment. Hypovolemia may be present in patients experiencing poor oral intake or emesis and could manifest with hemodynamic instability such as tachycardia or hypotension. However, these abnormalities should raise concern for abdominal sepsis or developing septic shock.

Leukocytosis or thrombocytopenia is further evidence of the degree of inflammation present. Electrolyte abnormalities, acute kidney injury, and lactic acidosis are also common in more advanced disease. C-reactive protein and other inflammatory markers may correlate with the severity of acute diverticulitis. [13–17] The American Society of Colon and Rectal Surgeons supports the use of C-reactive protein (CRP) as part of routine laboratory investigations [13]. CRP greater that 150 mg/dL is associated with complicated diverticulitis. In the presence of free fluid on imaging, elevated CRP has been associated with increased mortality. [16] The trio of guarding on physical examination, elevated CRP, and leukocytosis detect complicated diverticulitis with a negative predictive value of 96% [17]. Though these findings apply to the diagnosis of diverticulitis, they are nonspecific, and other diagnosis must be ruled out. The differential diagnosis is broad and includes intestinal tract malignancies, bowel obstruction, inflammatory bowel disease, perforated gastric or duodenal ulcers, intestinal ischemia, and others.

Imaging

Advanced imaging has become standard of care in the evaluation of the patient with abdominal pain and is a necessary tool for guiding treatment. Computed tomography (CT) scan is the recommended imaging modality for patients with suspected diverticulitis or intra-abdominal sepsis. The sensitivity and specificity of CT imaging for diagnosing diverticulitis and other mimickers of the disease are around 95% for each [18]. CT can reveal the extent of disease and help guide management. Presence of phlegmon (Fig. 17.1) versus pericolonic abscess formation will help distinguish the need for percutaneous intervention. Large abscesses may be distinguished from free perforation (Fig. 17.2) which can aid in surgical decision-making.

Magnetic resonance imaging (MRI) can also be considered for patients in which CT imaging is contraindicated such as in patients with contrast dye allergies or, in some cases, pregnancy. The use of ultrasound has also been described and may be useful in identifying fluid collections associated with diverticulitis or to diagnose pelvic conditions that may mimic disease, particularly in women with pelvic and lower abdominal pain [19]. Ultrasound is less sensitive and specific and is not considered the goal standard in identifying diverticulitis and its complications [20].

Management

Accepted management for acute colonic diverticulitis ranges from expectant management in the outpatient setting to emergency surgery. Subtleties of management are dependent on the severity of presenting disease, physiologic condition of the patient, and disease progression.

Medical Management

Antibiotics are the mainstay of first-line therapy for patients presenting with any severity of diverticulitis. More recently, management without antibiotics has demonstrated no statistically significant difference in complications, time to recovery, or long-term recurrence compared to treatment with antibiotics in patients with low-grade, uncomplicated diverticulitis without systemic symptoms [21–23]. The ASCRS 2020 guidelines now support outpatient treatment without antibiotics in immunocompetent patient who meet low-grade diverticulitis criteria. [13]

Expectant management should be reserved for patients without systemic symptoms including fevers, tachycardia, hypotension, and without peritoneal signs on physical exam. Close clinical follow-up is recommended when expectant management is pursued.

For those patients with evidence of more complicated disease, including sepsis or systemic inflammatory response, antibiotics are indicated as first-line therapy. Patients who screen positive for sepsis by any parameter should be started on antibiotics, be provided resuscitative fluids in a timely fashion, and be screened for lactic acidosis as recommend in the 2016 surviving sepsis campaign [24]. For patients meeting the thresholds for antibiosis, a variety of options are considered acceptable by current standards and evidence-based practices. However, the use of clinical judgment regarding the patient's overall clinical picture is important. Antibiotic choice should include coverage of gram-negative organisms and should take into account local antibiograms for organism resistance patterns affecting the local population.

Duration of antibiotic therapy has been studied in multiple settings. The STOP-IT trial demonstrated that shorter course antibiotics (4 days vs 8 days) did not have significantly different outcomes in complications, such as abscess formation or recurrence, in patients who had undergone procedural source control [25]. Additional randomized controlled trials have shown no difference in patient outcomes in the treatment of uncomplicated diverticulitis with short course versus longer courses of intravenous antibiotics (4 days vs 7 days). [26] Furthermore, no difference has been found when comparing inpatient intravenous to outpatient oral antibiotics in patients with acute uncomplicated diverticulitis. [27, 28] Enteral antibiotics represent a viable alternative to parenteral administration in low-grade diverticulitis, saving patient's hospital days and healthcare dollars. The DIVER trial compared management of acute uncomplicated diverticulitis using oral versus parenteral antibiotics. Among 132 randomized patients, there was no difference in treatment failure between groups, but the outpatient group demonstrated significantly lower overall healthcare costs [27]. Generally, low-grade disease in immunocompetent patients may be treated with oral antibiotics in the outpatient setting. For more complex disease, admission and treatment with intravenous antibiotics is indicated.

Image-Guided Drainage

Symptoms of diverticulitis that prompt patients to seek emergency medical attention are often associated with more advanced inflammation and higher grade disease. Computed tomography is indicated to assess extent of acute colonic diverticulitis. Small abscesses, <3–4 cm, can be successfully managed with antibiotics alone. Contained perforations with larger, well-formed abscesses can safely be treated by percutaneous drainage if the patient does not have an indication for urgent laparotomy. Up to 80% of diverticulitis with localized abscess will resolve with a combination of antibiotic therapy and drainage [29]. Furthermore, larger abscess size does not preclude image-guided drainage therapy and does not correlate with treatment failure.

Surgical Management

Laparoscopic Peritoneal Lavage

Laparoscopic peritoneal lavage has been used for abdominal washout for abscesses that are large and not amenable to percutaneous drainage or in hemodynamically stable patients with moderate free fluid and evidence of perforation. In general, the goal with this minimally invasive approach is to avoid the need for stoma creation [30]. In the LADIES trial, the LOLA arm randomly assigned patients with feculent peritonitis to laparoscopic lavage versus resection. The study was terminated early by the safety monitoring for high rates of short-term morbidity in the lavage group [31, 32]. Therefore, the conclusions from this study are that lavage is not superior to standard sigmoidectomy for perforated diverticulitis. The SCANDIV trial assessed 199 patients with perforated diverticulitis, who were randomly assigned to laparoscopic lavage versus sigmoidectomy. There was not difference in mortality between groups, but the lavage group had a significantly higher rage of reoperation. [33] The expert panel for Society of Gastrointestinal and Endoscopic Surgeons in 2018 came to consensus that laparoscopic peritoneal lavage could be considered in certain patient populations, but noted the lower incidence of stoma formation may be offset by increased short-term morbidity and increased reoperation. [34] In 2018, the American Association for the Surgery of Trauma published guideline statements on acute colonic diverticulitis that recommended against the use of laparoscopic lavage in most cases [35].

Emergency Surgical Resection

Emergency laparotomy is indicated in patients with generalized peritonitis or when systemic symptoms of sepsis or septic shock are present. Diffuse peritoneal free fluid or free air have also been associated with high rates of failure of non-operative management, and emergency surgical resection may be required in up to 15% of acute cases of dieverticulitis [16, 26, 36]. Immediate therapy with antibiotics and crystalloid fluid resuscitation are important initial preparatory steps. Surgery should be considered urgent, and time to operation should minimized.

Patients who do not require emergent resection at admission but fail to resolve with nonoperative therapies are in the minority but should be considered for sigmoid resection during the same hospitalization. [13] These patients may continue to smolder without resolution of abdominal pain and development of abscess and phlegmon or demonstrate persistent intestinal ileus. Though there may be an absence of clinical deterioration, these patients have higher rates of readmission and recurrence and should be considered for resection during the index hospitalization.

Laparoscopic Vs Open Resection

Minimally invasive surgery has revolutionized a number of surgical operations, such as appendectomy and cholecystectomy. The advantages of laparoscopy have been well described. As laparoscopic technique has improved, laparoscopy for colon resection has gained popularity for a number of pathologies, including diverticular disease.

A number of clinical considerations should be considered when choosing between laparoscopic and open resection for diverticular disease, particularly in the acute setting. The patient's physiologic status, hemodynamics, and comorbidities are important factors in this decision. In general, laparoscopy is reserved for stable patients who can tolerate the physiologic stress of peritoneal insufflation, as well as potentially longer operation. Previous abdominal surgery, anticipated hostile abdominal adhesions, and intestinal dilation may also render a laparoscopic approach difficult to prohibitive. Retrospective comparison of laparoscopic and open sigmoid resection for acute diverticulitis in patients who have failed medical treatment for complicated disease shows that laparoscopic procedures may be associated with lower blood loss, less incidence of ileus, more rapid resumption of a general diet, shorter length of hospital stay, fewer overall complications, and lower mortality compared to open colectomy [37, 38]. The available literature is sparse and retrospective and therefore has limitations. However, it suggests that the laparoscopic approach to colectomy for acute diverticulitis should be considered in stable patients in centers where complex laparoscopic procedures are routine.

Robotic surgery has also become increasingly popular for treatment of diverticular disease. The outcomes of the studies reviewing the use of robotic surgery generally focus on comparison with laparoscopic procedures, rates of converting to open procedure, length of operation, and overall medical cost. [39–42] The body of literature investigating the benefits of robotic colectomy is retrospective but does reveal some promising data suggesting lower overall morbidities with robotic compared to laparoscopic resection. Little data exists investigating the robotic approach in acute inflammatory diverticulitis, however. More investigation is needed to further elucidate the benefits of this approach in the emergency surgical population.

Extent of Resection

When able, the entire sigmoid colon should be resected when operating for diverticulitis. As diverticuli may be pan-colonic; however, it is not necessary to remove uninvolved descending colon. The distal margin of resection is generally at the level of the sacral promontory if the rectal tissue is normal. The rectosigmoid junction can be identified by the splaying of tenia coli. If inflammation significantly involves the rectum, the distal margin may need to be deeper to the level of healthy tissue. [43, 44] The margins should be soft and viable, particularly if anastomosis is planned. Mobilization of the splenic flexure may be necessary in order to create a tension-free anastomosis, if restoration of intestinal continuity is planned.

Stomas and Intestinal Continuity

A number of studies have been conducted to elucidate the operative approach to urgent sigmoidectomy for diverticulitis. Historically, sigmoidectomy with end colostomy has been considered the standard of care. Initially described as a three-staged approach, current practice typically involves two stages with initial resection and colostomy formation and subsequent takedown with restoration of intestinal continuity [45]. More recently, multiple randomized controlled trials have investigated the limitation with which resection and primary colonic anastomosis, with or without defunctionalizing loop ileostomy, can be safely performed. The LADIES trial randomized 133 hemodynamically stable, immunocompetent patients under the age of 85, with purulent or feculent peritonitis,

to Hartman's procedure or sigmoidectomy and anastomosis. The latter group was further subdivided into defunctionalizing ileostomy or no stoma creation. The 1-year stoma-free survival was significantly greater in the primary anastomosis group, and no difference in short-term complications was noted. [31]

The ColonPerfRCT and DIVERTI trials compared treatment of purulent and feculent diverticulitis by Hartman's procedure with resection versus primary anastomosis and diverting ileostomy. They found no difference in short-term morbidity and mortality; however the 1-year stoma-free survival rates were much higher in the primary anastomosis group. Furthermore, the perioperative complications for the stoma reversal after Hartmann's was considerably higher than for reversal of diverting ileostomy, prompting early termination of the ColonPerfRCT trial. The DIVERTI trial was carried out to completion and found no difference in morbidity or mortality between the groups but the 18-month stoma reversal was significantly higher in those who underwent primary anastomosis with defunctionalizing ileostomy. [46, 47]

Overall, the decision to resect and divert versus perform primary anastomosis will depend on multiple factors. These may include physiologic status of the patient at the time of resection, degree of inflammation or contamination, quality of the tissue, and other patient comorbidities. With more current research support, the 2020 ASCRS guideline made a strong recommendation for sigmoid resection with colorectal anastomosis and creation of diverting loop ileostomy in appropriate patients [13]. In general, the decision for fecal stream diversion should be left up the clinical judgment of the surgeon.

Damage Control

Damage control laparotomy was first described in the trauma population for major life-threatening abdominal injuries. Over the past decade, the indication for damage control surgery has been extended into the emergency general surgery population, especially in the cases of severe intra-abdominal sepsis, abdominal compartment syndrome, and progressive intestinal ischemia. [48] This practice is another area in which literature supporting or opposing its use for non-traumatic indications is limited to retrospective studies. Some suggest that the benefit of damage control may include shorter OR time at index operation and consideration of restoring intestinal continuity at second-look operations. [48, 49] Far more data is needed for definitive conclusions to be drawn, but it is currently acceptable practice to perform damage control surgery in patients with high-grade diverticulitis who present in septic shock or have other conditions making quick source control and minimization of time under anesthesia a priority.

Diverticular Fistulae

Incidence of fistulizing diverticular disease is low but can complicate the management of acute diverticulitis. Though it can be related to benign disease, presence of either of this diagnosis should raise the suspicion for malignancy. Risk factors for colonic fistulae include chronic recurrent diverticulitis and smoking. [50, 51] These fistulae occur most commonly in the form of colovesicle fistula; however, colovaginal, colocutaneous, coloenteric, and colouterine fistulae have been described. The presence of pneumaturia, fecaluria, or feculent vaginal discharge can be distressing to the patient and warrant prompt intervention when able.

The general accepted treatment for patients suffering from diverticulitis with colonic fistula is resection once the acute episode of diverticulitis has resolved unless the physiologic condition of the patient mandates emergent intervention. Laparoscopic approach has become an acceptable approach; however, many surgeons continue to opt for open resection. Restoration of intestinal continuity is recommended when able, particularly if the operation is completed in the elective setting [52]. In the case of coloenteric fistulae, small bowel resection is usually mandatory. Colovesicle and colovaginal fistulae may be more complex. To address these fistulae, primary repair by direct suture of the bladder or vaginal wall is commonly performed. Creation of omental pedicle flaps or buttresses have also been described but not well studied. In the case of colovesicle fistula, postoperative management includes maintenance of a Foley catheter for 7–14 days post repair. Cystogram is obtained prior to removal to ensure integrity of the urinary tract has been restored. It may be necessary to seek additional surgical expertise in complex cases involving the gynecologic or urinary tract. [52]

Perioperative Considerations

Bowel Prep

Though there is a paucity of literature in support of preoperative bowel preparation specific to diverticulitis, literature strongly supports bowel preparation for the general colorectal population. Several randomized controlled studies and retrospective cohorts in the general colorectal population have revealed that a bundle which include preoperative mechanical bowel preparation with oral antibiotics significantly reduce anastomotic leaks, hospital readmissions, and surgical site infections. [53–55] These findings have been substantiated over the years, and it is now the accepted standard of care to provide both bowel preparation and antibiotics prior to elective colectomy. When able, this practice should be incorporated into use for semi-elective or semi-urgent cases.

Ureteral Stents

The use of prophylactic ureteral stents to avoid or recognize ureteral injury is a controversial topic and literature supporting or opposing its use is limited. Much of the available literature suggests that prophylactic ureteral stenting aids only in recognition of ureteral injury but does not prevent injury from occurring. [56, 57] The SAGES consensus guidelines published in 2018 confer a weak recommendation for selective use based on patient characteristics and preoperative imaging in the elective setting [34]. However, there are currently no recommendation for the routine use of stenting in the urgent or emergent setting.

There are currently no randomized control trials investigating the efficacy of prophylactic ureteral stent placement for prevention or identification of ureteral injury in emergency settings. More recently some retrospective data based on NSQIP data has made a weak correlation between prophylactic ureteral stent placement for diverticular disease and a lower incidence of ureteral injury [58]. However, as with all retrospective data, the quality of evidence remains weak, and there are no strong recommendations for or against their use.

The argument against the use of stents is based on the risks of urinary tract-related complications such as infection, iatrogenic injury with ureteral stent placement, and increased length of operating room time. [59] Until more literature is available, the general accepted recommendation is to use ureteral stenting in select cases, based on surgeon discretion.

Post Recovery and Elective Surgical Resection

Elective Resection

Elective resection for diverticulitis has been a point of controversy for many years and continues to evolve. Historically, reflex elective resection after any given episode, or even multiple recurrent episodes of diverticulitis, was generally discouraged. Rather the number of recurrent episodes, degree of inflammation, and abscess dimensions were considered as part of the decision-making pathway for elective colectomy. More recently, the nonoperative approach has come under some scrutiny as more studies have revealed data supporting resectional treatment on an elective basis for patient who have recovered from a course of complicated diverticulitis. Diverticulitis recurrence has been reported between 9% and 61% [13].

Uncomplicated Diverticulitis

Patients who have successful nonoperative treatment of uncomplicated diverticulitis have relatively low rates of recurrence. The risk of subsequent complicated diverticulitis, or need for emergent surgery with stoma creation, is not increased. Elective surgery after successful treatment of a single episode of uncomplicated diverticulitis is not recommended. The risk of recurrent diverticulitis after a single episode is relatively low, though subsequent admissions for recurrent diverticulitis do confer an increased risk of further recurrences. [60–63] For patients with multiple episodes of recurring disease, elective colectomy should be considered on an individual basis and with consideration of patient's general condition and comorbidities. The risk of anastomotic leak and the need for stoma creation, among other perioperative complications, should be weighed against the morbidity of readmission, time lost from work, and other quality of life indicators.

Diverticulitis with Abscess

Large retrospective studies have shown the recurrence rate after a single episode of diverticulitis with abscess to be significantly higher than patients without abscess formation [60, 61]. Additionally, there is evidence to suggest that these patients recur with higher-grade disease and larger abscesses and need urgent resection more often when the initial occurrence required percutaneous abscess drainage. Recurrence rate in this circumstance is approximately 74%. [62] Given these risks, patients with abscess, particularly if treated by percutaneous drainage during the index episode, may be considered for elective colectomy after the resolution of the acute episode of diverticulitis. The lengthening body of data suggesting that diverticulitis recurs at higher rates and with more morbidity than previously suggested has led the ASCRS to change their recommendation to consider elective resection after successful treatment of diverticular abscess in the 2020 Clinical Practice Guidelines [13]. Consideration of the patient's overall physiologic condition and consideration of the patient's age and comorbidities should always be considered in the surgical planning and decision-making.

Colonoscopy

For the majority of patients, nonoperative management of an acute episode of uncomplicated diverticulitis achieves resolution of symptoms. The recurrence rate for uncomplicated diverticulitis has been reported between 13 and 33%. [64] Thus it can often be managed expectantly. The risk of occult malignancy in this population has been reported between 0.7 and 1.3%, compared to complicated diverticulitis where occult

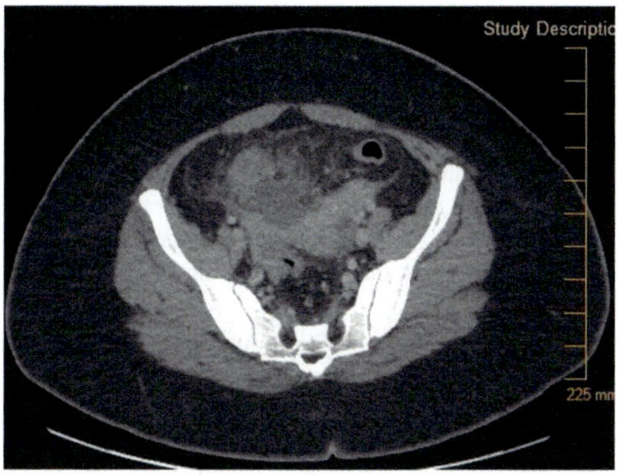

Fig. 17.3 CT showing pericolonic and mesenteric stranding with phlegmon and no drainable fluid collection

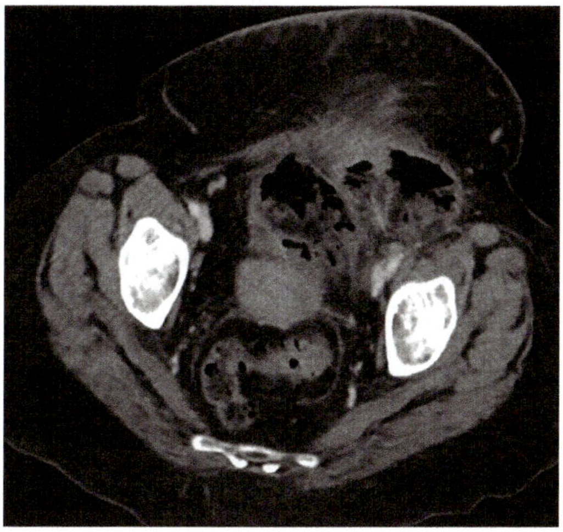

Fig. 17.4 CT abdomen showing perforation of colon into abdominal wall, free fluid, and pneumoperitoneum

malignancy increases to between 7.9 and 11% [65, 66]. Thus, in patients suffering from diverticulitis complicated by abscess formation, purulent or feculent peritonitis, or abscess formation, colonoscopy should be performed in the post-acute phase for full inspection of the length of the colon to rule out occult malignancy. Chronic inflammatory changes may be seen for several weeks (Fig. 17.3); therefore endoscopic exam should wait until 6 weeks after the resolutions of the acute inflammatory episode (Figs. 17.4 and 17.5).

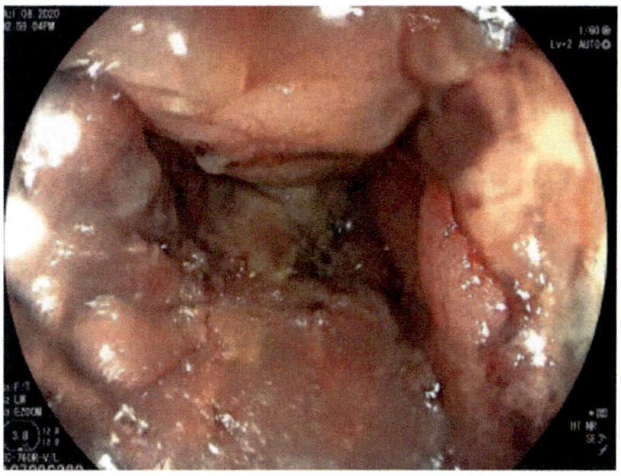

Fig. 17.5 Colonoscopy showing sigmoid colon with chronic inflammatory change

Summary

Diverticular disease has become increasingly prevalent in the United States and other countries due to dietary and lifestyle habits. Historically, diverticulitis was treated as a surgical emergency and mandated major open abdominal surgery which often resulted in the creation of an end colostomy. In the modern era, evidence-based practices have evolved as clinical research has expanded knowledge on the natural history of the disease, increasing the threshold for surgical intervention and need for stoma creation. Advances in percutaneous drainage techniques as a form of septic source control have decreased the need for emergent surgical resection in the inpatient setting and allowed for shorter hospitalizations. Much of this has transferred the burdens of the treatment of acute diverticulitis to the outpatient setting.

When the benefits of elective surgery are combined with the ability to perform preoperative bowel preparation with oral antibiotics, patients are at greatly reduced risk of the morbidities and mortality associated with anastomotic leak, surgical site infection, and prolonged hospital course. Additionally, laparoscopic techniques are becoming increasingly routine, offering the benefits of minimally invasive surgery.

Despite the advances in medical management of acute diverticulitis having increased the threshold for emergency laparotomy, patients continue to present with high grade disease requiring colectomy. However, even emergency surgical intervention has evolved as more studies show the benefits of restoration of intestinal continuity in lieu of the Hartmann's procedure. Novel approaches such as the use of damage control techniques continue to push the management of diverticulitis into a new era.

References

1. Humes DJ, Spiller RC. Review article: the pathogenesis and management of acute colonic diverticulitis. Aliment Pharmacol Ther. 2014;39:359–70.
2. Li D, Baxter NN, McLeod RS, Moineddin R, Wilton AS, Nathens AB. Evolving practice patterns in the management of acute colonic diverticulitis: a population-based analysis. Dis Colon Rectum. 2014:571397–405.
3. Hinchey EJ, Schaal PG, Richards GK. Treatment of perforated diverticular disease of the colon. Adv Surg. 1978;12:85–109.
4. Kaiser AM, Jiang JK, Lake JP, Ault G, Artinyan A, Gonzalez-Ruiz C, Essani R, Beart RW Jr. The management of complicated diverticulitis and the role of computed tomography. Am J Gastroenterol. 2005;100(4):910–7.
5. Shafi S, Aboutanos M, Brown CVR, Ciesla D, Cohen MJ, Crandall ML, Inaba K, Miller PR, Mowery NT, the American Association for the Surgery of Trauma Committee on Patient Assessment and Outcomes. Measuring anatomic severity of disease in emergency general surgery. J Trauma Acute Care Surg. 2014;76(3):884–7.
6. Savage SA, Klekar CS, Priest EL, Crandall ML, Rodriguez BC, Shafi S and the AAST Patient Assessment Committee. "Validating a new grading scale for emergency general surgery diseases." J Surg Res 2015;196(2):264–269.
7. Shafi S, Priest EL, Crandall ML, Klekar CS, Nazim A, Aboutanos M, Agarwal S, Bhattacharya B, Byrge N, Dhillon TS, Eboli DJ, Fielder D, Guillamondegui O, Gunter O, Inaba K, Mowery NT, Nirula R, Ross SE, Savage SA, Schuster KM, Schmoker RK, Siboni S, Siparsky N, Trust MD, Utter GH, Whelan J, Feliciano DV, Rozycki G, the AAST Patient Assessment Committee. Multicenter validation of the American Association for the Surgery of Trauma grading system for acute colonic diverticulitis and its use for emergency general surgery quality improvement program. J Trauma Acute Care Surg. 2015;80(3):405–11.
8. Ebersole J, Medvecz AJ, Connolly C, Sborov K, Matevish L, Wile G, Gondek S, Gunter O, Guillamondegui O, Dennis B. Comparison of American Association for the Surgery of Trauma grading scale with modified Hinchey classification in acute colonic diverticulitis: a pilot study. J Trauma Acute Care Surg. 2020;88(6):770.
9. Weizman AV, Nguyen GC. Diverticular disease: epidemiology and management. Can J Gastroenterol. 2011;25:385–9.
10. Young-Fadok T. Diverticulitis. N Engl J Med. 2018;379(17):1635–42.
11. Feuerstein JD, Falchuk KR. Diverticulosis and diverticulitis. Mayo Clin Proc. 2016;91(8):1094–104.
12. Bharucha AE, Parthasarathy G, Ditah I, et al. Temporal trends in the incidence and natural history of diverticulitis: a population-based study. Am J Gastroenterol. 2015;110:1589–96.
13. Hall J, Hardiman K, Lee S, et al. The American Society of Colon and Rectal Surgeons clinical practice guidelines for the treatment of left-sided colonic diverticulitis. Dis Colon Rectum. 2020;63(6):728–47.
14. Hogan J, Sehgal R, Murphy D, O'Leary P, Coffey JC. Do inflammatory indices play a role in distinguishing between uncomplicated and complicated diverticulitis? Dig Surg. 2017;34:7–11.
15. Kechagias A, Rautio T, Kechagias G, Mäkelä J. The role of C- reactive protein in the prediction of the clinical severity of acute diverticulitis. Am Surg. 2014;80:391–5.
16. Mäkelä JT, Klintrup K, Takala H, Rautio T. The role of C-reactive protein in prediction of the severity of acute diverticulitis in an emergency unit. Scand J Gastroenterol. 2015;50:536–41.
17. Bolkenstein HE, van de Wall BJ, Consten EC, van der Palen J, Broeders IA, Draaisma WA. Development and validation of a diagnostic prediction model distinguishing complicated from uncomplicated diverticulitis. Scand J Gastroenterol. 2018;53:1291–7.
18. Alshamari M, Norrman E, Geijer M, Jansson K, Geijer H. Diagnostic accuracy of low-dose CT compared with abdominal radiography in non-traumatic acute abdominal pain: prospective study and systematic review. Eur Radiol. 2016;26:1766–74.
19. Kameda T, Kawai F, Taniguchi N, Kobori Y. Usefulness of transabdominal ultrasonography in excluding adnexal disease. J Med Ultrason (2001). 2016;43:63–70.
20. Nielsen K, Richir MC, Stolk TT, et al. The limited role of ultrasound in the diagnostic process of colonic diverticulitis. World J Surg. 2014;38:1814–8.
21. Chabok A, Påhlman L, Hjern F, Haapaniemi S, Smedh K, AVOD Study Group. Randomized clinical trial of antibiotics in acute uncomplicated diverticulitis. Br J Surg. 2012;99:532–9.
22. Isacson D, Smedh K, Nikberg M, Chabok A. Long-term follow-up of the AVOD randomized trial of antibiotic avoidance in uncomplicated diverticulitis. Br J Surg. 2019;106:1542–8.

23. Daniels L, Ünlü Ç, de Korte N, et al. Dutch Diverticular Disease (3D) Collaborative Study Group. Randomized clinical trial of observational versus antibiotic treatment for a first episode of CT-proven uncomplicated acute diverticulitis. Br J Surg. 2017;104:52–61.
24. Rhodes A, Evans LE, Alhazzani W, et al. Surviving sepsis campaign: international guidelines for management of sepsis and septic shock: 2016. Intensive Care Med. 2017;43(3):304–77. https://doi.org/10.1007/s00134-017-4683-6.
25. Sawyer RG, Claridge JA, Nathens AB, Rotstein OD, Duane TM, Evans HL, Cook CH, O'Neill PJ, Mazuski JE, Askari R, Wilson MA, Napolitano LM, Namias N, Miller PR, Dellinger EP, Watson CM, Coimbra R, Dent DL, Lowry SF, Cocanour CS, West MA, Banton KL, Cheadle WG, Lipsett PA, Guidry CA, Popovsky K, STOP-IT Trial Investigators. Trial of short-course antimicrobial therapy for intraabdominal infection. N Engl J Med. 2015;372(21):1996–2005.
26. Schug-Pass C, Geers P, Hügel O, Lippert H, Köckerling F. Prospective randomized trial comparing short-term antibiotic therapy versus standard therapy for acute uncomplicated sigmoid diverticulitis. Int J Color Dis. 2010;25:751–9.
27. Biondo S, Golda T, Kreisler E, et al. Outpatient versus hospitalization management for uncomplicated diverticulitis: a prospective, multicenter randomized clinical trial (DIVER Trial). Ann Surg. 2014;259(1):38–44.
28. Mege D, Yeo H. Meta-analyses of current strategies to treat uncomplicated diverticulitis. Dis Colon Rectum. 2019;62(3):371–8.
29. Lambrichts DPV, Bolkenstein HE, van der Does DCHE, et al. Multicentre study of non-surgical management of diverticulitis with abscess formation. Br J Surg. 2019;106:458–66.
30. Toorenvliet BR, Swank H, Schoones JW, Hamming JF, Bemelman WA. Laparoscopic peritoneal lavage for perforated colonic diverticulitis: a systematic review. Color Dis. 2010;12:862–7.
31. Lambrichts DPV, Vennix S, Musters GD, et al. Hartmann's procedure versus sigmoidectomy with primary anastomosis for perforated diverticulitis with purulent or faecal peritonitis (LADIES): a multicentre, parallel-group, randomised, open-label, superiority trial. Lancet Gastroenterol Hepatol. 2019;4(8):599–610.
32. Vennix S, Musters GD, Mulder IM, Swank HA, Consten EC, Belgers EH, van Geloven AA, Gerhards MF, Govaert MJ, van Grevenstein WM, Hoofwijk AG, Kruyt PM, Nienhuijs SW, Boermeester MA, Vermeulen J, van Dieren S, Lange JF, Bemelman WA, Ladies trial collaborators. Laparoscopic peritoneal lavage or sigmoidectomy for perforated diverticulitis with purulent peritonitis: a multicentre, parallel-group, randomised, open-label trial. Lancet. 2015;386(10000):1269–77.
33. Schultz JK, Yaqub S, Wallon C, et al. Laparoscopic lavage versus primary resection for acute perforated diverticulitis: The SCANDIV randomized clinical trial. JAMA. 2015;314(13):1364–75.
34. Francis NK, Sylla P, Abou-Khalil M, et al. EAES and SAGES 2018 consensus conference on acute diverticulitis management: evidence-based recommendations for clinical practice. Surg Endosc. 2019;33(9):2726–41.
35. Schuster KM, Holena DN, Salim A, et al. American Association for the Surgery of Trauma emergency general surgery guideline summaries 2018: acute appendicitis, acute cholecystitis, acute diverticulitis, acute pancreatitis, and small bowel obstruction. Trauma Surg Acute Care Open. 2019;4(1):e000281.
36. Ballian N, Rajamanickam V, Harms BA, Foley EF, Heise CP, Greenberg CC, Kennedy GD. Predictors of mortality after emergent surgery for acute colonic diverticulitis: analysis of National Surgical Quality Improvement Project data. J Trauma Acute Care Surg. 2013;74(2):611–6.
37. Letarte F, Hallet J, Drolet S, et al. Laparoscopic emergency surgery for diverticular disease that failed medical treatment: a valuable option? Results of a retrospective comparative cohort study. Dis Colon Rectum. 2013;56(12):1395–402.
38. Turley RS, Barbas AS, Lidsky ME, Mantyh CR, Migaly J, Scarborough JE. Laparoscopic versus open Hartmann procedure for the emergency treatment of diverticulitis: a propensity-matched analysis. Dis Colon Rectum. 2013;56(1):72–82.
39. Halabi WJ, Kang CY, Jafari MD, et al. Robotic-assisted colorectal surgery in the United States: a nationwide analysis of trends and outcomes. World J Surg. 2013;37(12):2782–90.
40. Raskin ER, Keller DS, Gorrepati ML, Akiel-Fu S, Mehendale S, Cleary RK. Propensity-Matched Analysis of Sigmoidectomies for Diverticular Disease. *JSLS*. 2019;23(1).
41. Ogilvie JW Jr, Saunders RN, Parker J, Luchtefeld MA. Sigmoidectomy for diverticulitis-a propensity-matched comparison of minimally invasive approaches. J Surg Res. 2019;243:434–9.
42. Al Natour RH, Obias V, Albright J, et al. A propensity score matched comparison of intracorporeal and extracorporeal techniques for robotic-assisted sigmoidectomy in an enhanced recovery pathway. J Robot Surg. 2019;13(5):649–56.
43. Thaler K, Baig MK, Berho M, et al. Determinants of recurrence after sigmoid resection for uncomplicated diverticulitis. Dis Colon Rectum. 2003;46(3):385–8.
44. Benn PL, Wolff BG, Ilstrup DM. Level of anastomosis and recurrent colonic diverticulitis. Am J Surg. 1986;151:269–71.
45. Cirocchi R, Afshar S, Di Saverio S, et al. A historical review of surgery for peritonitis secondary to acute colonic diverticulitis: from Lockhart-Mummery to evidence-based medicine. World J Emerg Surg. 2017;12:14.
46. Oberkofler CE, Rickenbacher A, Raptis DA, et al. A multicenter randomized clinical trial of primary anas-

tomosis or Hartmann's procedure for perforated left colonic diverticulitis with purulent or fecal peritonitis. Ann Surg. 2012;256(5):819–27.
47. Bridoux V, Regimbeau JM, Ouaissi M, et al. Hartmann's procedure or primary anastomosis for generalized peritonitis due to perforated diverticulitis: a prospective multicenter randomized trial (DIVERTI). J Am Coll Surg. 2017;225(6):798–805.
48. Tartaglia D, Costa G, Camillò A, Castriconi M, Andreano M, Lanza M, Fransvea P, Ruscelli P, Rimini M, Galatioto C, Chiarugi M. Damage control surgery for perforated diverticulitis with diffuse peritonitis: saves lives and reduces ostomy. World J Emerg Surg. 2019;14:19.
49. Sohn M, Iesalnieks I, Agha A, Steiner P, Hochrein A, Pratschke J, Ritschl P, Aigner F. Perforated diverticulitis with generalized peritonitis: low stoma rate using a "damage control strategy". World J Surg. 2018;42(10):3189–95.
50. DeLeon MF, Sapci I, Akeel NY, Holubar SD, Stocchi L, Hull TL. Diverticular colovaginal fistulas: what factors contribute to successful surgical management? Dis Colon Rectum. 2019;62(9):1079–84.
51. Badic B, Leroux G, Thereaux J, Joumond A, Gancel CH, Bail JP, Meurette G. Colovesical fistula complicating diverticular disease: a 14-year experience. Surg Laparosc Endosc Percutan Tech. 2017;27(2):94–7.
52. Keady C, Hechtl D, Joyce M. When the bowel meets the bladder: optimal management of colorectal pathology with urological involvement. World J Gastrointest Surg. 2020;12(5):208–25.
53. Scarborough JE, Mantyh CR, Sun Z, Migaly J. Combined mechanical and oral antibiotic bowel preparation reduces incisional surgical site infection and anastomotic leak rates after elective colorectal resection: an analysis of colectomy-targeted ACS NSQIP. Ann Surg. 2015;262(2):331–7.
54. Ohman KA, Wan L, Guthrie T, et al. Combination of oral antibiotics and mechanical bowel preparation reduces surgical site infection in colorectal surgery. J Am Coll Surg. 2017;225(4):465–71.
55. 2017 European Society of Coloproctology (ESCP) Collaborating Group. Association of mechanical bowel preparation with oral antibiotics and anastomotic leak following left sided colorectal resection: an international, multi-centre, prospective audit. Colorectal Dis. 2018;20(Suppl 6):15–32.
56. Bothwell WN, Bleicher RJ, Dent TL. Prophylactic ureteral catheterization in colon surgery: a year review. Dis Colon Rectum. 1994;37:330–4.
57. Kuno K, Menzin A, Kauder HH, Sison C, Gal D. Prophylactic ureteral catheterization in gynecologic surgery. Urology. 1998;52:1004–8.
58. Coakley KM, Kasten KR, Sims SM, Prasad T, Heniford BT, Davis BR. Prophylactic ureteral catheters for colectomy: a national surgical quality improvement program-based analysis. Dis Colon Rectum. 2018;61(1):84–8.
59. Merola J, Arnold B, Luks V, et al. Prophylactic ureteral stent placement vs no ureteral stent placement during open colectomy. JAMA Surg. 2018;153(1):87–90.
60. Rose J, Parina RP, Faiz O, Chang DC, Talamini MA. Long-term outcomes after initial presentation of diverticulitis. Ann Surg. 2015;262:1046–53.
61. Aquina CT, Becerra AZ, Xu Z, et al. Population-based study of outcomes following an initial acute diverticular abscess. Br J Surg. 2019;106:467–76.
62. Devaraj B, Liu W, Tatum J, Cologne K, Kaiser AM. Medically treated diverticular abscess associated with high risk of recurrence and disease complications. Dis Colon Rectum. 2016;59:208–15.
63. Hupfeld L, Burcharth J, Pommergaard HC, Rosenberg J. Risk factors for recurrence after acute colonic diverticulitis: a systematic review. Int J Color Dis. 2017;32(5):611–22.
64. Hall JF, Roberts PL, Ricciardi R, et al. Long-term follow-up after an initial episode of diverticulitis: what are the predictors of recurrence? Dis Colon Rectum. 2011;54:283–8.
65. Sharma PV, Eglinton T, Hider P, Frizelle F. Systematic review and meta-analysis of the role of routine colonic evaluation after radiologically confirmed acute diverticulitis. Ann Surg. 2014;259:263–72.
66. Meyer J, Orci LA, Combescure C, et al. Risk of colorectal cancer in patients with acute diverticulitis: a systematic review and meta-analysis of observational studies. Clin Gastroenterol Hepatol. 2019;17:1448–56.

Intestinal Ischemia

18

Eric M. Campion, Melanie Hoehn, and Clay Cothren Burlew

An 82 y/o F presented to the emergency department with the acute onset of diffuse abdominal pain. It was associated with some nausea but no vomiting or diarrhea. She had a history of severe PAD and had undergone a previous carotid endarterectomy. On exam she was noted to have a BP of 105/65 and a HR of 112. Her WBC was 14 and her lactate was 2.9. Her abdominal exam revealed mild to moderate distention with some tenderness but no signs of peritonitis. She went immediately to the CT scan where she was noted to have evidence of severe aortic and branch vessel disease resulting in a severe stenosis of her celiac, an occlusion of her SMA, and a stenotic IMA. There was some mild small bowel thickening but no evidence of necrosis or perforation. She was taken to the interventional suite where an angio confirmed the arterial disease and a SMA stent was placed. She was admitted for serial abdominal exams. Her pain resolved and her diet was slowly advanced. She was discharged post procedure day #3.

Intestinal ischemia represents a unique challenge to the practicing emergency general surgeon. It is a rare but time-sensitive and potentially devastating condition that requires prompt diagnosis and treatment for optimal outcome. Intestinal ischemia, or mesenteric ischemia, is an emergency condition in which the intestinal oxygen supply does not meet its metabolic needs leading to ischemia and eventually necrosis. The overall incidence of intestinal ischemia is difficult to ascertain due to low autopsy rates. A historic study from Sweden with a high autopsy rate identified 12.9 cases/100,000/year from 1970 to 1982 [1]. A more recent study from Finland identified 7.3 cases per 100,000 per year from 2009 to 2013 [2]. While rare, it has a high mortality with reports of historic mortality of up to 80% [3]. Modern data have shown a decline in in-hospital mortality down to 21% [4]. While a significant improvement, this still is one of the most lethal conditions to present to most general surgeons. In order for an optimal outcome, mesenteric ischemia must be on the differential for every patient with acute abdominal pain and ruled out rapidly when the symptoms are consistent with the diagnosis.

Anatomy

The superior mesenteric artery arises from the abdominal aorta 1–2 cm distal to the celiac axis. The first branch of this artery is the pancreaticoduodenal artery. This artery is of particular importance as it is able to provide collateral flow through the gastroduodenal artery to the celiac axis when occlusions of the superior mesenteric artery (SMA) develop slowly. The middle colic

E. M. Campion · M. Hoehn · C. C. Burlew (✉)
Department of Surgery, Denver Health Medical Center, Denver, CO, USA
e-mail: Eric.Campion@dhha.org; melanie.hoehn@dhha.org; Clay.Cothren@dhha.org

M. D. Zielinski, O. Guillamondegui (eds.), *The Acute Management of Surgical Disease*,
https://doi.org/10.1007/978-3-031-07881-1_18

artery is the next branch which provides blood flow to the proximal colon. After this branch, the SMA abruptly narrows. Clots traveling through the SMA often lodge at either the origin of the middle colic artery or at the early jejunal branches. Occlusion proximal to the middle colic artery (approximately 70% of cases) will frequently lead to ischemia of the majority of the small bowel and ischemia of the right half of the colon. This is typically lethal without urgent revascularization. In the remaining 30% of patients, emboli lodge distal to the middle colic resulting in fewer areas of ischemic intestine. The need for revascularization at these sites depend on how distal the clot lodged and amount of bowel at risk. Less frequently due to its distal location, the inferior mesenteric artery (IMA) can be involved resulting in colonic ischemia. This is more commonly due to diffuse atherosclerotic disease rather than emboli and can lead to an ischemic colitis involving the sigmoid and parts of the descending colon. The rectum is typically spared due to its robust collateralization including blood supply outside the mesenteric vascular system.

Pathophysiology

Intestinal ischemia can have several different underlying pathophysiologic etiologies. The most common is acute arterial embolism accounting for 50% of cases [5]. This is classically associated with atrial fibrillation but can occur from other cardiac causes such as mural thrombus and endocarditis or from an atherosclerotic aorta. The SMA is the most common clinically relevant site involved due to lack of significant collaterals. Embolism to the SMA typically lodges between 3 and 10 cm distal to the SMA takeoff thus possibly sparring the proximal jejunum and colon [6]. This leads to acute ischemia of a large portion of the small bowel and produces significant acute abdominal pain that is classically "pain out of proportion to exam." This pain typically begins suddenly and is not well localized. Patients tend to have relatively benign abdominal exam with minimal to no tenderness during the early stages. Some patients may have an audible bruit on auscultation, but this is not a sensitive finding. As the bowel moves from ischemia to necrosis, signs of peritonitis occur. At this point, the ischemia is often not reversible and bowel needs to be resected. The amount of bowel at risk for necrosis depends on how distally the clot has lodged. A high index of suspicion early in the disease course is paramount to diagnose and treat intestinal ischemia before bowel necrosis occurs (Fig. 18.1).

Acute occlusion of a chronically diseased vessel is the second most common type of mesenteric ischemia, representing 20–35% of cases [5]. Acute on chronic intestinal ischemia can be particularly difficult to diagnose as the symptoms are varied and potentially more subtle. Atherosclerotic mesenteric ischemia typically occurs at the proximal SMA. Plaque rupture can lead to acute thrombosis of a chronic lesion. Classically, atherosclerotic stenosis leads to symptoms of chronic mesenteric ischemia due to narrowed blood flow; a subset of patients with

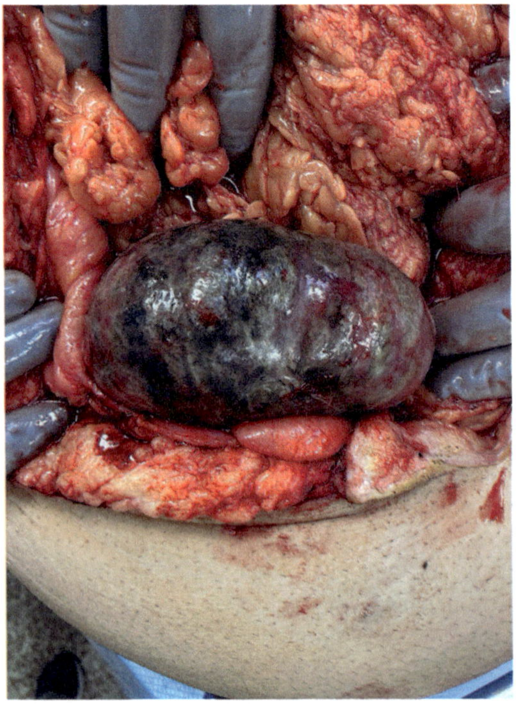

Fig. 18.1 Ischemic bowel

clinically silent atherosclerotic narrowing exists making a close evaluation of preoperative imaging essential in choosing the appropriate treatment modality. Chronic intestinal ischemia originates from atherosclerosis in proximal mesenteric arteries and over time leads to development of collaterals that can provide some perfusion to the intestine during acute thrombosis of a chronic atherosclerotic lesion. This can cloud the clinical presentation and lead to a delayed diagnosis of acute ischemia. Symptoms range from severe pain out of proportion to exam to diffuse and vague abdominal pain, diarrhea(often bloody), or vomiting. Additionally, they may present in a more subacute fashion with necrosis developing over days rather than hours and can have relatively normal lab values(lactate and white blood cell count). The amount of bowel that is threatened can span from devastating pan-intestinal ischemia to small patchy areas due to collateralization of blood flow and intestinal tolerance to low flow. Patients presenting with acute abdominal symptoms should be queried for a history of postprandial pain, food fear, and weight loss.

Mesenteric venous thrombosis (MVT) is an uncommon but potentially devastating condition and accounts for 5–15% of mesenteric ischemic events [6]. This occurs when there is clotting of the major venous outflow of the bowel leading to impaired circulation, ischemia, and eventually necrosis. This can occur secondary to inflammatory conditions in the vicinity of the major veins of the mesentery or can be due to a hypercoagulable state. MVT involves the superior mesenteric vein in the vast majority of cases and is described as the target sign on CT [6]. Prolonged occlusion of the venous outflow at this level leads to infarction of the ileum, jejunum, and, less commonly, the duodenum. Non-specific abdominal pain is the primary symptom of MVT. This pain can be insidious and wide ranging in severity. Unfortunately, the pain can be mistakenly attributed to the inflammatory cause of the thrombosis allowing thrombosis to go unrecognized. As with all intestinal ischemia, a high index of suspicion is critical to making the diagnosis in a timely manner.

Nonocclusive mesenteric ischemia occurs when a low flow state causes inadequate perfusion of the bowel to meet its demands. This can occur from a variety of causes such as a low flow state secondary to shock from another cause. Again, a high index of suspicion is key as patients are often already critically ill and further deterioration or a lack of appropriate response to resuscitation can easily be attributed to other causes. Other rare causes of ischemia include vasculitis and arterial dissection.

Diagnostic Workup

The diagnostic workup of a patient with intestinal ischemia begins with the clinician recognizing it as a diagnostic possibility. The most common presenting symptom is acute abdominal pain (95%) followed by nausea (44%), vomiting (35%), and diarrhea(35%) [7]. As with all patients presenting with acute abdominal pain, a through history and physical examination is essential. Any patient with acute onset of severe abdominal pain should raise suspicion for the diagnosis. Details of the onset of the pain, timing, and location can be helpful to narrow the differential diagnosis. History of a predisposing condition such as atrial fibrillation, recent myocardial infarction, and prior arterial embolus should serve as red flags for acute embolic mesenteric ischemia secondary to an embolus. Symptoms of chronic mesenteric ischemia should be sought (pain after eating, chronic nausea or vomiting, early satiety, weight loss, and food fear) as these may be suggestive of acute on chronic ischemia. A history of peripheral arterial disease or coronary disease should also raise suspicion. Additionally, a history of prior venous thrombosis or known thrombophilia disorder would suggest the possibility of mesenteric venous thrombosis. Nonocclusive mesenteric ischemia typically presents with a low flow state with associated shock. In these cases, the ischemia is typically not the presenting symptom unless the patient has had a delay to medical care.

Physical examination is often non-specific but can be helpful in a number of ways. Classically,

signal on the antimesenteric border being reassuring. If malperfusion is identified, the next step depends on the etiology, chronicity, and anatomic location of the occlusion. In the absence of a preoperative CTA, an on table angiogram can give information about the etiology as well as the location of the occlusion. Both will affect the approach for revascularization. The SMA should be surgically exposed unless it can be assured to have adequate flow (Fig. 18.3). Soft tissue overlying the SMA is divided with care taken to not injure the SMV which lies to the right.

In the most common scenario, arterial embolization, the preferred approach is a surgical embolectomy. After obtaining proximal and distal control, an arteriotomy is made. This approach is best performed transversely if the vessel feels soft and healthy. A #3 or #4 Fogarty catheter is passed distally as well as proximally into the aorta and inflated while it is retracted. Once the thrombus is removed, the artery is closed with double armed Prolene suture. If questions remain about the adequacy of distal flow, arteriography is warranted. The bowel must be thoroughly inspected. If blood flow is not adequately restored, then an alternate approach such as a bypass or proximal stent must be undertaken.

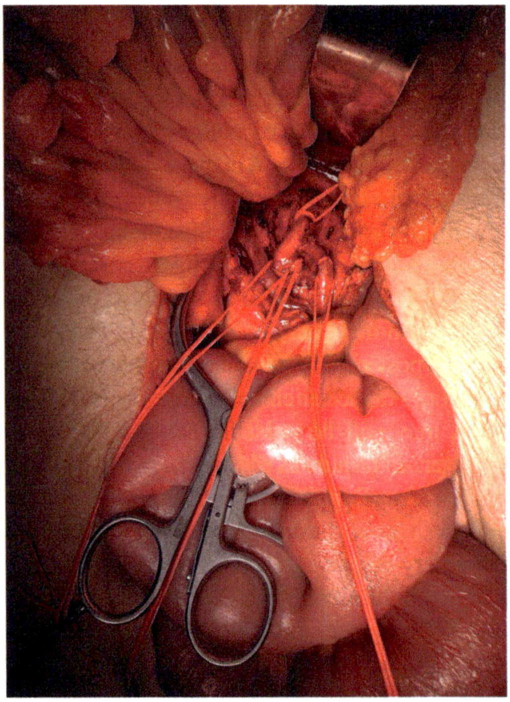

Fig. 18.3 Surgical exposure of the superior mesenteric artery

SMA bypass can be used if adequate inflow cannot be restored. This is frequently the case in the setting of atherosclerotic acute on chronic disease. This can be performed utilizing a vein or externally supported prosthetic graft. In the emergency setting, the right common iliac artery is used more frequently, but the infrarenal aorta, supraceliac aorta, or either iliac artery can be used. The atherosclerotic disease burden as well as the patients' ability to tolerate aortic clamping all factor into the decision. Vein graft is ideal for resisting infection in the setting of bowel necrosis, but is more prone to kinking but with a 3-year patency approaching 80–90%. There is no difference in complications or patency between the approaches [13, 14].

Even during the conduct of a laparotomy, endovascular stenting can potentially offer an advantage. This can be approached in the traditional manner from the femoral, brachial, or radial approach. Another option is a retrograde SMA stent of the underlying lesion. When thrombectomy fails, it is most commonly due to atherosclerosis of the proximal SMA at the origin. This area is amenable to stenting and has acceptable patency rates, particularly when covered stents are used [15]. The sheath and the stent can be placed directly through the exposed SMA. This has the theoretical advantage of a shorter "clamp time" as well as no prosthetic use in the setting of contamination. Complications, reintervention, and mortality rates are similar to those of mesenteric bypass in the setting of AMI [16].

Once blood flow is reestablished, any obviously necrotic bowel is resected, while bowel of questionable viability is preserved when possible. A planned second look is essential to reevaluate the bowel until viability of the remaining bowel is assured.

In situations where intestinal ischemia is suspected yet the clinical symptoms do not warrant immediate laparotomy, an urgent endovascular approach can be utilized to restore intestinal perfusion. The decision to defer laparotomy should be based on an overall clinical picture that suggests a low likelihood of bowel necrosis. This is based on a benign clinical exam, normal or only mildly elevated lactate and WBC, and symptoms that are not acutely worsening. Serial abdominal examinations and serial laboratory evaluation are mandatory until symptoms resolve. If there is suspicion of bowel necrosis, operative exploration with laparotomy or laparoscopy is warranted.

The specific technical considerations of endovascular intervention are based on the location and underlying pathology of the lesion. Percutaneous thrombectomy can be employed in patients with a true embolic etiology, but this scenario is rare, as most will require laparotomy. In the setting of laparotomy for embolic disease, open thrombectomy is a fast definitive way to establish flow, but the percutaneous approach is being used with increased frequency. Endovascular solutions are much particularly appealing in acute on chronic or subacute ischemia where laparotomy may be avoided. Depending on the lesion's chronicity, this may involve some component of percutaneous pharmacomechanical thrombectomy in addition to stenting of the underlying lesion. SMA stenting is well established with newer data suggesting patency rates similar to bypass; however, they do have a significant reintervention of 40% at 3 years [17] (Fig. 18.4).

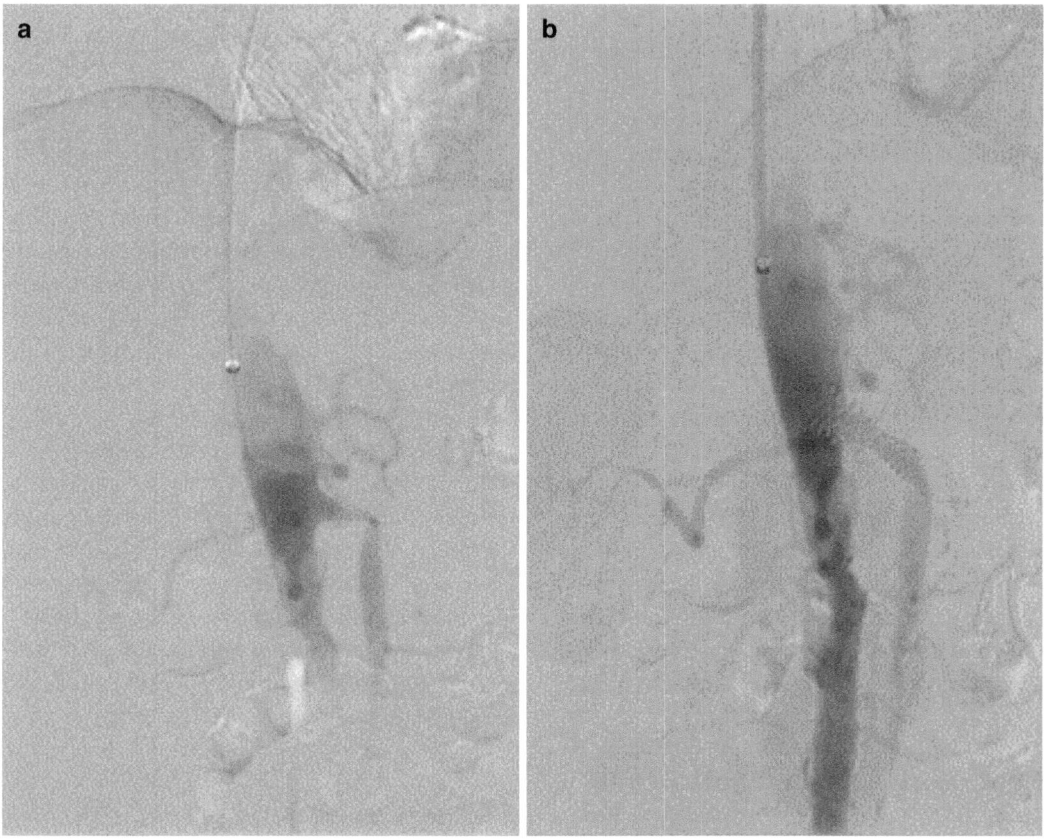

Fig. 18.4 Superior mesenteric artery with high-grade stenosis before (**a**) and after stent placement (**b**)

Venous Mesenteric Ischemia

The patient with mesenteric ischemia is evaluated and resuscitated in a similar manner to arterial ischemia above. Heparin is initiated immediately on making the diagnosis. Clinical exam, laboratory values, and imaging findings are carefully evaluated to determine if operative evaluation of the bowel is required. A history of genetic hypercoagulable disorder, leukocytosis, lactic acidosis, and bowel wall thickening on CT scan have been shown to be predictors for resection. Bowel rest and NG tube decompression are employed for nonoperative management. Serial abdominal examinations and laboratory evaluation is employed to identify evolving bowel ischemia. If necrosis of the bowel is suspected, open or laparoscopic evaluation should occur without delay. Anticoagulation with unfractionated heparin is the mainstay of early treatment. This is then transitioned to anticoagulation with warfarin (INR 2–3), low molecular weight heparin, or other full anticoagulation agent. While a large number of these patients improve without requiring a bowel resection, there remains a high rate of readmission for abdominal pain. All patients should be evaluated for a hypercoagulable disorder [18].

In severe acute cases that remain refractory to management with unfractionated heparin, or when a significant amount of intestine is thought to be at risk, endovascular treatment can be considered. This decision is made based on imaging findings and the patient's clinical course. This is challenging as access to the portovenous system is limited. The most common approach is via a transjugular or transhepatic approach with lysis catheters. The techniques are similar to the arterial approach involving percutaneous thrombectomy and the direct infusion of thrombolytics.

Nonocclusive Mesenteric Ischemia

The diagnosis of NOMI is challenging and traditionally requires digital subtraction angiography; however MDCT is gaining acceptance [19]. Findings include diffuse arterial spasm, poor filling of distal branches, or "pruning," reflux of contrast in to the aorta, slow portovenous filling, and improvement with the administration of papaverine (Fig. 18.5). Traditionally, NOMI is treated by aggressively resuscitating the patient in shock, restoring systemic perfusion, and treating the underlying pathology. Signs of ischemic bowel are sought and surgical evaluation of the bowel is undertaken if there is concern for necrosis. Any obviously necrotic bowel is resected, and questionable bowel is left behind for a planned second-look laparotomy. Re-exploration continues until no further questionable bowel is identified at which time the abdomen is closed. There is increased interest in intra-arterial papaverine infusion; a recent study has shown a significant improvement in mortality from 97% to 66% with vasodilator infusion, but it remains a highly lethal condition [20].

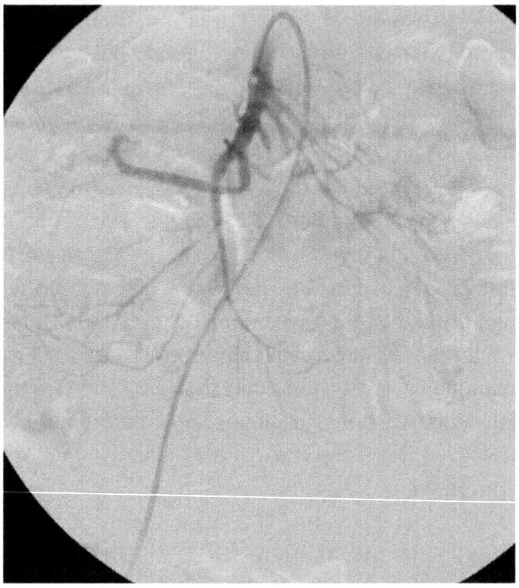

Fig. 18.5 Mesenteric angiogram in a patient with nonocclusive mesenteric ischemia showing diffuse vessel spasm, "pruning," and poor distal filling of the branches of the superior mesenteric artery

Further Considerations

In the setting of embolic disease, the patient needs a full workup including a CTA of the chest, abdomen, and pelvis as well as an echocardiogram to identify a potential source. No specific imaging is necessary for follow-up after a thrombectomy; however, lifelong anticoagulation should be considered. If a stent or a bypass is performed, then the patient should be treated for their underlying peripheral arterial disease. Antiplatelet medications are the mainstay of treatment. These patients also require surveillance imaging within 1 month of the procedure, then at 6 months and 12 months, and then annually thereafter.

References

1. Acosta S. Epidemiology of mesenteric vascular disease: clinical implications. Semin Vasc Surg. 2010;23(1):4–8.
2. Karkkainen JM, Lehtimaki TT, Manninen H, Paajanen H. Acute mesenteric ischemia is a more common cause than expected of acute abdomen in the elderly. J Gastrointest Surg. 2015;19(8):1407–14.
3. Jrvinen O, Laurikka J, Salenius JP, Tarkka M. Acute intestinal ischaemia. A review of 214 cases. Ann Chir Gynaecol. 1994;83(1):22–5.
4. Zettervall SL, Lo RC, Soden PA, Deery SE, Ultee KH, Pinto DS, et al. Trends in Treatment and Mortality for Mesenteric Ischemia in the United States from 2000 to 2012. Ann Vasc Surg. 2017;42:111–9.
5. Clair DG, Beach JM. Mesenteric ischemia. N Engl J Med. 2016;374(10):959–68.
6. Bala M, Kashuk J, Moore EE, Kluger Y, Biffl W, Gomes CA, et al. Acute mesenteric ischemia: guidelines of the World Society of Emergency Surgery. World J Emerg Surg. 2017;12:38.
7. Park WM, Gloviczki P, Cherry KJ Jr, Hallett JW Jr, Bower TC, Panneton JM, et al. Contemporary management of acute mesenteric ischemia: Factors associated with survival. J Vasc Surg. 2002;35(3):445–52.
8. Memet O, Zhang L, Shen J. Serological biomarkers for acute mesenteric ischemia. Ann Transl Med. 2019;7(16):394.
9. Kärkkäinen JM, Lehtimäki TT, Saari P, Hartikainen J, Rantanen T, Paajanen H, et al. Endovascular therapy as a primary revascularization modality in acute mesenteric ischemia. Cardiovasc Intervent Radiol. 2015;38(5):1119–29.
10. Aschoff AJ, Stuber G, Becker BW, Hoffmann MH, Schmitz BL, Schelzig H, et al. Evaluation of acute mesenteric ischemia: accuracy of biphasic mesenteric multi-detector CT angiography. Abdom Imaging. 2009;34(3):345–57.
11. Sindall ME, Davenport DL, Wallace P, Bernard AC. Validation of the American Association for the Surgery of Trauma grading system for acute mesenteric ischemia-More than anatomic severity is needed to determine risk of mortality. J Trauma Acute Care Surg. 2020;88(5):671–6.
12. Alvi AR, Khan S, Niazi SK, Ghulam M, Bibi S. Acute mesenteric venous thrombosis: improved outcome with early diagnosis and prompt anticoagulation therapy. Int J Surg. 2009;7(3):210–3; Epub 2009 Mar 28.
13. Scali ST, Ayo D, Giles KA, Gray S, Kubilis P, Back M, et al. Outcomes of antegrade and retrograde open mesenteric bypass for acute mesenteric ischemia. J Vasc Surg. 2019;69(1):129–40.
14. McMillan WD, McCarthy WJ, Bresticker MR, Pearce WH, Schneider JR, Golan JF, et al. Mesenteric artery bypass: objective patency determination. J Vasc Surg. 1995;21(5):729–40; discussion 40–1.
15. Girault A, Pellenc Q, Roussel A, Senemaud J, Cerceau P, Maggiori L, Huguet A, Corcos O, Ben Abdallah I, Castier Y. Midterm results after covered stenting of the superior mesenteric artery. J Vasc Surg. 2021:S0741-5214(21)00343-8.
16. Andraska E, Haga L, Li X, Avgerinos E, Singh M, Chaer R, et al. Retrograde open mesenteric stenting should be considered as the initial approach to acute mesenteric ischemia. J Vasc Surg. 2020;72(4):1260–8.
17. Barnes JA, Columbo JA, Ponukumati AS, Zwolak RM, Olive FT, Goodney PP, et al. Long-term outcomes of mesenteric stenting and analysis of in-stent restenosis duplex velocity criteria. Ann Vasc Surg. 2020;68:226–33.
18. Andraska E, Haga L, Reitz K, Li X, Ramos R, Avgerinos E, et al. Acute superior mesenteric venous thrombosis results in high rates of readmission and morbidity. J Vasc Surg Venous Lymphat Disord. 2020;8(5):748–55.
19. Kammerer S, Schuelke C, Berkemeyer S, et al. The role of multislice computed tomography (MSCT) angiography in the diagnosis and therapy of non-occlusive mesenteric ischemia (NOMI): Could MSCT replace DSA in diagnosis? PLoS One. 2018;13(3):e0193698. Published 2018 Mar 1.
20. Winzer R, Fedders D, Backes M, Ittermann T, Gründling M, Mensel B, et al. Local intra-arterial vasodilator infusion in non-occlusive mesenteric ischemia significantly increases survival rate. Cardiovasc Intervent Radiol. 2020;43(8):1148–55.

Perforated Peptic Ulcer

19

Stephens Daniel, John Zietlow, and Scott Zietlow

Case Report

A 68-year-old female with a history of rheumatoid arthritis on steroids and NSAIDS presents to the emergency department with acute onset of severe epigastric pain that awoke her from sleep. CT abdomen/pelvis was obtained which revealed free air, likely from the duodenum. The patient was taken to the operating room and underwent an open abdominal exploration with modified graham patch repair of a 1 cm perforated duodenal ulcer.

Introduction

Perforated peptic ulcer (PPU) is a life-threatening emergency associated with peptic ulcer disease (PUD) . Although perforation is less common than bleeding, complications associated with PUD, with a perforation to bleeding ratio of approximately 1:6, it is the most common indication for emergency operation in PUD and causes about 40% of all ulcer-related deaths [1]. Approximately 5% of patients with PUD will perforate [2]. While the exact mechanism of PUD resulting in PPU is not well defined, it is broadly described as an imbalance between acid, pepsin, and mucosal defense barriers. Some studies describe a 90-day mortality rate of up to 30% [3, 4]. Risk factors for perforation include nonsteroidals, *Helicobacter pylori (H. pylori)*, and physiologic stress [5]. The total cost of PUD in the USA is estimated at USD 5.65 billion dollars/year [6]. While PUD and PPU rates are decreasing in the developed world, their incidence remains a significant issue in the developing world.

Epidemiology

PUD annually affects 4 million people worldwide. The lifetime prevalence of perforation is estimated at 2–14% [7]. The overall prevalence of PUD has drastically declined over the last 50 years. The decline can be attributed to antisecretory medications, along with eradication of *H. pylori*, which is one of the most common infections worldwide [8]. Furthermore, *H. pylori* is prevalent in up to 50–80% of patients with PPU due to its physiologic effects on the gastrointestinal system, causing increased gastric acid secretion and decreased mucosal defense mechanisms [9]. The first major decline was noted in 1977 with the introduction of histamine H_2 receptors antagonists. In the 1980s, proton pump inhibitors (PPI) further decreased the disease burden, along

S. Daniel (✉) · J. Zietlow · S. Zietlow
Department of Surgery, Mayo Clinic,
Rochester, MN, USA
e-mail: stephens.daniel@mayo.edu;
zietlow.john@mayo.edu; zietlow.scott@mayo.edu

M. D. Zielinski, O. Guillamondegui (eds.), *The Acute Management of Surgical Disease*,
https://doi.org/10.1007/978-3-031-07881-1_19

with need for surgical management. Finally, a better understanding of *H. pylori* pathophysiology and eradication led to even further decline. Initially, the efficacy of the standard *H. pylori* treatment (PPI and two antibiotics, such as clarithromycin plus amoxicillin or metronidazole) was 90%. However, due to novel strains and increased resistance over the years, it has now reduced the efficacy rate to around 70% [10].

Medical management of PUD is critical and includes minimizing nonsteroidal anti-inflammatory drugs (NSAIDS), along with smoking and alcohol cessation. NSAIDS are widely used for the analgesic, anti-inflammatory, anti-pyretic effects and, for certain conditions (rheumatoid arthritis, osteoarthritis, pericarditis, other chronic disease states), are required for prolonged periods. It is also well-known that NSAIDS increase the risk of PPU [11]. Smoking has a twofold impact on increased risk of PPU, as it inhibits bicarbonate secretion from the pancreas, increasing the acidity in the duodenum while also inhibiting the body's healing ability for ulcers that are already present.

Overall, the current prevalence of PUD in western civilization is approximately 0.2–0.5%. In contrast, Asian countries have approximately a 2–3% prevalence due to higher *H. pylori* incidence, but also attributed to higher incidence of screening endoscopies for gastric cancer [12]. In the developing world, patients tend to be young, male, smokers, while in developed countries, patients tend to be elderly with multiple comorbidities and associated use of NSAIDs or steroids [13].

Diagnosis

A detailed history and physical exam are paramount in diagnosing patients with PPU. It is one of the most easily diagnosed acute abdominal conditions, provided that the symptoms are known and appreciated [14]. A broad differential for acute abdominal pain should be utilized, including but not limited to abdominal aortic aneurysm, aortic dissection, appendicitis, Boerhaave's syndrome, cholecystitis, foreign body ingestion, mesenteric ischemia, neoplasm, perforated viscus (other than stomach or duodenum), and small bowel obstruction. History should include previous diagnosis of PUD, previous or current *H. pylori* infection, NSAID use, smoking or illicit drug use, steroid use, and previous medical and surgical history. Specific questions about pain, including location, severity, worsening or alleviating factors, and radiation, are also important.

Patients with PPU disease will commonly present with sudden and severe epigastric pain. Over time, this localized pain can spread to the left upper quadrant, right upper quadrant, and back or even become generalized. Associated symptoms include syncope, cool extremities nausea, vomiting, early satiety, fevers, and chills. On physical exam, abdominal rigidity, guarding, and rebound tenderness may be present. It should be noted that physical exam findings may be suppressed or missing in patients who are obese, immunocompromised, pediatric, elderly, or those on steroids. The classic triad that hallmarks peptic ulcer perforation is sudden onset of abdominal pain, tachycardia (the earliest vital sign change), and abdominal rigidity [15]. Patients may eventually develop local or diffuse peritonitis and can develop sepsis with tachypnea, hypotension, and fever. However, typical symptoms may only be present in 2/3 of the patients presenting with PPU [16].

Imaging is an important adjunct in diagnosing PPU. An upright plain x-ray is a reasonable initial test, but it will miss up to 25% of patients with free air [17]. Patients with peritonitis may not tolerate erect X-rays, and thus a left lateral decubitus X-ray is an alternative for patient comfort. CT scan with IV and oral contrast has a sensitivity rate greater than 98% for PPU diagnosis [18]. An added benefit of obtaining a CT scan is the ability to rule out other causes of acute abdominal pathology that may not require operative intervention, such as acute pancreatitis. CT scan findings suspicious for perforation include pneumoperitoneum, bowel wall thickening, unexplained intraperitoneal fluid, mesenteric fat stranding, and presence of extraluminal water-soluble contrast (if given) [19]. Careful note of contained versus non-contained perforation is critical in the decision-making of operative versus a trial nonoperative management. If free air is not seen on imaging but suspicion remains high for perforation, imaging with water-soluble contrast (via either oral or nasogastric tube) can be performed [20]. Regardless of the imaging modality, an active leak of enteric contrast confirms the diagnosis. However, the lack of a leak does not preclude it, as a perforation may have sealed spontaneously.

Routine lab tests including CBC, BMP, and type and screen should be obtained. Blood amylase and lipase can also be obtained to assist with differential diagnosis for acute pancreatitis. Any patient with vital sign abnormalities concerning for sepsis should be worked up with the addition of an arterial blood gas (ABG) and lactate. As part of the septic workup, blood cultures should be obtained, along with ruling out other sources of sepsis. Broad-spectrum antibiotics should be started and not necessarily delayed for cultures.

Risk Scores

Perforated peptic ulcers (gastric or duodenal) have significant morbidity and mortality, especially in those patients with significant comorbidities. The American College of Surgeons (ACS), American Society of Anesthesiologists (ASA), and APACHE scoring systems have been used to estimate overall morbidity and mortality rates for patients. Specific to PPU, multiple grading systems have been used, including the Boey and Peptic Ulcer Perforation (PULP), for risk stratification to estimate the severity of PPU and predict outcomes [21–23]. The American Association for the Surgery of Trauma (AAST) developed a set of standardized definitions to further clarify the severity of PPU (Table 19.1) [24]. As disease severity increased, the rate of laparoscopic repair decreased, while the laparotomy rate increased [25]. Furthermore, as expected, the worse the AAST grade, the higher incidence of

Table 19.1 AAST grading system [24]

AAST grade	Description	Clinical criteria	Imaging criteria (CT findings)	Operative criteria	Pathologic criteria
I	Micro-perforation without peritonitis	Discomfort in the epigastric region	Extraluminal gas with no associated inflammatory changes	Preservation of normal anatomy with dissection required to identify the perforation	Perforation with minimal bowel wall inflammation
II	Contained perforation with localized peritonitis	Tenderness confined to the right upper quadrant (RUQ)	Extraluminal gas contained in a walled off collection or the retroperitoneum	Presence of inflammation and stigmata of perforation with contained collection	Perforation with bowel wall inflammation
III	Perforation with localized peritonitis and localized fluid collection in lesser sac or RUQ	Tenderness confined to the RUQ	Perforation with associated collection that is not contained in a anatomic space or abscess but not disseminated	Inflammation and contamination of peritoneal cavity confined to the RUQ	Perforation with bowel wall inflammation
IV	Free perforation with peritonitis	Diffuse peritonitis	Perforation with disseminated air and fluid	Perforation with disseminated succus or purulent peritonitis	Perforation with bowel wall inflammation
V	Perforation with duodenal destruction ± penetration into adjacent organs and generalized peritonitis	Diffuse peritonitis	Perforation with disseminated air and fluid with loss of local anatomic planes at the site of perforation	Perforation with disseminated succus or purulent peritonitis and erosion into adjacent structures	Destructive erosion of involved structures

postoperative complications, such as postoperative dehiscence, pneumonia, and acute kidney injury.

Management

Perforated peptic ulcer, especially with associated sepsis, is a medical/surgical emergency requiring rapid management [26]. All patients with perforated peptic ulcer require, at a minimum, prompt surgical consultation, volume resuscitation, antibiotics, proton pump inhibitor, and nasogastric decompression. Furthermore, many patients will benefit from intensive care monitoring. Goals for initial resuscitation include mean arterial pressure (MAP) >/− 65 mmHg, urine output >/− 0.5 mL/kg/h, and lactate normalization. Operative intervention should *not* be delayed for ongoing resuscitation.

Trial of Nonoperative Therapy

A significant number of ulcers are observed to seal spontaneously at the time of exploration, and therefore, in highly selected individuals, a trial of nonoperative management may be acceptable. Appropriate candidates for a trial of nonoperative management are those who are younger and those with relatively minor symptoms. Older (>70 years of age), immunocompromised, or obese patients are more likely to fail nonoperative management [27]. Volume of intraperitoneal air and fluid may be another marker for failure [28, 29]. Contained retroperitoneal perforations that lack signs of free intraperitoneal rupture and peritonitis may also be appropriate for this approach. If initial imaging is performed without enteral contrast, repeat imaging with contrast may be reassuring in these patients.

Our practice is to continue nasogastric tube decompression for at least 24–48 h. High-quality repeat imaging with upper gastrointestinal contrast that distends the upper GI tract and confirms ulcer seal should be considered prior to tube removal and diet advancement. Patients should also be placed on PPI therapy.

ICU level monitoring and treatment according to Surviving Sepsis Campaign is warranted in many patients, regardless of initial approach [30–32]. Patients with perforated peptic ulcers will require significant volume resuscitation and treatment of associated electrolyte and renal abnormalities. Persistent tachycardia and supraventricular arrythmias may be a sign of uncontrolled leak.

Adequate source control via surgical intervention or drainage, along with antimicrobial therapy, is critical in the management of PPU. Broad-spectrum antibiotics should be initiated to treat gram-negative, gram-positive, and anaerobic bacteria. Consideration of antifungal treatment should be given to patients who are immunocompromised. De-escalation or modification of the empiric antimicrobial treatment should be completed to avoid microbial resistance and should be based on hospital antibiograms [33]. Duration of antibiotics is not well defined in this patient population.

Failure of nonoperative management, with conversion to operative treatment, must be clearly defined, as delay to operative treatment is associated with increased mortality. Recognizing and accepting a failure is paramount. Ongoing or worsening symptoms, sepsis, or radiologic evidence should prompt exploration.

Operative Management

Patients who are not candidates for a trial of nonoperative therapy or those who fail should promptly undergo surgical management. This should not be delayed for further resuscitation. Studies have shown that the time from perforation to operative intervention is independently associated with increased mortality, as much as 6% increased risk of death per hour delay in surgery [34, 35]. Patients should have adequate IV access, and consideration should be given for central IV access, arterial access, and bladder decompression. Specific operative management is highly dependent on ulcer location, size of the defect, tissue quality, and local conditions. In addition to source control, consideration may be given to feeding gastrostomy, jejunostomy, or even nasojejunal feeding tube that can be placed and confirmed intraoperatively. Acid-reducing/drainage operations have nearly been abandoned in the acute setting due to high morbidity and mortality. Rare exceptions may be considered for patients with known absolute inability to tolerate PPI, inability to cease NSAIDs, nonsmokers, or those with negative *H. pylori.*

Perforated Duodenal Ulcers

The duodenal bulb is the most common location. This is followed by the pyloric channel. Rarely perforations may occur in the third or fourth portions of the duodenum. Smaller ulcers, less than 2 cm, are generally managed with a combination of closure with omental or falciform ligament patching. Intraoperative leak test can be considered. Drainage tubes remain controversial. Our practice is generally to leave drains in all but the smallest repairs, as postoperative access in the case of leak can be challenging. However, they do not prevent infections. Conflicting data exists on use of drains and is surgeon specific and dependent on local conditions and comfort with surgical repair [36].

A rare phenomenon associated with perforated duodenal ulcers is a synchronous posterior "kissing" duodenal ulcer with hemorrhage. Treatment of these includes repair of ulcer, with either ligation of gastroduodenal artery (GDA) or embolization as adjuncts [37].

Large duodenal perforations remain challenging to manage, and there is no clear best practice. Options include attempt at repair with omental patch or serosal patch. However, frequently, more extensive procedures are required due to the large nature of the perforation, location in relation to the ampulla, and local tissue conditions. Pyloric exclusion with loop gastrojejunostomy is one option for the high-risk perforation. Other less common options include jejunal serosal patch, Roux en-Y duodenojejunostomy, and retrograde duodenostomy. In these challenging cases, wide drainage with Malecot catheters placed into defects and closed suction drains are imperative, as postoperative leak is common and morbid. Though not without its own risks, percutaneous biliary drainage of the duodenum is sometimes a useful adjunct for postoperative leaks that cannot be treated with reoperation.

Illustration

Perforated Gastric Ulcers

In contrast to duodenal ulcers, gastric ulcers carry significantly higher risk of underlying malignancy. Typically, these are an adenocarcinoma, but occasionally are gastrointestinal stromal tumors (GISTs) or mucosa-associated lymphoid tissue (MALT) [38]. Therefore, tissue biopsy at the time of operation is appropriate when feasible, based on local conditions. If not, follow-up endoscopic assessment within 8 weeks is prudent. Occasionally, preoperative imaging may suggest underlying mass or metastases, but a definitive radiologic diagnosis is frequently obscured by inflammatory changes.

Ulcers of the greater curve can be treated with similar methods of closure with patching, as described above. Stapled resection is also appropriate. Ulcers located on the lesser curve are more challenging to treat due to the left gastric artery distally and proximity to the gastroesophageal junction proximally. Distal ulcers that are not amenable to simple repair may require distal gastrectomy or antrectomy.

Though marginal ulceration is a far more common complication after Roux-en-Y gastric bypass (RYGB), perforations of peptic ulcers may present in the remnant stomach. The remnant stomach, in theory, is a low pressure/low volume viscus, diverted of upper GI secretions. These may be treated appropriately with gastrostomy tube placement by CT guidance. Imaging must delineate a gastric remnant perforation from a gastric pouch perforation. Additionally, one must consider the possibility of gastro-gastric fistula.

Damage Control Surgery

In critically ill patients, source control is the primary goal. PPU may progress to septic shock with progressive organ dysfunction, hypothermia, hypotension, coagulopathy, and acidosis. Thus, in this patient population, a staged approach to surgical treatment may be warranted with temporary abdominal closure and aggressive resuscitation in the intensive care setting. However, committing a patient to an open abdomen is not without risk for complications such as enteroatmospheric fistula. Once the patient is appropriately resuscitated and hemodynamically stable (usually over the next 24–48 h), the abdomen can be reexplored and closed.

Laparoscopic Surgery

Minimally invasive approaches are safe and appropriate to attempt with similar outcomes to open surgery when repair is straightforward [39]. Rate of conversion to open surgery is acceptable and associated with larger, more complex ulcers. When the preoperative diagnosis is uncertain, laparoscopy may be an appropriate first step if it can be performed in a timely fashion. Surgical judgment and experience will dictate the mode of surgical intervention.

Adjuncts to Nonoperative Management and Emerging Therapies

Given the high operative mortality, a number of procedures have been evaluated as adjuncts to nonoperative management. These include endoscopic drainage via NOTES approach or omental patching, as well as a variety of endoscopic suturing, clipping, and stenting [40]. Small series have shown some promise in selected patients, but should only be performed in the setting of clinical trial with appropriate consent [41]. Endoscopic techniques may be more useful for postoperative complications, such as stricture, or perhaps leak, especially those not amenable to reoperation.

Postoperative Management

Duration of NGT should be guided by local conditions at the time of exploration. While a conservative approach to PPU patients postoperatively is common, there are studies that suggest an enhanced recovery after surgery (ERAS) pathway is acceptable in the appropriate patient population (i.e., simple repair of PDU) [42].

In the setting of diffuse peritonitis or contamination, or in the setting of a tenuous repair, postoperative imaging may be reassuring prior to drain removal and diet advancement.

H. pylori Testing

In the setting of perforated peptic ulcer, *H. pylori* testing can be performed by tissue biopsy at the time of exploration, by fecal antigen, or by IgG blood levels. Breath test is generally not feasible in this acute setting. Fecal antigen will diagnose active infection, but post-surgical patients may suffer from ileus, preventing sampling. Positive IgG test will only indicate exposure, but will not delineate active from previous infection.

Drain Management

Drains should be placed at the discretion of the surgeon, based on local conditions and comfort with quality of repair or surgical approach [43]. However, there is no clear evidence to support the placement of drains. Our general approach is frequently to leave a drain near the site of the repair or anastomosis if there is any concern for postoperative leak. We perform postoperative contrast study and remove the drain when the patient tolerates oral intake without concerning change in drainage quality or character.

Repeat endoscopy to ensure healing and rule out underlying malignancy is appropriate, several weeks following surgery [44].

Conclusion

Peptic ulcer disease, and specifically PPU, remains a significant healthcare problem, which can consume considerable financial resources, regardless of whether operative or nonoperative management is utilized. Management may involve various subspecialties including surgeons, gastroenterologists, and radiologists. Successful management of patients with PPU involves prompt recognition, resuscitation when required, appropriate antibiotic therapy, and timely surgical and/or radiological treatment.

References

1. Søreide K, Thorsen K, Harrison EM, Bingener J, Møller MH, Ohene-Yeboah M, Søreide JA. Perforated peptic ulcer. Lancet. 2015;386:1288–98.
2. Lau JY, Sung J, Hill C, Henderson C, Howden CW, Metz DC. Systematic review of the epidemiology of complicated peptic ulcer disease: incidence, recurrence, risk factors and mortality. Digestion. 2011;84(2):102–13. https://doi.org/10.1159/000323958. Epub 2011 Apr 14.
3. Chung KT, Shelat VG. Perforated peptic ulcer—an update. World J Gastrointest Surg. 2017;9(1):1–12. https://doi.org/10.4240/wjgs.v9.i1.1.
4. Bas G, Eryilmaz R, Okan I, Sahin M. Risk factors of morbidity and mortality in patients with perforated peptic ulcer. Acta Chir Belg. 2008;108(4):424–7. https://doi.org/10.1080/00015458.2008.11680254.
5. Byrne BE, Bassett M, Rogers CA, Anderson ID, Beckingham I, Blazeby JM, Association of Upper Gastrointestinal Surgeons for the National Emergency Laparotomy Project Team. Short-term outcomes after emergency surgery for complicated peptic ulcer disease from the UK National Emergency Laparotomy Audit: a cohort study. BMJ Open. 2018;8(8):e023721. https://doi.org/10.1136/bmjopen-2018-023721.
6. Sonnenberg A, Everhart JE. Health impact of peptic ulcer in the United States. Am J Gastroenterol. 1997 Apr;92(4):614–20.
7. Bertleff MJ, Lange JF. Perforated peptic ulcer disease: a review of history and treatment. Dig Surg. 2010;27(3):161–9. https://doi.org/10.1159/000264653. Epub 2010 Jun 22.
8. Marshall BJ, Warren JR. Unidentified curved bacilli in the stomach of patients with gastritis and peptic ulceration. Lancet. 1984;1(8390):1311–5. https://doi.org/10.1016/s0140-6736(84)91816-6.
9. Gisbert JP, Khorrami S, Calvet X, Gabriel R, Carballo F, Pajares JM. Meta-analysis: proton pump inhibitors vs. H2-receptor antagonists—their efficacy with antibiotics in Helicobacter pylori eradication. Aliment Pharmacol Ther. 2003;18(8):757–66. https://doi.org/10.1046/j.1365-2036.2003.01766.x.
10. Lanas A, Chan FKL. Peptic ulcer disease. Lancet. 2017;390(10094):613–24. https://doi.org/10.1016/S0140-6736(16)32404-7. Epub 2017 Feb 25.
11. García Rodríguez LA, Jick H. Risk of upper gastrointestinal bleeding and perforation associated with individual non-steroidal anti-inflammatory drugs. Lancet. 1994;343(8900):769–72. https://doi.org/10.1016/s0140-6736(94)91843-0. Erratum in: Lancet 1994 Apr 23;343(8904):1048.
12. Yeo SH, Yang CH. Peptic ulcer disease associated with Helicobacter pylori infection. Korean J Gastroenterol. 2016;67(6):289–99. https://doi.org/10.4166/kjg.2016.67.6.289.
13. Windsor JA, Hill AG. The management of perforated duodenal ulcer. N Z Med J. 1995;108(994):47–8.
14. Cope Z, Silen W. Cope's Early diagnosis of the acute abdomen, twenty-first edition. Oxford University Press. 106–107. 2005.
15. Anbalakan K, Chua D, Pandya GJ, Shelat VG. Five year experience in management of perforated peptic ulcer and validation of common mortality risk prediction models - are existing models sufficient? A retrospective cohort study. Int J Surg. 2015;14:38–44. https://doi.org/10.1016/j.ijsu.2014.12.022. Epub 2015 Jan 2.
16. Thorsen K, Glomsaker TB, von Meer A, Soreide K, Soreide JA. Trends in diagnosis and surgical management of patients with perforated peptic ulcer. Gastrointest Surg. 2011;15:1329–35.
17. Grassi R, Romani S, Pinto A, Romano L. Gastroduodenal perforations: conventional plain film, US, and CT findings in 166 consecutive patients. Eur J Radiol. 2004;
18. Kim SH, Shin SS, Jeong YY, Heo SH, Kim JW, Kang HK. Gastrointestinal tract perforation: MDCT findings according to the perforation sites. Korean J Radiol. 2009;10(1):63–70. https://doi.org/10.3348/kjr.2009.10.1.63.
19. Tarasconi A, Coccolini F, Biffl WL, et al. Perforated and bleeding peptic ulcer: WSES guidelines. World J Emerg Surg. 2020;15:3. https://doi.org/10.1186/s13017-019-0283-9.
20. Malhotra AK, Fabian TC, Katsis SB, Gavant ML, Croce MA. Blunt bowel and mesenteric injuries: the role of screening computed tomography. J Trauma. 2000;48:991–1000.

21. Boey J, Choi S, Alagaratnam T, Poon A. Risk stratification in perforated duodenal ulcers. Ann Surg. 1987;
22. Møller MH, Engebjerg MC, Adamsen S, Bendix J, Thomsen RW. The P eptic U lcer P erforation (PULP) score: a predictor of mortality following peptic ulcer perforation. A cohort study. Acta Anaesthesiologica Scandinavica. 2012;56(5):655–62.
23. Thorsen K, Soreide JA, Soreide K. Scoring systems for outcome prediction in patients with perforated peptic ulcer. Scand J Trauma Resusc Emerg Med. 2013;21:25.
24. Tominaga, Gail T, Staudenmayer, KL, Shafi, S, Schuster, KM, Savage, SA, Ross, Steven, Muskat, Peter, Mowery, Nathan T, Miller, Preston, Inaba, Kenji, Cohen, Mitchell Jay, Ciesla, David, Brown, Carlos V.R., Agarwal, Suresh, Aboutanos, Michel B., Utter, Garth H., Crandall, Marie, American Association for the Surgery of Trauma Committee on Patient Assessment. The American Association for the Surgery of Trauma grading scale for 16 emergency general surgery conditions, J Trauma Acute Care Surg: 2016;81(3);593–602. doi: https://doi.org/10.1097/TA.0000000000001127.
25. Tan S, Wu G, Zhuang Q, Xi Q, Meng Q, Jiang Y, Han Y, Yu C, Yu Z, Li N. Laparoscopic versus open repair for perforated peptic ulcer: A meta analysis of randomized controlled trials. Int J Surg. 2016;33(Pt A):124–32. https://doi.org/10.1016/j.ijsu.2016.07.077. Epub 2016 Aug 5.
26. Ross JT, Matthay MA, Harris HW. Secondary peritonitis: principles of diagnosis and intervention. BMJ. 2018;361:k1407.
27. Crofts TJ, Park KG, Steele RJ, Chung SS, Li AK. A randomized trial of nonoperative treatment for perforated peptic ulcer. N Engl J Med. 1989;320:970–3.
28. Oriuchi N, Nakajima T, Mochiki E, Takeyoshi I, Kanuma T, Endo K, Sakamoto J. A new, accurate and conventional five-point method for quantitative evaluation of ascites using plain computed tomography in cancer patients. Jpn J Clin Oncol. 2005;35(7):386–90. https://doi.org/10.1093/jjco/hyi109. Epub 2005 Jun 23.
29. Ishiguro T, Kumagai Y, Baba H, et al. Predicting the amount of intraperitoneal fluid accumulation by computed tomography and its clinical use in patients with perforated peptic ulcer. Int Surg. 2014;99(6):824–9. https://doi.org/10.9738/INTSURG-D-14-00109.1.
30. Singer M, Deutschman CS, Seymour CW, Shankar-Hari M, Annane D, Bauer M, Bellomo R, Bernard GR, Chiche JD, Coopersmith CM, Hotchkiss RS, Levy MM, Marshall JC, Martin GS, Opal SM, Rubenfeld GD, van der Poll T, Vincent JL, Angus DC. The third international consensus definitions for sepsis and septic shock (Sepsis-3). JAMA. 2016;315:801–10.
31. Levy MM, Evans LE, Rhodes A. The surviving sepsis campaign bundle: 2018 update. Intensive Care Med. 2018;44:925–8. https://doi.org/10.1007/s00134-018-5085-0.
32. Dellinger RP, Levy MM, Rhodes A, et al. Surviving sepsis campaign: international guidelines for management of severe sepsis and septic shock, 2012. Intensive Care Med. 2013;39:165–228. https://doi.org/10.1007/s00134-012-2769-8.
33. Solomkin JS, Mazuski JE, Bradley JS, Rodvold KA, Goldstein EJ, Baron EJ, O'Neill PJ, Chow AW, Dellinger EP, Eachempati SR, Gorbach S, Hilfiker M, May AK, Nathens AB, Sawyer RG, Bartlett JG. Diagnosis and management of complicated intra-abdominal infection in adults and children: guidelines by the Surgical Infection Society and the Infectious Diseases Society of America. Clin Infect Dis. 2010;50:133–64.
34. Boyd-Carson H, Doleman B, Cromwell D, Lockwood S, Williams JP, Tierney GM, Lund JN, Anderson ID, National Emergency Laparotomy Audit Collaboration. Delay in source control in perforated peptic ulcer leads to 6% increased risk of death per hour: a Nationwide cohort study. World J Surg. 2020;44(3):869–75. https://doi.org/10.1007/s00268-019-05254-x.
35. Buck DL, Vester-Andersen M, Moller MH. Danish clinical register of emergency S. surgical delay is a critical determinant of survival in perforated peptic ulcer. Br J Surg. 2013;100:1045–9.
36. Schein M. To drain or not to drain? The role of drainage in the contaminated and infected abdomen: an international and personal perspective. World J Surg. 2008;32:312–21. https://doi.org/10.1007/s00268-007-9277-y.
37. Stabile BE, Hardy HJ, Passaro E. 'Kissing' duodenal ulcers. Arch Surg. 1979;114(10):1153–6. https://doi.org/10.1001/archsurg.1979.01370340059010.
38. Selinger CP, Cochrane R, Thanaraj S, Sainsbury A, Subramanian V, Everett S. Gastric ulcers: malignancy yield and risk stratification for follow-up endoscopy. Endosc Int Open. 2016;4(6):E709–14. https://doi.org/10.1055/s-0042-106959.
39. Cirocchi R, Soreide K, Di Saverio S, Rossi E, Arezzo A, Zago M, Abraha I, Vettoretto N, Chiarugi M. Meta-analysis of perioperative outcomes of acute laparoscopic versus open repair of perforated gastroduodenal ulcers. J Trauma Acute Care Surg. 2018;85(2):417–25. https://doi.org/10.1097/TA.0000000000001925.
40. Bingener J, Loomis EA, Gostout CJ, Zielinski MD, Buttar NS, Song LM, Baron TH, Ghahfarokhi LS, Rajan E. Feasibility of NOTES omental plug repair of perforated peptic ulcers: results from a clinical pilot trial. Surg Endosc. 2013;27(6):2201–8. https://doi.org/10.1007/s00464-012-2740-3. Epub 2013 Jan 26.
41. Malkov IS, Zaynutdinov AM, Veliyev NA, Tagirov MR, Merrell RC. Laparoscopic and endoscopic management of perforated duodenal ulcers. J Am Coll Surg. 2004;198(3):352–5. https://doi.org/10.1016/j.jamcollsurg.2003.10.015.
42. Mohsina S, Shanmugam D, Sureshkumar S, Kundra P, Mahalakshmy T, Kate V. Adapted ERAS pathway

vs. standard Care in Patients with perforated duodenal ulcer-a randomized controlled trial. J Gastrointest Surg. 2018;22(1):107–16. https://doi.org/10.1007/s11605-017-3474-2. Epub 2017 Jun 26.
43. Okumura K, Hida K, Kunisawa S, et al. Impact of drain insertion after perforated peptic ulcer repair in a Japanese nationwide database analysis. World J Surg. 2018;42:758–65. https://doi.org/10.1007/s00268-017-4211-4.
44. Yerxa J, Agarwal S. Current problems in surgery: surgical management of peptic ulcer disease, vol. 57; 2020. p. 2.

Acute Pancreatitis: Nonoperative and Operative Management

20

Isaac W. Howley and Martin A. Croce

Case Presentation

A 41-year-old man was transferred to the tertiary center intensive care unit for management of acute necrotizing pancreatitis and two recent bouts of hematemesis. He had suffered multiple bouts of acute pancreatitis over the past 2 years, secondary to hypertriglyceridemia which was only partially controlled by fenofibrate. Upper endoscopy revealed old blood products and a small ulcer in the posterior wall of the stomach. Contrast-enhanced CT scan demonstrated an enlarged hypoattenuating pancreas with extravasation of contrast from his gastroduodenal artery, which was coil embolized by interventional radiology. Two days later, he suffered a large bout of hematemesis with a cardiac arrest but was successfully resuscitated by CPR and massive transfusion. Once stabilized, he was taken for a repeat CT scan, demonstrating extravasation near the left gastric artery. In angiography immediately afterward no extravasation was seen, but the left gastric artery was empirically embolized.

He had another large-volume upper GI bleed 3 days later. He was taken to the operating room, where he underwent upper endoscopy, unfortunately limited by a large amount of clot in the stomach. As endoscopic and angiographic options had been exhausted; a laparotomy was performed. The anterior wall of the stomach was opened widely, blood was evacuated from the stomach, and the posterior wall was opened, incorporating a fistulous tract into the retroperitoneum. Blood and necrotic pancreas were evacuated from the retroperitoneum, but no active bleeding was found. The stomach was closed, and the patient returned to the intensive care unit. Three hours later, he developed a recurrent upper gastrointestinal hemorrhage and profound hypotension. A Zone 1 REBOA was placed, and the patient was immediately transferred back to the operating room, where his laparotomy was re-opened. There was active bleeding from the approximate location of the splenic artery, which was suture ligated. More bleeding was coming from the area of the gastroduodenal artery, and the previous embolization coils were visualized from within the pancreatic bed. Suture ligation failed to stop the bleeding. Vascular surgery was consulted and placed a stent graft in the com-

I. W. Howley (✉) · M. A. Croce
Department of Surgery, University of Tennessee Health Science Center, Memphis, TN, USA
e-mail: ihowley@uthsc.edu; mcroce@uthsc.edu

M. D. Zielinski, O. Guillamondegui (eds.), *The Acute Management of Surgical Disease*,
https://doi.org/10.1007/978-3-031-07881-1_20

mon hepatic artery, covering the origin of the gastroduodenal artery and arresting the hemorrhage. The patient's retroperitoneum and stomach were packed, and the abdomen was temporarily closed. He was re-explored on postoperative day 2, with closure of the stomach and abdomen. He was discharged home 3 weeks later and has not had additional bleeding episodes in 3 years of follow-up.

Workup

Patients with acute pancreatitis almost always present with severe epigastric pain radiating to the back. The pain may be localized to either side or may be in the midline and is typically associated with significant tenderness to palpation and guarding, although without the diffuse tenderness, rigidity, or rebound tenderness characteristic of peritonitis. Nausea and nonbilious emesis are frequent associated symptoms; less commonly, patients in whom pancreatitis has caused a localized gastric ileus may also have distention focused in the left upper quadrant. The date of onset of symptoms should be elicited and clearly recorded in the medical record; this may be difficult to discern in a patient who has been transferred to a tertiary center with altered mental status or under sedation, but is of crucial importance in understanding the maturation and evolution of pancreatic inflammatory processes, as will be discussed below.

All patients in whom pancreatitis is suspected should have a biochemical workup including a comprehensive metabolic panel, a complete blood count, amylase, and lipase. In patients with the correct historical and examination findings, lipase or amylase levels at least three times the upper limit of normal are diagnostic of acute pancreatitis. Transaminitis feature in some predictive scoring models for severe pancreatitis, as will be discussed below. However, the most crucial use of hepatic function tests is to rule out concurrent biliary pathology. Three to 5% of patients with gallstone pancreatitis may present with concurrent choledocholithiasis or even cholangitis [1, 2]; as with any other patient, true cholangitis is an emergent condition and requires prompt biliary drainage, typically endoscopic retrograde cholangiopancreatography (ERCP), for source control. Rarely, severe pancreatic edema may cause extrinsic compression of the common bile duct with direct hyperbilirubinemia and alkaline phosphatemia, which should be relieved by biliary stenting. A lactate level should be measured to assess end-organ perfusion. Any patient with signs of physiologic compromise (e.g., acute kidney injury (AKI), lactemia, unexplained hypoxia) should undergo a contrast-enhanced computed tomography scan (CECT) of the abdomen and pelvis contrast to assess for pancreatic necrosis. CECT may also reveal a pancreatic or periampullary tumor, although in the setting of acute pancreatic and peripancreatic edema, this is more often a vague suggestion than a clearly demarcated finding. Additionally, CECT may be useful in those patients with a suspicious history but normal laboratory values, especially if they have had pain for more than a few days, as amylase and lipase levels may have returned to normal before the patient presented to medical attention.

In addition to measuring the severity and assessing for complications of pancreatitis, the initial workup should attempt to determine the etiology of pancreatitis. A significant majority of acute pancreatitis is caused by alcohol abuse or by mechanical obstruction of the pancreatic duct by an impacted gallstone. The exact pathophysiologic mechanism of alcoholic pancreatitis remains unclear, but given the intractable nature of alcohol addiction, many of these patients suffer recurrent bouts of acute pancreatitis. Other, less common causes of pancreatitis include hyperlipidemia, medications, autoimmune disease, ERCP (pancreatitis is the most common complication, occurring 3.5% of the time [3]), pancreatic ductal obstruction by a pancreatic duct calculus or tumor, trauma, congenital abnormalities such as pancreas divisum, and the sting of the *Tityus trinitatis* scorpion native to Trinidad. A significant proportion of pancreatitis is idiopathic. Treatment for the precipitating factors does not lessen the severity or shorten the duration of a bout of pancreatitis, but the etiology should be determined whenever possible to prevent future occurrences.

Alcohol use, medication history, recent ERCP, prior cholecystectomy, and exposure to Trinidadian scorpion bites should be assessed by history. To discriminate between different etiologies, all patients presenting with a first episode of acute pancreatitis should have a right upper quadrant ultrasound to rule out cholelithiasis. Additionally, a serum triglyceride level should be sent, as hypertriglyceridemia is a treatable condition.

For patients presenting with recurrent pancreatitis known to be secondary to alcohol abuse, we forgo an involved workup if a patient presents with a subsequent bout of mild pancreatitis. However, in those patients who have recurrent pancreatitis without an obvious etiology, uncommon causes should be investigated—anatomic abnormalities such as pancreas divisum can be seen on magnetic resonance cholangiopancreatography (MRCP), or an elevated serum IgG4 level suggests autoimmune pancreatitis. Consultation with gastroenterology may be useful in determining the etiology if the common causes have been ruled out.

Severity Scoring: Schemata for Prognostication and Classification

After making the diagnosis of acute pancreatitis, the next factor the surgeon must determine is the severity of the pancreatitis episode—whether the patient is in for a painful but short-lived episode which will self-resolve within a few days or is on their way to multisystem organ dysfunction or failure, with or without pancreatic necrosis that may lead to any of a variety of intra-abdominal complications. Over the past several decades, several schemata have been developed to predict which patients are at elevated risk of death or a complicated hospital course. More recently, as the acute care surgery literature has grown, new classification systems have allowed patients' disease processes to be stratified, allowing similar patients to be identified for prospective research or treatment algorithms and allowing for meaningful comparisons in retrospective studies.

In 1974, Ranson et al. analyzed biochemical data from 300 patients at Bellevue Hospital and identified 9 factors (age, WBC, glucose, AST, and LDH at admission; hematocrit drop, BUN increase, calcium, PaO_2, base deficit, and fluid requirement at 48 h), which were associated with mortality or prolonged intensive care unit (ICU) stay [4]. The Glasgow criteria, published a decade later, simplified this to eight data points, with slightly different cutoff values (age, WBC, glucose, AST or ALT or LDH, BUN, calcium, PaO_2, albumin) (Table 20.1) [5, 6]. In the decades since then, multiple other scores have been used to predict the severity of acute pancreatitis, including general critical illness survival scores such as APACHE-II, as well as numerous pancreatitis-specific scores including the Japanese Severity Score (JSS) [7], Pancreatitis Outcome Prediction (POP) [8], Panc 3 [9], Bedside Index for Severity in Acute Pancreatitis (BISAP) [10], and the

Table 20.1 Ranson score for severity of alcoholic pancreatitis and Glasgow criteria for pancreatitis of any etiology. Increasing scores are associated with increased mortality and resource utilization

	Ranson	Glasgow
At admission	Age >55 years	
	WBC >16,000/μL	
	LDH >350 μ/L	
	AST >250 μ/L	
	Glucose >200 mg/dL	
48 hours from admission	Drop in hematocrit >10%	PaO_2 <60 mmHg
	BUN increase >5 mg/dL	Age >55
	Calcium <8 mg/dL	WBC >15,000/μL
	PaO_2 < 60 mmHg	Calcium <8 mg/dL
	Base deficit >4 mEq/L	BUN >45 mg/dL
	Fluid resuscitation >6 L	LDH >600 μ/L
		Albumin <3.2 g/dL
		Glucose >180 mg/dL

Harmless Acute Pancreatitis Score [11]. A head-to-comparison of these scoring systems, as well as APACHE-II and the SIRS criteria, found that no scoring system provided more than moderate accuracy at predicting organ failure >48 h, with the highest performing model being the JSS with AUCs of 0.84 and 0.74 in two different patient cohorts [12]. In our practice, we do not routinely calculate any of the available predictive scores, although when deciding whether to admit patients to a monitored setting, we do look closely at the early markers of organ failure which constitute the components of the various scores.

In addition to these biochemical- and physiologic-based indices, Balthazar et al. described the computed tomography severity index (CTSI, commonly referred to as the Balthazar score) in 1990 [13]. The CTSI assigns 0 to 4 points based on the extensiveness of edema and fluid collections and 0 to 6 points for increasing degrees or necrosis, for a total possible score of 10. This correlates closely with the Ranson score [14], and its chief contribution is not that it supersedes physiologic and biochemical criteria, but rather that it showed as early as 1990 that CECT can predict the clinical course of acute pancreatitis.

Given the plethora of possible complications from pancreatitis, as will be discussed in detail later in this chapter, discussion of the disease can quickly become impossible if different people use different words to describe different subsets of the disease process or, even worse, if people use the same words to describe different processes. To prevent this imprecision in the literature, a group of 40 physicians from 6 specialties and 15 countries gathered in Atlanta, Georgia, in 1992 to set common definitions for presentations of acute pancreatitis [15]. Equally importantly, they recommended abandonment of terms which they felt to be particularly ambiguous, including "phlegmon" and "hemorrhagic pancreatitis." The article's discussion benefitted from advances in the understanding of acute pancreatitis from CT imaging. Their clearly described set of definitions was widely adopted, allowing for much clearer clinical and especially research communication. However, the recommended changes to terminology were applied inconsistently, and additional clinical entities were reported that were not adequately captured by the terminology from the Atlanta classification system [16, 17]. Additionally, improvements in CT imaging technology and management strategies led to a greater understanding of the disease process.

An Internet-based, collaborative, iterative revision process was begun in 2012, involving 11 national and international pancreatic associations. The resulting revised Atlanta classification (RAC) schema was published in 2012 (Table 20.2) [18]. The RAC divides acute pancreatitis into two types, *interstitial edematous pancreatitis (IEP)* and *necrotizing pancreatitis (NP;* Figs. 20.1a and 20.1b, *respectively).* IEP is differentiated from NP on the basis of CECT findings; the edematous but perfused pancreatic tissue in IEP appears similar in color to splenic tissue, while NP shows significant hypoattenuation of the pancreatic parenchyma or peripancreatic tissues. The RAC defines three levels of severity, with *severe* defined as persistent single- or multiple-organ failure (a modified Marshall score of ≥2 for >48 h) [19], *moderately severe* defined as transient organ failure (<48 h) and/or local or systemic complications (e.g., an exacerbation of a chronic lung illness or a non-ST elevation myocardial infarction), and *mild* defined as lacking in organ failure or other complications. For IEP, the RAC defines two additional morphologic features – *acute peripancreatic fluid collections* (occurring with the 4 weeks of symptom onset, with homogeneous fluid density and no definite encapsulating wall), which either resolve or turn into *pseudocysts* (typically more than 4 weeks after symptom onset, with homogeneous fluid density and a clear capsule). For NP, they defined two analogous morphologic entities, *acute necrotic collections* (intra- and/or extra-pancreatic, with heterogeneous density but no encapsulating wall) which typically mature into *walled-off necrosis*, a process that typically takes at least 4 weeks from symptom onset.

In 2012–2013, the American Association for the Surgery of Trauma (AAST) Patient Assessment Committee created uniform grading systems for the severity of emergency general

Table 20.2 Morphologic features of acute pancreatitis based on the revised Atlanta criteria [18]

Morphologic feature	CECT appearance	Morphologic feature	CECT appearance
Interstitial edematous pancreatitis	Acute edema and stranding of the pancreatic parenchyma and surrounding tissues, with homogeneous enhancement of parenchyma by IV contrast	Necrotizing pancreatitis	Inflammation associated with pancreatic parenchymal or peripancreatic necrosis, with areas of lack of enhancement
Acute pancreatic fluid collection	Seen within first 4 weeks of onset; peripancreatic fluid without associated peripancreatic necrosis. Homogeneous fluid, confined by normal tissue planes, without intrapancreatic extension or definable encapsulating wall	Acute necrotic collection	Usually seen within first 4 weeks of onset; fluid collection(s) with variable amounts of solid and liquid contents, associated with pancreatic parenchymal or pancreatic necrosis. No encapsulating wall
Pancreatic pseudocyst	Usually seen at least 4 weeks from onset; well-circumscribed, usually regular oval- or spherical-shaped homogeneous fluid collection without solid components but with a defined, completely encapsulating wall	Walled-off necrosis	Usually seen at least 4 weeks from onset; heterogeneous, liquid, and solid density collection associated with necrosis, completely encapsulated by a well-defined wall

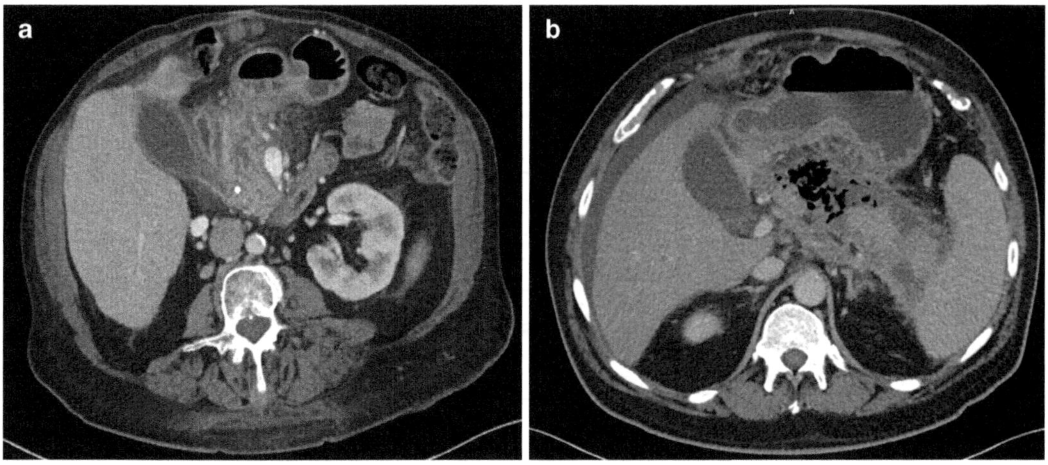

Fig. 20.1 (**a**) Computed tomography image of interstitial edematous pancreatitis. A biliary stent is in place in the common bile duct traversing the edematous head of the pancreas. (**b**) Computed tomography image of necrotizing pancreatitis. Air is noted within the necrotic pancreas

surgery (EGS) conditions, including acute pancreatitis. These are intended not as clinical tools, like for the Ranson score and the Glasgow criteria, nor as communication standards like the RAC, but rather as research and quality improvement tools analogous to the AAST's Organ Injury Scales (OIS) from the field of traumatology. Like the OIS, the EGS scores were intended to be graded on a five-point ordinal scale. For each EGS disease process, grades I and II are confined to the organ with either minimal or severe abnormality, grade III has local extension, grade IV has regional extension, and grade V has widespread or systemic extension of the disease process [20]. The definitions of the five grades for 16 EGS diseases, including acute pancreatitis, were subsequently described in 2016 (Table 20.3) [21]. The AAST EGS score correlates closely with the Ranson score, the modified Glasgow criteria, and the BISAP score and has similar to slightly better receiver operating characteristics [22].

($p < 0.0001$) of patients reported colicky pain during the interval. In a large database analysis, deferred cholecystectomy is associated with an odds ratio of 2.27 for readmission [29]. In our practice at an urban safety-net hospital, our patients are frequently lost to follow-up; same-admission cholecystectomy ensures that they receive appropriate care.

Medical Management of Moderate and Severe Pancreatitis

The medical management of moderate and severe pancreatitis differs quantitatively, rather than qualitatively, from that of mild pancreatitis. By definition, these patients have local complications and/or at least transient organ failure, so they generally require consideration of procedures to manage the local complications or critical care evaluation and support for organ failure. As with any other disease process, patients with signs of organ failure at the time of initial evaluation should be admitted to an intensive care unit; the difference between transient (moderate pancreatitis) and persistent (severe pancreatitis) organ failure may only become evident after 48 hours, but appropriate monitoring and standard goal-directed resuscitation will help avoid persistent organ failure.

Nutrition management, like for mild pancreatitis, should emphasize enteral nutrition. Traditional teaching has emphasized avoiding oral alimentation for fear that this will encourage additional pancreatic enzyme secretion. Even for necrotizing pancreatitis, however, enteral nutrition is associated with two- to fourfold lower incidences of morbidity (infected necrosis, multi-organ failure, need for surgical debridement) and mortality than the use of total parenteral nutrition [30, 31]. Specialty guidelines recommend oral nutrition to be started within 72 h of admission, with all possible attempts made to keep the patient on oral or enteral alimentation [32]. Severe inflammation of the pancreas and lesser sac frequently causes a regional ileus of the stomach and duodenum; in these patients, enteral nutrition should be delivered through a nasoduodenal or nasojejunal feeding tube, positioned to administer the feeds distal to the Ampulla of Vater. This may require endoscopic placement, but is still preferable to parenteral nutrition. Even for patients with stable, low-level vasopressor requirements—relatively common in patients with severe pancreatitis—enteral nutrition should be cautiously provided, monitoring for signs of feeding intolerance or mesenteric ischemia [33]. Pancreatic exocrine insufficiency is common, and pancreatic enzyme supplementation should be administered to patients with significant diarrhea or steatorrhea.

Many patients with pancreatitis will have received CT scans of the abdomen and pelvis at the discretion of emergency department staff prior to surgical consultation. While cross-sectional imaging is unnecessary for most patients with mild pancreatitis, those patients with leukocytosis, lactemia, or organ dysfunction should undergo CECT. The use of IV contrast is necessary to differentiate between necrotizing and interstitial edematous pancreatitis. In either situation, the acute management of peripancreatic fluid collections should be expectant. Fluid collections in interstitial edematous pancreatitis frequently resolve without management. While collections are less likely to resolve in necrotizing pancreatitis, early intervention has been strongly associated with increased mortality (75% within 14 days of admission, 45% from 15 to 29 days of admission, and 8% at 30+ days) [34]. This delay allows a rind to form around the collection and is associated with lower mortality even in the setting of infected necrosis or persistent organ failure. Patients with signs of infection should undergo repeat CT scans as they are at risk for pancreatic and peripancreatic infections. In the absence of clinical changes, frequent serial CECTs should be avoided during this period as they are unlikely to change management. Rarely, patients with significant pancreatic necrosis on imaging may remain clinically well; they may be discharged home with close follow-up and appropriate discharge instructions to seek medical attention with any sign of complications, e.g., fevers or significant emesis.

The main clinical significance of necrosis is the possibility that it will become secondarily infected, requiring drainage through any of several modalities. Infected necrosis has been the subject of a large amount of research and changes in clinical practice over the past decade. Until the early 2000s, guidelines for the management of necrotizing pancreatitis recommended prophylactic IV antibiotic administration in an attempt to prevent secondary infection [35–37]. More recent and more methodologically sound research has consistently reported an absence of benefit [38–40], and such use is no longer recommended [32, 41], especially since prophylactic use may select for antibiotic resistance when infection does occur. Nonetheless, this remains a common practice among American gastroenterologists and primary care physicians [42], and the consulting surgeon should recommend the cessation of prophylactic antibiotics.

Determining whether pancreatic necrosis is infected requires clinical judgment. As with any other infection, the gold standard to determine if an acute necrotic collection or walled-off necrosis is infected is to obtain a tissue culture, either via percutaneous or endoscopic fine needle aspiration (FNA), with or without placement of a percutaneous drain. Unfortunately, if a collection is not already infected, aspiration or drainage brings a theoretical risk of introducing bacteria into a ready substrate for infection, thus creating the infection that it was meant to diagnose. Short of a tissue culture, the next best way to diagnose infection is by CT appearance. The one and only pathognomonic feature of infected pancreatic necrosis is gas within the collection. Since even sterile pancreatitis is an intense inflammatory process, all mature walled-off collections—pseudocysts or walled-off necrosis—will form a contrast-enhancing rind such as is otherwise seen around an intra-abdominal abscess. Regardless of the radiologist's interpretation, these collections should not be considered infected unless there are locules of gas within them.

Assessment and Management of Infected Pancreatic Necrosis

Since instrumentation of a necrotic collection brings a risk of introducing infection, it should be reserved for situations with high pre-test probability of finding infection. This often requires significant restraint on the part of the surgeon, as other physicians involved in a patient's care may exert significant pressure to sample or drain collections that may not be infected. Patients with severe pancreatitis are often critically ill for weeks and are at risk of all the usual infections among the critically ill, including urinary tract infections, pneumonia, central line-associated bloodstream infections, and septic thrombophlebitis. The patient with signs of infection—most frequently fever and worsening leukocytosis—should undergo a standard infectious workup, including two sets of peripheral blood cultures, urinalysis and urine culture, and chest X-ray with or without bronchoalveolar lavage as indicated. A CECT of the abdomen and pelvis should be obtained; new locules of gas appearing within pancreatic necrosis make the diagnosis of infected necrosis. In the absence of gas, pancreatic necrosis should only be cultured in the setting of persistent or recurrent bacteremia without an obvious alternative source.

While sterile asymptomatic pancreatic necrosis should be cautiously ignored, infected pancreatic necrosis frequently requires management via invasive procedure. For most of the twentieth century, the only viable option for managing infected necrosis was open necrosectomy, a highly invasive operation with complication rates reported as 30–95% and mortality rates of 11–39% [43–50]. In the current era, there are four potential modalities through which drainage of pancreatic necrosis may be performed—in order of increasing invasiveness: percutaneous drainage, endoscopic debridement, video-assisted retroperitoneal drainage surgery (VARDS), and open pancreatic necrosectomy via laparotomy. As with most therapeutic options in emergency general surgery, the least invasive appropriate option should generally be attempted first, but ultimately the patient's physiology and anatomy dictate the optimal course of therapy.

This philosophical guidance is encapsulated in the step-up approach to pancreatitis, as described in the landmark PANTER study by van Santvoort et al. in 2010 [51]. Eighty-eight patients with acute pancreatitis, either pancreatic or peripancreatic necrosis, and evidence or strong suspicion of infection were randomized to either open necrosectomy or a step-up approach. All surgical interventions were delayed for at least a month following hospital admission when possible. The step-up approach consisted of either percutaneous (41/43 patients) or endoscopic transgastric drainage (2/43 patients); these patients were observed for 72 h following drainage. If there was no improvement, additional drainage was performed, via repeat percutaneous or endoscopic methods if possible (19 patients, 44%), or else via surgical necrosectomy (26 patients, 60%), either VARDS (24 patients) or via laparotomy (2 patients without appropriate retroperitoneal access). Neither mortality (19% step-up, 16% primary necrosectomy) nor duration of stay (50 vs. 60 day median) differed between groups, but the step-up group had significantly lower rates of new-onset organ failure (5% vs. 19%), incisional hernia (3% vs. 11%), new-onset diabetes (7% vs. 17%), pancreatic exocrine insufficiency (3% vs. 15%), and new ICU admissions (7% vs. 18%).

While percutaneous and, to a lesser extent, endoscopic drainage had already been reported by numerous publications, the PANTER trial firmly established their role as the first procedure for source control in infected pancreatic necrosis. While percutaneous drainage is performed by an interventional radiologist, the surgeon should be involved in the planning. As will be discussed below, an appropriately placed percutaneous drain is an important guide during VARDS should such an operation become necessary, allowing the surgeon to find the main area of necrosis while avoiding the other retroperitoneal structures of the left upper quadrant. The surgeon should review the patient's CT with the interventional radiologist prior to drainage, with all efforts made to identify a horizontal percutaneous window via the left retroperitoneum.

Endoscopic drainage and debridement appear to have significant advantages over surgical drainage. The major downsides of the procedure are the relatively uncommon skillset required—endoscopic ultrasound and advanced endoscopy are not available at many hospitals. Even if appropriately skilled endoscopists are available, the necrotic collection must be in close proximity to the stomach to allow for endoscopic access. Given these specifications, the scientific literature on endoscopic debridement consists of even smaller studies than that for surgical debridement. If the procedure can be performed, it appears to cause a much smaller inflammatory response than open surgery, with a concomitant decrease in multi-system organ failure [52]. Additionally, since the necrotic collection is accessed from within the GI tract, persistent drainage of pancreatic fluid is essentially physiologic and does not create pancreatic fistulae as can minimally invasive or open surgical debridement. The desirability of allowing necrotic collections to mature for at least a month—in other words, to become walled-off necrosis by the RAC definition—is even higher for endoscopic debridement than for surgical debridement. One of the authors has managed a patient who had undergone attempted endoscopic debridement before the necrotic collection had matured; the insufflation spread infected pancreatic necrosis and gastrointestinal flora throughout the peritoneal cavity, leading to recurrent and ultimately fatal intra-abdominal abscesses.

Technique for Video-Assisted Retroperitoneal Debridement Surgery (VARDS)

VARDS is indicated if the patient remains clinically sick despite appropriate placement of a percutaneous drain. The procedure works best for walled-off necrosis within the normal location of the pancreas; it is difficult to debride much inferiorly along the left paracolic gutter and nearly impossible to do so along the right paracolic gutter. Additionally, a percutaneous drain should be placed via the left flank prior to VARDS.

We position the patient supine with a bump under the left flank and the percutaneous drain prepped into the field. A 5 cm horizontal incision is made below the costal margin at the posterior axillary line. The drain site may be included in the incision, or else the drain should be identified in its subcutaneous course at the level of the abdominal wall. Using electrocautery, dissection is carried out through the oblique muscles of the abdominal wall and into the retroperitoneal space, taking care to follow the percutaneous drain into the walled-off necrosis. Often some portion of the necrotic pancreas can be removed blindly with gentle sweeps of a Yankauer suction device, creating a working space within the cavity. As the cavity is too deep to allow direct visualization and too small to permit the angulation necessary for coordinated minimally invasive techniques, a right-angled thoracoscope connected to a laparoscopic tower allows for both visualization and a working channel through which an atraumatic grasper can be used for debridement. An empty sponge-stick holder or a Yankauer suction tip can also be inserted into the cavity alongside the thoracoscope, allowing debridement much like as for a video-assisted thoracoscopic (VATS) decortication. The cavity should be repeatedly lavaged with saline, improving visualization and removing liquid components of the necrosis.

The most dangerous complication of VARDS is bleeding, particularly from the splenic artery or vein. This risk can be minimized through prudent technique. Any tissue which seems still attached to the cavity should be left in place; tearing intact, hyperemic tissue quickly leads to nuisance bleeding that impedes visualization. Much worse, intact tissue which is forcibly torn from the walls of the cavity may be adherent to the wall of a named vessel, bringing the potential for catastrophic bleeding deep within a cavity with limited visualization. Even major venous bleeding can typically be controlled with packing. For major arterial bleeding, open surgical control via laparotomy is both time-consuming and likely to be unsuccessful, as the friable edges of the splenic artery within an area of walled-off necrosis cannot be durably repaired using vascular techniques. Even suture ligation of the splenic artery or a dorsal pancreatic branch may fail when bathed in pancreatic fluid. Most arterial bleeding, however, can be temporized with aggressive packing, allowing time for the patient to undergo angiographic embolization. For this reason, it is prudent to communicate with interventional radiology or vascular surgery prior to beginning the procedure, to make sure that angiographic interventions can be readily performed.

As long as catastrophic bleeding does not interrupt the operation, debridement should continue until no more tissue can safely be removed. At this point, a large Axiom or Abramson drain should be inserted into the cavity. We prefer Abramson drains, as they are made of relatively soft material and thus may be less likely to erode into nearby bowel or blood vessels. Depending on the size and geometry of the now-debrided cavity, one or two drains should be placed, with the fascia closed around them if possible and the skin reapproximated. Both types of drains have irrigation channels as well as a suction channel; irrigation through each drain with 50 mL per hour of normal saline for a few days, with suction applied to the main channel at 80–100 mmHg, may help clean up residual pus and bacteria. Depending on the character of the drain output, an attempt should be made to remove Abramson or Axiom drains within a week to avoid erosion into vital structures. If significant drainage continues, interventional radiology can be consulted to replace the drains with softer pigtail catheters via the Seldinger technique with fluoroscopic guidance, reducing the chance of erosion and gastrointestinal fistula.

Technique for Open Necrosectomy

While nonoperative management and minimally invasive procedures have reduced the need for open necrosectomy in the modern era, there continue to be patients whose infected necrosis is not anatomically amenable to these therapies or for whom these therapies prove inadequate. Open necrosectomy continues to be a crucial technique for source control and shows no sign of obsolescence. While technically more simple than other drainage procedures, knowing when to perform open necrosectomy requires significant clinical judgment. And since there is significant postoperative mortality from the procedure, yet more clinical judgment, surgical critical care expertise, and clinical resources are needed to shepherd patients through the perioperative period. For these reasons, open necrosectomy is likely best performed at tertiary centers that can provide these resources.

Patients who require open necrosectomy have intense acute inflammatory responses and large areas of necrosis, frequently extending into areas of the retroperitoneum that are inaccessible to other drainage techniques, such as the paracolic gutters. Normal anatomy is nearly always distorted, and anatomic structures such as blood vessels and bowel wall may be both friable and impossible to differentiate from the thickened rind of the necrotic collection by normal techniques of visualization and palpation. For these reasons, a recent CECT should be reviewed before proceeding to the operating room, with special attention paid to which areas require debridement and where these lie in relation to important structures such as the colon, porta hepatis, gastroduodenal artery, and splenic artery.

The inflammatory rind of pancreatic necrosis collections typically adheres densely to the posterior wall of the stomach, obliterating the lesser sac. In trauma and surgical oncology, the body and tail of the pancreas are typically accessed by dividing the gastrocolic ligament; this may not be possible for pancreatic necrosectomy. Similarly, medial visceral rotation of the spleen and pancreatic tail cannot typically be accomplished as the avascular plane behind the spleen has been obliterated; should this maneuver be attempted and the splenic artery be avulsed, it may be impossible to gain control of the vessel. When the lesser sac cannot be used for access, there are two safe alternative routes to the pancreas in the setting of infected necrosis. The first is via the gastrohepatic ligament, taking care to avoid the left gastric artery and any replaced or accessory left hepatic arteries seen on preoperative CT imaging. The alternative route, giving better access into the inferior reaches of the retroperitoneum, is transgastric. An anterior gastrotomy is created using electrocautery for approximately 8 cm. A posterior gastrotomy is then created with electrocautery, dividing both the wall of the stomach and the adherent anterior wall of the necrotic collection. To provide hemostasis and prevent the collection from becoming walled off from the stomach again, we run a continuous 3-0 polydioxanone (PDS) suture around the posterior gastrotomy (Fig. 20.2).

Regardless of which route is used into the necrotic collection, we find that the operation is best performed with the assistance of a Bookwalter self-retaining retractor. Heavy body wall and Richardson retractors are used to keep open a generous upper midline or full laparotomy incision. Malleable retractors are placed into the necrotic collection, either retracting the lesser curve of the stomach caudally in the case of gastrohepatic ligament access or else holding apart the anterior gastrotomy in the case of transgastric access.

Debridement follows the same principles as discussed above for VARDS. Cultures should always be sent; these are typically polymicrobial infections, but cultures will allow for targeted antimicrobial treatment of fungal and antibiotic-resistant bacterial flora. Suction should be used where possible. For debridement of more solid necrosis, an empty sponge stick holder is used to gently remove only those tissues that readily give way. Aggressive debridement of firmly adherent tissues is likely to cause significant oozing from still-viable hyperemic tissue and may lead to disastrous arterial injuries. Should a named artery be injured, it is neither possible nor advisable to attempt vascular repair, as the suture line is unlikely to survive being bathed in infected fluid full of pancreatic enzymes. If possible, major arterial bleeding can be staunched via ligation using large figure-of-eight sutures; if this is not possible, the cavity should be tightly packed and the patient taken emergently for angiographic embolization.

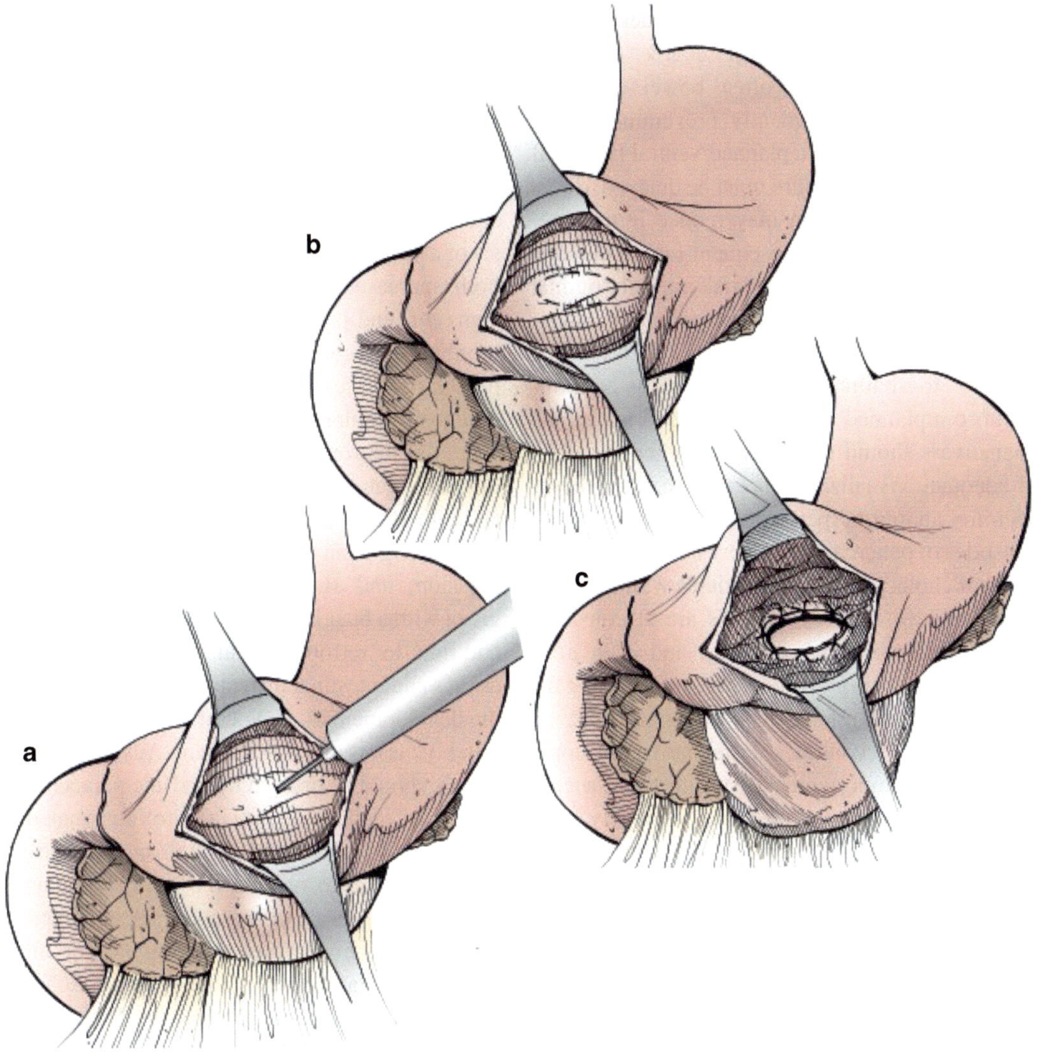

Fig. 20.2 Technique for cystgastrostomy (**a**) After performing an anterior gastrotomy, the necrotic collection is identified by palpation and its location is confirmed by aspiration. (**b**) An elliptical area of the posterior gastric wall, directly overlying the necrotic collection, is excised with electrocautery. (**c**) The edges of the cystgastrotomy are sutured for hemostasis and to prevent premature closure [58]

Drains should be left in the necrotic collection. When the necrosis has been debrided by the transgastric route, drainage may be performed directly into the GI tract, with one nasogastric tube directed through the posterior gastrotomy into the necrotic collection and another nasogastric tube left in the stomach or passed slightly beyond the pylorus. In the case of transperitoneal access, Axiom or Abramson drains should be left in the cavity, which may be used for irrigation in addition to suction as described above. We make every attempt to avoid unnecessary contact between these drains and the GI tract; they can be directed through the abdominal wall in the bilateral upper quadrants, coming in contact only with the well-vascularized and relatively erosion-resistant wall of the lesser curve of the stomach.

Necrosectomy often benefits from repeat laparotomy. In the case of significant bleeding requiring packing with or without embolization, this is mandatory. Even if hemorrhage is not a concern, a second look may allow for further demarcation of necrosis and additional debridement. These patients often have a large degree of intra-abdominal edema and often bowel dilatation from dysmotility, frequently preventing fascial closure and requiring a planned ventral hernia. If abdominal fascial closure must be delayed, direct peritoneal resuscitation may reduce intraperitoneal edema, facilitate subsequent fascial closure, and minimize the associated risk intra-abdominal complications such as abscess and enterocutaneous fistula [53, 54].

Prior to abdominal wall closure or commitment to a planned ventral hernia, two additional maneuvers should be performed when possible. If adequate visualization is possible, a cholecystectomy should be performed to prevent further episodes of pancreatic duct obstruction and future risks of cholecystitis. Even patients with different etiologies for their pancreatitis are at considerable risk for biliary pathology, and even after complete recovery from pancreatitis, the gallbladder will be relatively inaccessible by even open surgical techniques, let alone laparoscopy. Even more importantly, distal feeding access should always be obtained. If a relatively mild postoperative course is anticipated, this may be accomplished by guided placement of a nasojejunal tube. For most patients requiring open necrosectomy, a surgical jejunostomy tube at some distance from the pancreas is the safest and most durable option.

Other Local Complications of Pancreatitis

In addition to infected collections, necrotizing pancreatitis and severe interstitial edematous pancreatitis cause a variety of intra-abdominal complications. In our experience, these account for a significant portion of the abdominal surgery that severe pancreatitis patients require. Even in the PANTER trial of van Sanvoort et al., a third of excluded patients met exclusion criteria for prior laparotomies or acute complications requiring laparotomy [51]. Should any of the complications below occur, consideration should be given to performing open necrosectomy, cholecystectomy, and distal feeding access at the same time, as subsequent safe surgical access may become impossible.

Abdominal compartment syndrome (ACS) may occur, typically within the first few days of an episode of acute pancreatitis, as a side effect of massive fluid resuscitation. While intra-abdominal hypertension is common, the diagnosis of abdominal compartment syndrome requires both increased intra-abdominal pressures and signs of end-organ malperfusion, most commonly oliguria and acute kidney injury. Elevated peak airway pressures are a clue to ACS, but its diagnosis requires measurement of bladder pressure after neuromuscular blockade. In the setting of end-organ malperfusion attributed to intra-abdominal hypertension, a bladder pressure ≥25 mmHg is an absolute indication for decompression, and strong consideration should be given with a bladder pressure of 20–24 mmHg. In addition to retroperitoneal and bowel edema, ascites and intestinal distention may play a role in the development of ACS, both of which are most reliably assessed by CT scan. Any significant ascites should be drained by bedside paracentesis with ultrasound guidance. Gastrointestinal distention may be relieved enough by nasogastric decompression to obviate the need for laparotomy. In the absence of these factors, decompressive laparotomy with temporary abdominal closure with a Barker ("poor man's VAC") or AbThera dressing (3M, Maplewood, MN) is indicated. If significant resuscitation continues following decompression, bladder pressures should be rechecked every 4 or 6 h. While uncommon, abdominal compartment syndrome may recur with a temporary abdominal closure device in place; in this case, the temporary closure dressing should be replaced either as a sterile procedure in the ICU or else in the operating room.

The local inflammation surrounding the pancreas may cause thrombosis in arteries or veins. Venous thrombosis may occur in the portal vein, superior mesenteric vein, or splenic vein and is typically detected as an incidental finding in a CECT. Complete obstruction of venous outflow from the small intestine causes fatal mesenteric venous ischemia. For this reason, patients with proximal mesenteric venous thrombosis should be treated with full anticoagulation. Given the risks of hemorrhage or other acute complications requiring emergent invasive procedures, heparin infusion is the safest method of anticoagulation until the patient has reached the convalescent stage of illness and preparations are being made for discharge, at which point they can be transitioned to enoxaparin or warfarin. We typically avoid the use of direct oral anticoagulants, due to difficulty in reversing their effect should the patient require further invasive procedures.

Arterial thrombosis typically presents in a more dramatic fashion. The middle colic artery is the first major branch of the superior mesenteric artery and lies adjacent to the enlarged inflamed pancreas, making it the most commonly affected vessel. This leads to infarction and necrosis of the transverse colon, typically presenting hours later with peritonitis due to perforation. If the patient has already undergone laparotomy and re-intervention is deemed to be absolutely contraindicated, percutaneous drainage may suffice to convert the necrotic colon into a controlled colocutaneous fistula. Most patients, however, should undergo laparotomy. The mesentery of the transverse colon may be inaccessible within a hardened inflammatory mass, precluding a standard bowel resection. The liquefied, necrotic transverse colon should be resected, with bleeding points controlled with suture ligation. Drains should be left in place, with proximal diversion via ileostomy. Small bowel may be necrosed as well as, or instead of, colon.

In addition to mesenteric arterial thrombosis leading to necrosis, pancreatitis may cause bowel perforation through direct erosion into the wall of adjacent portions of the GI tract, primarily the stomach and duodenum. A perforation contained within the retroperitoneum may be managed conservatively, as this is anatomically the same as endoscopic drainage. However, if this causes peritonitis, severe sepsis, or accelerated organ failure, it should be treated with necrosectomy and management of the perforation even in the setting of acute necrosis (less than 4 weeks from onset). The second, third, and fourth portions of the duodenum are directly adjacent to the pancreas and are some of the most inaccessible portions of the GI tract, especially when acute inflammation obliterates normal dissection planes. Simply identifying the perforation may be difficult. Techniques we have used to identify the location have included intraoperative endoscopy and foregut insufflation or instillation of dilute methylene blue via a nasogastric tube. Prior to using any of these techniques, the proximal jejunum should be gently occluded with an atraumatic bowel clamp to prevent gaseous distention of the distal GI tract, which may preclude fascial closure. The perforation itself is unlikely to be amenable to primary repair; even if it can be adequately exposed, any suture line will be bathed in pancreatic fluid and is nearly guaranteed to break down. Instead, drainage and resection to a margin away from the pancreatic necrosis should be performed, with diversion similarly located beyond the reach of pancreatic fluid. For distal duodenal perforations, this may require a segmental resection with a lateral duodenojejunostomy.

Blood vessels in proximity to the pancreas are at risk for mural erosion, leading to potentially dramatic hemorrhage into the retroperitoneum. This is a greater concern for arteries than veins, as the higher pressure makes arteries more susceptible to pseudoaneurysm formation whereas a vein is more likely to thrombose. The highest risk vessels are the gastroduodenal artery and splenic artery, as they are in close proximity to the pancreas, although severe necrosis may engulf the entirety of the celiac axis (Fig. 20.3). This may

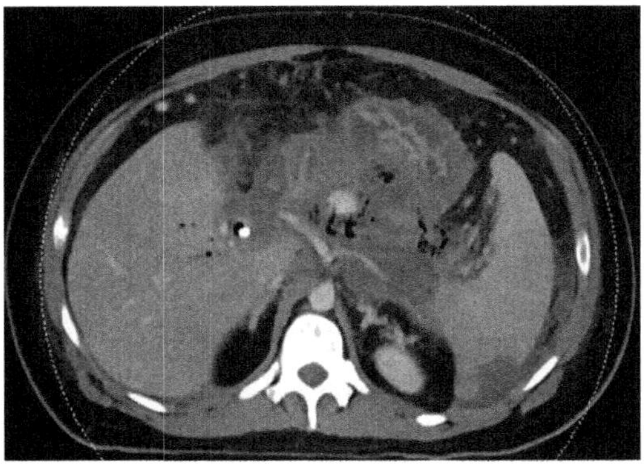

Fig. 20.3 Contrast-enhanced CT of a patient with necrotizing pancreatitis, showing pancreatitis engulfing the celiac axis with active extravasation within the walled-off collection. Patient was ultimately managed with a hybrid open and endovascular operation to control hemorrhage from the splenic and gastroduodenal arteries

present as an upper gastrointestinal bleed via either hemobilia or concomitant gastrointestinal fistulization. Alternatively, the bleeding may be contained within the retroperitoneum or may evacuate into the peritoneal cavity. Direct surgical control is an unappealing option, as it is typically difficult to visualize the bleeding vessel within a necrotic collection. Even if the bleeding location can be visualized, vascular repair is unlikely to offer durable hemostasis as the suture line will be bathed in pancreatic fluid; even if the friable vessel wall can be repaired with suture, the vessel is likely to thrombose or rupture again. The first-line treatment for hemorrhagic pancreatitis is angiographic embolization in a more proximal portion of the affected vessel. Should this prove ineffective, direct surgical control is the only remaining option. This should be performed in conjunction with vascular surgery or interventional radiology in a hybrid operating room or with a C-arm, as angiography can be invaluable in locating the bleeding vessel and additional attempts at embolization can be made during a combined operation. We have successfully used resuscitative endovascular balloon occlusion of the aorta (REBOA) placed in Zone 1 (descending thoracic aorta) to temporize an exsanguinating patient for transport to the operating room. If there is any unavoidable delay in transporting the patient to the operating room, femoral arterial access can be obtained at bedside in addition to large-bore venous access for resuscitation. An existing femoral arterial line can be rapidly converted to a vascular sheath for REBOA deployment or angiographic access in the operating room.

Chronic Complications of Acute Pancreatitis

The persistent critical illness which accompanies severe pancreatitis brings its own panoply of respiratory, renal, neuropsychiatric, and other complications which are beyond the scope of this chapter. Pancreatitis itself may cause both systemic metabolic complications and local anatomic complications.

The normal pancreas has both endocrine and exocrine functions; both may be affected by severe pancreatitis, particularly if necrosis and debridement obliterate a significant portion of the pancreatic parenchyma. Glycemic control is the most critical of the pancreatic endocrine functions; other pancreatic hormones have more subtle effects that are difficult to separate from chronic pain and dysmotility, are difficult or impossible to replace if their deficiencies can be measured, and receive far less attention in the clinical setting or the scientific literature. Insulin deficiency, however, leads to diabetes in a significant number of patients. A recent systematic review reported a 23% prevalence of new-onset diabetes within a year of the first episode of acute pancreatitis and a 30% prevalence for those patients with severe pancreatitis. For those patients followed for 60 months after their first episode of pancreatitis, the diabetes prevalence reached 40% [55]. A review of pancreatic exocrine insufficiency in acute pancreatitis gave a pooled prevalence of 62% during the initial hospital admission, and 35% had continued exocrine insufficiency in follow-up. Severe vs. mild and necrotizing vs. interstitial edematous pancreatitis were associated with higher rates. The included studies measured exocrine insufficiency using a variety of direct and indirect laboratory assays, contributing to high heterogeneity in the meta-analysis [56]. It is not clear whether all such patients required pancreatic enzyme supplementation or what the clinical sequelae were beyond this. The only clear takeaway is that both endocrine and exocrine insufficiency occur in a large minority of patients; they should be assessed in the surgical clinic, with appropriate referrals made to endocrinology, gastroenterology, and high-quality primary care as needed.

Pseudocysts are the most frequent chronic anatomic complication of acute pancreatitis. They arise from a disruption of the pancreatic duct or a major branch and can occur after interstitial edematous or necrotizing pancreatitis. A pseudocyst is a collection of pancreatic fluid that has been walled off by the patient's immune system. While peripancreatic fluid collections are relatively common in interstitial edematous pancreatitis, they do not become pseudocysts for at least 4 weeks, as it generally takes this long for a wall to form around the collection. Many peripancreatic collections seen on imaging early in the course of pancreatitis will resolve; even formed pseudocysts frequently become smaller or resolve without intervention. While pseudocysts frequently lead to surgical consultation, they only warrant treatment when they compress the stomach or small intestine sufficiently to cause early satiety or obstructive symptoms. The first line of treatment is endoscopic cyst gastrostomy or cyst duodenostomy, which should be guided by endoscopic ultrasound. This is a similar but simpler procedure than endoscopic necrosectomy; one to three plastic stents connecting the cyst to the GI tract are usually enough to allow drainage, and once drained the cavity typically scars down and obliterates.

In rare circumstances where the pseudocyst is anatomically inaccessible, surgical drainage may still be necessary. Depending on the location of the pseudocyst, a cyst gastrostomy, cyst duodenostomy, or cyst jejunostomy using a Roux limb or a loop of proximal jejunum may be indicated. Similar to transgastric necrosectomy, the uninvolved margin of the stomach or small bowel is incised and retracted, exposing the side of the GI tract in connection with the pseudocyst. An 18-gauge needle is used to aspirate pseudocyst fluid, confirming its location. The involved wall of the stomach or small bowel is then divided with electrocautery, and the contiguous wall of the cyst and GI tract are sutured with a running continuous polydioxanone suture for hemostasis. If the pseudocyst is to be accessed through the transverse mesocolon, the cyst is opened into the peritoneal cavity, and an anastomosis is made to the appropriately mobilized loop of jejunum. A recent small randomized controlled trial of endoscopic versus surgical drainage demonstrated equal efficacy with higher physical and mental health scores among patients undergoing endoscopic drainage, as well as hospital charges less than half as much as for surgical drainage [57], confirming endoscopy's role as first-line therapy.

Less frequently, patients may develop disconnected duct syndrome. This occurs when pancreatic necrosis, with or without debridement, obliterates the body or head of the pancreas, resulting in a persistent pancreatic fistula from a retained, functional pancreatic tail. If the pancreatic fistula fails to resolve after several months of expectant management and imaging demonstrates a persistent pancreatic tail, this may be managed by distal pancreatectomy. Given the extensive scarring found in this situation, this is typically a more challenging and morbid operation than the distal pancreatectomy performed for trauma or cancer.

Conclusions

Despite advances in interventional radiology and endoscopy, and despite accumulating evidence favoring more conservative approaches to pancreatic debridement in the last two decades, acute pancreatitis remains an important disease process in general surgery. Its management requires several of the core competencies of the acute care surgeon, including surgical critical care, coordinating a multidisciplinary team, and the ability to perform both minimally and maximally invasive surgeries when needed. While most patients with even severe pancreatitis do not need surgical management, those that do require some of the most complex pre-, intra-, and postoperative decision-making in all the general surgery subspecialties.

References

1. Chang L, Lo SK, Stabile BE, Lewis RJ, de Virgilio C. Gallstone pancreatitis: a prospective study on the incidence of cholangitis and clinical predictors of retained common bile duct stones. Am J Gastroenterol. 1998;93(4):527–31.
2. Oria A, Alvarez J, Chiappetta L, Spina JC, Hernandez N, Iovaldi M, et al. Choledocholithiasis in acute gallstone pancreatitis. Incidence and clinical significance. Arch Surg. 1991;126(5):566–8.
3. Dumonceau JM, Andriulli A, Elmunzer BJ, Mariani A, Meister T, Deviere J, et al. Prophylaxis of post-ERCP pancreatitis: European Society of Gastrointestinal Endoscopy (ESGE) guideline—updated June 2014. Endoscopy. 2014;46(9):799–815.

J, et al. Exocrine pancreatic insufficiency following acute pancreatitis: systematic review and meta-analysis. Dig Dis Sci. 2019;64(7):1985–2005.
57. Varadarajulu S, Bang JY, Sutton BS, Trevino JM, Christein JD, Wilcox CM. Equal efficacy of endoscopic and surgical cystogastrostomy for pancreatic pseudocyst drainage in a randomized trial. Gastroenterology. 2013;145(3):583–90.e1.
58. Traverso LW, Clark CJ. Pancreatic cystenterostomy: technique and rationale for pseudocyst treatment. In: Fischer JE, Jones DB, Pomposelli FB, Upchurch GR, Klimberg VS, Schwaitzberg SD, et al., editors. Fischer's mastery of surgery. 6th ed. Philadelphia: Lippincott Williams & Wilkins; 2012. p. 1424–31.

Enterocutaneous Fistula

21

James P. Byrne, Benjamin Braslow, and Mariela Rivera

Case Report

72-y/o man presented with a recto-urethral fistula in the setting of prostate cancer status post-open radical prostatectomy. To repair this urinary fistula, he underwent pelvic exenteration, ileal conduit formation, and an end sigmoid colostomy. This procedure was complicated by a midline wound dehiscence and the development of a high-output enterocutaneous fistula within the confines of the wound. He developed severe electrolyte derangements and skin irritation prompting. He required volume resuscitated and correction of his electrolytes. The volume of effluent from his ECF was medically optimized with anti-diarrheal medications, and his skin irritation improved with topical therapy and the maintenance of a well-sealed wound manager. He was placed on TPN. He was eventually discharged to rehab with intent to limit oral intake with full parenteral nutritional support. During follow-up, he reported continued watery output from his fistula, averaging about 1 liter per day with frequent wound manager leakage issues now handled by his wife at home. He was able to tolerate limited soft foods in addition to his ongoing TPN support. There was no output from his colostomy or rectum. His most recent labs revealed a normal WBC, stable electrolytes, and a pre-albumin of 23. He continued to report good function of his urostomy site although he endorsed issues with appliance leaking into his fistula wound. After a thorough discussion of the risks and benefits of the procedure, informed consent was obtained for a planned enterocutaneous fistula takedown via a midline incision 9 months after the enterocutaneous fistula was diagnosed.

At exploration, the patient had an extensive lysis of adhesions with ECF takedown with resection of the involved small bowel. Ongoing lysis of adhesions looking for downstream obstructions revealed dense adhesive disease. Through meticulous sharp lysis of adhesions, multiple bowel

J. P. Byrne · B. Braslow (✉)
Department of Surgery, Pennsylvania Presbyterian Medical Center, Division of Traumatology, Emergency General Surgery and Surgical Critical Care, Perelman School of Medicine, University of Pennsylvania, Philadelphia, PA, USA
e-mail: James.Byrne@pennmedicine.upenn.edu; benjamin.braslow@pennmedicine.upenn.edu; benjamin.braslow@uphs.upenn.edu

M. Rivera
Department of Surgery, Mayo Clinic, Rochester, MN, USA
e-mail: rivera.mariela@mayo.edu

M. D. Zielinski, O. Guillamondegui (eds.), *The Acute Management of Surgical Disease*,
https://doi.org/10.1007/978-3-031-07881-1_21

loops were mobilized out of the pelvis and the small bowel was run from ligament of Treitz through the resected ECF to the ileocecal valve beyond the existing ileal–ileal anastomosis from his ileal conduit creation. Due to extensive de-serosalization, the decision to resect the involved small bowel including the dilated appearing prior small bowel anastomosis was made. A stapled iso-peristaltic side-to-side small bowel anastomoses was created to restore intestinal continuity. He remained NPO with an NGT to suction until his ostomy was functional by post-operative day 9; his diet was advanced as tolerated. A calorie count was started once he was tolerating a regular diet, he was eating enough by calorie counts and his TPN was discontinued. He was dismissed to a skilled nursing facility for ongoing rehabilitation needs.

Overview

Enterocutaneous fistulas (ECFs), defined as the abnormal connection between the bowel and skin, are among the most challenging problems that acute care surgeons face in clinical practice. They frequently arise as the consequence of complex underlying disease processes, require thoughtful and resource-intensive multidisciplinary care, and are often difficult to surgically treat. While improved approaches to treating sepsis, nutritional support, wound care, and surgical technique have resulted in improved outcomes, fistula-related mortality remains in the range of 5–15% [1–5]. Resolution of the fistula without surgery is uncommon (15–40%) [3–6] and the rate of successful healing after operative intervention is 75–90% [3–5, 7]. This chapter will provide a stepwise approach to ECF management by classifying the pathology, reviewing management priorities, and highlighting key considerations when planning for definitive management of this intimidating problem.

Classification and Risk Factors

ECFs are classified based upon their anatomy, etiology, and physiologic impact on the patient [8]. In understanding these factors, the best approach to management can be planned.

Anatomy

An ECF is categorized anatomically by which segment of the gastrointestinal (GI) tract it originates. For example, gastrocutaneous, enterocutaneous, and colocutaneous refer to fistulas that arise from the stomach, small intestine, and colon, respectively. While the term "enterocutaneous" most strictly refers to fistulas between the small bowel and the skin, it is frequently used to describe any fistula arising from the GI tract. While dependent on local practice and referral patterns, retrospective series show small bowel fistulas are most common (70–90%), followed by colonic (15–25%) and gastric (0–8%) [4, 5, 9].

Etiology

Etiologic classification of ECFs is based on the underlying disease processes and circumstances under which they arose (Table 21.1). The majority of ECFs occur as the consequence of prior surgery (85–90%), while spontaneous fistulas are less common (10–15%) [1, 2, 4, 5]. Spontaneous ECFs are most likely to occur in the presence of inflammatory bowel disease (most commonly

Table 21.1 Causes of enterocutaneous fistula

Etiology	Frequency[a]
Post-operative	85–90%
Spontaneous	10–15%
Inflammatory bowel disease	35–50%
Malignancy	9%
Foreign body (mesh)	6%
Radiation	5%
Diverticular disease	5%

[a]Multiple conditions may be present in the same patient; therefore, frequencies add up to greater than 100%

Crohn's disease) or malignancy, often following percutaneous drainage for control of spontaneous perforation [5, 6]. For patients undergoing surgery, factors that predispose to post-operative fistula formation include inflammatory bowel disease, malignancy, prior radiation therapy, malnutrition, presence of infection, and prior operations performed in the emergency setting [6].

The mnemonic "FRIEND" is helpful to remember risk factors for fistula formation and/or persistence: **F**oreign body (e.g., presence of mesh), **R**adiation, **I**nflammation or **I**nfection, **E**pithelialized tract (shorter/wider tracts less favorable), **N**eoplasm, **D**istal obstruction [6]. The presence of these factors also predicts that a fistula is unlikely to heal spontaneously.

Physiology (Output)

ECFs are also classified by volume of fistula output [6, 8]. Output has traditionally been grouped into three categories: low output (<200 mL per day), moderate output (200–500 mL per day), and high output (>500 mL per day). Fistulas that originate from the proximal GI tract are more likely to be high output. Patients with high-output fistulas are more likely to present with significant electrolyte imbalances, dehydration, and malnutrition due to the loss of GI fluids rich in electrolytes, minerals, and protein. High-output fistulas are also less likely to be amenable to spontaneous closure without surgical intervention.

Diagnosis and Stabilization

The diagnosis of ECF is made clinically. Early recognition and medical stabilization are essential. The diagnosis of an ECF may be obvious in some, manifesting as frank dehiscence of an anastomosis or serosal injury into the surgical wound, or as feculent output from a percutaneous drain placed for source control. In others, the manifestation of an ECF might be preceded by some period of faltering clinical progress after surgery, mounting signs of sepsis, and physiologic derangement. The presence of risk factors discussed in the previous section should raise clinical suspicion. Others present with a subcutaneous or intra-abdominal fluid collection after surgery. Ultimately, the result is the same: leakage of enteric content, whether bile-tinged succus or feculent material, into a drain, a wound or through a defect in the skin.

Once the diagnosis of ECF is made, attention and resources should be directed at addressing four potentially life-threatening clinical problems [6, 8]: (1) resuscitation and correction of electrolyte imbalances, (2) treatment of sepsis, (3) protecting the skin and controlling fistula output, and (4) ensuring adequate nutrition.

Initial Resuscitation and Electrolyte Replacement

Patients presenting with ECF frequently show evidence of intravascular volume depletion and electrolyte abnormalities. Therefore, an initial priority in the acute phase of management is the accurate assessment of volume status and thoughtful fluid resuscitation. Physical examination may reveal clinical signs of dehydration, such as dry mucus membranes and decreased skin turgor. Vital sign findings such as tachycardia or relative hypotension reflect hypovolemia. Laboratory findings consistent with acute kidney injury (AKI) of a pre-renal nature (increased serum BUN:Cr ratio and decreased urinary fractional excretion of sodium), in addition to oliguria, are common findings. Generous fluid replacement should be given with frequent reassessment of these measures to ensure a trajectory toward improvement.

Equally important are the correction of electrolyte abnormalities and replacement of ongoing losses. Electrolytes that most often require supplementation are sodium, potassium, and magnesium [10]. The volume of fistula output should be monitored accurately and replaced every 4–6 h, initially on a 1:1 basis, during the acute phase of care. Replacement fluids should reflect the composition of the GI effluent being lost. For example, normal saline with supplemental potassium (e.g., NS + 10 mEq/L KCl) is recommended for replacement of losses from small bowel fistulas [8, 10]. Ringer lactate can be a reasonable option to replace fistula output. The addition of bicarbonate may be required in more proximal fistulas involving duodenal or pancreatic losses [8].

Treatment of Sepsis

Sepsis is a leading cause of fistula-related mortality, accounting for between 40 and 90% of in-hospital deaths in retrospective series [1, 4, 5]. Therefore, evaluating for signs and sources of infection is the primary goal in the acute phase of care for patients presenting with ECF and must be conducted in parallel to fluid resuscitation. Patients manifesting signs of sepsis or septic shock should be managed in accordance with latest guidelines from the Surviving Sepsis Campaign [11]. Empiric antimicrobial therapy with broad spectrum coverage of intra-abdominal organisms, with consideration to local antibiograms, should be started early based on clinical suspicion. Critically ill patients should be transferred to an intensive care setting where critical care personnel and monitoring are available. Shock may require support with vasopressors.

Anatomic source control is then prioritized. For patients presenting systemically unwell with signs of peritonitis, urgent surgical intervention with laparotomy is required for the purpose of drainage, exteriorization of the leak, or proximal diversion [8]. Where surgery is not indicated, CT scan is the investigation modality of choice for identification of abscess, which should then be drained by percutaneous approach when feasible. It is important to be aware that manipulation of septic foci may provoke transient bacteremia exacerbating systemic signs of sepsis and so patient monitoring and supports should be planned accordingly [6]. Culture data taken at the time of source control procedures should be reviewed frequently for consideration of de-escalating and narrowing antibiotic coverage.

Skin Protection and Wound Management

Controlling the fistula effluent is an essential component of care in patients with ECFs and must be carefully planned. Enteric fluids, particularly those arising from the proximal GI tract rich in bicarbonate, are irritating and caustic to the skin. Failure to protect the integrity of the skin can result in significant pain and distress to the patient, and risk of secondary soft tissue infection. Therefore, a wound care specialist or enterostomal therapist should be consulted early to determine a successful management strategy appropriate to the unique patient [6, 8]. This is particularly important in the case of high-output fistulas and those involving complex wounds. Doing so will facilitate ongoing nursing care and lay the groundwork for longer-term, outpatient management.

Common strategies for management of fistula output include skin barriers and pouches. Simple gauze dressings may suffice for low-output fistulas. A sump drain can occasionally be used in conjunction with a wound management system to directly drain effluent from the fistula opening. Vacuum-assisted closure (VAC) systems have recently gained favor. While no randomized evidence exists, a recent systematic review of retrospective studies found a median fistula closure rate of 65% with VAC therapy [12]. Fistula output is an important predictor of closure with VAC, ranging from 86% in low-output to 42% in high-output fistulas. Median time to closure approached 60 days. In the largest study of patients with high-output fistulas, 40% did not improve with VAC therapy and required surgical correction [13].

Entero-atmospheric fistulae, defined as fistulas that occur in the setting of an open abdomen, present unique challenges. Management of the fistula is complicated by the presence of exposed small bowel in the field of a larger wound. Such fistulas often require intensive wound care using multiple modalities, including improvised collection systems for controlling the fistula effluent in combination with VAC therapy. Caution must be taken, however, as the authors have experienced new fistula formation with VAC therapy when applied directly to intra-abdominal granulation tissue. Regardless of the strategy selected to control the fistula output, the ultimate goal is to divert the effluent away from the skin to allow for wound formation with minimal bacterial contamination.

Nutritional Support

Malnutrition is present in many patients presenting with ECF due to poor oral intake, ongoing enteric losses, and the hypercatabolic state of sepsis [6]. Developing an effective nutrition strategy tailored to the patient is essential to support their metabolic needs and ability to heal. Once initial resuscitation and management of sepsis is underway, the patient's current nutritional state should be assessed. Physical examination might reveal a clinical picture of cachexia while peripheral edema might suggest protein malnutrition. Total body weight and body mass index should be measured to determine the patient's deviation from baseline. Laboratory measures of nutrition should be drawn, including albumin, pre-albumin, and transferrin. Liver function tests and triglycerides should be measured in anticipation of need for parenteral nutrition.

Nutritional support and monitoring should be planned with inpatient nutrition specialists. In most of the patients with active fistulas, daily caloric and protein requirements approach 30 kcal/kg and 1.5–2.5 g/kg, respectively [6, 8]. It is common that patients are unable to achieve these requirements by mouth although, if possible, early enteral nutrition should be undertaken to prevent intestinal mucosal atrophy thereby supporting the immune function of the gut [6]. If the effluent increases and puts wound healing at risk, then enteral nutrition may not be possible. This is particularly true for fistulas present higher in the gastrointestinal tract such as the duodenum or jejunum. Oral solutions rich in electrolytes (high sodium) and glucose can be helpful in replacing fluid and electrolyte losses [2]. If indicated, whether due to inadequate oral intake or malnourished state, supplemental parenteral nutrition should be started to achieve nutritional goals. This should be done with caution and consideration to the risk of refeeding syndrome, which is greatest in critically ill chronically malnourished patients. Where refeeding syndrome is a concern, hypocaloric feeding with close monitoring and replacement of electrolytes (phosphate, magnesium, potassium) and vitamins (especially thiamine) may be required [14]. In patients with intestinal discontinuity, proximal fistulas with <75 cm bowel length, or where fistula output is very high (>1.5 L), enteral nutrition might not be feasible [10]. Even when enteral nutrition is possible, intestinal absorption may be impaired. In these cases, total parenteral nutrition may be necessary.

Monitoring progress with respect to nutritional recovery should be done by measuring patient weight and serum nutritional markers at least weekly in the early phase of care [10]. Determining the endpoint is not straightforward. Nutritional support, including supplemental or total parenteral nutrition, is continued until either the fistula has closed, or the patient's nutritional state has improved to where surgical intervention is deemed appropriate. Evidence suggests that nutritional status is a potent predictor of outcome in patients undergoing surgery for ECF, with mortality approaching zero in those with albumin >3.5 g/dL [15]. A period of weight gain and correction of albumin, pre-albumin, and transferrin to normal ranges is therefore ideal.

Investigations

Laboratory Workup

Laboratory investigations obtained at presentation should include a complete blood count (CBC) and basic metabolic panel (BMP) with "extended electrolytes" including calcium, magnesium, and phosphate. Liver function tests (LFTs), serum triglycerides, pre-albumin, and transferrin should also be included. AKI with evidence of pre-renal azotemia (elevated BUN:Cr ratio) is common as evidence of dehydration. Urine electrolyte studies with low calculated fractional excretion of sodium (FeNa <1%) confirm pre-renal AKI likely secondary to hypovolemia in these patients. Electrolyte imbalances are common and should be corrected aggressively. Albumin, pre-albumin, and transferrin provide a baseline assessment of nutrition. Pre-albumin specifically has a short half-life (2–3 days) and responds quickly to correction of catabolism with nutritional replacement. Transferrin has an intermediate half-life (8–9 days) and is both a reflection of systemic inflammation and iron status. However, according to a recent guideline published by The American Society for Parenteral and Enteral Nutrition (ASPEN) regarding nutritional support of adult patients with ECF: although serum protein level monitoring was common in the 1980s–1990s, it is now accepted that the values lack sensitivity and specificity in making a diagnosis of malnutrition. Decreased plasma concentrations of serum albumin, transferrin, retinol binding protein, and pre-albumin may be more a consequence of ECF-related inflammation rather than a true marker of nutritional status. While not an appropriate nutrition assessment parameter, low serum protein concentrations may still have valuable clinical prognostic significance regarding spontaneous ECF closure or the ability to heal an anastomosis at time of surgical ECF takedown [16]. LFTs provide a baseline sense of liver synthetic function and are required in preparation for parenteral nutrition, as are triglycerides. LFTs, triglycerides, and electrolytes should be monitored closely upon beginning parenteral nutrition.

Where sepsis is a concern, it is important to remember to obtain cultures from all possible infectious sources, including surgical or percutaneous drainage procedures, central lines, and urine. This should be done prior to administering antibiotics when possible.

Imaging

Imaging studies are performed to elucidate fistula anatomy and aid in planning for definitive management. This should be done when the patient has been medically stabilized. Abdominal CT has largely replaced fluoroscopic fistulogram as the radiologic study of choice. CT scans are often able to demonstrate the fistula tract anatomy, the segment of the GI tract from which it arises, as well as identifying undrained sources of sepsis, distal obstruction, or associated pathology [8]. Coordination with the radiologist performing the study is helpful, particularly with regard to planning timing of the study with regard to luminal contrast. An upper GI contrast study can be used to assess transit time and distance along the GI tract to the fistula. Fistulogram, performed by injecting water-soluble contrast directly into a well-epithelialized fistula opening, can be helpful in confirming the presence of communication with the GI tract but often does not delineate anatomy as well as CT. Magnetic resonance imaging enterography can be helpful in patients with inflammatory bowel disease where there is suspicion for complex fistula or strictures [10].To rule out colonic obstruction, colonoscopy or hypaque enema should be considered.

Medical Management

The aim of medical management of ECFs is to reduce fistula output. In doing so, wound care, fluid balance, and nutritional support can be optimized. Medical treatments to control fistula output fall into three broad categories: (1) antimotility agents, (2) somatostatin analogues, and (3) antisecretory agents (Table 21.2) [17].

Table 21.2 Medical strategies for reducing fistula output

Medication	Dose, route, and frequency
Antimotility agents	
Loperamide	4 mg PO TID every 6 h before food
Diphenoxylate/atropine	2.5–5 mg/0.025–0.05 mg PO every 6 h before food
Codeine	15–30 mg PO every 6 h before food
Tincture of opium	6 mg PO undiluted every 6 h before food
Antisecretory agents	
Pantoprazole	40 mg IV BID
Somatostatin analogues	
Octreotide	100 mcg SC TID

TID Three times daily, *BID* Twice daily

Antimotility agents that are commonly used are opioid derivatives. These medications are taken by mouth, ideally before consuming food for optimal effect. Loperamide (brand name Imodium) is the first agent used. In one study of high-output ileostomies, while both loperamide and codeine decreased output, loperamide resulted in improved electrolyte balance and fewer side effects [18]. For high-output fistulas, we recommend beginning at the maximal dose of 4 mg PO every 6 h. Diphenoxylate/atropine (brand name Lomotil) can be added and up titrated to 5 mg diphenoxylate (two tablets) every 6 h. Where possible, the liquid formulations of loperamide and diphenoxylate/atropine should be avoided due to the cathartic effects of propylene glycol and sorbitol content respectively. While codeine and tincture of opium can be added in high-output fistulas, their use is limited by central nervous system side effects (namely, sedation). While higher doses of loperamide (40 mg daily) and codeine (240 mg daily) have been described in the management of high-output fistulas [2, 5], slow up-titration and caution should be used at higher-than-recommended doses.

Proton pump inhibitors have been shown to decrease intestinal output and improve water absorption [19]. Intravenous agents avoid challenges with respect to limited absorption of the medication. Therefore, it is recommended that intravenous proton pump inhibitors (e.g., pantoprazole) are used in the initial phase of care in patients with high-output fistulas [17].

The addition of a somatostatin analogue (e.g., octreotide) is recommended after a brief period of stabilization on other antimotility and antisecretory medications [17]. Recent meta-analyses of randomized-controlled trials have concluded that use of a somatostatin analogue (typically octreotide 100 mcg SC TID) results in significant reduction in fistula output and shorter time to closure [20, 21]. However, the current evidence does not confirm a significant improvement in fistula closure rates [17]. Current recommendations support a 72-hour trial of octreotide in patients with high-output fistulas [2, 5]. If reduced output is achieved, this treatment is continued.

Operative Management

The decision to undertake surgical correction of ECFs is based on an understanding of patient and disease factors that make non-operative management unlikely to succeed (Table 21.3). Fistulas that are high output, with short/wide defects, which arose in the presence of intestinal disease, irradiated bowel, or distal obstruction, are unlikely to close without surgery [2, 6, 10]. A trial of non-operative management with intensive wound care, nutritional support, and medical therapies to decrease fistula output is appropriate. This time period may last several weeks to months, during which associated wounds are allowed to heal and sources of infection are resolved. Ultimately, only 15–40% of fistulas close without surgery [3–6].

Surgery for intestinal fistula is often complex and highly morbid. This is, in part, due to the patient population often having experienced complicated courses from prior surgery, frequently in the setting of significant underlying comorbidity. In one series from a high-volume US center, patients undergoing definitive surgical treatment of ECFs had a mean of 6 previous abdominal surgeries, 80% had required parenteral nutrition, with only 40% being functionally independent [9]. The majority of patients (75–80%) are referred from other institutions for definitive surgery [2, 9]. Therefore, it is essential to review available records and obtain sufficient imaging to fully understand the patient's surgical history and unique anatomy. Operative duration

Table 21.3 Predictors of success or failure of non-operative fistula closure

Favorable	Unfavorable
Long, narrow fistula tract	Short, wide fistula tract
Intestinal continuity	Discontinuity or distal obstruction
Low fistula output	High fistula output
Good nutritional status	Poor nutritional status
No sepsis	Intra-abdominal sepsis
Absence of systemic illness	Systemic illness adversely affecting healing
No intrinsic intestinal disease	Inflammatory bowel disease, malignancy, radiation enteritis

is longer than 8 h in 25% of patients and peri-operative blood transfusion is required in 70% [9]. In-hospital complications from definitive ECF surgery occur in more than 80%, with systemic sepsis (35%) and surgical site infection (30%) being common [9, 22]. One in 4 require mechanical ventilation for more than 48 hours [9]. Peri-operative mortality is approximately 5–7% [2, 22] with 15% deceased within 1 year of surgery [9].

The optimal timing for surgery is a matter of clinical judgment. Ideally, patients should be free of sepsis, well-nourished, and their surgical wounds healed [23]. Sufficient time should have elapsed from the previous operation to have allowed intra-abdominal inflammation to have settled and re-peritonealization to have occurred [24]. The abdomen should be soft and supple to examination. This may take several months. The median time from previous surgery or diagnosis of ECF to definitive surgery is 8–9 months in large retrospective series [2, 5, 9, 25].

Definitive surgery for ECF requires careful planning. It is wise not to schedule other major operations on the same day, as operations for ECF are frequently "all-day cases" [8]. The potential for difficulty in closing fascia should be anticipated and a surgeon experienced in abdominal wall reconstruction should be involved in advance where necessary. If distal small bowel or colonic obstruction was identified in previous imaging, it should be address during fistula take-down surgery. Entry into the abdominal cavity is through an incision placed so as to avoid injury to underlying bowel. This process might be complicated by the presence of mesh from prior surgery—this should be fully excised. Extensive and meticulous lysis of adhesions is then performed to mobilize the intestine sufficiently. Care must be taken to identify and repair injuries to the serosa during this process. The bowel must be followed along its entire length from proximal to distal at the level of the rectum. Downstream obstruction must be excluded or addressed surgically. The fistula should be clearly defined. The segment of bowel from which the fistula arises should be excised back to healthy tissue or segmentally resected, and GI continuity is re-established [24]. There is no clear evidence to support the technique for anastomosis, hand sewn, or stapled. Definitive closure of the abdominal wall defect is then undertaken. Fascial closure is achieved in only 70% of patients and component separation or use of mesh is often required [9, 22].

Recurrence of fistula is unfortunately common, occurring in 10–20% [9, 22]. The use of mesh in closure of the abdominal wall is a strongly predictive factor in recurrence.

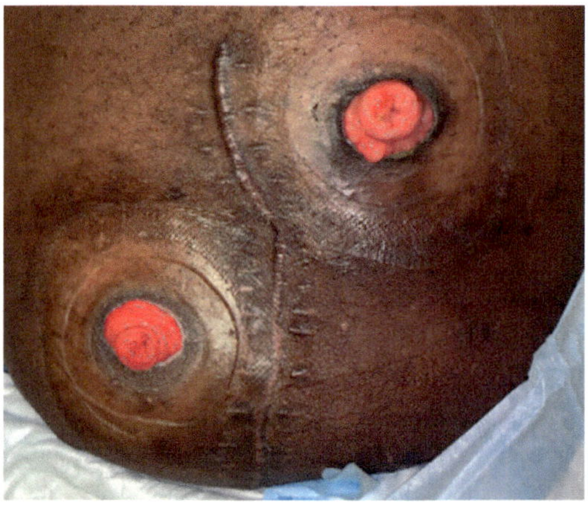

References

1. Quinn M, Falconer S, McKee RF. Management of Enterocutaneous Fistula: outcomes in 276 patients. World J Surg. 2017;41(10):2502–11.
2. Datta V, Engledow A, Chan S, Forbes A, Cohen CR, Windsor A. The management of enterocutaneous fistula in a regional unit in the United Kingdom: a prospective study. Dis Colon Rectum. 2010;53(2):192–9.
3. Martinez JL, Luque-de-Leon E, Mier J, Blanco-Benavides R, Robledo F. Systematic management of postoperative enterocutaneous fistulas: factors related to outcomes. World J Surg. 2008;32(3):436–43; discussion 44.
4. Draus JM Jr, Huss SA, Harty NJ, Cheadle WG, Larson GM. Enterocutaneous fistula: are treatments improving? Surgery. 2006;140(4):570–6; discussion 6-8.
5. Hollington P, Mawdsley J, Lim W, Gabe SM, Forbes A, Windsor AJ. An 11-year experience of enterocutaneous fistula. Br J Surg. 2004;91(12):1646–51.
6. Evenson AR, Fischer JE. Current management of enterocutaneous fistula. J Gastrointestinal Surg. 2006;10(3):455–64.

7. Lynch AC, Delaney CP, Senagore AJ, Connor JT, Remzi FH, Fazio VW. Clinical outcome and factors predictive of recurrence after enterocutaneous fistula surgery. Ann Surg. 2004;240(5):825–31.
8. Schecter WP, Hirshberg A, Chang DS, Harris HW, Napolitano LM, Wexner SD, et al. Enteric fistulas: principles of management. J Am Coll Surg. 2009;209(4):484–91.
9. Owen RM, Love TP, Perez SD, Srinivasan JK, Sharma J, Pollock JD, et al. Definitive surgical treatment of enterocutaneous fistula: outcomes of a 23-year experience. JAMA Surg. 2013;148(2):118–26.
10. Gribovskaja-Rupp I, Melton GB. Enterocutaneous fistula: proven strategies and updates. Clin Colon Rectal Surg. 2016;29(2):130–7.
11. Howell MD, Davis AM. Management of sepsis and septic shock. JAMA. 2017;317(8):847–8.
12. Misky A, Hotouras A, Ribas Y, Ramar S, Bhan C. A systematic literature review on the use of vacuum assisted closure for enterocutaneous fistula. Colorectal Dis. 2016;18(9):846–51.
13. Wainstein DE, Fernandez E, Gonzalez D, Chara O, Berkowski D. Treatment of high-output enterocutaneous fistulas with a vacuum-compaction device. A ten-year experience. World J Surg. 2008;32(3):430–5.
14. Koekkoek K, van Zanten ARH. Nutrition in the ICU: new trends versus old-fashioned standard enteral feeding? Curr Opin Anaesthesiol. 2018;31(2):136–43.
15. Fazio VW, Coutsoftides T, Steiger E. Factors influencing the outcome of treatment of small bowel cutaneous fistula. World J Surg. 1983;7(4):481–8.
16. Kumpf VJ, de Aguilar-Nascimento JE, Graf JI, et al. 2017 ASPEN-FELANPE clinical guidelines. Nutrition support of adult patients with Enterocutaneous fistula. JPEN. 2017;41(1):104–12.
17. Parli SE, Pfeifer C, Oyler DR, Magnuson B, Procter LD. Redefining "bowel regimen": pharmacologic strategies and nutritional considerations in the management of small bowel fistulas. Am J Surg. 2018;216(2):351–8.
18. King RF, Norton T, Hill GL. A double-blind crossover study of the effect of loperamide hydrochloride and codeine phosphate on ileostomy output. Aust N Z J Surg. 1982;52(2):121–4.
19. Jeppesen PB, Staun M, Tjellesen L, Mortensen PB. Effect of intravenous ranitidine and omeprazole on intestinal absorption of water, sodium, and macronutrients in patients with intestinal resection. Gut. 1998;43(6):763–9.
20. Rahbour G, Siddiqui MR, Ullah MR, Gabe SM, Warusavitarne J, Vaizey CJ. A meta-analysis of outcomes following use of somatostatin and its analogues for the management of enterocutaneous fistulas. Ann Surg. 2012;256(6):946–54.
21. Coughlin S, Roth L, Lurati G, Faulhaber M. Somatostatin analogues for the treatment of enterocutaneous fistulas: a systematic review and meta-analysis. World J Surg. 2012;36(5):1016–29.
22. Connolly PT, Teubner A, Lees NP, Anderson ID, Scott NA, Carlson GL. Outcome of reconstructive surgery for intestinal fistula in the open abdomen. Ann Surg. 2008;247(3):440–4.
23. Marinis A, Gkiokas G, Argyra E, Fragulidis G, Polymeneas G, Voros D. "Enteroatmospheric fistulae"—gastrointestinal openings in the open abdomen: a review and recent proposal of a surgical technique. Scand J Surg. 2013;102(2):61–8.
24. Slade DA, Carlson GL. Takedown of enterocutaneous fistula and complex abdominal wall reconstruction. Surg Clin North Am. 2013;93(5):1163–83.
25. Bannon MP, Heller SF, Rivera MR, Leland AL, Schleck CD, Harmsen WS. Reconstructive operations for enteric and colonic fistulas: low mortality and recurrence in a single-surgeon series with long follow-up. Surgery. 2019;165(6):1182–92.

veillance data for group A streptococcal infections [2–6]. At the current U.S. population (329,000,000; http://worldpopulationreview.com/countries/united-statespopulation/), this incidence would equate to between 1000 and 1500 cases annually, grossly underestimating the true incidence. Recent studies using large national datasets provide a much higher incidence of NSTI, estimating between 8.7 and 10.3 infections per 100,000 persons (28,500–33,600 cases) in 2018 [7].

Mortality from NSTI remains significant but has been decreasing over time (see Table 22.1), the decline believed to be related improved recognition, decreased time to operative debridement, and advances in resuscitation [1, 7–10]. In 30 studies of NSTI from 1980 through 1999 including 945 patients, the average mortality was 28% [1]. More recent data demonstrate a much lower mortality, closer to 10% [8, 9, 11, 12]. In seven more recent studies between 2007 and 2018 including 252 patients all undergoing surgery in less than 24 h of presentation (frequently less than 12 h), average mortality was 9% [13, 14].

Admission for the treatment of NSTI is associated with significant hospital cost, likelihood of requiring readmission, and long-term impact on patient quality of life [7, 11, 15]. Estimated mean cost for an index hospitalization for NSTI between 2010 and 2015 is $45,500 to $50,500 per admission [7, 11]. Patients with NSTI who survive to discharge have a 90-day readmission risk of 28%, the majority unplanned [7]. Mean cost of readmission in 2015 was greater than $23,000.

Table 22.1 Mortality trends in published series of necrotizing soft tissue infections

Publication dates:	Number of studies	Number of cases	Number of deaths	Percent mortality
1980–1990	17	375	118	31.7%
1991–2000	15	628	167	26.6%
2001–2010	37	2670	565	21.2%
2011–2014	11	2508	394	15.7%
Total 1980–2014	**80**	**6181**	**1245**	**20.1%**

Pathophysiology, Bacteriology, and Terminology

Necrotizing soft tissue infections differ from other non-necrotizing skin and soft tissue infections by the presence of devitalized and necrotic tissue [1]. The tissue necrosis provides a unique pathophysiologic environment, feeding bacterial microorganisms while simultaneously limiting the immunological response [1]. The infections tend to have rapid tissue involvement with progressive destruction, resulting in risk of limb loss and death [10].

Necrotizing soft tissue infections may be caused by a diverse array of microbiologic etiologies and have variable clinical presentations, thus contributing to the variety of terms used to describe these conditions. Necrotizing infection may involve any of the soft tissue layers, alone or in combination. Necrotizing cellulitis is an infection of the dermis and subcutaneous fat, necrotizing fasciitis is an infection of the deep fascial layers, and necrotizing myositis and myonecrosis are infections of the muscle layers. Each of the tissue layers has variable resistance to infection that contributes to the relative frequency of which layer becomes infected. Intact, well-perfused dermis and subcutaneous layers and muscle have relatively higher resistance to most infections and are involved less frequently than the fascia. The deep fascia has tentative blood supply and lymphatic drainage with necrotizing fasciitis accounting for 50–75% of all infections [1, 10, 16].

Necrotizing soft tissue infections may be grouped by bacterial pathogenesis, originally proposed by Giulliano and colleagues and since extended and variably defined in the literature [2, 6, 17–19]. We prefer to group infections into three types, based upon bacterial species and pathogenesis. Type 1 infections are polymicrobial in nature, typically arise from a more chronic, indolent source and subsequently enter and spread across fascial planes. The great majority of cases of necrotizing fasciitis are type 1 infections. Fourier's gangrene represents a subset of type 1 necrotizing fasciitis that involves the perineum, perianal, periurethral, or genital area. Patients with type 1 necrotizing infections are typically comprised of both aerobic and anaerobic and may have gram-positive and gram-negative bacteria, with on average more than 4 species isolated [1, 20]. Most patients with type 1 necrotizing infections have significant medical comorbidities placing them at risk such as diabetes and morbid obesity [8].

Type 2 infections are monomicrobial infections caused by gram-positive, aerobic cocci either virulent Streptococcal species (most commonly *S pyogenes*) or community-acquired methicillin-resistant *Staphylococcus aureus* (CA-MRSA) [19, 21]. The pathogenesis and presentation of these infections are significantly related to toxin production by these bacteria which allow them to invade and disrupt healthy tissue, particularly the dermis. These infections can be very rapidly progressive. *S pyogenes* may cause a necrotizing cellulitis, a necrotizing fasciitis, or a necrotizing myonecrosis with or without a clearly defined portal of entry [19].

Type 3 infections are also monomicrobial infections, caused by either gram-positive or gram-negative bacilli. As in type 2 infections, pathogenesis and disease presentation are related to toxin production by the bacteria and are rapidly progressive. These infections may be caused by *Clostridia, Bacillus, Vibrio, Aeromonas,* and *Eikenella* species. Of type 3 infections, those caused by Clostridia species are most common in the United States.

Of the Clostridial species, *C. perfringens* is the most common pathogen, accounting for 70–80% of all Clostridial infections. Clostridium is a spore-forming obligate anaerobic bacteria that produce potent extracellular toxins including α toxin (phospholipase C) and θ toxin (perfringolysin) that cause microvascular thrombosis and ischemia, hemolysis, and impede migration of polymorphonuclear leukocytes. Under appropriate conditions, Clostridial growth is extremely rapid with doubling time of approximately 8 min [10]. Its rapid growth under anaerobic conditions produces large amounts of non-CO_2 gases that collect in tissue, the rationale for the frequently used term of "gas gangrene." While most cases of Clostridial NSTI are initiated by some inciting trauma, cases can occur spontaneously. Spontaneous *C. septicum* infections have been associated with leukemia and gastrointestinal malignancy [10].

NSTI Severity Stratification and Prediction of Mortality

NSTI severity stratification is complex due to the diversity of bacteriology and clinical presentation, the complexity of quantitatively assessing extent of tissue involvement, the variable nature of systemic involvement that may dramatically change from pre-debridement to post-debridement, and the relative infrequency of the disease. To date, no accepted standard exists to stratify NSTI severity. Numerous non-therapy-related factors have been shown to be independently associated with mortality using regression analysis. These factors can be categorized into four groups, comorbidity, organ system dysfunction, patient physiology, and bacteriology as outlined in Table 22.2. The Fournier's Gangrene Severity Index (FGSI) combines nine different physiologic and laboratory variables to estimate overall mortality. A FGSI threshold score of 9 performed reasonably well in one study (71% sensitive, 90% specific) [22], but has not been validated in multicenter studies. Three additional severity stratification systems have been studied and applied to NSTIs and are discussed below, the American Association for the Surgery of Trauma (AAST) grading scale for including skin and skin structure infection (SSTI), the modified Sequential Organ Failure Assessment (mSOFA) score, and the Acute Physiology and Chronic Health Evaluation II (APACHE II) score.

AAST NSTI Grade: In 2016, the AAST created an anatomic-based grading system for several emergency general surgery conditions, including SSTI [23]. While the AAST anatomic severity grading scale for SSTI has been shown to correlate with outcomes [24], it has not been validated in any multicenter fashion and lacks many components shown to correlate to mortality [11, 14, 20, 25, 26].

mSOFA: The degree of organ dysfunction at presentation has previously been shown to inde-

Table 22.2 Factors independently associated with mortality in NSTI

Comorbidity:		**Organ dysfunction:**	
– Age [3, 11, 20, 26, 29, 31, 82, 83] – Liver disease [3, 11, 26] – Pulmonary disease [3, 11] – Cancer [3, 25]	– > 1 comorbidity [31] Heart disease [84] – Immunocompromised [83]	– AKI [3, 11, 20, 26, 29, 31, 82, 83] Coagulopathy [11, 26, 31] – SOFA/organ dysfunction [20, 27]	
Patient physiology:		**Bacteriology**	
– Shock [3, 11, 25, 29]	– WBC/bandemia [25, 26, 82, 84]	– Extent of infection [20, 30]	
– Lactate [8, 20, 85]	– Hypothermia [82]	– Bacteremia [26]	
– APACHE II [8, 29, 30]	– Heart rate [82]	– Pathogen including	
		• Aeromonas [25, 26] • Vibrio [25]	• Clostridia [84] • Strep Toxic Shock [83]

pendently correlate with mortality in NSTI [20]. More recently, using mSOFA (SOFA with bilirubin excluded) score to quantitate organ dysfunction, NSTI patients with an mSOFA of ≥3 on admission were demonstrated to have a higher mortality risk, required greater ventilator use, required prolonged intensive care, and had a lower return of renal function [27]. A similar association of mSOFA score with mortality has been demonstrated in other studies [12, 28].

APACHE II: The APACHE II is frequently used in critically ill populations to stratify and assign mortality risk and has been used in several NSTI studies to risk stratify. As its name implies, it includes both physiologic parameters and measures of medical comorbidities to provide a combined numerical score. The APACHE II score includes several of the physiologic and comorbidity variables shown to be independently associated with mortality in NSTI. APACHE II has been shown to independently correlate with mortality from NSTI in several studies [8, 29, 30] with reasonably good predictive performance (area under the receiver-operating characteristic curve = 0.86) [8].

Table 22.3 Clinical features strongly suggestive of NSTI—hard signs *(In at-risk patients, these findings should prompt operative exploration)*

1.	Pain disproportionate to the findings on physical exam
2.	Tense edema
3.	Bullae
4.	Skin ecchymosis/necrosis
5.	Cutaneous anesthesia over area
6.	Systemic toxicity
7.	Progression despite appropriate antibiotic therapy
8.	Soft tissue gas on exam or radiographic imaging

Diagnosis of NSTI

Establishing the early diagnosis of NSTI is significantly important to patient outcome as numerous studies demonstrate that delays in operative intervention worsen outcome [10, 13, 16, 20, 31, 32] and misdiagnosis is independently associated with operative delay [9]. Unfortunately, the diagnosis is frequently difficult to establish. In retrospective series of patients with NSTI, the correct diagnosis is made on admission a minority of the time; the majority being diagnosed with either cellulitis or abscess [25, 32–34].

Several clinical findings strongly suggestive of NSTI should be considered "hard signs" (see Table 22.3) and prompt operative exploration unless other etiologies of findings can be firmly established. However, many of these findings develop late in the clinical course and are present less than 50% of NSTI cases [10, 16]. The presence of gas in the soft tissue is also very specific for NSTI and is more readily detected on imaging than on physical exam. CT and MRI are both more sensitive for the detection of gas in tissues than plain imaging [10, 16]. However, we must emphasize that the absence of gas does not eliminate NSTI as a diagnosis and very severe infections may be present without this finding. Gas within tissues results from the production of poorly diffusible gases during anaerobic metabolism. The product of both aerobic metabolism and fermentation is carbon dioxide, a gas that is rapidly diffusible through tissues. Thus, potentially highly virulent pathogens such as *Streptococcus pyogenes* may produce very severe infections without the finding of gas in tissues.

Several laboratory values have been shown to be predictive of NSTI and can aid in the diagnosis as shown in Table 22.4 [10, 16]. In general, these values add specificity and should increase one's clinical suspicion for NSTI if present, but they lack sensitivity. The use of laboratory parameters in addition to clinical findings does appear to improve individual clinical diagnostic ability [35]. To improve the diagnostic accuracy for NSTI, Wong and colleagues combined several laboratory values to create a composite score to patients into low, medium, and high risk for NSTI. The Laboratory Risk Indicator for Necrotizing Fasciitis Score, or LRINEC score, utilizes six laboratory parameters including CRP, WBC, hemoglobin, sodium, creatinine, and glucose to create a composite score [33]. In the authors original study, a LRINEC score of 6 demonstrated good positive and negative predictive power. However, the enthusiasm originally generated for the use of the LRINEC score has been tempered by case reports of severe NSTI with scores of 0 and an inability to validate its sensitivity and specificity [36–40].

Ultimately, the diagnosis of NSTI may only be made once an incision is created. Surgical exploration is indicated if clinical suspicion is high and considering that the consequences of delay are catastrophic. Early surgical consultation is essential and taking the approach of "ruling out" NSTI rather than "ruling in" is warranted considering the high mortality of this infectious process.

Table 22.4 Laboratory values predictive of the presence of NSTI (these factors generally add specificity but lack sensitivity)

1.	White blood cell count >14 × 10^9/L
2.	Serum sodium concentration <135 mmol/L
3.	BUN >15 mg/L
4.	C-reactive protein (CRP) ≥150 mg/L

Treatment

In patients with NSTI, three factors are strongly associated with outcome, particularly patients with shock:

1. Time to appropriate resuscitation
2. Time to appropriate empiric antibiotic therapy
3. Time to operative debridement.

Resuscitation: For patients with NSTI and shock, like all patients with septic shock, appropriate resuscitation improves outcomes [41–43]. Aggressive resuscitation should be undertaken for preoperative preparation, continue into the operating theater, and post-operatively as required. As the time to operative debridement is strongly associated with outcome, quantitative fluid resuscitation, rapid and ongoing correction of coagulopathy, and vasoactive support as needed should be all be undertaken in a manner to limit delay to the operating room.

Empiric antibiotic therapy: Initiating appropriate antibiotic therapy early in the course also significantly alters outcomes. For patients with soft tissue infection and septic shock, selection of appropriate antibiotics that cover the pathogens involved greatly increases survival (OR ~10) compared with inappropriate selection [44]. Additionally, the time to initiation also has a significant impact on survival with roughly a 14% increase in mortality for each hour from onset of hypotension to antibiotic therapy. Selection of appropriate empiric antibiotic therapy should be directed toward the likely pathogens involved which can be determined by the clinical setting and course, inciting pathophysiology, and previous exposure to antibiotics [10, 16].

Distinguishing NSTIs as either type 1 polymicrobial infections that typically arise from a preexisting, indolent source versus a more rapidly progressive type 2 or type 3 infection where very rapid growth and toxin production contribute significantly to the clinical course is an important first step. Type 1 infections, such as Fournier's gangrene, are polymicrobial by definition and typically involve gram-positive and gram-negative bacteria as well as aerobic, facultative aerobic, and anaerobic bacteria. Generally, if there is no prior antibiotic exposure or known colonization or history of CA-MRSA, then multiple single-agent or combination choices provide adequate therapy as shown in Table 22.5 [10, 16, 34].

Table 22.5 Recommended empiric antibiotics for type I NSTI

Effective single-agent regimens:
– Piperacillin-tazobactam, imipenem-cilastatin, meropenem, ertapenem, ticarcillin-clavulanic acid, and tigecycline
Combinations regimens—many available:
– 2nd/3rd generation cephalosporins +/− fluoroquinolone in combination with anaerobic agents—metronidazole or clindamycin
Increasing resistance among Enterobacteriaceae may limit the use of:
– *Ampicillin-sulbactam, Ciprofloxacin, Levofloxacin*
CA-MRSA Colonization or clinical history suggestive of CA-MRSA
– *Consider adding vancomycin, linezolid, daptomycin, or clindamycin*

Patients with rapidly progressive type 2 and type 3 infections likely benefit from combination, high-dose antibiotic therapy with beta-lactam class and with anti-ribosomal class agents. The improved outcome with this combination therapy is believed to be related to two separate phenomena in these clinical settings (1) inhibition of bacterial toxin production by anti-ribosomal agents and (2) failure of cell-wall active agents with high inoculum infections due to downregulation of penicillin binding proteins in stationary phase. This has been demonstrated for both gram-positive and gram-negative pathogens [10, 45]. Anti-ribosomal antibiotics shown to inhibit toxin production and/or improve efficacy differ for gram-positive and gram-negative pathogens:

- gram-positive bacteria—clindamycin or linezolid
- gram-negative bacteria—tetracycline class antibiotics

An understanding of the clinical scenario and result of gram stain may be required to correctly target these aggressive infections. Table 22.6 below provides a summary of these pathogens and their characteristics.

Antibiotic therapy should be tailored to the cultures as results return. No high-quality data exist to make strong recommendations regarding the length of antibiotic treatment. Our practice is to continue antibiotics until hemodynamics

Table 22.6 Rapidly progressive NSTI: characteristics and pathogens

Metabolism	Anaerobic and facultative anaerobic	Obligate aerobic and fermentation	
Radiographic findings	Gas in tissue	No gas in tissues	
Gram stain	Gram-positive rods	Gram-positive cocci	Gram-negative rods
Pathogens and clinical syndromes	Clostridium species – Necrotizing myonecrosis.	Group A Streptococcus – Necrotizing cellulitis – Necrotizing myonecrosis	Vibrio – Salt water/shellfish exposure – Bullous skin necrosis, myonecrosis
			Aeromonas – Fresh water exposure – Necrotizing cellulitis, fasciitis, myonecrosis
		Staphylococcus aureus – Necrotizing cellulitis, fasciitis	Eikenella – Human bite wounds
			Pasteurella – Dog/cat bites

improve and the wound bed appears healthy. We do not continue them until the wounds are fully covered and healed.

Operative debridement: While resuscitation and appropriate antibiotic therapy have significant impact on outcome, operative debridement is the mainstay supporting positive outcomes, with time to debridement having a strong correlation with outcome [10, 13, 16, 20, 31, 32]. Debridement should be undertaken as soon as the diagnosis is established or strongly suspected and the patient appropriately resuscitated and stabilized. Graded recommendations for time to debridement target less than 12 hours from diagnosis [13].

Surgery and Debridement Technique

Index debridement: The cornerstone of operative debridement is to gain source control by removal of all necrotic tissue, provide drainage for all infected fluid collections, and prevention of fluid recollection. No high-quality data exist to guide the determination of when adequate debridement has been reached. Early reports emphasized wide debridement of involved tissues as a requirement for positive outcomes [46, 47] and debridement of all overlying skin, subcutaneous fat, fascia and, in some cases, musculoskeletal elements has become the traditional approach by many surgeons [48, 49]. With improvements in overall mortality from NSTI, focus has expanded to include preservation of function and decreasing morbidity. Surgical approach has evolved to skin-sparing technique which focuses on debridement of only the involved tissues and preserving overlaying skin and subcutaneous tissue [48–52].

As described by Wong et al., the degree of tissue involvement may be classified into three zones [52]. Zone 1 is necrotic tissue, zone 2 tissue remains viable but is involved with infection and inflammation, zone 3 is healthy, uninvolved tissue. Zone 1 tissue must be fully excised and skin in this zone demonstrates the "hard findings" of NSTI, hemorrhagic bullae, dermal hemorrhage, cutaneous anesthesia, and frank dermal gangrene. Zone 2 tissue is potentially salvageable and requires significant judgment and understanding of the pathophysiology of the infectious process.

Necrotizing infections that have a component of necrotizing fasciitis travel along fascial planes beyond the direct involvement of overlying skin and subcutaneous tissues. Collateral blood flow to skin from the dermal and subdermal plexus allow preservation of overlying tissue [50, 51]. The skin-sparing technique includes using curvilinear incisions and stairstep bridging incisions, debriding underlying fascia, and evacuating all purulent fluid, while preserving skin perforators to ensure viability of skin flaps. The technique has been shown to improve outcomes without increasing complications [48]. Progressive tensioning is a technique that has been described to limit the enlargement of the wound defect caused by removal of necrotic fascia to aid in wound healing [50].

Repeat debridement: Re-examination of the surgical wounds and repeat debridement as indicated at bedside or in the operating theater is also an important aspect of management of NSTI [1, 10, 16]. The optimal time interval to re-examination and repeat debridement has not been established by studies and is likely altered by the aggressiveness of the infectious process, clinical response to the index debridement, and comorbid factors of the patient. Most authors recommend re-examination and debridement within 24 h, with this time interval independently associated with improved outcome [53].

Adjunctive Therapies

Several adjunctive therapies have been proposed and studied in specific clinical scenarios of NSTI including hyperbaric oxygen therapy (HBO), Reltecimod (see below), steroids, and intravenous immunoglobulin. Adjunctive therapies, by definition, are provided in addition to the accepted standard therapies of NSTI including resuscitation, antibiotic therapy, and timely and adequate surgical debridement and source control.

Reltecimod: A synthetic octapeptide with homology to portions of the T lymphocyte receptor CD28 that blocks binding of superantigens from gram-positive organisms to the receptor and impairs endotoxin mediated T-cell activation. A phase 2 human trial demonstrated significant improvement in resolution of organ dysfunction in the treatment groups [54]. In a recently completed multicenter, phase 3 randomized controlled trial, treatment with Reltecimod achieved success in the composite endpoint for the per-protocol analysis but not the modified intent to treat analysis (primary endpoint). Treatment did result in significant improvements in resolution of organ dysfunction in both the per-protocol and modified intent to treat analyses [12]. This medication is under review by the FDA at the time of writing this chapter.

Hyperbaric oxygen therapy: The administration of oxygen under high atmospheric positive pressure in the treatment of "gas phlegmon" was first described by Brummelkamp in 1961 [55]. Hyperoxia has significant theoretic benefits in-vitro including enhancement of leukocyte-killing activity, suppression of bacterial growth and bactericidal effects of some anaerobic bacteria, enhanced antibiotic efficacy, and suppression of clostridial alpha toxin production [56]. Some animal data of Clostridial NSTI support the benefit of HBO [57, 58]. Studies in humans have all been observational in nature providing mixed results, with no controlled prospective trials available [59–63]. With the limited human data, meta-analyses, reviews, and guidelines do not strongly support HBO use, providing recommendations from "may be beneficial/considered" to "not recommended" [10, 34, 59–68]. Studies of the National Inpatient Sample demonstrate that HBO is used in only a very small minority of patients with NSTI, roughly 1% overall [69, 70].

Steroids: Short-course, high-dose steroid therapy has been advocated by some authors for the treatment of *Streptococcal pyogenes* (Group A Streptococcus—GAS) toxic shock syndrome in the setting of skin infections, though data are limited. Short courses of high-dose steroids have proven to improve outcomes in meningitis, a setting in which an exuberant inflammatory response contributes to adverse outcomes [71]. High-dose, short-course steroids have also been shown to improve time to resolution in uncomplicated erysipelas [72]. Specifically, 30 mg of prednisolone tapered over several days shortened the time to resolution, antibiotic therapy, hospital stay with no difference in relapse, recurrence, or complications [72, 73]. Guidelines for treatment of cellulitis state that steroids may be considered as a weak recommendation [74]. A few case reports and case series are reported with favorable outcome [75–79]. To date, no significant observational data or controlled studies are available.

Intravenous immunoglobulin: Similar to the rationale supporting potential efficacy of steroids in GAS toxic shock syndrome, intravenous immunoglobulin (IVIG) has been proposed as an adjunctive therapy. Several case reports describe the use of IVIG in settings of toxic shock syndrome including cases of necrotizing fasciitis with good results [10, 80]. However, case series provide conflicting outcomes [80]. One randomized, controlled trial of IVIG for toxic shock syndrome has been published, though it was stopped early with only 21 patients due to slow enrollment. The study was underpowered to demonstrate mortality benefit but did reach significance with decrease in sepsis-related organ failure at days 2 and 3 [81]. Three contemporary observational or national surveillance trials do support the use of IVIG in this setting, though the total cohort size is small [64]. More controlled and randomized data do exist regarding IVIG in a more broadly defined septic shock setting, though these data remain conflicting as well [80]. Considering this data, guidelines provide recommendations to consider IVIG in the setting of toxic shock syndrome but not in other NSTIs [10, 64].

Conclusion

Necrotizing soft tissue infections comprise a group of life-threatening infections with highly variable clinical presentations. Initially considered rare infections, recent studies have demonstrated a much higher incidence. NSTIs have a unique pathophysiology and have a diverse microbiological etiology which is used to classify them by types and guide antibiotic selection. Patients may present with a variety of physiologic derangements from non-toxic to fulminant septic shock with organ dysfunction. Time to appropriate resuscitation, empiric antibiotics administration, and operative debridement are strongly associated with clinical outcome. Early diagnosis of NSTI is critical to improving survival. Several hard signs are highly suggestive of NSTI including disproportionate pain, tense edema, bullae, skin ecchymosis or necrosis, cutaneous anesthesia, soft tissue gas on imaging, systemic toxicity, or progressive clinical worsening despite appropriate antibiotic treatment. These signs should prompt surgical exploration. The index operation is critical to gaining source control by debridement of involved tissues while maintaining uninvolved skin and subcutaneous tissue in a skin-sparing technique. Often a second-look wound exploration is utilized to ensure source control. Adjunctive therapies including steroids and IVIG have been utilized with overall mixed results; however, a new specific immunomodulator is showing promise.

References

1. May AK. Skin and soft tissue infections. Surg Clin North Am. 2009;89(2):403–20, viii.
2. Bonne SL, Kadri SS. Evaluation and management of necrotizing soft tissue infections. Infect Dis Clin N Am. 2017;31(3):497–511.
3. Mills MK, Faraklas I, Davis C, Stoddard GJ, Saffle J. Outcomes from treatment of necrotizing soft-tissue infections: results from the National Surgical Quality Improvement Program database. Am J Surg. 2010;200(6):790–6; discussion 6–7.
4. Nelson GE, Pondo T, Toews KA, Farley MM, Lindegren ML, Lynfield R, et al. Epidemiology of invasive group a streptococcal infections in the United States, 2005-2012. Clin Infect Dis. 2016;63(4):478–86.
5. Sarani B, Strong M, Pascual J, Schwab CW. Necrotizing fasciitis: current concepts and review of the literature. J Am Coll Surg. 2009;208(2):279–88.
6. Hakkarainen TW, Kopari NM, Pham TN, Evans HL. Necrotizing soft tissue infections: review and current concepts in treatment, systems of care, and outcomes. Curr Probl Surg. 2014;51(8):344–62.
7. May AK, Talisa VB, Wilfret DA, Bulger E, Dankner W, Bernard A, et al. Estimating the impact of necrotizing soft tissue infections in the United States: incidence and re-admissions. Surg Infect. 2020;
8. Gunter OL, Guillamondegui OD, May AK, Diaz JJ. Outcome of necrotizing skin and soft tissue infections. Surg Infect. 2008;9(4):443–50.
9. Kongkaewpaisan N, Hwabejire J, Lee JM, Narueponjirakul N, Meier K, Mendoza A, et al. Necrotizing soft tissue infection: time is crucial, and the admitting service matters. Surg Infect. 2020;21:828–33.
10. May AK, Stafford RE, Bulger EM, Heffernan D, Guillamondegui O, Bochicchio G, et al. Treatment of complicated skin and soft tissue infections. Surg Infect. 2009;10(5):467–99.
11. Al-Qurayshi Z, Nichols RL, Killackey MT, Kandil E. Mortality risk in necrotizing fasciitis: national prevalence, trend, and burden. Surg Infect. 2020;21:840–52.
12. Bulger EM, May AK, Robinson BRH, Evans DC, Henry S, Green JM, et al. A novel immune modulator for patients with necrotizing soft tissue infections (NSTI): results of a multicenter, phase 3 randomized controlled trial of Reltecimod (AB 103). Ann Surg. 2020;272:469–78.
13. Gelbard RB, Ferrada P, Yeh DD, Williams BH, Loor M, Yon J, et al. Optimal timing of initial debridement for necrotizing soft tissue infection: a practice management guideline from the Eastern Association for the Surgery of Trauma. J Trauma Acute Care Surg. 2018;85(1):208–14.
14. Zhao JC, Zhang BR, Shi K, Zhang X, Xie CH, Wang J, et al. Necrotizing soft tissue infection: clinical characteristics and outcomes at a reconstructive center in Jilin Province. BMC Infect Dis. 2017;17(1):792.
15. Hakkarainen TW, Burkette Ikebata N, Bulger E, Evans HL. Moving beyond survival as a measure of success: understanding the patient experience of necrotizing soft-tissue infections. J Surg Res. 2014;192(1):143–9.
16. May AK. Skin and soft tissue infections: the new surgical infection society guidelines. Surg Infect. 2011;12(3):179–84.
17. Garcia NM, Cai J. Aggressive soft tissue infections. Surg Clin North Am. 2018;98(5):1097–108.
18. Giuliano A, Lewis F Jr, Hadley K, Blaisdell FW. Bacteriology of necrotizing fasciitis. Am J Surg. 1977;134(1):52–7.
19. Stevens DL, Bryant AE. Necrotizing soft-tissue infections. N Engl J Med. 2017;377(23):2253–65.
20. Elliott DC, Kufera JA, Myers RA. Necrotizing soft tissue infections. Risk factors for mortality and strategies for management. Ann Surg. 1996;224(5):672–83.
21. Miller LG, Perdreau-Remington F, Rieg G, Mehdi S, Perlroth J, Bayer AS, et al. Necrotizing fasciitis caused by community-associated methicillin-resistant Staphylococcus aureus in Los Angeles. N Engl J Med. 2005;352(14):1445–53.
22. Corcoran AT, Smaldone MC, Gibbons EP, Walsh TJ, Davies BJ. Validation of the Fournier's gangrene

severity index in a large contemporary series. J Urol. 2008;180(3):944–8.
23. Tominaga GT, Staudenmayer KL, Shafi S, Schuster KM, Savage SA, Ross S, et al. The American Association for the Surgery of Trauma grading scale for 16 emergency general surgery conditions: disease-specific criteria characterizing anatomic severity grading. J Trauma Acute Care Surg. 2016;81(3):593–602.
24. Ray-Zack MD, Hernandez MC, Younis M, Hoch WB, Soukup DS, Haddad NN, et al. Validation of the American Association for the Surgery of Trauma emergency general surgery grade for skin and soft tissue infection. J Trauma Acute Care Surg. 2018;84(6):939–45.
25. Hsiao CT, Weng HH, Yuan YD, Chen CT, Chen IC. Predictors of mortality in patients with necrotizing fasciitis. Am J Emerg Med. 2008;26(2):170–5.
26. Huang KF, Hung MH, Lin YS, Lu CL, Liu C, Chen CC, et al. Independent predictors of mortality for necrotizing fasciitis: a retrospective analysis in a single institution. J Trauma. 2011;71(2):467–73.
27. Bulger EM, May A, Bernard A, Cohn S, Evans DC, Henry S, et al. Impact and progression of organ dysfunction in patients with necrotizing soft tissue infections: a multicenter study. Surg Infect. 2015;16(6):694–701.
28. Bulger EM, May A, Dankner W, Maislin G, Robinson B, Shirvan A. Validation of a clinical trial composite endpoint for patients with necrotizing soft tissue infections. J Trauma Acute Care Surg. 2017;83(4):622–7.
29. Kao LS, Lew DF, Arab SN, Todd SR, Awad SS, Carrick MM, et al. Local variations in the epidemiology, microbiology, and outcome of necrotizing soft-tissue infections: a multicenter study. Am J Surg. 2011;202(2):139–45.
30. Yilmazlar T, Ozturk E, Alsoy A, Ozguc H. Necrotizing soft tissue infections: APACHE II score, dissemination, and survival. World J Surg. 2007;31(9):1858–62.
31. Liu YM, Chi CY, Ho MW, Chen CM, Liao WC, Ho CM, et al. Microbiology and factors affecting mortality in necrotizing fasciitis. J Microbiol Immunol Infect. 2005;38(6):430–5.
32. Wong CH, Chang HC, Pasupathy S, Khin LW, Tan JL, Low CO. Necrotizing fasciitis: clinical presentation, microbiology, and determinants of mortality. J Bone Joint Surg Am. 2003;85-A(8):1454–60.
33. Wong CH, Khin LW, Heng KS, Tan KC, Low CO. The LRINEC (laboratory risk indicator for necrotizing fasciitis) score: a tool for distinguishing necrotizing fasciitis from other soft tissue infections. Crit Care Med. 2004;32(7):1535–41.
34. Stevens DL, Bisno AL, Chambers HF, Dellinger EP, Goldstein EJ, Gorbach SL, et al. Practice guidelines for the diagnosis and management of skin and soft tissue infections: 2014 update by the infectious diseases society of America. Clin Infect Dis. 2014;59(2):147–59.
35. Chan T, Yaghoubian A, Rosing D, Kaji A, de VC. Low sensitivity of physical examination findings in necrotizing soft tissue infection is improved with laboratory values: a prospective study. Am J Surg. 2008;196(6):926–30.
36. Chao WN, Tsai SJ, Tsai CF, Su CH, Chan KS, Lee YT, et al. The laboratory risk indicator for necrotizing fasciitis score for discernment of necrotizing fasciitis originated from Vibrio vulnificus infections. J Trauma Acute Care Surg. 2012;73(6):1576–82.
37. Holland MJ. Application of the laboratory risk indicator in Necrotising fasciitis (LRINEC) score to patients in a tropical tertiary referral Centre. Anaesth Intensive Care. 2009;37(4):588–92.
38. Hsiao CT, Chang CP, Huang TY, Chen YC, Fann WC. Prospective validation of the laboratory risk indicator for necrotizing fasciitis (LRINEC) score for necrotizing fasciitis of the extremities. PLoS One. 2020;15(1):e0227748.
39. Neeki MM, Dong F, Au C, Toy J, Khoshab N, Lee C, et al. Evaluating the laboratory risk indicator to differentiate cellulitis from necrotizing fasciitis in the emergency department. West J Emerg Med. 2017;18(4):684–9.
40. Wilson MP, Schneir AB. A case of necrotizing fasciitis with a LRINEC score of zero: clinical suspicion should trump scoring systems. J Emerg Med. 2013;44(5):928–31.
41. Castellanos-Ortega A, Suberviola B, Garcia-Astudillo LA, Holanda MS, Ortiz F, Llorca J, et al. Impact of the surviving sepsis campaign protocols on hospital length of stay and mortality in septic shock patients: results of a three-year follow-up quasi-experimental study. Crit Care Med. 2010;38(4):1036–43.
42. Jones AE, Brown MD, Trzeciak S, Shapiro NI, Garrett JS, Heffner AC, et al. The effect of a quantitative resuscitation strategy on mortality in patients with sepsis: a meta-analysis. Crit Care Med. 2008;36(10):2734–9.
43. Lee SJ, Ramar K, Park JG, Gajic O, Li G, Kashyap R. Increased fluid administration in the first three hours of sepsis resuscitation is associated with reduced mortality: a retrospective cohort study. Chest. 2014;146(4):908–15.
44. Kumar A, Ellis P, Arabi Y, Roberts D, Light B, Parrillo JE, et al. Initiation of inappropriate antimicrobial therapy results in a fivefold reduction of survival in human septic shock. Chest. 2009;136(5):1237–48.
45. Liu JW, Lee IK, Tang HJ, Ko WC, Lee HC, Liu YC, et al. Prognostic factors and antibiotics in Vibrio vulnificus septicemia. Arch Intern Med. 2006;166(19):2117–23.
46. Bilton BD, Zibari GB, McMillan RW, Aultman DF, Dunn G, McDonald JC. Aggressive surgical management of necrotizing fasciitis serves to decrease mortality: a retrospective study. Am Surg. 1998;64(5):397–400.
47. McHenry CR, Piotrowski JJ, Petrinic D, Malangoni MA. Determinants of mortality for necrotizing soft-tissue infections. Ann Surg. 1995;221(5):558–63.
48. Tom LK, Maine RG, Wang CS, Parent BA, Bulger EM, Keys KA. Comparison of traditional and skin-sparing approaches for surgical treatment of necrotizing soft-tissue infections. Surg Infect. 2020;21(4):363–9.

49. Tom LK, Wright TJ, Horn DL, Bulger EM, Pham TN, Keys KA. A skin-sparing approach to the treatment of necrotizing soft-tissue infections: thinking reconstruction at initial debridement. J Am Coll Surg. 2016;222(5):e47–60.
50. Kranker LM, Curry EE, Perry TL. Response to Tom et al., comparison of traditional and skin-sparing approaches for surgical treatment of necrotizing soft-tissue infections. Surg Infect. 2020;21(5):474–5. https://doi.org/10.1089/sur.2019.263.
51. Perry TL, Kranker LM, Mobley EE, Curry EE, Johnson RM. Outcomes in Fournier's gangrene using skin and soft tissue sparing flap preservation surgery for wound closure: an alternative approach to wide radical debridement. Wounds. 2018;30(10):290–9.
52. Wong CH, Yam AK, Tan AB, Song C. Approach to debridement in necrotizing fasciitis. Am J Surg. 2008;196(3):e19–24.
53. Okoye O, Talving P, Lam L, Smith J, Teixeira PG, Inaba K, et al. Timing of redebridement after initial source control impacts survival in necrotizing soft tissue infection. Am Surg. 2013;79(10):1081–5.
54. Bulger EM, Maier RV, Sperry J, Joshi M, Henry S, Moore FA, et al. A novel drug for treatment of necrotizing soft-tissue infections: a randomized clinical trial. JAMA Surg. 2014;149(6):528–36.
55. Brummelkamp WH. The importance of administration of oxygen under atmospheric positive pressure in the treatment of gas phlegmon. Ned Tijdschr Geneeskd. 1961;105:2430–2.
56. Kaide CG, Khandelwal S. Hyperbaric oxygen: applications in infectious disease. Emerg Med Clin North Am. 2008;26(2):571–95, xi.
57. Demello FJ, Haglin JJ, Hitchcock CR. Comparative study of experimental Clostridium perfringens infection in dogs treated with antibiotics, surgery, and hyperbaric oxygen. Surgery. 1973;73(6):936–41.
58. Stevens DL, Bryant AE, Adams K, Mader JT. Evaluation of therapy with hyperbaric oxygen for experimental infection with Clostridium perfringens. Clin Infect Dis. 1993;17(2):231–7.
59. Devaney B, Frawley G, Frawley L, Pilcher DV. Necrotising soft tissue infections: the effect of hyperbaric oxygen on mortality. Anaesth Intensive Care. 2015;43(6):685–92.
60. George ME, Rueth NM, Skarda DE, Chipman JG, Quickel RR, Beilman GJ. Hyperbaric oxygen does not improve outcome in patients with necrotizing soft tissue infection. Surg Infect. 2009;10(1):21–8.
61. Shaw JJ, Psoinos C, Emhoff TA, Shah SA, Santry HP. Not just full of hot air: hyperbaric oxygen therapy increases survival in cases of necrotizing soft tissue infections. Surg Infect. 2014;15(3):328–35.
62. Shupak A, Shoshani O, Goldenberg I, Barzilai A, Moskuna R, Bursztein S. Necrotizing fasciitis: an indication for hyperbaric oxygenation therapy? Surgery. 1995;118(5):873–8.
63. Wilkinson D, Doolette D. Hyperbaric oxygen treatment and survival from necrotizing soft tissue infection. Arch Surg. 2004;139(12):1339–45.
64. Cocanour CS, Chang P, Huston JM, Adams CA Jr, Diaz JJ, Wessel CB, et al. Management and novel adjuncts of necrotizing soft tissue infections. Surg Infect. 2017;18(3):250–72.
65. Endorf FW, Cancio LC, Klein MB. Necrotizing soft-tissue infections: clinical guidelines. J Burn Care Res. 2009;30(5):769–75.
66. Levett D, Bennett MH, Millar I. Adjunctive hyperbaric oxygen for necrotizing fasciitis. Cochrane Database Syst Rev. 2015;1:CD007937.
67. Wang C, Schwaitzberg S, Berliner E, Zarin DA, Lau J. Hyperbaric oxygen for treating wounds: a systematic review of the literature. Arch Surg. 2003;138(3):272–9; discussion 80.
68. Willy C, Rieger H, Vogt D. Hyperbaric oxygen therapy for necrotizing soft tissue infections: contra. Chirurg. 2012;83(11):960–72.
69. Psoinos CM, Flahive JM, Shaw JJ, Li Y, Ng SC, Tseng JF, et al. Contemporary trends in necrotizing soft-tissue infections in the United States. Surgery. 2013;153(6):819–27.
70. Soh CR, Pietrobon R, Freiberger JJ, Chew ST, Rajgor D, Gandhi M, et al. Hyperbaric oxygen therapy in necrotising soft tissue infections: a study of patients in the United States Nationwide inpatient sample. Intensive Care Med. 2012;38(7):1143–51.
71. van de Beek D, de Gans J, McIntyre P, Prasad K. Corticosteroids for acute bacterial meningitis. Cochrane Database Syst Rev. 2007;(1):CD004405.
72. Bergkvist PI, Sjobeck K. Antibiotic and prednisolone therapy of erysipelas: a randomized, double blind, placebo-controlled study. Scand J Infect Dis. 1997;29(4):377–82.
73. Bergkvist PI, Sjobeck K. Relapse of erysipelas following treatment with prednisolone or placebo in addition to antibiotics: a 1-year follow-up. Scand J Infect Dis. 1998;30(2):206–7.
74. Stevens DL, Bisno AL, Chambers HF, Everett ED, Dellinger P, Goldstein EJ, et al. Practice guidelines for the diagnosis and management of skin and soft-tissue infections. Clin Infect Dis. 2005;41(10):1373–406.
75. Alwattar BJ, Strongwater A, Sala DA. Streptococcal toxic shock syndrome presenting as septic knee arthritis in a 5-year-old child. J Pediatr Orthop. 2008;28(1):124–7.
76. Chiu CH, Ou JT, Chang KS, Lin TY. Successful treatment of severe streptococcal toxic shock syndrome with a combination of intravenous immunoglobulin, dexamethasone and antibiotics. Infection. 1997;25(1):47–8.
77. May AK, Daniels TL, Obremskey WT, Kaiser AB, Talbot TR 3rd. Steroids in the treatment of group A streptococcal necrotizing soft tissue infection. Surg Infect. 2011;12(1):77–81.
78. Shoji F, Yoshino I, Osoegawa A, Yano T, Maehara Y. Toxic shock syndrome following thoracic surgery for lung cancer: report of a case. Surg Today. 2007;37(7):587–9.
79. Stegmayr B, Bjorck S, Holm S, Nisell J, Rydvall A, Settergren B. Septic shock induced by group A strep-

tococcal infection: clinical and therapeutic aspects. Scand J Infect Dis. 1992;24(5):589–97.
80. Raithatha AH, Bryden DC. Use of intravenous immunoglobulin therapy in the treatment of septic shock, in particular severe invasive group A streptococcal disease. Indian J Crit Care Med. 2012;16(1):37–40.
81. Darenberg J, Ihendyane N, Sjolin J, Aufwerber E, Haidl S, Follin P, et al. Intravenous immunoglobulin G therapy in streptococcal toxic shock syndrome: a European randomized, double-blind, placebo-controlled trial. Clin Infect Dis. 2003;37(3):333–40.
82. Anaya DA, Bulger EM, Kwon YS, Kao LS, Evans H, Nathens AB. Predicting death in necrotizing soft tissue infections: a clinical score. Surg Infect. 2009;10(6):517–22.
83. Golger A, Ching S, Goldsmith CH, Pennie RA, Bain JR. Mortality in patients with necrotizing fasciitis. Plast Reconstr Surg. 2007;119(6):1803–7.
84. Anaya DA, McMahon K, Nathens AB, Sullivan SR, Foy H, Bulger E. Predictors of mortality and limb loss in necrotizing soft tissue infections. Arch Surg. 2005;140(2):151–7.
85. Yaghoubian A, de Virgilio C, Dauphine C, Lewis RJ, Lin M. Use of admission serum lactate and sodium levels to predict mortality in necrotizing soft-tissue infections. Arch Surg. 2007;142(9):840–6.

Acute Perianal Disease

23

Kerri A. Ohman, Kellie E. Mathis, and Paul E. Wise

Introduction

Perianal disease is a common problem that can present with several etiologies and appearances. Acute variations of these problems include perianal abscess and fistula, which is most commonly related to cryptoglandular disease but may be the first manifestation of Crohn's disease; hemorrhoids, which may present with bleeding, thrombosis, or prolapsing tissue; anal fissure, which can be acute or chronic and associated with pain; or a number of other infections or acute pathology. It is important to be able to do a thorough examination to properly diagnose and treat patients with these conditions. A patient may seem to have a common or straightforward history but may actually have an underlying diagnosis of Crohn's disease, malignancy, or an undrained abscess that may be missed without appropriate and directed questioning or a thorough examination or imaging. Basic tenets of management can vary from supportive care/expectant management to a quick incision and drainage to far more complex and definitive surgical interventions, with therapy tailored uniquely to each patient.

K. A. Ohman (✉) · P. E. Wise
Section of Colon and Rectal Surgery, Department of Surgery, Washington University School of Medicine in St. Louis, St. Louis, MO, USA
e-mail: ohmank@wustl.edu; wisepe@wustl.edu

K. E. Mathis
Mayo Clinic, Rochester, MN, USA
e-mail: mathis.kellie@mayo.edu

Case Report

A 23-year-old man with no known past medical history presents to the emergency department with a chief complaint of perianal pain for 24 h. Upon further questioning, he denies other relevant symptoms such as abdominal pain, change in bowel habits, or weight loss and denies family history of inflammatory bowel disease. His temperature is 37 °C, heart rate 90, and blood pressure 110/80. He appears well but is unable to sit in a chair without discomfort. On external examination, you detect a tender fullness approximately 1 cm from the anal verge in the left posterolateral perianal tissue that is fluctuant without significant overlying cellulitis. Digital rectal examination (DRE) is performed, and no intra-anal fluctuance, lesions, or other masses are detected. After consenting the patient, you perform an incision and drainage to evacuate the abscess. No antibiotics are indicated as he has no overlying cellulitis, signs of undrained collections, or sepsis. He follows up in clinic in the next few weeks with complete resolution of his

M. D. Zielinski, O. Guillamondegui (eds.), *The Acute Management of Surgical Disease*,
https://doi.org/10.1007/978-3-031-07881-1_23

symptoms and no evidence of ongoing infection or drainage on examination.

Six months later, he presents again with a perianal abscess at the same location. He notes new complaints of increased perianal drainage, vague abdominal pain, abnormal bowel movements with new diarrhea, and weight loss over the last few weeks. On examination, an external opening is found in the left posterolateral perianal tissue at the site of the prior abscess. On DRE, a scant amount of purulent fluid is expressed through the external opening. Given clinical suspicion for fistula-in-ano, he is taken to the operating room for an exam under anesthesia. Anoscopy is performed and an internal opening is noted in the posterior midline. A probe is passed through the tract and you can palpate external and internal sphincter, confirming your suspicion of a transsphincteric fistula. You place a draining seton and refer him for evaluation for Crohn's disease, including consideration of colonoscopy and cross-sectional imaging.

Perianal Abscess and Fistula

Introduction

Perianal abscess is one of the most common etiologies of acute perianal disease, and while it may arise as an isolated problem, it may be the first manifestation of other perianal pathology or later develop into a fistula-in-ano. The majority of perianal abscesses arise from cryptoglandular disease, which is also the leading cause of fistula-in-ano, but there are other less common etiologies that may present similarly (Fig. 23.1a). An abscess may arise secondary to inflammatory bowel disease (IBD), trauma, malignancy, or less common infectious etiologies. In young adults such as in the Case Report, a perianal abscess may be the first symptom or presentation of Crohn's disease. It is important to perform a thorough history and physical examination in patients presenting with acute abscess, assessing for other systemic symptoms such as weight loss, abdominal pain, or change in bowel habits (or personal or family history of IBD). Trauma may lead to an undrained abscess, possibly in the setting of a retained foreign body, impalement injury, or previous surgery including procedures such as hemorrhoidectomy or episiotomy during childbirth.

Less common etiologies such as malignancy or the more rare infectious etiologies (e.g., tuberculosis, Actinomyces, Lymphogranuloma venereum) should remain on the differential diagnosis to be thorough and complete. Patients with acute or chronic complaints of perianal pain may have an associated malignancy such as an advanced anal squamous cell carcinoma or low rectal adenocarcinoma, so a thorough examination with DRE should be routinely performed. While even less common, lymphoma and leukemias may present as a perianal abscess as well.

Work-Up

The history and physical examination is paramount to an accurate diagnosis and therefore treatment. It is important to assess prior history of abscess or prior perianal procedures or repairs, assess for personal or family history of IBD and continence. If the patient otherwise appears well and non-toxic, laboratory tests such as a complete blood count and electrolyte panel are not indicated. In patients appearing ill or toxic with more concerning signs on examination, laboratories may help guide your resuscitation and antibiotic therapy.

Routine imaging is not indicated unless there is suspicion for a more complicated abscess or fistula. CT may be helpful if the diagnosis is uncertain or if the patient has pain out of proportion to examination without any clear features on physical exam. Pelvic MRI may be considered in patients with a recurrent abscess or with features suspicious for a more complex abscess such as concern for supralevator or bilateral extension or an occult abscess or in those patients with confounding disease processes such as Crohn's or known or suspected malignancies. Ultrasound

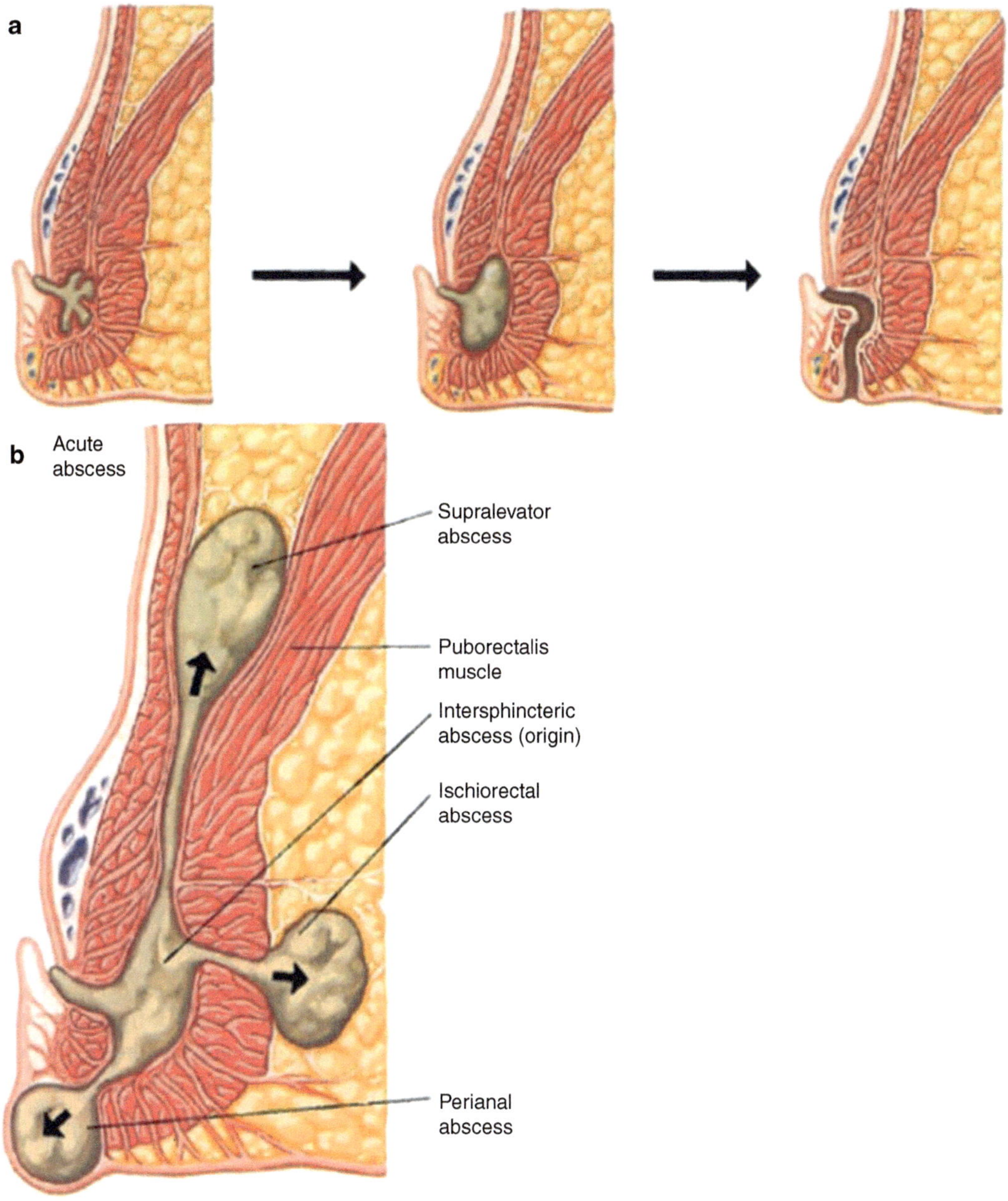

Fig. 23.1 Anatomy of anorectal abscess and fistula-in-ano development. (**a**) Cryptoglandular theory of inflammation of anal crypt leading to anorectal abscess formation and later fistula development. (**b**) Perianal abscess is superficial and may be treated with simple I&D compared to more complex abscess formation such as supralevator and ischiorectal abscesses, which may not be detectable on external examination alone. (These images were originally published in CIBA Clinical Symposia, Volume 37 (6), Authors Robert D. Fry, MD and Ira J. Kodner, MD, Illustrator John A. Craig, MD, "Anorectal Disorders," Plate 9, Copyright Elsevier 1985)

with either transanal or transcutaneous techniques is very user dependent and should not be routinely used unless the examiner is comfortable and skilled with this technique as the examiner may miss an undrained collection. Furthermore, transanal ultrasound may be uncomfortable and not well tolerated by the patient.

Examination

On perianal examination, an area of erythema or induration that will likely be fluctuant and tender to touch. Based on time of presentation, the patient may have either partially or completely evacuated the abscess cavity, but it is important to ensure that the abscess cavity is completely drained or it will re-accumulate. DRE should be routinely performed to ensure that there are no other undrained abscesses or pathology, as a patient with an intersphincteric or supralevator abscess (Fig. 23.1b) may not have findings on external assessment. You may palpate a fluctuant area in the anal canal or elicit pain and tenderness on examination.

In patients with more complex abscesses such as intersphincteric abscess or supralevator abscess, obtaining the correct diagnosis is important as a simple superficial perianal incision and drainage (I&D) may be inadequate and inappropriate therapy. Similarly, patients with more complex fistulous disease should be identified and referred to a specialist after drainage of the abscess.

It is estimated that 16–25% of patients will develop a fistula-in-ano after I&D of a perianal abscess [1–3], and patients with Crohn's disease are more than twice as likely to progress to fistula formation [2]. An internal opening to a fistula may be identifiable on digital exam, which may be palpable as a soft but firm fullness in the anal canal. Goodsall's rule (Fig. 23.2a), initially published in 1900, may point toward the direction of the internal opening. Based on Goodsall's rule, if the external opening lies posterior to a line drawn transversely across the anal verge, the fistula is likely to track posteriorly and open onto the posterior midline. If the external opening is anterior to this line, the fistula tracks directly into the anal canal. The exception is for anterior fistulas that are more than 3 cm from the anal verge as they may have a more indirect course. Of note, recent literature has challenged its predictive accuracy, so it is important to not base surgical planning on the rule alone [4–6].

Anal fistulas are defined as "simple" or "complex." While the terms are not standardized, complex fistulas include those that are high transsphincteric, suprasphincteric, or extrasphincteric, those occurring anteriorly in women, or any that increase the risk of fecal incontinence following fistulotomy. Fistulas due to Crohn's disease or malignancies or those that arise from trauma or other iatrogenic procedures are also considered complex. The Parks classification of anal fistula described the four main routes in which fistulas may track: intersphincteric, transsphincteric, suprasphincteric, and extrasphincteric (Fig. 23.2b) [7].

If the patient is able to tolerate DRE, anoscopy may be considered to assess for other internal pathology or the location of the internal opening.

Pathology

Cultures are not routinely indicated. If abnormal pathology is observed on exam, a biopsy should be sent to evaluate for IBD, malignancy, and other pathologies.

Non-operative Management

I&D is the mainstay of therapy for an acute perianal abscess and may be performed at the bedside if the patient is able to tolerate it. If not, this may require I&D in the operating room (see below). Ideally, the I&D opening will be made as close to the dentate line as possible so that any resultant fistula will be as superficial as possible. Whether the abscess is fully unroofed and packed versus drained with a punctate incision and placement of a mushroom-type catheter is based on the experience and preference of the practitioner. Antibiotics are not routinely indicated unless the patient is immunocompromised, shows signs of systemic illness or sepsis, if there is significant cellulitis, or if the abscess is unable to be fully drained. Antibiotics have been suggested to be utilized to prevent fistula formation, but the quality of evidence is low and there was no protective effect observed on a randomized, double-blinded,

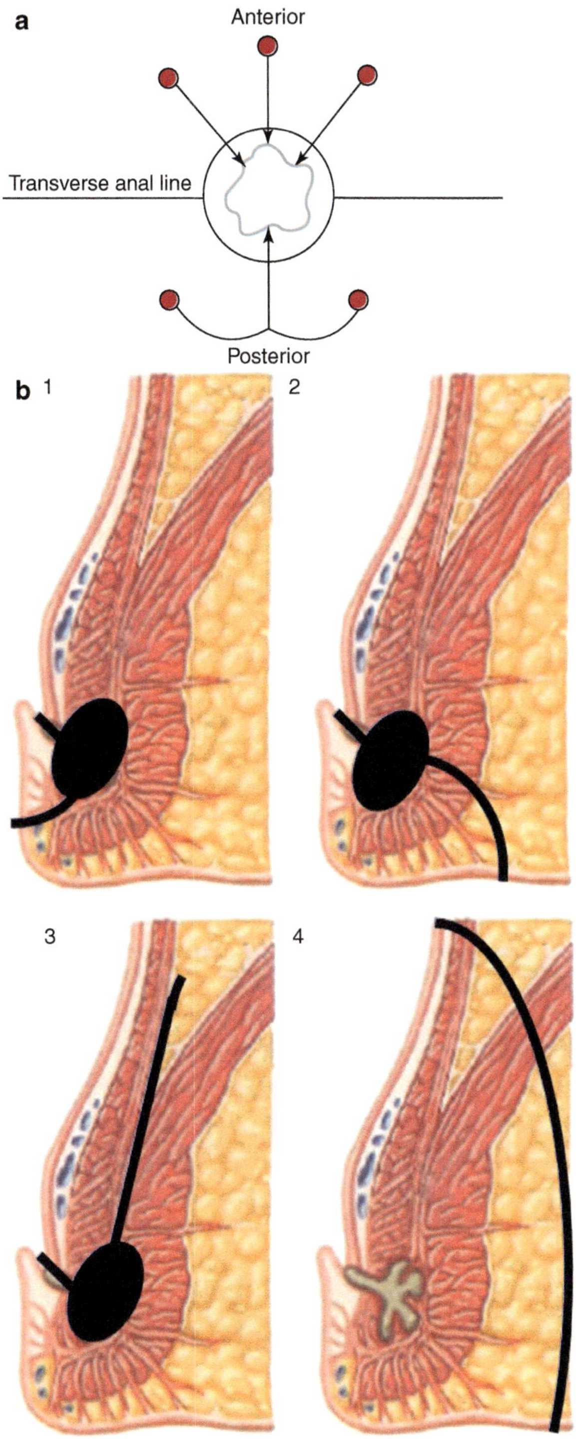

Fig. 23.2 Fistula-in-ano. (**a**) Goodsall's rule. External openings to the fistula that open anterior to the transverse anal line are associated with a radial tract to the anal canal whereas external openings that open posterior to the transverse anal line will have a curvilinear passage and open in the posterior midline in the anal canal. (**b**) Parks classification of fistula-in-ano: (1) intersphincteric, (2) transsphincteric, (3) suprasphincteric, (4) extrasphincteric. (These were modified and originally published in CIBA Clinical Symposia, Volume 37 (6), Authors Robert D. Fry, MD and Ira J. Kodner, MD, Illustrator John A. Craig, MD, "Anorectal Disorders," Plate 9, Copyright Elsevier 1985)

multicenter trial [8, 9]. If antibiotics are indicated, patients may be treated with a short course of amoxicillin-clavulanate or ciprofloxacin and metronidazole; an intravenous correlate may be utilized if the patient requires operative drainage. Wound culture should be considered for immunocompromised patients or those with recurrent abscesses.

Operative Management

Examination under anesthesia (EUA) should be performed for patients with a recurrent abscess, an abscess too painful for bedside I&D, or those with suspicion for a fistula. A simple linear or cruciate incision may be used to evacuate (± packing) the cavity. Mushroom (e.g., Pezzer or Malecot, Fig. 23.3) catheters are not routinely needed if the cavity is adequately drained and not too large. It is important to note that while a superficial abscess may be drained through the perianal skin, those with a submucosal, intersphincteric, or supralevator abscess will require internal drainage for adequate source control. These patients should be seen and evaluated by a specialist if available. Drainage of an intersphincteric abscess may be by internal sphincterotomy as part of the fistulotomy. External drainage may be considered but that risks development of a fistula. The origin of a supralevator abscess dictates its management. If the abscess arises from superior extension of an intersphincteric abscess, it should be drained internally by internal sphincterotomy or transanal drainage catheter into the cavity. If the abscess arises from superior extension of an ischiorectal abscess, it should be drained externally as close to the dentate line as possible. In the event of a horseshoe abscess, which is typically a deep posterior anal space abscess that progresses either unilaterally or bilaterally into the ischiorectal spaces—hence, a "horseshoe" appearance—the modified Hanley procedure is indicated. The modified Hanley is sphincter-preserving and involves drainage of the posterior anal space with seton placement and debridement and drainage of the lateral tracts and extension. Of note, a supralevator abscess may be associated with intra-abdominal pathology (e.g., diverticulitis, appendicitis, etc.).

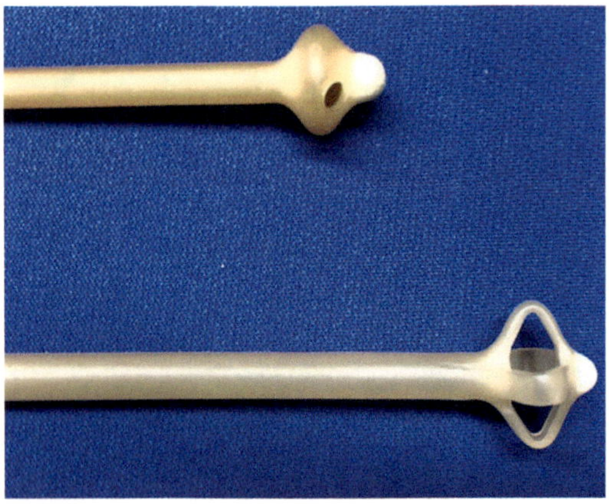

Fig. 23.3 Mushroom catheters such as the Pezzer catheter (above) and Malecot catheter (below) may be employed for larger cavities to promote adequate drainage and are more comfortable and easier for patients to manage than traditional packing. Excess tubing length may be trimmed for patient comfort. The drain is typically removed after the drainage has stopped, typically within a week after placement

If drainage persists beyond 6–12 weeks, the patient should undergo an EUA to assess for a fistula. However, if on index presentation the patient presents with an abscess and a concomitant fistula-in-ano, fistulotomy may be performed for a simple fistula if there is low risk of incontinence or complication [10, 11]. If there is any concern, a draining seton should be left instead.

In patients with a fistula where the internal opening can be identified, either a draining seton or a primary fistulotomy can be considered. A draining seton is a loosely placed silastic band or suture placed through the external opening to the internal opening and is around the subcutaneous tissue and sphincter musculature; it is loose to promote abscess drainage and fibrosis of the tract. Fistulotomy is a definitive treatment for simple anal fistulas and is successful in healing more than 90% of patients with high patient satisfaction scores [12, 13]. Primary fistulotomy may be employed for submucosal, intersphincteric, or low transsphincteric fistulas; however, if there is a significant burden of sphincter overlying the fistula, if the fistula is complicated, if there is concern for IBD, or if the patient has pre-operative incontinence, fistulotomy should not be performed and a seton should be placed across the tract instead. The patient should be referred to a specialist for further evaluation and to consider advanced procedures such as ligation of intersphincteric fistula tract [LIFT], endorectal or cutaneous advancement flap, or fistula plug.

Outcomes

There is no "perfect" procedure for a fistula-in-ano. Fistulotomy for any non-subcutaneous fistula mandates partial division of the sphincter with subsequent risk of fecal incontinence, with rates varying from 6.9% to 45% of patients experiencing at least some degree of impairment in fecal continence [14–18]. Cutting setons, which work by draining the abscess and slowly dividing the sphincter by tightening the seton over time with subsequent healing of the fistula tract, also carry the risk of incontinence, with a rate of 12% [19]. While it is not specified if the incontinence is to flatus, liquid stool, or solid stool, any form can certainly be distressing for the patient. Furthermore, the fistula may eventually recur, with patients with complex or previous fistulas being at highest risk [14].

Advanced procedures such as the LIFT procedure or endorectal advancement flap do not involve dividing the sphincter musculature but have varied success rates. In a recent systematic review and meta-analysis, endorectal advancement flap had an overall success rate of 69.9%; patients with a cryptoglandular etiology had a success rate of 74.6% and patients with Crohn's disease had a success rate of 61% [20]. The overall success rate for patients after LIFT was 68.9%; patients with cryptoglandular etiology had an overall success rate of 69.1% and those with Crohn's disease had a success rate of 53% [20]. Given the risk of failure and complications related to these procedures, these procedures should be performed by a specialist after appropriate informed consent.

Hemorrhoids

Introduction

Hemorrhoids are a common anorectal complaint, leading to nearly 4 million office and emergency department visits yearly as well as varying degrees of impact in quality of life for patients [21]. All patients have hemorrhoidal tissue, but in some patients the hemorrhoidal cushions can become symptomatic, likely from a combination of bowel habit issues, sphincter dysfunction, and/or excessive straining. Hemorrhoids are normal vascular cushions in the anal canal, consisting of submucosal, fibrovascular, and arteriovenous sinusoids thought to have a role in sensation, sampling, facilitating anal continence, and protecting the anal sphincter. Hemorrhoidal complexes are typically found in the left lateral, right anterolateral, and right posterolateral positions of the anal canal. Hemorrhoids are further classified as internal or external based on their relationship to the dentate line. Internal hemorrhoids are proximal to the dentate line, external hemorrhoids are distal, and mixed hemorrhoids extend both proximally and distally. This distinction is important in determining therapy because distal to the dentate line, the anoderm is innovated by somatic nerves and is more sensitive to pain, whereas sensation above the dentate line is from parasympathetic and sympathetic nerves.

Internal hemorrhoids more commonly present with painless bleeding or itching and are classified based on their degree of prolapse (Table 23.1). These are thought to become symptomatic from vascular congestion and mucosal prolapse. Factors that increase intra-abdominal pressure such as obesity, pregnancy, or abnormal bowel

Table 23.1 Classification and treatment of internal hemorrhoids

Grade	Presentation	Treatment
1	No prolapse	Dietary and lifestyle optimization
2	Prolapse that spontaneously reduces	Dietary and lifestyle optimization; rubber band ligation or other office-based measures; hemorrhoidectomy in select patients
3	Prolapse that requires manual reduction	Dietary and lifestyle optimization; rubber band ligation; hemorrhoidectomy
4	Prolapse that cannot be reduced	Dietary and lifestyle optimization; hemorrhoidectomy

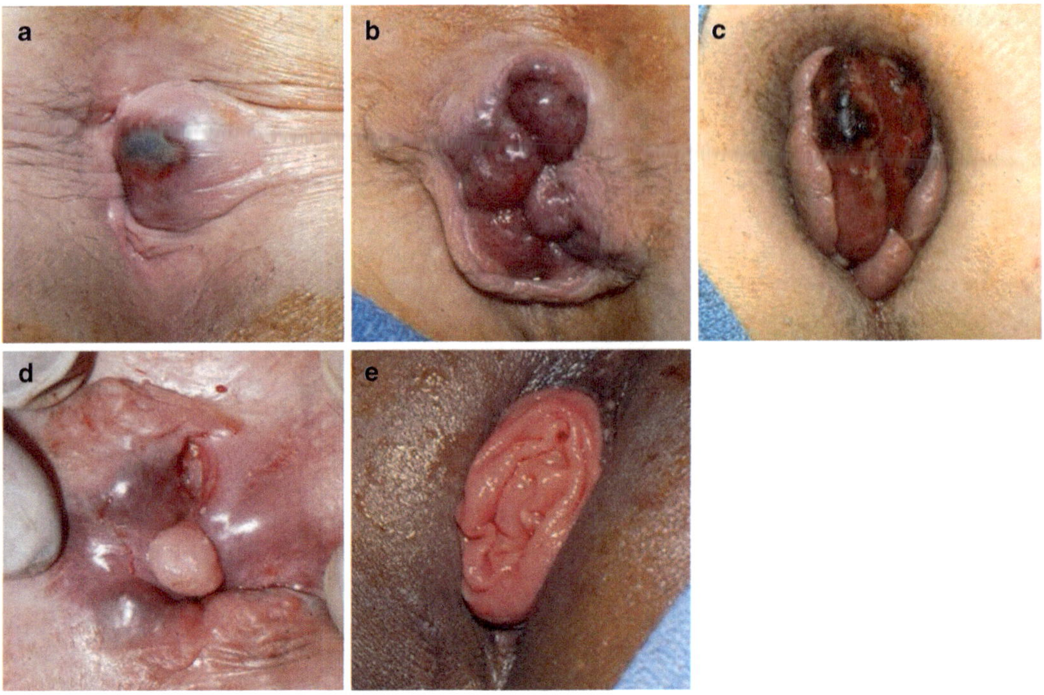

Fig. 23.4 Acute anorectal pathology. (**a**) Thrombosed external hemorrhoid; (**b**) prolapsed internal hemorrhoids; (**c**) incarcerated and thrombosed internal hemorrhoids; (**d**) chronic anal fissure; (**e**) rectal prolapse. (Images courtesy of Dr. Richard Devine)

habits with straining can cause subsequent engorgement and decreased venous return of the hemorrhoidal cushions, leading to vascular congestion [22]. Mucosal prolapse may be due to abnormal sphincter musculature or loss of supporting tissue, either due to trauma or aging. As support is lost, the mucosa prolapses, and the veins become distended [23].

Symptomatic external hemorrhoids are usually thrombosed presenting with a spontaneously developing, exquisitely tender, blue/purple perianal lump (Fig. 23.4a). Anal skin tags may be found as a residual lesion after resolution of a thrombosed external hemorrhoid.

Work-Up

Abnormal bowel habits such as constipation and diarrhea with prolonged straining are commonly elicited in the history. Dietary patterns such as fiber and water intake should be assessed as those will be the mainstay of prevention or symptom minimization in the future. Patients may complain of painless bleeding, possibly associated with a bowel movement or straining, itching, and possible prolapse of tissue. Symptomatic external hemorrhoids are often acute and painful. Before proceeding with any therapy for hemorrhoidal disease, patients must be assessed for sphincter dysfunction (including past surgeries and trauma from vaginal delivery) and baseline continence to both gas and stool. Patients with rectal bleeding and other indications for colon cancer screening should undergo colonoscopy as part of their evaluation. The updated guidelines now recommend beginning screening at age 45 [24]. For other patients, an individualized risk assessment should be performed to guide the need for additional or repeat testing with sigmoidoscopy or colonoscopy.

Examination

External exam and DRE should be performed to rule out any other intra-anal pathology or distal rectal masses. For patients with prolapsing hemorrhoids who do not easily exhibit the prolapse on exam, having patients use the commode to strain to reproduce their degree of prolapse may be helpful (Fig. 23.4b). For incarcerated prolapsing internal hemorrhoids, visual inspection for strangulation (i.e., ischemic changes ± necrosis) should be performed to determine the safety of reduction (versus need for more urgent excision) (Fig. 23.4c). Anoscopy can help assess which column is symptomatic (based on prolapse or friability or active bleeding) and therapeutic if the equipment is available to perform rubber band ligation (for non-strangulated internal hemorrhoids only).

Pathology

Specimens during excisional hemorrhoidectomy should be sent to pathology to review for any underlying dysplasia or malignancy.

Non-operative Management

Therapy for symptomatic internal hemorrhoids is guided by the degree of prolapse, but all patients benefit from dietary and lifestyle optimization. Patients should be instructed to increase dietary fiber to 20–35 g daily or take a fiber supplement such as psyllium. With that, it is important to increase water or any non-caffeinated and non-alcohol beverage intake to 64 ounces daily to prevent constipation. Patients should minimize straining and time on the toilet.

There are a number of office-based therapies, but most are employed in specialty offices, such as infrared photocoagulation or sclerotherapy. Elastic band ligation is a common procedure that can be utilized in patients with grade 1 and 2 and in select grade 3 internal hemorrhoids. It is performed by grasping and ligating the hemorrhoid at the apex, above the dentate line, thus correcting prolapse and decreasing the blood flow to the hemorrhoid. Before the band is placed, the patient should be asked if they feel pain or tenderness when the hemorrhoid is grasped. Typically, only 1–3 bands should be placed during a session given the risk of bleeding, urinary retention, and vasovagal reactions. Local anesthetic can be injected into the swollen hemorrhoid to prevent the band from slipping off. The band creates ischemia to the hemorrhoid, with the tissue sloughing off within the course of a week. Bleeding is an expected consequence, but can be a significant post-procedure risk, occurring up to a week after band placement (which should be avoided in patients on therapeutic anticoagulation). While rare, pelvic sepsis may occur and is characterized by fever, pain, and sometimes urinary retention. Patients should be resuscitated with IV fluids, started on IV antibiotics, and monitored with a low threshold to return to the OR for debridement.

Operative Management

Surgical excision should be offered to patients who have failed or cannot tolerate office-based procedures, have grade 3 or 4 hemorrhoids, incarcerated/strangulated hemorrhoids, or mixed internal and external hemorrhoids [25]. Hemorrhoidectomy is the most successful procedure but also carries with it an increased risk of complications as well as a significant burden of pain compared to other techniques [26].

For an excisional hemorrhoidectomy, patients undergo either monitored anesthetic care (MAC) or general anesthesia and are placed in either prone jack-knife or lithotomy position with a perineal/perianal block performed at the start of the case. DRE and anoscopy are then performed to assess and confirm which columns will be excised. With the use of a retractor, a clamp is used to grasp the hemorrhoid and lift it gently off of the underlying sphincter musculature. An elliptical incision around the external aspect of the hemorrhoid is made which is elevated off the sphincter complex. The pedicle/hemorrhoid apex internally is ligated with a 2-0 or 3-0 Chromic or other dissolvable suture to guide hemostasis and the hemorrhoid is then excised using electrocautery. Tension and retraction are obtained by using a lap pad or a gauze in the opposite hand, aiding in dissecting the hemorrhoid off of the internal and external sphincters. The defect is either closed with a running absorbable suture or left open. Locked stitches can be helpful in obtaining hemostasis and small bites of internal sphincter may also be taken to help decrease the dead space in the defect. It is imperative to maintain significant skin bridges of at least 1 cm^2 between hemorrhoidectomy specimens to prevent anal canal stenosis. If a medium-size Hill–Ferguson retractor is able to be passed after hemorrhoidectomy that would indicate a minimal risk of anal stenosis. For strangulated/necrotic grade 4 internal hemorrhoids, all necrotic tissue must be excised, thus complicating the ability to preserve anoderm and increasing the risk for postoperative anal stenosis.

Other techniques include stapled hemorrhoidopexy and transanal hemorrhoidal dearterialization, reserved more for chronic as opposed to acute hemorrhoidal symptoms. Briefly, stapled hemorrhoidopexy involves utilizing an end-to-end stapling device to circumferentially staple and resect hemorrhoidal tissue above the dentate line using a single fire. Patients experience less postoperative pain but the procedure has a higher risk of recurrence [27]. Additionally, the procedure should not be performed for patients with concurrent symptomatic external disease as the procedure only treats the internal component. Transanal hemorrhoidal dearterialization is performed using an anoscope with a doppler to locate and subsequently ligate feeding arteries and is associated with less pain that conventional excisional hemorrhoidectomy [28]. Mucopexy may also be performed at this time to treat the prolapsing columns but patients with grade 4 disease may require an additional procedure.

Special Scenarios

In the setting of symptomatic thrombosed external hemorrhoids, if the patient is unable to tolerate the pain and discomfort and it is within 3–4 days after the acute thrombosis, surgical excision of the overlying skin and clot evacuation will improve and expedite resolution of pain. If it is after that time frame, surgical intervention will not impact healing as the thrombosis has organized and contracted, and non-operative therapy is recommended (Table 23.2). In certain instances, if the OR is not available or preferred by the patient, after local blockade, an incision and enucleation of the clot can be performed to relieve patient and pressure with the understanding that there is an increased risk of recurrence.

Strangulated hemorrhoids are prolapsed internal hemorrhoids that have thrombosed and possibly necrosed. These patients often present with severe anal pain and non-reducible hemorrhoids with gross evidence of thrombosis, ischemia, and/or necrosis. Urgent hemorrhoidectomy is the mainstay of treatment. If hemorrhoids are acutely incarcerated and unable to be reduced, hemorrhoidectomy is indicated.

Table 23.2 Non-operative therapy for symptomatic thrombosed external hemorrhoids

Recommendation
Increase dietary fiber to 20–35 g daily or begin fiber supplementation and increase water intake to 64 ounces daily
Avoid straining and prolonged toileting
Sitz baths with warm water three times daily and after bowel movements
Consider topical therapies (lidocaine ointment or mixed hydrocortisone/lidocaine ointment) but do not apply steroid longer than 1 week given risk of contact dermatitis
Consider anti-spasmodics such as topical nitroglycerin or calcium channel blockers
Oral pain medications such as acetaminophen and NSAIDs as needed; narcotics should be utilized selectively due to constipating side effects

Outcomes

Urinary retention is the most common complication after hemorrhoidectomy, and the judicious use of fluids in the operating room, avoiding postoperative constipation, and pain control are important for prevention [29]. It is important to ensure that patients can urinate and are properly informed prior to discharge. Bleeding is also a common complication, as bands can fall off or erode and sutures can break or separate. Delayed bleeding can be observed 7–10 days postoperatively. Anal stenosis can occur after hemorrhoidectomy if there are insufficient skin bridges between suture lines. Dilation is often ineffective and patients may require as anocutaneous advancement flap to surgically treat the stenosis. Fecal incontinence may also occur either due to an injury from retraction, injury to the nerves or sphincter musculature, or due to loss of the hemorrhoidal cushions.

Anal Fissure

Introduction

Anal fissure refers to a tear in the anoderm of the anal canal, typically extending from the dentate line to the anal verge, and is typically associated with abnormal bowel habits, especially constipation. The hallmark symptom is anal pain, and many patients can recall the acute onset of pain during defecation that caused the anal fissure. Pain may last minutes to hours and is worse with and after bowel movements; anorectal bleeding may also be present and confuse the diagnosis for hemorrhoids. Fissures occur most commonly in the posterior midline from the stress created from the anorectal angle, but they may be present anteriorly or simultaneously both anteriorly and posteriorly. Lateral fissures are atypical and should raise clinical concern for diseases processes such as Crohn's disease, malignancy, or infectious processes such as syphilis, tuberculosis, or HIV. Acute fissures are defined as symptoms lasting less than 6–8 weeks and are likely to heal with only dietary modification, resolution of bowel habit changes, and supportive local care. Chronic anal fissures, lasting more than 6–8 weeks, are less likely to heal with conservative measures.

Work-Up

Patients will likely be able to recall the acute pain of the fissure and may recall straining or passing a hard stool. Pain or spasm may last up to several hours and there may be occasional anorectal bleeding, usually manifesting as a streak of blood on the toilet paper (versus the more typical dripping of blood in the toilet water associated with symptomatic internal hemorrhoids). Chronicity and severity of symptoms often dictate therapy.

Examination

Patients may not be able to tolerate DRE due to pain, but it is important to perform a thorough external examination to rule out any other obvious pathology. Begin by gently separating the buttocks to see the entire anoderm and overcome any local muscle spasm. An external sentinel skin tag may be present in patients with a chronic anal fissure. A cotton swab or Q-Tip can be used to lightly probe the perianal tissue to elicit tenderness and locate the position of the fissure. While most fissures are in the posterior midline, it is important to be mindful that atypical fissures can occur elsewhere and are more likely associated with other disease processes, as mentioned above. Many patients will not tolerate DRE or anoscopy given the anorectal pain and spasm, but if an internal examination is tolerated, increased sphincter tone is commonly noted. If anoscopy is tolerated, in an acute fissure, a longitudinal tear in the anoderm is visible. In a chronic fissure, an external sentinel tag at the apex is often present along with exposed internal anal sphincter muscle and a hypertrophied anal papilla (Fig. 23.4d).

Pathology

Specimens are not required for patients with typical or acute fissures; however, in patients with atypical fissures or with clinical concern for a more advanced disease process, biopsy should be considered for diagnosis, rule out cancer, and subsequently tailoring appropriate treatment.

Non-operative Management

Non-operative management is the first-line therapy for typical acute fissures as they are well tolerated and with minimal side effects. Sitz baths provide symptomatic relief and relax sphincter spasm, and fiber supplementation with a bulking agent along with increased water intake to 64 ounces daily may heal fissures alone. Topical anesthetics (e.g., lidocaine 2–5%) and OTC non-narcotic pain medications can help with discomfort associated with these fissures.

If there is no symptomatic relief from those measures, a topical compounded ointment such as nitroglycerin (0.2%) or a calcium channel blocker such as diltiazem (2%) or nifedipine (0.2–0.3%) may be employed. These topical agents have been associated with healing rates that vary widely from 49% to 89% [30–32]. Headaches may occur in patients utilizing nitroglycerin ointment up to 30%, leading to cessation of its use.

Botulinum toxin (Botox) injections, while less efficacious than surgical sphincterotomy, should be considered in patients who have failed topical agents and are at increased risk of fecal incontinence. Results typically last 3 months and can be repeated at least once if symptoms or the fissure recur.

Operative Management

Lateral internal sphincterotomy remains the gold standard for chronic anal fissure and can be performed as a first-line therapy in select patients. It can be performed in an open or closed technique with the mainstay of therapy involving dividing the lateral internal sphincter muscle to the apex of the fissure or until the palpable band of hypertrophied sphincter muscle is released in the lateral anal canal. Sphincterotomy at the site of the fissure may lead to a keyhole deformity. Sphincterotomy risks fecal incontinence if there is prior sphincter damage due to previous procedure or trauma including vaginal deliveries. Patients who fail sphincterotomy may be candidates for more advanced procedures such an anocutaneous advancement flap to cover the fissure.

Outcomes

For the initial management of a patient with an anal fissure, non-operative therapy and topical agents are low risk and should be utilized first for most patients. Botox injections have variable success, with reports ranging from 33% to 96% in the literature with no evidence of dose-dependent efficacy [33]. Lateral internal sphincterotomy has the highest rates of healing compared to other therapies with rate of healing up to 96% [34, 35].

Rectal Prolapse

Introduction

Rectal prolapse is a pelvic floor disorder in which the rectum has loss of or weakened attachments that normally keep it fixated in the pelvis, causing the rectum to protrude through the anal canal. Prolapse can either be complete (full-thickness), partial (mucosal only), or occult (does not extend beyond the anus), and common symptoms include mucous discharge or seepage or frank fecal incontinence, rectal bleeding, rectal bulge, difficulty evacuating, and anal or rectal pain or pressure. Symptoms may also be similar to the presentation of internal hemorrhoids. On examination, it is important to distinguish the orientation of the mucosal folds—prolapsing hemorrhoids have radial mucosal folds whereas rectal prolapse has circular folds of mucosa—as they require different therapies (Fig. 23.4b, e). Rectal prolapse is more common in women than men [36], occurring only rarely children [37].

Work-Up and Examination

The history should raise concern for rectal prolapse, and the physical examination is key in confirming the diagnosis. The patient should try to elicit prolapse by straining and this can be aided by the use of a commode to simulate defecation. It is important to note how much prolapse is present. Examination will also commonly reveal a patulous anus with decreased sphincter tone. Proctoscopy may show distal rectal inflammation and/or a solitary rectal ulcer. In a patient with additional vaginal vault or urinary symptoms, urogynecologic exam should be performed and urodynamics should be considered. These patients may require a multidisciplinary team for appropriate repair.

Some patients present acutely with incarcerated or strangulated rectal prolapse. If reduction of incarcerated prolapse is not successful or if the prolapse is strangulated, the patient will need to proceed with emergent surgery. A transabdominal approach should be avoided in these cases, favoring a transanal approach known as a perineal proctectomy to resect the ischemic tissue.

Non-operative Management

The mainstay of treatment for rectal prolapse is operative repair, but in those patients who are too high risk or minimally symptomatic, non-operative management may be entertained with the understanding that non-operative therapy can only palliate but not resolve prolapse. Fiber and stool softeners may help regulate bowel movements and prevent diarrhea and constipation, common precipitating factors for rectal prolapse. Pelvic floor physical therapy may help with continence issues.

Patients must be counseled on appropriate techniques for manual reduction. Lying in Trendelenburg position with gentle pressure on the prolapse may reduce the rectum back into the pelvic cavity alone. If that is not successful, table sugar can be placed topically on the prolapse to decrease the edema and thus facilitate reduction [38].

Operative Management

For the acute rectal prolapse that is either incarcerated and unable to be reduced and/or strangulated, perineal proctectomy (Altemeier) is the procedure of choice. Altemeier initially described his technique in 1952, and the procedure remains widely used today in the acute setting and for patients who are weak, debilitated, and/or with severe co-morbidities and thus at increased risk from a transabdominal procedure [39]. A perineal approach minimizes contaminating the abdominal cavity in the setting of strangulation or perforation (which is difficult to reduce from above via a transabdominal procedure regardless). The procedure can be performed without general anesthesia (e.g., spinal anesthesia) in patients at increased risk. However, the procedure can also safely be performed for many patients under general anesthesia and in prone jack-knife position. The buttocks are gently taped apart and a self-retaining retractor may also be utilized for exposure. A circumferential incision is made with electrocautery 2–5 cm proximal to the dentate line and continued through all layers of the rectal wall and to the mesorectal fat with continuous attention to meticulous hemostasis. An energy device such as a LigaSure can be utilized to then divide the mesorectum circumferentially. The anterior cul-de-sac is then entered, and tension is placed on the prolapsed segment to determine the extent of resection needed to eliminate any redundancy of the rectum and distal colon. The mesorectum is divided circumferentially until the point of modest tension to ensure viability of the anastomosis while resecting sufficient intestine to prevent recurrence, and the remaining mesentery is divided flush to the bowel wall. Levatorplasty of the levator ani musculature may be considered. The bowel is then incised with electrocautery on the posterior aspect and 3-0 Vicryl (or silk, if preferred) full-thickness stay sutures are placed from the proximal and distal

tion may lead to the development of anogenital warts, which may be present on the external genitalia, perineum, anal canal, or surrounding skin. The condyloma are typically soft papules or plaques and may be single or multiple; they may vary in appearance from simple and flat to cauliflower-shaped and fungating. Diagnosis is typically made by physical examination alone, but biopsy can be performed if the diagnosis is unclear.

Patients with external warts should be assessed for risk factors for other STIs including HIV and other immunocompromised states. The urethral orifice and anal canal should also be examined in patients with external warts; women should also undergo speculum examination.

While genital warts may spontaneously resolve in up to 30% of patients, patients should be offered treatment given the risk of the disease enlarging or the growth of new lesions [50]. Treatment ranges from topical medications to surgical removal with excision and fulguration. Patients with a small burden of disease may elect to proceed with topical therapy rather than surgery. Topical prescription agents that patients may use to treat at home include Imiquimod, Podophyllotoxin, and Sinecatechins [49]. Patients may also elect to undergo ablation with either cryotherapy, trichloroacetic acid, or surgical removal with excision and/or fulguration [49]. Surgery is best suited for patients with large condyloma or a more extensive burden of disease. Representative specimens should be sent to pathology to rule out any underlying dysplasia or malignancy.

Pilonidal Disease

Introduction

Pilonidal disease results from traumatization and injury of the skin and hair follicles in the natal cleft resulting from trapping of hairs and local injury. While many patients are asymptomatic, some may develop a granulomatous foreign body-type reaction and subsequently develop areas of acute induration and infection.

Work-Up

Patients may complain of a lump with occasional drainage (serous or purulent) or may be entirely asymptomatic. It is important to assess the degree of discomfort and interference with the patient's life as the definitive surgical therapy can often be quite uncomfortable and can often be more uncomfortable and painful than the disease itself. Patients who have developed an abscess may experience worsening pain, increased drainage, fever, and erythema or induration of the affected region. It is important to note how many procedures the patient has undergone (either I&D or even attempts at definitive surgery) to help understand the burden of disease for the patient.

Examination

Pits are commonly observed in the midline intergluteal cleft with associated induration lateral to the midline in acutely infected cysts. Additional draining sinuses and tunneling tracts may also be present. The area should be palpated to assess for an abscess—key physical exam findings such as an area of fluctuance or induration with associated erythema or tenderness should point to that diagnosis.

Non-operative Management

Definitive surgical therapy can often be quite painful and lead to large wounds for the patient to heal, so patients who are asymptomatic or only mildly symptomatic may elect for non-operative management. Risk factor modification can be helpful in prevention of acute abscess. Patients are encouraged to avoid prolonged sitting and clip or removal the hair in the affected area. Weight loss can also help in the obese patient.

Operative Management

For an infected pilonidal cyst, I&D of the abscess is the mainstay of therapy. Definitive therapy should not be proceeded with in the case of an acute infection but patients may elect to undergo definitive therapy later, with options that range from more to less invasive. Excisional therapy of the cyst and sinus tracts is commonly performed and may lead to a large wound to manage. It is surgeon preference whether to excise all tracts down to the level of the sacrococcygeal fascia or to unroof and debride the tracts without a full excision. The wound can subsequently be left open to close by secondary intention with packing with gauze dampened with normal saline one to two times daily, marsupialized to decrease the overall wound size but still leave it open to drainage, closed primarily with the risk of abscess, or closed with a flap technique, which is a more advanced procedure.

Pit picking is a less invasive procedure than can be performed in the clinic or the operating room and entails excising the epithelial lining of central pits to a margin of skin typically less than 1 mm as well as the associated lateral fistula tracts. All retained hair is evacuated and the wound is either closed or left open. The procedure is less invasive than a complete excision, thus decreasing wound morbidity, pain, and time to recovery for the patient. Some patients may require an additional procedure if still symptomatic. The overall risk of complication and recurrence is low, and as the procedure is well tolerated in an office setting, if additional procedures are required it is at low risk to the patient [51, 52].

Outcomes

Wound morbidity is a challenge for patients with pilonidal disease. While wounds may heal more quickly when primary closure is employed, there is a greater risk of recurrence of disease if the wound is not left open [53]. While the overall reported incidence of recurrence is rare, estimated at 8%, healing by secondary intention may lead to a 58% lower risk of recurrence compared to a closed wound [54]. It is important to take in account wound morbidity as well as risk of recurrence when managing patients with pilonidal disease.

Foreign Body

Description

Rectal foreign bodies can be a challenge to manage, as they can be caused by a variety of objects and lead to variable degrees of rectal trauma. Placement may be voluntary or forced, and it is important to remain sensitive to the patient and the circumstances. While it is more common for foreign bodies to be introduced voluntarily through sexual practice, it is important to be aware that foreign bodies may arise also involuntarily through rape or through body-packing of substances, for example. Patients may feel uncomfortable disclosing this information, and their presentation may be delayed by hours to days due to fear or embarrassment.

Work-Up and Examination

As patients may be reluctant to disclose all details, direct questioning may help in obtaining an accurate history. Eliciting duration of symptoms and timing of placement may be helpful in triaging injury or ischemic or perforation risk. Physical examination is helpful in determining if the patient has a benign or peritonitic abdomen, and DRE may be diagnostic or even therapeutic (although this should be avoided until the nature and safety of the item is confirmed to avoid injury to the patient or provider). However, absence of foreign body on DRE does not exclude its presence as it may have migrated more proximally. Plain radiographs may help locate the foreign body and evaluate for pneumoperitoneum. CT scan should not be routinely performed but can be considered when there is suspicion for a radiolucent foreign body.

Management

Patients who have signs of sepsis or perforation should be resuscitated, given appropriate antibiotics, and undergo emergent surgical intervention. Stable patients may be observed first to see if the foreign body will pass distally but there should be a low threshold to proceed with extraction.

Most foreign bodies can be removed transanally [55]. Adequate patient relaxation is imperative and can be achieved with intravenous sedation and perianal nerve blockade. Lithotomy is the preferred position for adequate access to the perineum and abdomen. After relaxation, it may be easier to grasp the foreign body either digitally or with a clamp or forceps. Blunt objects may create a seal around the rectum. Passing a foley catheter or insufflating air with a colonoscope above the object to break the seal may aid in removal. Using endoscopic techniques including snare or obstetrical tools such as forceps or vacuum devices have also been employed in extracting foreign bodies [56, 57].

In the event of a sharp object, blind or manual extraction should not be attempted due to the risk of injury, both to surgeon and to the patient. Sharp objects may cause significant trauma and have increased risk of rectal perforation and warrant extraction under direct visualization. In the unique setting of body-packing, in which drug-filled packets are placed into a body cavity such as the rectum to conceal the paraphernalia, sharp instrumentation should be avoided as they risk injuring the packet and causing systemic absorption of the agent, possibly leading to overdose and death. Patients should undergo endoscopy after foreign body extraction to rule out injury and ensure viability to the rectum, especially after a sharp or difficult-to-remove object has been extracted.

Objects that are more proximal in the rectum or in the sigmoid colon may require a combined perineal and abdominal approach [55]. The assistant can press on the abdomen to help guide the foreign body to the pelvis. If those techniques are unsuccessful, a small laparotomy may be required. In the absence of perforation or injury, a colotomy is not required as the foreign body can be manipulated down to the pelvis with the guidance of the surgeon below. If this is unsuccessful, a colotomy can be made to extract the specimen. Proximal diversion is not required in the absence of perforation or gross spillage.

Summary and Key Points

Management of acute perianal disease often presents a diagnostic challenge to the provider, and accurate diagnosis is key to tailoring appropriate therapy for the patient.

- Perianal abscess is successfully treated by I&D, but if there is recurrence, be mindful of a potential fistula and the need for subsequent definitive procedures.
- Acute anal fissure can usually be successfully managed non-operatively, but may require Botox or sphincterotomy if these interventions fail as the fissure becomes more chronic.
- Most patients presenting with hemorrhoidal complaints can be managed by non-operative therapy; however, those with strangulated or incarcerated hemorrhoids require definitive excisional hemorrhoidectomy. Thrombosed external hemorrhoids may require excision if non-operative therapy fails.
- Rectal prolapse can often be manually reduced; sugar may be employed to decrease edema. In the event of incarceration and strangulation, perineal proctectomy is indicated.
- STIs require thoughtful consideration of possible etiologies and etiology-directed treatments.
- For an infected pilonidal cyst, I&D is recommended. Definitive therapy should be avoided in the setting of acute infection.

References

1. Ho YH, et al. Randomized controlled trial of primary fistulotomy with drainage alone for perianal abscesses. Dis Colon Rectum. 1997;40(12):1435–8.
2. Sahnan K, et al. Persistent fistula after anorectal abscess drainage: local experience of 11 years. Dis Colon Rectum. 2019;62(3):327–32.
3. Sahnan K, et al. Natural history of anorectal sepsis. Br J Surg. 2017;104(13):1857–65.
4. Gunawardhana PA, Deen KI. Comparison of hydrogen peroxide instillation with Goodsall's rule for fistula-in-ano. ANZ J Surg. 2001;71(8):472–4.
5. Cirocco WC, Reilly JC. Challenging the predictive accuracy of Goodsall's rule for anal fistulas. Dis Colon Rectum. 1992;35(6):537–42.

6. Barwood N, et al. Fistula-in-ano: a prospective study of 107 patients. Aust N Z J Surg. 1997;67(2–3):98–102.
7. Parks AG, Gordon PH, Hardcastle JD. A classification of fistula-in-ano. Br J Surg. 1976;63(1):1–12.
8. Mocanu V, et al. Antibiotic use in prevention of anal fistulas following incision and drainage of anorectal abscesses: a systematic review and meta-analysis. Am J Surg. 2019;217(5):910–7.
9. Sözener U, et al. Does adjuvant antibiotic treatment after drainage of anorectal abscess prevent development of anal fistulas? A randomized, placebo-controlled, double-blind, multicenter study. Dis Colon Rectum. 2011;54(8):923–9.
10. Vogel JD, et al. Clinical practice guideline for the management of anorectal abscess, fistula-in-ano, and rectovaginal fistula. Dis Colon Rectum. 2016;59(12):1117–33.
11. Malik AI, Nelson RL, Tou S. Incision and drainage of perianal abscess with or without treatment of anal fistula. Cochrane Database Syst Rev. 2010;7:CD006827.
12. Hall JF, et al. Outcomes after operations for anal fistula: results of a prospective, multicenter, regional study. Dis Colon Rectum. 2014;57(11):1304–8.
13. Abramowitz L, et al. The outcome of fistulotomy for anal fistula at 1 year: a prospective multicentre French study. Color Dis. 2016;18(3):279–85.
14. Garcia-Aguilar J, et al. Anal fistula surgery. Factors associated with recurrence and incontinence. Dis Colon Rectum. 1996;39(7):723–9.
15. Abbas MA, Jackson CH, Haigh PI. Predictors of outcome for anal fistula surgery. Arch Surg. 2011;146(9):1011–6.
16. Rosa G, et al. Fistula in ano: anatomoclinical aspects, surgical therapy and results in 844 patients. Tech Coloproctol. 2006;10(3):215–21.
17. van Koperen PJ, et al. Long-term functional outcome and risk factors for recurrence after surgical treatment for low and high perianal fistulas of cryptoglandular origin. Dis Colon Rectum. 2008;51(10):1475–81.
18. Visscher AP, et al. Long-term follow-up after surgery for simple and complex cryptoglandular fistulas: fecal incontinence and impact on quality of life. Dis Colon Rectum. 2015;58(5):533–9.
19. Ritchie RD, Sackier JM, Hodde JP. Incontinence rates after cutting seton treatment for anal fistula. Color Dis. 2009;11(6):564–71.
20. Stellingwerf ME, et al. Systematic review and meta-analysis of endorectal advancement flap and ligation of the intersphincteric fistula tract for cryptoglandular and Crohn's high perianal fistulas. BJS Open. 2019;3(3):231–41.
21. Sandler RS, Peery AF. Rethinking what we know about hemorrhoids. Clin Gastroenterol Hepatol. 2019;17(1):8–15.
22. Schubert MC, et al. What every gastroenterologist needs to know about common anorectal disorders. World J Gastroenterol. 2009;15(26):3201–9.
23. Haas PA, Fox TA Jr, Haas GP. The pathogenesis of hemorrhoids. Dis Colon Rectum. 1984;27(7):442–50.
24. Wolf AMD, et al. Colorectal cancer screening for average-risk adults: 2018 guideline update from the American Cancer Society. CA Cancer J Clin. 2018;68(4):250–81.
25. Shanmugam V, et al. Rubber band ligation versus excisional haemorrhoidectomy for haemorrhoids. Cochrane Database Syst Rev. 2005;(3):CD005034.
26. MacRae HM, McLeod RS. Comparison of hemorrhoidal treatments: a meta-analysis. Can J Surg. 1997;40(1):14–7.
27. Jayaraman S, Colquhoun PH, Malthaner RA. Stapled hemorrhoidopexy is associated with a higher long-term recurrence rate of internal hemorrhoids compared with conventional excisional hemorrhoid surgery. Dis Colon Rectum. 2007;50(9):1297–305.
28. Popov V, et al. Doppler-guided transanal hemorrhoidal dearterilization versus conventional hemorrhoidectomy for treatment of hemorrhoids—early and long-term postoperative results. BMC Surg. 2019;19(1):4.
29. Toyonaga T, et al. Postoperative urinary retention after surgery for benign anorectal disease: potential risk factors and strategy for prevention. Int J Color Dis. 2006;21(7):676–82.
30. Sanei B, Mahmoodieh M, Masoudpour H. Comparison of topical glyceryl trinitrate with diltiazem ointment for the treatment of chronic anal fissure: a randomized clinical trial. Acta Chir Belg. 2009;109(6):727–30.
31. Ezri T, Susmallian S. Topical nifedipine vs. topical glyceryl trinitrate for treatment of chronic anal fissure. Dis Colon Rectum. 2003;46(6):805–8.
32. Nelson RL, et al. Non surgical therapy for anal fissure. Cochrane Database Syst Rev. 2012;2012(2):CD003431.
33. Bobkiewicz A, et al. Botulinum toxin injection for treatment of chronic anal fissure: is there any dose-dependent efficiency? A meta-analysis. World J Surg. 2016;40(12):3064–72.
34. Nelson RL. Anal fissure (chronic). BMJ Clin Evid. 2014;2014:0407.
35. Arslan K, et al. Lateral internal sphincterotomy versus 0.25% isosorbide dinitrate ointment for chronic anal fissures: a prospective randomized controlled trial. Surg Today. 2013;43(5):500–5.
36. Kairaluoma MV, Kellokumpu IH. Epidemiologic aspects of complete rectal prolapse. Scand J Surg. 2005;94(3):207–10.
37. Cares K, El-Baba M. Rectal prolapse in children: significance and management. Curr Gastroenterol Rep. 2016;18(5):22.
38. Myers JO, Rothenberger DA. Sugar in the reduction of incarcerated prolapsed bowel. Report of two cases. Dis Colon Rectum. 1991;34(5):416–8.
39. Altemeier WA, Giuseffi J, Hoxworth P. Treatment of extensive prolapse of the rectum in aged or debilitated patients. AMA Arch Surg. 1952;65(1):72–80.
40. Riansuwan W, et al. Comparison of perineal operations with abdominal operations for full-thickness rectal prolapse. World J Surg. 2010;34(5):1116–22.

41. Ris F, et al. Altemeier's procedure for rectal prolapse: analysis of long-term outcome in 60 patients. Color Dis. 2012;14(9):1106–11.
42. Habr-Gama A, et al. Rectal procidentia treatment by perineal rectosigmoidectomy combined with levator ani repair. Hepato-Gastroenterology. 2006;53(68):213–7.
43. Glasgow SC, et al. Recurrence and quality of life following perineal proctectomy for rectal prolapse. J Gastrointest Surg. 2008;12(8):1446–51.
44. Byrne CM, et al. Long-term functional outcomes after laparoscopic and open rectopexy for the treatment of rectal prolapse. Dis Colon Rectum. 2008;51(11):1597–604.
45. de Bruijn H, et al. Long-term outcome of laparoscopic rectopexy for full-thickness rectal prolapse. Tech Coloproctol. 2019;23(1):25–31.
46. Postillon A, et al. Long-term outcomes of robotic ventral mesh rectopexy for external rectal prolapse. Surg Endosc. 2020;34(2):930–9.
47. Chun SW, et al. Perineal rectosigmoidectomy for rectal prolapse: role of levatorplasty. Tech Coloproctol. 2004;8(1):3–8; discussion 8–9.
48. Nguyen XH, et al. Case series: incarcerated massive rectal prolapse successfully treated with Altemeier's procedure. Int J Surg Case Rep. 2018;51:309–12.
49. Workowski KA, Bolan GA. Sexually transmitted diseases treatment guidelines, 2015. MMWR Recomm Rep. 2015;64(Rr-03):1–137.
50. Yanofsky VR, Patel RV, Goldenberg G. Genital warts: a comprehensive review. J Clin Aesthet Dermatol. 2012;5(6):25–36.
51. Gips M, et al. Minimal surgery for pilonidal disease using trephines: description of a new technique and long-term outcomes in 1,358 patients. Dis Colon Rectum. 2008;51(11):1656–62; discussion 1662–3.
52. Di Castro A, et al. Minimally invasive surgery for the treatment of pilonidal disease. The Gips procedure on 2347 patients. Int J Surg. 2016;36(Pt A):201–5.
53. McCallum IJ, King PM, Bruce J. Healing by primary closure versus open healing after surgery for pilonidal sinus: systematic review and meta-analysis. BMJ. 2008;336(7649):868–71.
54. McCallum I, King PM, Bruce J. Healing by primary versus secondary intention after surgical treatment for pilonidal sinus. Cochrane Database Syst Rev. 2007;(4):CD006213.
55. Lake JP, et al. Management of retained colorectal foreign bodies: predictors of operative intervention. Dis Colon Rectum. 2004;47(10):1694–8.
56. Johnson SO, Hartranft TH. Nonsurgical removal of a rectal foreign body using a vacuum extractor. Report of a case. Dis Colon Rectum. 1996;39(8):935–7.
57. Singaporewalla RM, Tan DE, Tan TK. Use of endoscopic snare to extract a large rectosigmoid foreign body with review of literature. Surg Laparosc Endosc Percutan Tech. 2007;17(2):145–8.

Complications After Metabolic and Bariatric Operations

24

Kimberly A. Davis and Dirk C. Johnson

Complications After Metabolic and Bariatric Operations

A 45-year-old woman with a past surgical history significant for laparoscopic Roux-en-Y gastric bypass 6 years earlier presents with diffuse abdominal pain and distension for 24 h. She has had similar intermittent symptoms over the past year, but this episode has lasted for longer than her typical duration. She has lost over 105 pounds from her heaviest with a current BMI of 29. Computed tomography demonstrates small bowel dilatation of the Roux limb with swirling of the associated mesenteric vessels. Emergent laparoscopic exploration by the on-call acute care surgeon showed the Roux limb had herniated through a defect formed by the potential space between the transverse mesocolon, retroperitoneum, and the Roux limb mesentery. The small bowel was repositioned and the defect was closed with running suture. She had an uneventful recovery.

K. A. Davis
Division of General Surgery, Trauma and Surgical Critical Care, Surgery, Yale School of Medicine, New Haven, CT, USA
e-mail: kimberly.davis@yale.edu

D. C. Johnson (✉)
Yale University, School of Medicine, New Haven, CT, USA
e-mail: dirk.johnson@yale.edu

Obesity has long been as significant negative health predictor. In recent years, it has gained increasing recognition international as major public health issues. With this recognition, our options for management have expanded from purely medical and behavioral options to include surgical therapies. Sporadic reports of weight loss operations date back to the tenth century but the rise of modern bariatric surgery did not begin until the 1990s [1]. Since then, its usage has steadily increased with over a quarter of a million being performed annual. Bariatric surgery is highly effective. It leads to sustained weight loss, improvement of obesity-related comorbidities and mortality, and improvement of quality of life.

Historically bariatric surgery was performed with open techniques, but the field was revolutionized in 1994 when the first laparoscopic procedure was performed setting the stage for the exponential growth in its usage worldwide. It continues to be one of the fasting growing segments of the surgical care. Being able to recognize and treat the complications that are bound to develop afterward, as with all medical procedures, is essential for acute care surgeons. Fortunately, many standard general surgical principles are applicable to these patients, but specific conditions related to the various bariatric operations should influence the differential diagnoses considered. Additionally, altered postsurgical anatomy may impact management priorities and options in many instances.

M. D. Zielinski, O. Guillamondegui (eds.), *The Acute Management of Surgical Disease*,
https://doi.org/10.1007/978-3-031-07881-1_24

Common of Operations

The two major physiologic underpinnings produce long-term weight loss after metabolic and bariatric procedures. Operations can be classified as restrictive, malabsorptive, or a combination of both. Restrictive procedures reduce gastric volume available to store ingested food. Malabsorptive procedures exclude a length of small bowel from the absorptive process, thereby allowing food to bypass the excluded segment. There are some significant hormonal changes related to all bariatric operations which are poorly understood due to conflicting results of studies. These changes may contribute to the weight loss or simple be a result of the operation [2].

Biliopancreatic diversion with or without duodenal switch (BPD/DS), laparoscopic adjustable gastric banding (LAGB), Roux-en-Y gastric bypass (RYGB), and sleeve gastrectomy are the most commonly bariatric operation performed. These four established options have shifted dramatically in relative popularity in the past two decades. The latter two account for over 90% cases in recent years with SG gaining market share annually while RYGB is waning. LAGB and BPD/DS account for less than 5% of procedures in the USA annually [3]. SG evolved into an independent bariatric procedure after first being described as the first stage of planned biliopancreatic diversion and has been recommended for over a decade.

SG is favored due to technical ease, short learning curve, and similar rapid initial weight loss and impact on weight-related conditions as RYGB. There is greater long-term excess weight loss with malabsorptive procedures like RYBG but the clinical significance of this advantage continues to be debated. Although RYGB is still considered "the gold standard," SG now accounts for over half of the weight loss operations performed in the USA.

The only pure malabsorptive operation is the traditional biliopancreatic diversion which is rarely performed insolation or as a primary weight loss operation. Instead, it is most often combined with a SG and dubbed duodenal switch. The DS and RYGB combine both malabsorptive and restrictive principles to achieve weight loss. The gastric band, in contrast, is a purely restrictive procedure.

The LAGB is the safest but least effective option for weight loss and resolution of comorbid conditions. BPD is the highest risk operation but most effective. SG has low morbidity and mortality, good results in reduction of excess weight although less than RYGB and BPD/DS. The RYGB has similar impact on comorbidities and short-term morbidity and mortality rates as SG but has longer operative times and long-term risks [4].

General Postoperative Surgical Complications

Bariatric patients are at risk for typical postoperative complications of abdominal operations like myocardial infarctions, pulmonary embolism, surgical site infections, and incisional hernias. The nature of the operation and required patient characteristic for metabolic and bariatric operations are inherent risk factures for many of these. Pulmonary embolism (PE) risk tracks with BMI and increased for open as compared to laparoscopic operations. The rate is low but PE is the most common cause of perioperative mortality after bariatric surgery. PE is frequently identified in patients that have other postoperative complications. Diabetes and obesity are also risk factures for surgical site infections and hernias. Incisional hernias are significantly higher in open operations than in the now much more common laparoscopic procedures.

Nutritional Deficiencies

The nutritional consequences of bariatric procedures could potentially hinder the clinical benefits of this therapeutic option. The anatomic alterations make patients susceptible to developing nutritional deficiencies of nutrients, both micro and macro, and series disease states such as anemia, osteoporosis, protein malnutrition. Most obese patients have nutritional deficits prior to surgery, the most importantly vitamin D and iron, which should be identified and addressed. However, these issues can persist in the postoperative patients and impact perioperative management of subsequent operations.

Protein malnutrition, associated with malabsorptive procedures, is the most severe macronutrient complication. The incidence of protein calorie malnutrition is up to 20% after BPD/DS and is also seen in 10% of patients after RYGB, particularly when the Roux limb is longer than 150 cm. Vitamins D and B-12 deficiencies are the most common which is why these patients are routinely prescribed postoperative supplementation. Decreased absorption of vitamin D increases the risk of osteoporosis due to secondary hyperparathyroidism. The loss of acidification by the anatomic rearrangement inactivates intrinsic factor and negatively impacts iron and B-12 levels [5].

While less common in SG and LAGB, maladaptive eating behaviors can also leave patients with protein malnutrition. Clinical signs are edema, hearing loss, and hypoalbuminemia. Dumping syndrome, which occurs in 5–10% of patients, and hypoglycemia which is much more rare (<1%) can be seen after RYGB but also after SG. Life-long monitoring of nutritional status and supplementation of minerals and vitamins as needed can prevent deficiencies after bariatric surgery [6].

Cholecystitis and Symptomatic Cholelithiasis

Bariatric surgery predisposes patients to develop gallstones [7]. Changes in entero-hepatic circulation, gallbladder emptying, and hormones may lead to formation of stones or make formerly silent stones become symptomatic. The development of symptomatic cholelithiasis is related to the amount and speed of weight loss. Patients may have pain which is not postprandial or other atypical symptoms because of rearranged anatomy, delayed transmissions from the signaling apparatus for gallbladder contraction. The risks of biliary symptoms after bariatric operations are highest 3–18 months after surgery, paralleling the period of peak weight loss. Some bariatric surgeons perform cholecystectomy at the time of weight loss operation while others suppress stone formation with ursodeoxycholic acid for 6 months postoperatively [8].

If gastrointestinal anatomy is preserved, standard management of biliary disease applies. Common procedures for biliary colic or cholecystitis such as laparoscopic cholecystectomy with or without intraoperative cholangiogram can be performed with little trouble. Cholangiography should be performed routinely in patients with malabsorptive procedures where postoperative endoscopic access the common bile duct would be difficult. Inspection of the bariatric surgical anatomy while in the operating room to ensure there are no other pathologies is recommended.

Procedure-Specific Postoperative Surgical Complications

Biliopancreatic Diversion With or Without Duodenal Switch

Both technical difficulty and high potential morbidity have been identified as impediments to wider adoption of BPD despite the best long-term results for both weight loss and resolution of comorbidities. The classic BPD required two anastomoses but was modified to require just one and combined with a SG.

Due to sporadic use, it is difficult to draw definitive conclusions about the risk of complications. A recent review identified 12 studies for a meta-analysis which included less than 600 patients in total. A 5% complication rate was reported, with diarrhea being the most common acute complication. Staple line and anastomotic leaks, bowel obstruction, gastroesophageal reflux, bleeding, and hernias were reported. However, each was a relatively rare event occur in less than 1% of patients [9]. Excessive side effects or weight loss may require revision or reversal is can be challenging.

directly accessible from the stomach. A standard ERCP is not an option for stone extraction. Highly skilled endoscopists may be able to reach the ampulla via the roux limb with a pediatric colonoscope or specialized double-balloon endoscopy. Transhepatic cholangiography with percutaneous access with image guidance is an option for decompression. Surgical common bile duct exploration, or surgical assisted ERCP, the "rendezvous" procedure, where a surgeon laparoscopically accesses the excluded stomach remnant for the gastroenterologist to get to the ampulla of Vater with a standard side viewing ERCP scope, may be needed to remove the obstruction. A newer technique uses endoscopic ultrasound to access the gastric remnant with a metal stent thus creating a pathway for an otherwise standard ERCP.

Anastomotic Leaks

Anastomotic failure is the most feared complication of all bariatric procedures because it increases risk of other morbidities and mortality [19, 20]. The rate is reported around 2% for RYGB [4]. It leads to increases in hospital lengths of stay and may result in long-term issues like fistulae. Super morbidly obese patients (preoperative BMI >50 kg/m^2) and those having revision bariatric operations are most at risk for leaks [21–23]. Persistent tachycardia, shortness of breath, fevers, and abdominal pain are signs of a leak. Typically, leaks are an early complication presenting on average on postoperative day 3 [24]. Most bariatric patients are discharged by POD2 and the leak is often diagnosed in an emergency department. The only symptom may be tachycardia which should heighten suspicion of a leak and rapid investigation. Pulmonary and cardiac evaluation is essential as thromboembolic events are also possible. After these are ruled out, emergency return to the OR for either laparoscopic or open exploration is the next step. When choosing laparoscopy versus open approach hemodynamic status and surgeon comfort should be considered. There are three main goals: reduce contamination, control the leak, and feeding access. Closing the leak is not mandatory and may not be safe or possible. If a repair is undertaken, interrupted sutures and omental patching are recommended.

If hemodynamic status allows, other causes for tachycardia, such as hemorrhage, volume depletion, and sepsis from other causes (i.e., pneumonia), should guide the need for reoperation. An abdominal computed tomography (CT) with a small volume of oral contrast (100 cc) immediately prior to the scan will detect most leaks [24, 25]. Additionally, CT may rule in or out other diseases on the differential diagnosis. Evidence of an abscess, phlegmon, or fluid collection on CT should be treated as a leak even if no frank extravasation is identified. An upper GI series, while less sensitive, can be used as an alternative imaging modality. Neither CT nor upper GI series is sensitive for distal leaks at a jejuno-jejunal or jejunal-ileal anastomosis. There should be a low threshold for surgical exploration for patients with persistent tachycardia ($P > 120$), even without radiographic suggestion, if no other etiology of shock can be identified because 20–40% of leaks do not have radiographic signs. Negative laparoscopic exploration seems to have no impact on postoperative results [5]. In the absence of sepsis physiology, leaks can be managed with percutaneous image-guided drainage and bowel rest.

Leaks after bariatric operations are not unique to RYGB. All procedures with intestinal anastomosis have a reported leak rated with BPD/DS having the highest rate at nearly 5%. RYGB is next followed closely by SG at slightly above and below 2%, respectively. The intraluminal pressure of the intestine at the level of the leak leads to different management considerations and paradigms. The gastric pouch of RYGB has low-pressure system because the pylorus has been excluded. *Sleeve leaks*, on the other hand, occur in a high-pressure system and their management will be discussed later. For RYGB leaks, operative or non-operative simply controls effluent without definitive closure can effectively treat a alone in over 70% of cases [26]. Endoscopic placed clips, covered stents, or a vacuum dressings can help close chronic or persistent leaks lasting longer than 30 days [27]. Nutrition is an essential adjunct to healing leaks and preferably provided with distal enteral feeding. TPN may be necessary if distal feeding tube cannot be placed in the Roux limb, biliopancreatic limb, or common channel safely.

Hemodynamic instability in the postoperative period should raise high suspicion for a leak and be treated with as such with surgical exploration whether the diagnosis is confirmed or not. The operation should focus on control of contamination, drainage, and feeding access. Following surgery, the patient should receive 4 days of intravenous antibiotics and restriction of oral intake until the leak is sealed. Image-guided drainage is more appropriate for stable patients and may be supplemented with endoscopic interventions.

Hemorrhage

Among the most concerning of all postoperative complications is bleeding. Some report the rate around 10% but the vast majority resolve without reoperation [28, 29]. Potentially life-threatening bleeding requires establishment of adequate IV access and balanced blood component resuscitation with packed cells, plasma, and platelets supplemented with crystalloid. Progress is monitored with serial blood counts and vital signs. All anticoagulants must be stopped, and coagulopathies corrected.

Patients unresponsive to transfusions or who have continued hemodynamic instability need emergency exploration. Common sites of bleeding are the anastomoses, mesentery, omentum, and spleen. If no hemoperitoneum or bleeding source is identified evaluate intraluminal possibilities including the gastric remnant, biliopancreatic limb, and Roux limb as alternatives. Endoscopic examination and intervention can be done safely by an experienced endoscopist as first-line treatment with surgical support as a backup.

For patients with better clinical status determination of intraluminal and extraluminal sources of hemorrhage is key establishing management strategy. Intraluminal bleeding may be managed with resuscitation and urgent endoscopy gastroscopy. Extraluminal bleeding from staple lines, spleen, liver, or abdominal wall is managed surgically with laparoscopic or open evacuation of hemoperitoneum and establishing hemostasis. Hemorrhages can also be treated with endovascular therapies but should be used with extreme caution when the source is near the site of an anastomosis.

Marginal Ulcers

Marginal ulcers are a result of gastric acid injuring the jejunal mucosa at the gastro-jejunal anastomosis. Epigastric burning pain is the most frequent symptom and is present in over half of patients. The next most common presentation is bleeding, seen in 15% of patients [30]. Marginal ulceration is a postoperative complication occurring in 5% or more of RYGB patients [30, 31]. Typical peptic ulcers in the first portion of the duodenum are in the literature and should be considered during the work up [32]. Marginal ulcers may be associated with fistulas to either the gastric remnant or colon. Smoking, nonsteroidal anti-inflammatory drug use, or noncompliance with acid suppression therapy may be clues from the patients' history. Ischemia from anastomotic tension and *Helicobacter pylori* infection are also contributing factors to ulcer formation. Patients sometimes present with bleeding, but more often with nausea, abdominal pain, obstructive symptoms from anastomotic stenosis, or peritonitis due to perforation. Treatment with proton pump inhibitors for acid suppression and follow endoscopy after 6 weeks has a high rate of success. Nonsteroidal anti-inflammatory drugs should be avoided, *H. pylori* infections treated, and counseling for smoking cessation offered. Evaluation for gastro-gastric or gastro-colic fistula with UGI series or CT should be performed. When medical management of marginal ulcers fails or is not safe due to the condition of the patient, surgery may necessary. Patients with perforations, persistent pain, or recurrent bleeding even with maximal medical therapy may require operations. Patients with contained leaks on imaging may be managed with percutaneous drainage. However, those with uncontained perforation should undergo exploration. Stable patients can be referred to a bariatric center for revision of the gastrojejunostomy [33]. Unstable patients can have perforations covered with an omental patch, removal of contamination, and feeding tube placement. If the anastomosis is stenotic, the GJ revision should deferred to at a later operation when the patient is more stable.

Bleeding from marginal ulcers is relatively common but massive hemorrhage is rare [31]. A classic presentation with melena or bright red blood per rectum, hematemesis, and hemodynamic compromise is common. Management follows traditional algorithms consisting of large-bore intravenous access, correction of coagulopathies, fluid and balanced blood component resuscitation, and acid suppression. Bleeding from the GJA can be controlled with endoscopically with only a minority of patients requiring operative control of bleeding. When surgery is required, the ulcer should be resected entirely and the GJA revised in an unaffected area of the gastric pouch. Non-healing ulcers or large/dilated gastric pouches may need elective revision or referral to a bariatric center. After management of the acute issue, patients with marginal ulcers should be counseled against smoking and NSAID usage.

Anastomotic Strictures (Stenosis)

Stricture occurs when GJA orifice is narrowed from inflammation or ischemia. An accumulation of scar tissue blocks or slows food from passing through the gastric pouch to the small bowel. Patients report symptoms include of dysphagia, nausea, vomiting, or inability to tolerate food. Strictures can be either acute or chronic. If found in the immediately postoperative period, most strictures will resolve with non-operative care of bowel rest, intravenous fluids, and nutritional support. If they persist, endoscopic pneumatic dilation can be offered. Need for surgical revision is exceedingly uncommon.

Small Bowel Obstruction

Small bowel obstructions are a common condition requiring acute surgical care. RYGB patients may have standard small bowel obstructions related to internal hernias or postoperative adhesions but have potential for more unusual causes. They may have a stenosis of the GJA or more rarely stenosis of the JJA. Small bowel bezoars and intussusception (at the JJA) have also been identified as the points of obstruction after RYGB. Presentation may be misleading as vomiting may be absent or less impressive because the gastric pouch is too small to accumulate sufficient volume. Other typical symptoms like nausea, distension, bloating, and abdominal pain are often present. Adhesive bowel obstruction is more common after open procedures. Patients who have had laparoscopic RYGB internal hernias account for over half of small bowel obstructions [34].

Internal Hernia

RYGB postoperative anatomy creates three potential spaces for internal hernias. Herniation can occur at the level of the JJA through the mesenteric defect, under the afferent Roux limb (Peterson's defect) or through the transverse mesocolon if the GJA is retrocolic in position. Some bariatric surgeons close these defects prophylactically during the index operation. It reduces the rate of internal hernias but may increase incidence of adhesive disease and other complications. This practice remains a subject of debate [35].

Nonspecific and periodic symptoms make internal hernias a diagnostic challenge. They are a late complication after RYGB but can be catastrophic if associated with bowel ischemia. Patients may report sudden or rapid onset of epigastric or periumbilical pain. Their pain may intermittent or constant, often, exacerbated by eating. Late in the course, obstruction symptoms may predominate with obstipation and vomiting. In more insidious cases, providers may have ordered endoscopy or ultrasounds suspecting marginal ulcers or biliary disease delaying definitive treatment [36, 37]. Cross-sectional imaging is more helpful and may show mesenteric swirling, dilated bowel, or enlarged mesenteric lymph nodes [38]. However, CT is not sensitive in this population and may be interpreted falsely as negative in 30% or more of patients [39, 40]. Changes in hemodynamics and laboratory abnormalities are a late sign of vascular compromise.

Patients with a history of RYGB and confirmed or suspected small bowel obstruction laparoscopic exploration are generally best. Nasogastric decompression will not reduce and internal hernia and may perforate the jejunum [41]. It is helpful to know the patient's anatomy but is often not available. Examining the bowel retrograde, from the terminal ileum toward the obstruction, aids in identifying anatomy and appropriate direction to apply traction to reduce an internal hernia. A volvulus may be a part of the hernia and appear as a "knot" or twist of bowel loops. This can it more difficult to reduce the bowel through the defect. If the bowel is healthy and no resection is needed, the defect should be closed with permanent suture. Gangrenous or ischemic bowel should be resected. Reconstruction of remaining bowel is acceptable, even if short gut syndrome is a concern. Prior to closure, inspect for additional mesenteric defects. Most cases of internal hernia can be treated laparoscopically but converting to open is not uncommon.

Complications of Gastric Sleeve Surgery

Gastroesophageal Reflux Disease

Gastroesophageal reflux disease (GERD) is a very common long-term complication after bariatric surgery but is seen most often after SG. The pathophysiology is poorly understood and difficult to study. Many bariatric patients have preoperative GERD, which improves in many cases; others have de novo GERD postoperatively. There numerous anatomic and physiologic factors interacting, but most patients have relief with acid suppression by proton pump inhibitors. If operation is needed, the procedure of choice is conversion of SG to RYGB unless there is another anatomical problem such as a stricture, kink, or twist. Of note, patients should not expect additional weight loss by the conversion [42].

Bleeding

Bleeding after a SG is most often from the staple line, but splenic injuries may also occur. The management principles discussed above for RYBG apply.

Leaks

Leaks are less common after SG than RYGB likely because there are fewer suture lines. However, they can be more difficult to treat due to differences in endoluminal pressure related to the pyloric sphincter in addition to the lower esophageal sphincter. The superior margin of resection is the most susceptible to break down due to its blood supply. Tachycardia, dyspnea, and fever may be the only signs. Stenosis, kinking, and twisting of the SG can also decrease the caliber of the lumen increase the pressure and lead to a leak. These predisposing structural problems must be addressed when treating a leak. The risk of staple line failure is estimated around 2%.

Leaks in the first few days after surgery should be reexplored laparoscopically and repaired. Patients that show signs of a leak more than a week postoperatively with acceptable hemodynamics may be better treated with percutaneous drainage and endoscopic placement of covered stents. Some advocate placement of a stent long enough to cover both the lower esophageal and pyloric sphincters to decrease the pressure to and promote healing [43]. However, it is difficult to find devices sufficiently long and others have reported success with shorter devices. Unstable patients should go directly to the operating room for control of contamination and draining or repair if possible.

Stenosis, Twists, or Kinks

Like RYGB, SG can become stenotic either intrinsically or due to a kink or a twist. Pure stenoses occur infrequently and are seen less than 2% of patients [44–46]. Dysphagia or intolerance of oral intake, the primary symptoms of "stenosis," may actually be the result of a kink in the SG or a twist around the SG's longitudinal axis. These conditions collectively may affect nearly one in ten patients [47]. Endoscopy may miss the pathology because insufflation during scope advancement can reposition the anatomy. Static UGS may not demonstrate the abnormality if the kink or twist is dynamic and not present at the time of imaging. UGS with video fluoroscopy with real-time image interpretation is more sensitive to make the diagnosis.

Correction of focal stenoses without dynamic kinks or twists can generally be achieved with 2–3 serial balloon dilatations to result in an acceptable diameter [46]. Longer length of stenosis may require stenting for 6 weeks. Persistent strictures may benefit from a myotomy, which can be performed either endoscopic or laparoscopic [48]. When all other treatments for strictures have failed, conversion of SG to RYGB or total gastrectomy can be considered. Patients with kinks or twists receive little benefit from endoscopic treatment. There are a few reports of repeat balloon dilations to avoid an additional operation [44]. However, most patient's anatomy reverts to its abnormal position after the intervention is completed.

Conversion to a RYGB is their best option. Some of these cases are associated with leaks which influences the optimal timing of operative management. Control of contamination should be prioritized an operation delayed until inflammation has improved. Stenting for 6 weeks may temporize a leak and allow for a less formidable operative field for a conversion.

Conclusion

As bariatric operations continue to grow in popularity, surgeons will find themselves caring for increasing numbers of patients who have this in their past medical history. Most have permanent anatomy arrangements predisposing to certain complications. Acute care surgical care for post-bariatric surgery patients should not ignore common etiologies of acute surgical abdomen. These patients may still suffer from appendicitis, infectious or ischemic colitis, and pancreatitis. In many instances, the history of bariatric surgery has no bearing on work-up or treatment. On the other hand, some problems have different treatment options or additional concerns based on the new anatomy

Well-trained surgeons need to able to provide acute surgical care for bariatric patients. Surgeons not trained as bariatric providers can safely care for patients who have had bariatric surgery including many of the complications related to their weight loss procedures.

References

1. Faria GR. A brief history of bariatric surgery. Porto Biomed J. 2017;2(3):90–2.
2. Dimitriadis GK, Randeva MS, Miras AD. Potential hormone mechanisms of bariatric surgery. Curr Obes Rep. 2017;6(3):253–65.
3. Khorgami Z, et al. Trends in utilization of bariatric surgery, 2010-2014: sleeve gastrectomy dominates. Surg Obes Relat Dis. 2017;13(5):774–8.
4. Zilberstein B, Santo MA, Carvalho MH. Critical analysis of surgical treatment techniques of morbid obesity. Arq Bras Cir Dig. 2019;32(3):e1450.
5. Contival N, et al. Guiding the non-bariatric surgeon through complications of bariatric surgery. J Visc Surg. 2018;155(1):27–40.
6. Lupoli R, et al. Bariatric surgery and long-term nutritional issues. World J Diabetes. 2017;8(11):464–74.
7. Coupaye M, et al. Evaluation of incidence of cholelithiasis after bariatric surgery in subjects treated or not treated with ursodeoxycholic acid. Surg Obes Relat Dis. 2017;13(4):681–5.
8. Doulamis IP, et al. Concomitant cholecystectomy during bariatric surgery: the jury is still out. Am J Surg. 2019;218(2):401–10.
9. Shoar S, et al. Single anastomosis duodeno-ileal switch (SADIS): a systematic review of efficacy and safety. Obes Surg. 2018;28(1):104–13.
10. Zinzindohoue F, et al. Laparoscopic gastric banding: a minimally invasive surgical treatment for morbid obesity: prospective study of 500 consecutive patients. Ann Surg. 2003;237(1):1–9.
11. Keidar A, et al. Band slippage after laparoscopic adjustable gastric banding: etiology and treatment. Surg Endosc. 2005;19(2):262–7.
12. Wernick B, et al. Essential bariatric emergencies for the acute care surgeon. Eur J Trauma Emerg Surg. 2016;42(5):571–84.
13. Pieroni S, et al. The "O" sign, a simple and helpful tool in the diagnosis of laparoscopic adjustable gastric band slippage. AJR Am J Roentgenol. 2010;195(1):137–41.
14. Swenson DW, et al. Gastric band slippage: a case-controlled study comparing new and old radiographic

signs of this important surgical complication. AJR Am J Roentgenol. 2014;203(1):10–6.
15. Cherian PT, et al. Band erosion after laparoscopic gastric banding: a retrospective analysis of 865 patients over 5 years. Surg Endosc. 2010;24(8):2031–8.
16. Abu-Abeid S, et al. Treatment of intra-gastric band migration following laparoscopic banding: safety and feasibility of simultaneous laparoscopic band removal and replacement. Obes Surg. 2005;15(6):849–52.
17. Spann MD, et al. Endoscopic management of erosion after banded bariatric procedures. Surg Obes Relat Dis. 2017;13(11):1875–9.
18. Weiss H, et al. Gastroscopic band removal after intragastric migration of adjustable gastric band: a new minimal invasive technique. Obes Surg. 2000;10(2):167–70.
19. Edwards MA, et al. Anastomotic leak following antecolic versus retrocolic laparoscopic Roux-en-Y gastric bypass for morbid obesity. Obes Surg. 2007;17(3):292–7.
20. Almahmeed T, et al. Morbidity of anastomotic leaks in patients undergoing Roux-en-Y gastric bypass. Arch Surg. 2007;142(10):954–7.
21. Inabnet WB, et al. Early outcomes of bariatric surgery in patients with metabolic syndrome: an analysis of the bariatric outcomes longitudinal database. J Am Coll Surg. 2012;214(4):550–6; discussion 556–7.
22. Aurora AR, Khaitan L, Saber AA. Sleeve gastrectomy and the risk of leak: a systematic analysis of 4,888 patients. Surg Endosc. 2012;26(6):1509–15.
23. Westling A, Ohrvall M, Gustavsson S. Roux-en-Y gastric bypass after previous unsuccessful gastric restrictive surgery. J Gastrointest Surg. 2002;6(2):206–11.
24. Gonzalez R, et al. Diagnosis and contemporary management of anastomotic leaks after gastric bypass for obesity. J Am Coll Surg. 2007;204(1):47–55.
25. Sakran N, et al. Gastric leaks after sleeve gastrectomy: a multicenter experience with 2,834 patients. Surg Endosc. 2013;27(1):240–5.
26. Thodiyil PA, et al. Selective nonoperative management of leaks after gastric bypass: lessons learned from 2675 consecutive patients. Ann Surg. 2008;248(5):782–92.
27. Keith JN. Endoscopic management of common bariatric surgical complications. Gastrointest Endosc Clin N Am. 2011;21(2):275–85.
28. Doumouras AG, Saleh F, Hong D. 30-Day readmission after bariatric surgery in a publicly funded regionalized center of excellence system. Surg Endosc. 2016;30(5):2066–72.
29. Mehran A, et al. Management of acute bleeding after laparoscopic Roux-en-Y gastric bypass. Obes Surg. 2003;13(6):842–7.
30. Coblijn UK, et al. Development of ulcer disease after Roux-en-Y gastric bypass, incidence, risk factors, and patient presentation: a systematic review. Obes Surg. 2014;24(2):299–309.
31. Nguyen NT, et al. Gastrointestinal hemorrhage after laparoscopic gastric bypass. Obes Surg. 2004;14(10):1308–12.
32. El-Hayek K, et al. Marginal ulcer after Roux-en-Y gastric bypass: what have we really learned? Surg Endosc. 2012;26(10):2789–96.
33. Brethauer SA, et al. Systematic review on reoperative bariatric surgery: American Society for Metabolic and Bariatric Surgery Revision Task Force. Surg Obes Relat Dis. 2014;10(5):952–72.
34. Husain S, et al. Small-bowel obstruction after laparoscopic Roux-en-Y gastric bypass: etiology, diagnosis, and management. Arch Surg. 2007;142(10):988–93.
35. Nuytens F, et al. Closure of mesenteric defects is associated with a higher incidence of small bowel obstruction due to adhesions after laparoscopic antecolic Roux-en-y gastric bypass: a retrospective cohort study. Int J Surg. 2019;71:149–55.
36. Gandhi AD, Patel RA, Brolin RE. Elective laparoscopy for herald symptoms of mesenteric/internal hernia after laparoscopic Roux-en-Y gastric bypass. Surg Obes Relat Dis. 2009;5(2):144–9; discussion 149.
37. Alsulaimy M, et al. The utility of diagnostic laparoscopy in post-bariatric surgery patients with chronic abdominal pain of unknown etiology. Obes Surg. 2017;27(8):1924–8.
38. Iannuccilli JD, et al. Sensitivity and specificity of eight CT signs in the preoperative diagnosis of internal mesenteric hernia following Roux-en-Y gastric bypass surgery. Clin Radiol. 2009;64(4):373–80.
39. Iannelli A, Facchiano E, Gugenheim J. Internal hernia after laparoscopic Roux-en-Y gastric bypass for morbid obesity. Obes Surg. 2006;16(10):1265–71.
40. Parakh S, Soto E, Merola S. Diagnosis and management of internal hernias after laparoscopic gastric bypass. Obes Surg. 2007;17(11):1498–502.
41. Rogula T, Yenumula PR, Schauer PR. A complication of Roux-en-Y gastric bypass: intestinal obstruction. Surg Endosc. 2007;21(11):1914–8.
42. Felinska E, et al. Do we understand the pathophysiology of GERD after sleeve gastrectomy? Ann N Y Acad Sci. 2020;1482:26–35.
43. Galloro G, et al. A novel dedicated endoscopic stent for staple-line leaks after laparoscopic sleeve gastrectomy: a case series. Surg Obes Relat Dis. 2014;10(4):607–11.
44. Donatelli G, et al. Pneumatic dilation for functional helix stenosis after sleeve gastrectomy: long-term follow-up (with videos). Surg Obes Relat Dis. 2017;13(6):943–50.
45. Burgos AM, Csendes A, Braghetto I. Gastric stenosis after laparoscopic sleeve gastrectomy in morbidly obese patients. Obes Surg. 2013;23(9):1481–6.
46. Rebibo L, et al. Gastric stenosis after laparoscopic sleeve gastrectomy: diagnosis and management. Obes Surg. 2016;26(5):995–1001.
47. Nath A, et al. Dysphagia after vertical sleeve gastrectomy: evaluation of risk factors and assessment of endoscopic intervention. World J Gastroenterol. 2016;22(47):10371–9.
48. Dapri G, Cadière GB, Himpens J. Laparoscopic seromyotomy for long stenosis after sleeve gastrectomy with or without duodenal switch. Obes Surg. 2009;19(4):495–9.

personnel. All other personnel should minimize talking and keep a safe distance from the patient's bedside in order to allow essential personnel to do their jobs. Essential personnel for most emergent airway situations are the proceduralist, the backup proceduralist, the medication administration provider. The proceduralist is the individual who will be performing the airway procedure. The proceduralist should have familiarity with the procedure prior to performing it. In teaching settings, this person may have variable degrees of familiarity with the procedure, but less experience. In this situation, the backup proceduralist should be very closely supervising and guiding the primary proceduralist through the procedure. Even in the setting of experienced proceduralist, having experienced backup proceduralist has been associated with increased rates of successful intubation [1, 2]. Both proceduralists should have training and familiarity with placing surgical airways in the event that intubation or supraglottic airways fail. The medication administration provider is the nurse or physician who administers sedatives, paralytics, vasopressors, and any other medications required for the procedure. This role should be filled by someone familiar with the medications and medication administration. Depending on the setting, this may be a paramedic, registered nurse, advanced practice provider, or a physician.

Other personnel that are helpful if conditions allow include respiratory therapist, scribe, and procedural support assistant. Often, respiratory therapists are among the first members of the healthcare team at the patient's bedside in developing airway situations. The respiratory therapist is helpful in setting up the ventilator and putting the patient on the ventilator after intubation. They are often present prior to intubation administering supplemental oxygen, providing bag-valve mask ventilation, and performing other respiratory care interventions. While not essential to the procedure, having another team member perform these tasks frees the proceduralist to do other tasks. Scribes are helpful in documenting interventions, medications, and vital signs in real time. A procedural support assistant is a role that can have tremendous benefit to airway procedures, particularly surgical airway procedures. The procedural support assistant may be asked to perform a variety of roles. Retrieving supplies and equipment for surgical airway, setting up for a surgical airway procedure, and even assisting the proceduralist during a surgical airway are all potential tasks performed by the procedural support assistant. At the authors' institution, this role is filled by a dedicated procedure support nurse.

One note related to personnel that bears mentioning is the importance of personal protective equipment. Protection of the team should be of the utmost importance. This notion is especially true since the outbreak of the SARS-CoV-2 virus and COVID-19. Protection from both bloodborne and airborne infections is required. While it is tempting to forego PPE due to the speed of an airway emergency, it is important that all team members take the time to protect themselves. Appropriate personal protective equipment should be available. At a minimum, non-sterile gloves, surgical mask, and eye protection should be used for any intubation. For surgical airways, sterile gloves, surgical cap, and sterile gown should be also be included. For patients suspicious for airborne infections, consideration should be given to N95 mask or powered air-purifying respirators (PAPR).

Equipment

Preparation for emergent airway management should also include accumulating the appropriate equipment. Many places that perform emergency airway management with some frequency, like emergency departments and ICUs, keep all necessary equipment in a specially designated cart or bag. Airway carts or emergency airway bags ensure that last minute scrambles to find supplies or airway adjuncts are not needed. It is important that an emergency airway kit (whether a cart, a bag or some other method) includes non-invasive airway supplies, invasive airway supplies, airway adjuncts, and rescue airway devices. Specific airway devices will be discussed later in this chapter.

Non-invasive devices include nasal canula, preferably one that can also measure end-tidal

CO_2, nasopharyngeal airway devices (NPA), and oropharyngeal airway devices (OPA). Various sizes of NPAs and OPAs should be available to accommodate patients of different sizes. Various sizes of endotracheal tubes and supraglottic airway devices should be available as well. In addition to airway devices, adjuncts to aid intubation should be present. The gum-elastic bougie is an essential airway adjunct. Other important equipment includes syringes for cuff inflation, lubrication, end-tidal detection devices (qualitative and/or qualitative), and sterile scalpels. Many facilities utilize mats with outlines of the essential equipment needed for basic airway management (Fig. 25.1). These mats allow for proceduralists to rapidly identify if any essential equipment is missing.

One of the most essential pieces of equipment of airway management is the laryngoscope. Any useful emergency airway kit will have direct laryngoscopes. Straight and curved blades of various sizes should also be present. Video laryngoscopy has become increasingly popular. There are many types of video laryngoscopes. Some are small enough to fit in an emergency airway bag. Others are larger free-standing units and are stationed in locations where emergency airway procedures are frequently performed such as the emergency department trauma bay. For difficult airways, fiberoptic bronchoscopes may be employed. Using a fiberoptic scope allows one to pass an endotracheal tube over the scope and then, under video guidance, maneuver the bronchoscope through the oropharynx and beyond the vocal cords. At that point, the endotracheal tube is passed back over the scope into the trachea and inflated below the cords.

Medications

Medications are used for airway management to accomplish specific goals. Understanding these goals is important in selecting the most appropriate medications or when a medication is not needed. Medications for the purpose of intubation are intended to achieve two goals:

1. Creating good intubating conditions (i.e., muscle relaxation/paralysis)
2. Prevent patient recall of the procedure (i.e., sedation)

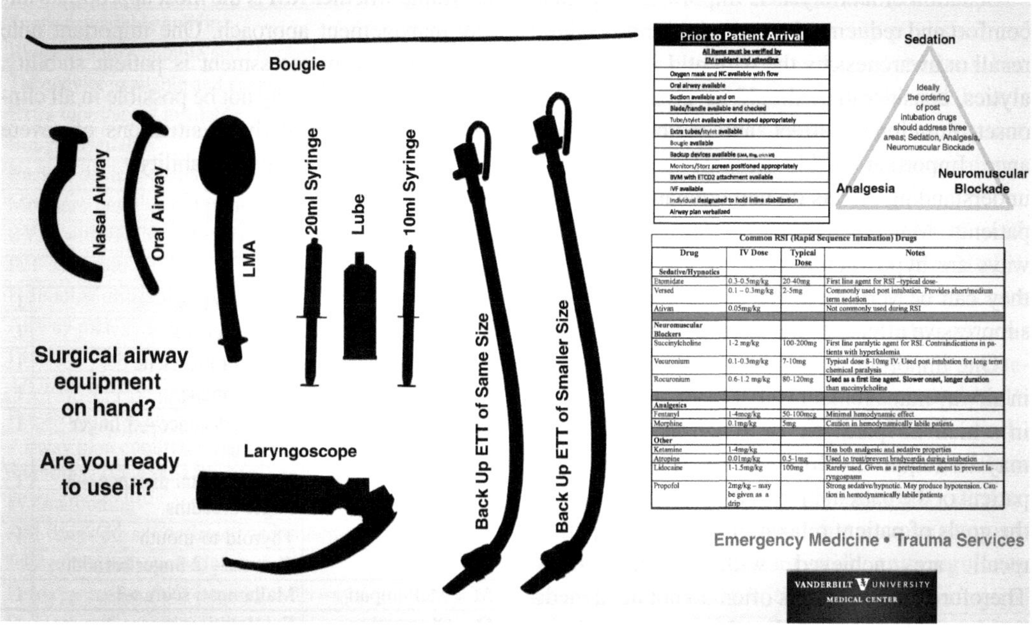

Fig. 25.1 Pre-arrival checklist

Airway Devices

There are four basic types of tubes that are used to manage airways.

1. Endotracheal tubes
2. Supraglottic devices
3. Tracheostomy tubes
4. Cricothyrotomy tubes

Within each category above, there are numerous variations of each tube. An exhaustive discussion of the many modifications of each device would be outside the scope of emergency airway management. Instead, what follows will be a general discussion of each basic category of airway device used in emergency airway management.

Endotracheal Tubes

For almost all emergency airway situations, the endotracheal tube is the default airway device. It is, far and away, the device with which providers have the most experience using. Difficult airway algorithms and difficult airway adjuncts focus extensively on assisting providers in achieving successful endotracheal intubation. Endotracheal tubes come in a wide range of sizes. The sizing of endotracheal tubes is based on the internal diameter of the tube in millimeters. Most adults can be successfully intubated using endotracheal tubes between 7.0 and 8.5 mm. Endotracheal tubes should be inserted far enough into the trachea to allow the entire cuff to rest below the vocal cords. Care should be taken to ensure the distal tip of the tube does not enter a mainstem bronchus. The depth of insertion will vary based on patient size but the typical adult is around 21–25 cm from incisors to vocal cords. Cuffs are manufactured with various shapes and sizes. Some cuffs are designed to distribute force across a broad area to prevent pressure necrosis on the trachea. Some cuffs are designed in a tapered fashion to prevent migration out of the airway. Many cuffs are designed to prevent drainage of oropharyngeal secretions into the airway and lungs. Cuffs should be inflated with enough air to allow contact with the trachea but not so much as to cause ischemia due to pressure.

Supraglottic Devices

In the event that an endotracheal intubation is not possible, a supraglottic airway may be an acceptable short-term alternative. Supraglottic devices sit with the ventilatory portion of the device above the glottic opening. These devices are considered short-term airway devices because they are not secured below the vocal cords and are therefore somewhat tenuous. There are a number of different products in this category of airway. They vary based on where the sealing mechanism rests (base of tongue vs perilaryngeal), cuffed vs uncuffed, protection against aspiration [9].

Two specific devices warrant special mention. The laryngeal mask airway (LMA) has been used for many years by anesthesiologists for select operative procedures. It consists of a mask surrounded by an inflatable cuff at the distal end of an airway tube. The distal end of the device encircles the laryngeal structures to create a bowl that allows for oxygenation and ventilation in a supraglottic position. There have been many modifications and additions to the standard LMA design over the years, but the functional principles are largely the same. In the prehospital setting, the King Airway (Ambu A/S, Ballerup, Denmark) is a very popular supraglottic airway device. It consists of an airway tube with oropharyngeal and esophageal cuffs. While the LMA can be used as a first line airway device, the King Airway is recommended for emergency use only in situations of failure to intubate or ventilate [10]. It is inserted blindly and is considered easy to insert, but it comes with a relatively high rate of airway obstruction.

Surgical Airway Tubes

Tubes for surgical airways, like the other airway devices, all have the same basic parts, but many unique alterations and modifications exist. Tubes designed to be used for surgical airways typically consist of a short airway tube and a skin-level flange that attaches to it and allows for the tube's securement and connection to the ventilator. The surgical airway tubes are more highly curved than endotracheal tubes due to the insertion point on the neck being much closer and more perpendicular to the trachea. The decreased distance from insertion point to airway requires some curve on the tube to allow it to sit properly in the airway.

Tracheostomy tubes are constructed of various materials depending on the intended use. Metal, typically stainless steel, tubes lack cuffs and adapters to allow for attachment to a ventilator. Therefore, tracheostomy tubes used for emergent surgical airways should be made of polyvinyl chloride (PVC), polyurethane, or silicone rather than metal. Tubes of constructed of these materials are softened by the patient's body temperature and are able to conform to the soft tissues of the patient's airway more effectively than metal tubes. However, these tubes are more rigid than endotracheal tubes made of similar materials because they are at higher risk of kinking.

There is much more variation in size in tracheostomy tubes than in endotracheal tubes. Most of the available devices for tracheostomy come in various inner diameter sizes like endotracheal tubes. With increasing inner diameter size also comes increasing airway tube length. The reason for the increasing length is that most tracheostomy tubes are not made to adjust the depth of insertion. The position of the cuff may vary along the length of the airway tube based on the specific product chosen; however, most are located within about 1 cm of the distal tip of the tracheostomy tube. Differences in patients' neck sizes requires some variation in the soft tissue portion of tracheostomy tubes. Therefore, some manufacturers have created tubes with increased length from cuff to flange. Not often seen in the setting of emergency airway management, some manufacturers have created tubes with longer airway tubes distal to the cuff to allow tubes to extend beyond areas of tracheal pathology like tracheomalacia. In the setting of emergency surgical airway, most proceduralists will use a cuffed tracheostomy tube. Cuffless tracheostomy tubes are typically not used in the setting of emergency airway management due to the need for controlled oxygenation and ventilation. Some tracheostomy tubes have an inner cannula within the tracheostomy tube itself. These inner cannulas can be removed and cleaned or discarded and replaced. Lastly, some tracheostomy tubes come fenestrated in which there is an opening in the posterior portion of the tube above the cuff [10].

Cricothyrotomy Tubes

Cricothyrotomy is much less common procedure than tracheostomy or endotracheal intubation. Additionally, cricothyrotomies are almost always short-term airways. For these two reasons, most cricothyrotomy tubes are essentially modifications of endotracheal tubes or tracheostomy tubes. In most adults, a cricothyrotomy tube is equivalent to a 6.0 endotracheal tube (6 mm inner diameter). In fact, a 6.0 endotracheal tube is frequently used as the airway tube for cricothyrotomies. A smaller tube is used in cricothyrotomies to decrease the risk of iatrogenic injury from the insertion procedure or the tube itself. With the cricothyroid membrane being just inferior to the vocal cords, there is an increased risk of injury to the structures in this area.

Cricothyroidotomy

When time is of the essence and orotracheal intubation cannot be performed, a cricothyroidotomy is the most expeditious and technically straightforward technique for definitive airway access. The only equipment required is a scalpel and a tube; an endotracheal tube or tracheostomy tube can be used. If available, a bougie can help facilitate expeditious tube placement. As the anatomy is more favorable than that of a tracheostomy, it can allow for less blood loss in the pursuit of a definitive airway [11–13].

It is ideal to prepare for a cricothyroidotomy prior to an intubation attempt, to ensure all equipment is available and patient positioning optimized. For an open cricothyroidotomy, the minimum necessary equipment is a scalpel and a tube, either a small (5.0 or 6.0) endotracheal tube or a tracheostomy tube. A bougie can help facilitate placement ("scalpel-finger-bougie technique"). If possible (and cervical spine injury not suspected), a shoulder roll can help optimize patient positioning for more favorable anatomy. As well, an assistant with a suction catheter can aid in visualization. Finally, any available light, whether overhead, a headlamp, or procedural lights can be of great assistance during such a procedure [13, 14].

If time allows, the neck is prepped with antiseptic solution. Though either a transverse or longitudinal incision may be made, the authors prefer a longitudinal incision in the midline of the neck over the trachea, as it is an extensible incision and helps avoid injury to the anterior jugular veins. This incision is carried down to the trachea at the level of the thyroid and cricoid cartilage. The cricothyroid membrane is incised to gain access to the lumen of the trachea. If a bougie is available, it may be inserted into the cricothyroid incision and the tube inserted over it. If no bougie is available, the handle of the scalpel may be used to hold the tracheal incision open and insert the available cuffed tube [11, 13, 14].

Once the tube is inserted into the airway, the cuff is inflated and connected to a bag-valve mask. Capnometry should be used to confirm airway placement if available. It is important to auscultate for breath sounds, as it is exceedingly common to intubate a mainstem bronchus if using a standard endotracheal tube for a cricothyroidotomy. Once the position is confirmed, the tube is secured.

Percutaneous cricothyroidotomy kits are also available. These allow for placement via the Seldinger technique. An incision is made over the thyroid and cricoid cartilages. A needle is inserted into the cricothyroid membrane and is exchanged over a wire for a cricothyroidotomy tube. As with an open cricothyroidotomy, the tube position should be confirmed using capnometry and auscultation, and the tube secured. In an animal model, this was found to be slower than an open cricothyroidotomy [15].

Once the patient is stabilized, it is ideal to revise a cricothyroidotomy to a tracheostomy, to limit the risk of subglottic stenosis and vocal cord impairment, unless extubation is anticipated [16, 17]. Training is vital for this procedure, as it is rarely performed, but with repetition, time to a secure airway is reduced [18]. Additionally, with training, anesthesiologists and paramedics could achieve similar time to placement and success rates, suggesting that comfort and experience with operative tracheostomy is not necessary to effective performance of cricothyroidotomy [19, 20].

Tracheostomy

When time allows, a tracheostomy is a more durable procedure to obtain a definitive airway with less long-term complication risk. The authors find this technique particularly useful for a patient who can be ventilated, either using Bag-Mask ventilation or a supraglottic airway device but cannot be intubated. This affords the extra time necessary to perform the procedure [21–26].

Like a cricothyroidotomy, a tracheostomy may be performed open via a tracheal incision, or percutaneous using the Seldinger technique [22]. The authors prefer a modified percutaneous technique which is described below. Performing a tracheostomy when able is advantageous as it provides a durable definitive airway without the need for revision. In addition, it is associated with a lower rate of subglottic stenosis than cricothyroidotomy [16, 17, 27, 28].

If possible, the patient is positioned on a shoulder roll to facilitate exposure. The neck is prepped using an antiseptic solution. An incision is made in the one fingerbreadth above the sternal notch. As with a cricothyroidotomy, the authors prefer a vertical incision to minimize the risk of venous injury. Using blunt dissection, the trachea is exposed and palpated. The endotracheal tube is retracted above the intended insertion site (this step is omitted if no endotracheal tube is in place). A needle is inserted between the first and second tracheal rings, and serially dilated over a wire to accommodate a tracheostomy tube. The balloon is inflated, the inner cannula inserted, and position is confirmed with capnometry. The tracheostomy device secured with suture and a tracheostomy tie [29].

If no percutaneous tracheostomy kit is available, an open tracheostomy may be performed. As with the percutaneous technique, an incision is made between the thyroid cartilage and the sternal notch. This is carried through the platysma and the strap muscles separated in the midline. The thyroid gland is then encountered. This may be retracted superiorly, inferiorly, or divided between ties as necessary to expose the trachea. A cricoid hook is used to retract the trachea superiorly to expose the rings. A tracheotomy is then made below the first tracheal ring and is dilated using a tracheal dilator. The tracheostomy tube is passed with an obturator, the balloon inflated, the obturator removed, inner cannula inserted, and position confirmed with capnometry. The device is secured with suture and a tracheostomy tie.

Post-procedure Management

Obtaining a secure airway in the emergent situation is often a stressful exercise for all involved. It is very easy to let one's guard down after inserting a tube into the trachea. However, neglecting to properly secure an airway device can lead to a second emergent situation. Depending on the airway device used and institutional practice, one may use an endotracheal tube holder, umbilical tape, tracheostomy ties, and/or sutures to secure a device in place. This helps to prevent unintended dislodgment of the tube to help support the patient through their illness [30].

It is important to ensure the patient is appropriately sedated and that restraints are used in a judicious fashion to reduce the risk of self-extubation or decannulation. Furthermore, the authors' institution has instituted a Compromised Tracheostomy Algorithm which includes a laminated sign in the patient's room which holds the obturator, details about the placement of the tracheostomy, and a checklist of mandatory supplies to be kept in the room (Fig. 25.2). Additionally, it includes emergency phone numbers for the Emergency Airway Team.

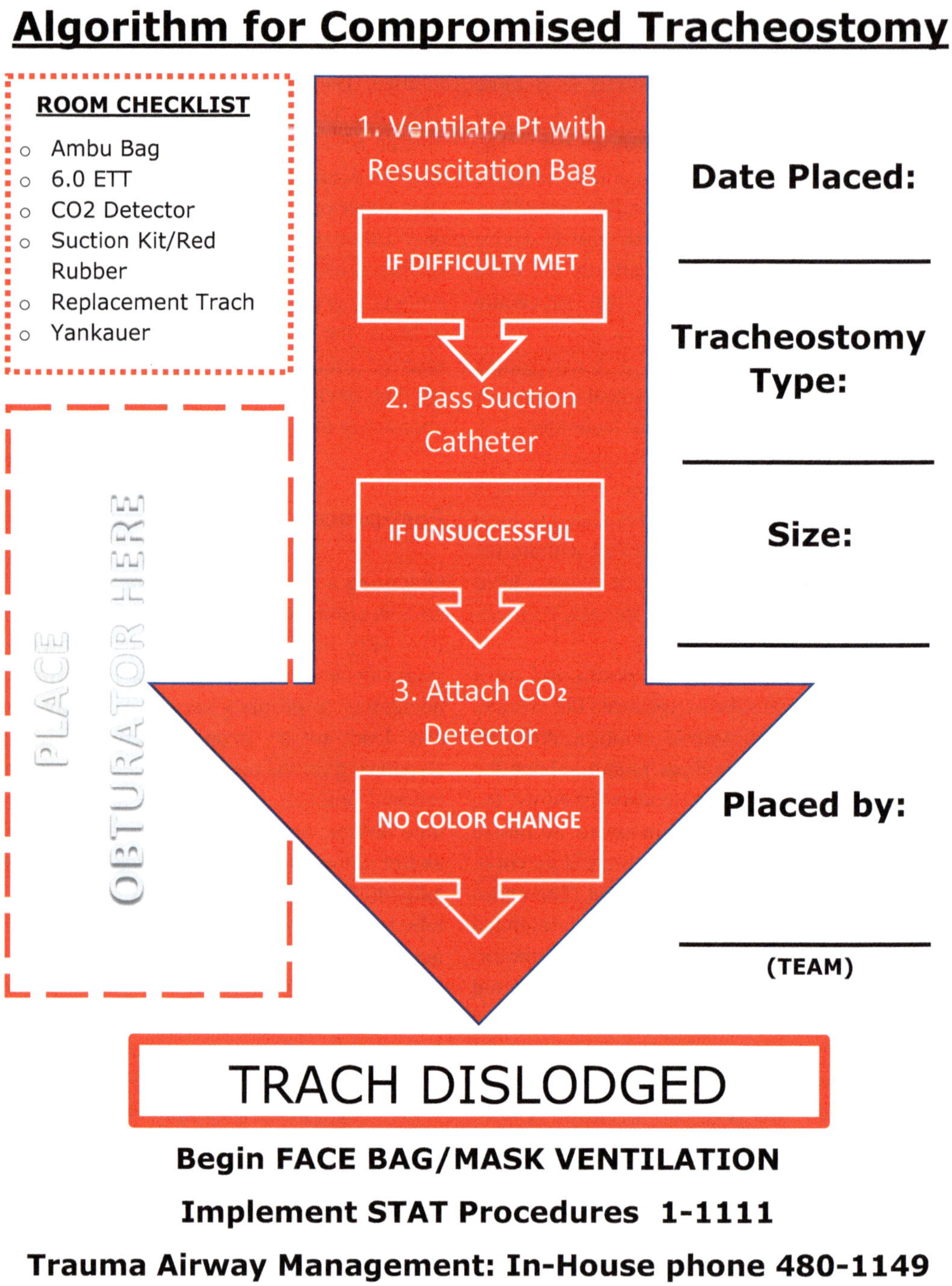

Fig. 25.2 Compromised tracheostomy checklist

Case Conclusion

The team prepares for the patient's arrival with its pre-arrival checklist and a detailed airway plan communicated between the team members. The patient is positioned optimally, and using a video laryngoscope, suction, and a bougie, the patient is intubated without desaturation. His facial injuries are identified on CT scan and repaired by the oral maxillofacial surgeons. The patient then has an uneventful recovery. This case highlights the complexity of emergency airway management as well as all the necessary steps for appropriate preparedness.

References

1. Kim JH, Kim YM, Choi HJ, Je SM, Kim E. Factors associated with successful second and third intubation attempts in the ED. Am J Emerg Med. 2013;31:1376–81.
2. Goto Y, Goto T, Okamoto H, Hagiwara Y, Watase H, Hasegawa K. Factors associated with successful rescue intubation attempts in the emergency department: an analysis of multicenter prospective observational study in Japan. Acute Med Surg. 2020;7:e462.
3. Ji SM, Moon EJ, Kim TJ, Yi JW, Seo H, Lee BJ. Correlation between modified LEMON score and intubation difficulty in adult trauma patients undergoing emergency surgery. World J Emerg Surg. 2018;13:33.
4. Haynes AB, Weiser TG, Berry WR, et al. A surgical safety checklist to reduce morbidity and mortality in a global population. N Engl J Med. 2009;360:491–9.
5. Jaber S, Jung B, Corne P, et al. An intervention to decrease complications related to endotracheal intubation in the intensive care unit: a prospective, multiple-center study. Intensive Care Med. 2010;36:248–55.
6. Smith KA, High K, Collins SP, Self WH. A preprocedural checklist improves the safety of emergency department intubation of trauma patients. Acad Emerg Med. 2015;22:989–92.
7. Weingart SD, Levitan RM. Preoxygenation and prevention of desaturation during emergency airway management. Ann Emerg Med. 2012;59:165–75.e1.
8. Taha SK, Siddik-Sayyid SM, El-Khatib MF, Dagher CM, Hakki MA, Baraka AS. Nasopharyngeal oxygen insufflation following pre-oxygenation using the four deep breath technique. Anaesthesia. 2006;61:427–30.
9. Sharma B, Sahai C, Sood J. Extraglottic airway devices: technology update. Med Devices (Auckl). 2017;10:189–205.
10. Kikuchi T, Kamiya Y, Ohtsuka T, Miki T, Goto T. Randomized prospective study comparing the laryngeal tube suction II with the ProSeal laryngeal mask airway in anesthetized and paralyzed patients. Anesthesiology. 2008;109:54–60.
11. McNiven ND, Pracy JP, McGrath BA, Robson AK. The role of Scalpel-bougie cricothyroidotomy in managing emergency Front of Neck Airway access. A review and technical update for ENT surgeons. Clin Otolaryngol. 2018;43:791–4.
12. Pracy JP, Brennan L, Cook TM, et al. Surgical intervention during a can't intubate can't oxygenate (CICO) event: emergency front-of-neck airway (FONA)? Clin Otolaryngol. 2016;41:624–6.
13. Melchiors J, Todsen T, Konge L, Charabi B, von Buchwald C. Cricothyroidotomy—the emergency surgical airway. Head Neck. 2016;38:1129–31.
14. MacIntyre A, Markarian MK, Carrison D, Coates J, Kuhls D, Fildes JJ. Three-step emergency cricothyroidotomy. Mil Med. 2007;172:1228–30.
15. Andresen ÅEL, Kramer-Johansen J, Kristiansen T. Percutaneous vs surgical emergency cricothyroidotomy: an experimental randomized crossover study on an animal-larynx model. Acta Anaesthesiol Scand. 2019;63:1306–12.
16. Cook TM, Woodall N, Harper J, Benger J. Major complications of airway management in the UK: results of the Fourth National Audit Project of the Royal College of Anaesthetists and the Difficult Airway Society. Part 2: intensive care and emergency departments. Br J Anaesth. 2011;106:632–42.
17. Macêdo MB, Guimarães RB, Ribeiro SM, Sousa KM. Emergency cricothyrotomy: temporary measure or definitive airway? A systematic review. Rev Col Bras Cir. 2016;43:493–9.
18. Shetty K, Nayyar V, Stachowski E, Byth K. Training for cricothyroidotomy. Anaesth Intensive Care. 2013;41:623–30.
19. Groom P, Schofield L, Hettiarachchi N, et al. Performance of emergency surgical front of neck airway access by head and neck surgeons, general surgeons, or anaesthetists: an in situ simulation study. Br J Anaesth. 2019;123:696–703.
20. Jacobson LE, Gomez GA, Sobieray RJ, Rodman GH, Solotkin KC, Misinski ME. Surgical cricothyroidotomy in trauma patients: analysis of its use by paramedics in the field. J Trauma. 1996;41:15–20.
21. Davidson SB, Blostein PA, Walsh J, Maltz SB, VandenBerg SL. Percutaneous tracheostomy: a new approach to the emergency airway. J Trauma Acute Care Surg. 2012;73:S83–8.

22. Cheung NH, Napolitano LM. Tracheostomy: epidemiology, indications, timing, technique, and outcomes. Respir Care. 2014;59:895–915; discussion 6–9.
23. Jonas N, Mulwafu W, Joubert J. Emergency percutaneous tracheostomy. S Afr J Surg. 2007;45:105–6.
24. Ben-Nun A, Altman E, Best LA. Emergency percutaneous tracheostomy in trauma patients: an early experience. Ann Thorac Surg. 2004;77:1045–7.
25. Klein M, Weksler N, Kaplan DM, Weksler D, Chorny I, Gurman GM. Emergency percutaneous tracheostomy is feasible in experienced hands. Eur J Emerg Med. 2004;11:108–12.
26. Ault MJ, Ault B, Ng PK. Percutaneous dilatational tracheostomy for emergent airway access. J Intensive Care Med. 2003;18:222–6.
27. Sise MJ, Shackford SR, Cruickshank JC, Murphy G, Fridlund PH. Cricothyroidotomy for long-term tracheal access. A prospective analysis of morbidity and mortality in 76 patients. Ann Surg. 1984;200:13–7.
28. Klotz R, Probst P, Deininger M, et al. Percutaneous versus surgical strategy for tracheostomy: a systematic review and meta-analysis of perioperative and postoperative complications. Langenbeck's Arch Surg. 2018;403:137–49.
29. Dennis BM, Eckert MJ, Gunter OL, Morris JA Jr, May AK. Safety of bedside percutaneous tracheostomy in the critically ill: evaluation of more than 3,000 procedures. J Am Coll Surg. 2013;216:858–65; discussion 65–7.
30. Akulian JA, Yarmus L, Feller-Kopman D. The role of cricothyrotomy, tracheostomy, and percutaneous tracheostomy in airway management. Anesthesiol Clin. 2015;33:357–67.

Non-operative Approaches to the Biliary Tree

26

Kevin D. Platt and Ryan J. Law

Introduction

While first-line treatment in patients with biliary disease often involves surgery, there remains a substantial role for less invasive options, particularly with the growing number of medically complex and aging patients who may not be surgical candidates. It is therefore prudent that surgeons be familiar with the available non-operative armamentarium for management of patients with biliary disease, which includes a growing number of percutaneous and endoscopic techniques which can serve as alternative or complimentary approaches to conventional management. Similarly, interventional radiologic and endoscopic interventions have had an expanding role in the management of adverse events from biliary surgery. In this chapter, we will review the most common biliary diseases requiring intervention: cholecystitis, choledocholithiasis, cholangitis, and bile leaks. We will focus on percutaneous and endoscopic techniques and highlight non-operative approaches in patients with surgically-altered gastrointestinal anatomy.

Section 1: Acute Biliary Disease

Cholecystitis

Acute cholecystitis is an infection of the gallbladder, most commonly (>90%) caused by gallstone disease (calculous) leading to cystic duct obstruction, with the minority of cases being related to bile stasis and hypoperfusion (acalculous) [1]. Overall, treatment consists of antibiotics and either cholecystectomy or non-surgical methods of gallbladder decompression. Please refer Chap. 15 for additional details regarding the clinical presentation, evaluation, and conventional surgical management.

While cholecystectomy remains the standard of care in the management of acute cholecystitis, in patients deemed unfit for surgery due to acute illness and/or significant medical comorbidities, there are a variety of non-operative approaches for consideration, including percutaneous cholecystostomy, transpapillary cystic duct stent placement, or endoscopic ultrasound (EUS)-guided gallbladder drainage. As described below, these approaches may serve as a bridge to future cholecystectomy or may be used as destination therapy.

K. D. Platt
Division of Gastroenterology and Hepatology, Department of Medicine, University of Michigan, Ann Arbor, MI, USA
e-mail: plattk@med.umich.edu

R. J. Law (✉)
Division of Gastroenterology and Hepatology, Department of Medicine, Mayo Clinic, Rochester, MN, USA

M. D. Zielinski, O. Guillamondegui (eds.), *The Acute Management of Surgical Disease*,
https://doi.org/10.1007/978-3-031-07881-1_26

Percutaneous Cholecystostomy

Percutaneous cholecystostomy (PC) was first introduced in 1980 [2]. The technique involves using ultrasonographic or computed tomographic guidance to puncture the gallbladder allowing subsequent wire-guided placement of a percutaneous pigtail catheter. This approach effectively resolves acute cholecystitis in approximately 90% of patients [3]. The use of PC has been on the rise, now accounting for nearly 3% of gallbladder procedures performed in the Medicare population [4].

The most frequent reported adverse event of PC is catheter dislodgement (8.6%). Other adverse events include hemorrhage, sepsis, bile leak, bowel perforation, and pneumothorax, occurring overall in <2% of procedures. Intraprocedural mortality is <0.5%. The 30-day mortality ranges from 10% to 15%, likely reflecting the medically complex population who undergo PC [3, 5].

Advantages of PC include a high rate of technical and clinical success. Additionally, the procedure can be performed at the bedside in critically ill patients with no need for general anesthesia, as is typically needed for surgical and advanced endoscopic techniques. The major disadvantage of this approach revolves around the external drainage system. Percutaneous drainage catheters require routine maintenance with catheter exchanges and are often complicated by inadvertent dislodgement and patient discomfort, which can adversely affect quality of life [6, 7].

There is a growing body of literature comparing outcomes of cholecystectomy and PC. The recently completed CHOCOLATE trial by Loozen et al. [8] compared laparoscopic cholecystectomy and PC in severely ill patients with acute calculous cholecystitis. In this study, 142 high operative risk patients (APACHE II score >7) with symptoms of acute cholecystitis were randomly assigned to either laparoscopic cholecystectomy or percutaneous catheter drainage. Mortality at 1-year did not significantly differ between the two cohorts (3% vs. 9%, $p = 0.27$), but the rates of major adverse events (65% vs. 12%, $p < 0.001$), need for re-intervention at 1-year (66% vs. 12%, $p < 0.001$), and recurrent biliary disease at 1-year (53% vs. 4.5%, $p < 0.001$) favored the cholecystectomy approach. While this study favored cholecystectomy, there remain questions of generalizability to real-world scenarios, as only 17% of screened patients were ultimately enrolled in the trial and very high risk patients (APACHE II scores ≥15) were excluded [9].

PC is often performed to serve as a bridge to definitive surgery; however, available data suggest >50% of patients who undergo percutaneous drainage do *not* ultimately undergo cholecystectomy [3, 10]. The rate of recurrent cholecystitis within 1 year of those patients who do *not* undergo interval cholecystectomy is up to 40% [11]. In patients who remain poor surgical candidates after percutaneous drainage, gallbladder drainage can be internalized via endoscopic techniques using transpapillary cystic duct stent placement [12] or EUS-guided gallbladder drainage [13].

Endoscopic Transpapillary Gallbladder Drainage (ERCP with Cystic Duct Stent Placement)

Transpapillary drainage of the gallbladder was first described in 1990 [14]. During endoscopic retrograde cholangiopancreatography (ERCP), the bile duct is cannulated, and a guidewire is passed into the biliary tree. The guidewire is then manipulated through the cystic duct and ultimately coiled in the gallbladder. A transpapillary double-pigtail plastic stent is then deployed with one pigtail in the gallbladder and the other pigtail in the duodenum, thus facilitating gallbladder decompression into the intestinal lumen (Fig. 26.1a, b). The procedure can be technically challenging as it requires selective guidewire access into the thin, tortuous and often obstructed cystic duct, as well as advancement of a stent through the cystic duct into the gallbladder lumen. Cystic duct patency, as determined by fluoroscopic visualization during contrast injection, is paramount in achieving successful guidewire passage and stent placement into the gallbladder. Lack of fluoroscopic visualization of the cystic duct most commonly occurs due to obstruction by a stone or, less commonly, from malignant

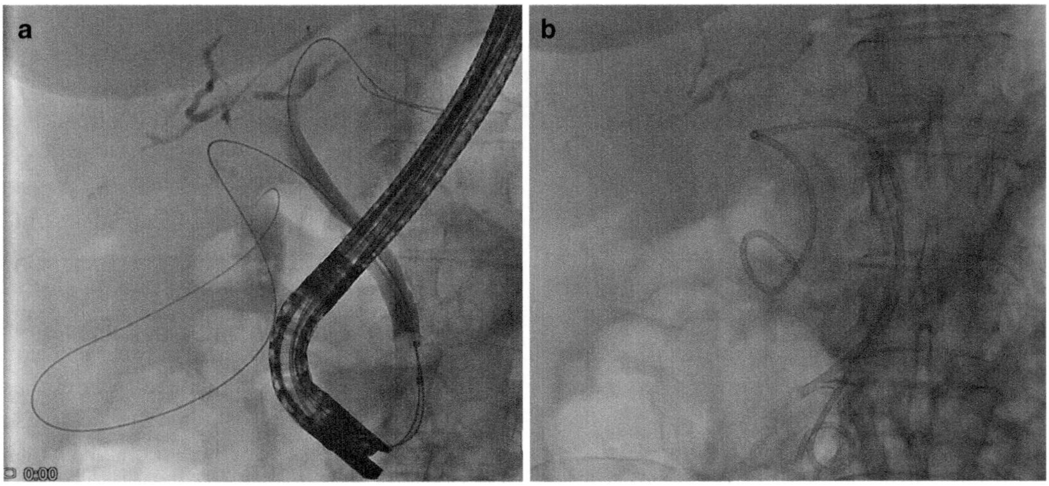

Fig. 26.1 Transpapillary gallbladder stent placement. (**a**) Following selective cannulation of the bile duct, a guidewire is passed into the cystic duct takeoff. The guidewire is manipulated through the Valves of Heister and ultimately coiled in the body of the gallbladder. A second guidewire is seen in the left hepatic duct. (**b**) Over the guidewire, a double-pigtail plastic stent is place with one pigtail in the gallbladder and the other in the duodenal lumen. A second plastic stent is seen in the common bile duct

obstruction. In such circumstances, access to the cystic duct will be extremely difficult, if not impossible [15]. Cholangioscopy using a digital, single operator cholangioscope (Spyglass DS; Boston Scientific, Marlborough, MA) or dedicated direct peroral cholangioscope may be helpful in identification of the cystic duct orifice [16]. Most commonly, double-pigtail plastic stents either 5–7 Fr in diameter and >12 cm in length are used.

When the procedure is technically successful, this method provides effective treatment in 90% of patients with acute cholecystitis [17]. The stent may be left indefinitely or can serve as bridge to surgery with removal prior to cholecystectomy [18]. Cystic duct stents can be left in place indefinitely—compared to common bile duct (CBD) stents—because they act as "wick" whereby bile flows around the stent, and thus patency of the stent is not imperative to maintain bile flow from the gallbladder [19]. As mentioned above, transpapillary cystic duct stents can also be used to facilitate removal of an indwelling PC tube after the tract has matured [12].

Adverse events can be seen in up to 10% of patients, including post-ERCP pancreatitis, stent migration, or post-sphincterotomy bleeding (if biliary sphincterotomy is performed) [18, 20]. In a recent review of 38 patients, technical success of first-attempt transpapillary drainage was observed in 84%, with 76% clinical success [20]. Recurrent cholecystitis was observed in 6 of 32 patients (18%), ranging from 23 to 865 days after the procedure. Recurrent cholecystitis is typically managed with antibiotics, stent exchange, EUS-guided gallbladder drainage, or cholecystectomy, if feasible.

There are advantages of transpapillary gallbladder drainage that make it attractive in certain patient populations, particularly those with advanced liver disease and coagulopathy. The procedure is done endoscopically, with no incisions required externally, and can be done without performing biliary sphincterotomy, thereby minimizing the risk of bleeding in patients with coagulopathy or those receiving systemic anticoagulation [21]. Furthermore, internal drainage is performed while leaving the anatomy untouched, without internal or external fistulous tracts, making transpapillary drainage the procedure of choice in patients with advanced liver disease with ascites and/or awaiting liver transplantation [22, 23].

EUS-Guided Gallbladder Drainage

EUS-guided gallbladder drainage (EUS-GBD) was first described in 2007 [24]. A linear-array therapeutic channel echoendoscope is passed transoral and positioned in the distal gastric antrum or duodenum to identify the gallbladder body. There are several techniques which can be utilized. The conventional method requires puncture of the gallbladder wall with an EUS-FNA needle, followed by bile aspiration and/or cholecystography using water-soluble contrast and fluoroscopy. A guidewire is passed through the needle and coiled within the gallbladder lumen. The tract is then dilated using electrocautery and/or balloon dilation. The stent, either a double-pigtail plastic stent, fully covered self-expandable metal stent (FCSEMS), or lumen-apposing metal stents (LAMS), can then be deployed under endosonographic and fluoroscopic guidance to appose the gallbladder and gastrointestinal lumen [25]. More recently, the gallbladder puncture and stent deployment are done with a LAMS that has an electrocautery tip without the need for guidewire placement and tract dilation (Fig. 26.2a, b). This approach minimizes over-the-wire device exchanges, allowing for a theoretically safer and more efficient procedure [26].

EUS-guided gallbladder drainage is associated with high technical (>90%) and clinical success (>90%) rates. Technical failure may occur due to inability to pass the guidewire, accidental guidewire loss, or stent maldeployment [27]. Adverse events have been reported at a frequency of 7–15% and include bleeding, recurrent cholecystitis, stent migration, stent occlusion, and pneumoperitoneum [28, 29]. When comparing the various stent options for EUS-GBD, data suggest that LAMS have the lowest rate of adverse events [28]. LAMS are specifically designed for transmural drainage, shaped like a barbell with two flanges to appose each luminal surface, thus carrying a very low risk of migration while also allowing for a larger inner lumen diameter than either plastic stents or FCSEMS.

Laparoscopic cholecystectomy may be technically difficult or impossible in certain patients following EUS-guided gallbladder drainage as this procedure creates a permanent fistula between the gallbladder and the adjacent gastrointestinal lumen. EUS-GBD is contraindicated in patients with gallbladder perforation, untreated large-volume ascites, or uncorrectable coagulopathy [30].

Several studies have compared percutaneous cholecystostomy and EUS-GBD [31, 32]. Results have shown no difference in technical or clinical success rates for the treatment of acute cholecystitis; however, these studies have shown statistically significant differences in time to

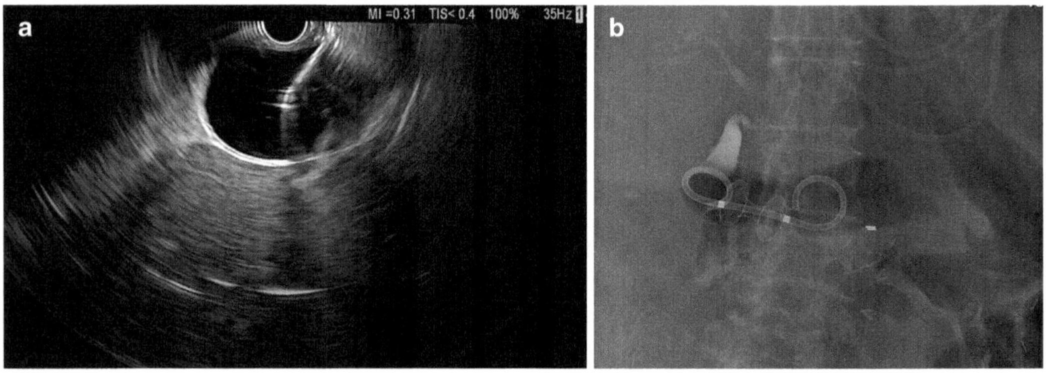

Fig. 26.2 Transmural EUS-guided gallbladder drainage. (**a**) From the antrum of the stomach or the proximal duodenum the gallbladder can be seen endosonographically. A cautery-enhanced catheter housing a lumen-apposing metal stent (LAMS) can then be passed into the gallbladder body. (**b**) The LAMS is then deployed thereby creating an anastomosis between the gallbladder and gastrointestinal lumen. A short double-pigtail stent is placed to minimize mucosal irritation from the stent and prevent stent migration/separation

resolution of cholecystitis, need for re-intervention, mean pain scores, adverse events, and hospital length of stay, favoring EUS-GBD [32]. More recently, a randomized trial (DRAC 1) of 80 patients comparing PC and EUS-GBD demonstrated that EUS-GBD significantly reduced 1-year adverse events, 30-day adverse events, and re-interventions with equivalent technical and clinical success rates [33].

In comparing the endoscopic approaches to manage acute cholecystitis, there are several retrospective studies comparing outcomes between transpapillary (cystic duct stent) and EUS-GBD. These have demonstrated that the EUS-guided approach is associated with better technical and clinical success with a trend toward lower adverse event rates and lower recurrence of cholecystitis [20, 34]. Furthermore, a recent meta-analysis including over 80 studies comparing transpapillary, EUS-guided, and percutaneous drainage found EUS-GBD to have better clinical success, with comparable adverse events between all groups [35].

Choledocholithiasis

Choledocholithiasis, or bile duct stones, generally results from migration of gallstones from the gallbladder into the biliary tree [36]. Less commonly, stones may develop de novo within the CBD. Small bile duct stones may spontaneously pass through the ampulla of Vater and into the duodenum which may cause intermittent symptoms or may result in no clinical symptoms at all. Symptomatic choledocholithiasis typically manifests with characteristic biliary pain with elevated liver enzymes. More serious sequelae of choledocholithiasis include obstruction of bile duct drainage leading to cholangitis and irritation of the pancreatic duct orifice leading to biliary pancreatitis. Choledocholithiasis is typically managed with endoscopic stone extraction, followed by interval cholecystectomy.

Among those with symptomatic cholelithiasis or acute cholecystitis, 10–20% have concomitant choledocholithiasis [37, 38]. The evaluation and management strategy differs depending on the pretest probability of bile duct stones (Table 26.1). The available data clearly support that patients at high risk for choledocholithiasis should undergo ERCP prior to cholecystectomy, while patients at low risk should proceed directly to cholecystectomy. Patients at intermediate risk should be referred for either EUS, magnetic resonance cholangiopancreatography (MRCP), or intraoperative cholangiography (IOC) [39]. All three of these modalities have high sensitivity and specificity for choledocholithiasis and can identify patients in need of endoscopic therapy, with the choice between them often based on local expertise and availability of resources.

ERCP is the first-line therapeutic modality for choledocholithiasis. Endoscopic sphincterotomy

Table 26.1 ASGE risk stratification of choledocholithiasis

Probability	Predictors of choledocholithiasis	Recommended management
High	1. CBD stone visualized on ultrasound or cross-sectional imaging or 2. Total bilirubin >4 mg/dL *and* dilated CBD (>6 or >8 mm in patients who have undergone cholecystectomy) or 3. Ascending cholangitis	ERCP
Intermediate	1. Abnormal liver biochemical tests or 2. Age >55 or 3. Dilated CBD	EUS vs MRCP
Low	None of the above	Cholecystectomy

ASGE Standards of Practice Committee, Buxbaum JL, Abbas Fehmi SM, et al. ASGE guideline on the role of endoscopy in the evaluation and management of choledocholithiasis. Gastrointest Endosc. 2019;89(7):1075–1105.e15 with stone extraction is successful in more than 90% of cases, with an overall adverse event rate of approximately 5%. Adverse events of ERCP of include pancreatitis (2–10%), bleeding (2%), perforation (<1%), and cholangitis (<1%) [40]. During this procedure, a duodenoscope is passed into the second portion of the duodenum where the ampulla can be identified. Selective bile duct cannulation is achieved using a catheter or sphincterotome. Contrast is then injected under fluoroscopy for cholangiography, allowing for delineation of biliary anatomy and identification of stones. A biliary sphincterotomy is performed using electrocautery. This small incision through the sphincter of Oddi enlarges the papillary opening permitting easier stone removal. Stones can then be extracted from the duct using a stone extraction balloon or a wire basket (Fig. 26.3a, b). An alternative technique to endoscopic sphincterotomy is balloon dilation of the intact biliary sphincter (endoscopic balloon sphincteroplasty) to enlarge the biliary orifice using hydrostatic dilating balloons (up to 10 mm). This approach may be best suited for removal of bile duct stones in patients at high risk for post-sphincterotomy bleeding (i.e., routine antithrombotic use) or those with unfavorable or surgically-altered anatomy which may preclude sphincterotomy [41, 42]. While historical data have suggested a higher rate of post-ERCP pancreatitis with endoscopic papillary balloon dilation, this risk appears to be mitigated with the use of larger balloons (>12 mm) held for longer duration (>30 s) [42, 43].

For larger stones (>1 cm), a partial sphincterotomy may be combined with large papillary balloon dilation, using a larger hydrostatic dilating balloon (12–20 mm) to further distend the ampullary orifice (Fig. 26.4) [44]. Alternatively, the stones may need to be fragmented using mechanical or intraductal lithotripsy. During mechanical lithotripsy, a wire basket is used to capture and crush the stone using mechanical force (Fig. 26.5) [45]. Intraductal electrohydraulic or laser lithotripsy can be performed using a cholangioscope, either passed through a duodenoscope into the bile duct (mother-baby system) or by transoral passage of a dedicated small caliber endoscope (direct peroral cholangioscope). An electrohydraulic probe (oscillating shock waves) or pulsed laser (beam of energy) is directed at the stones leading to fragmentation (Fig. 26.6). Fragment clearance can then be performed with standard stone extraction methods. Rarely, extracorporeal shock wave lithotripsy (ESWL) can be used as a last resort [46]. If complete stone removal is not

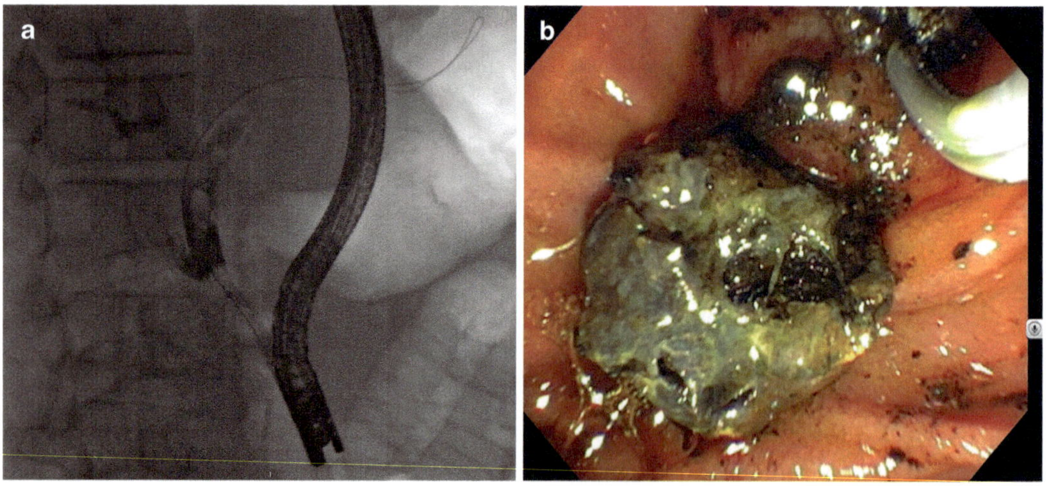

Fig. 26.3 Choledocholithiasis. (**a**) An occlusion cholangiogram demonstrating a large common hepatic duct stone with smaller stones noted in the right and left hepatic ducts. (**b**) Removal of a large bile duct stone into the duodenal lumen using a balloon extraction technique

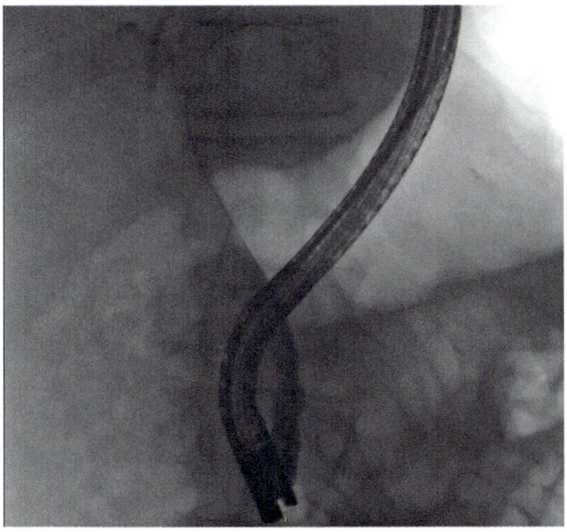

Fig. 26.4 Endoscopic large papillary balloon dilation. Fluoroscopic image of a large (>10 mm) dilating balloon is used to dilate the papillary orifice to aid in extraction of larger common bile duct stones

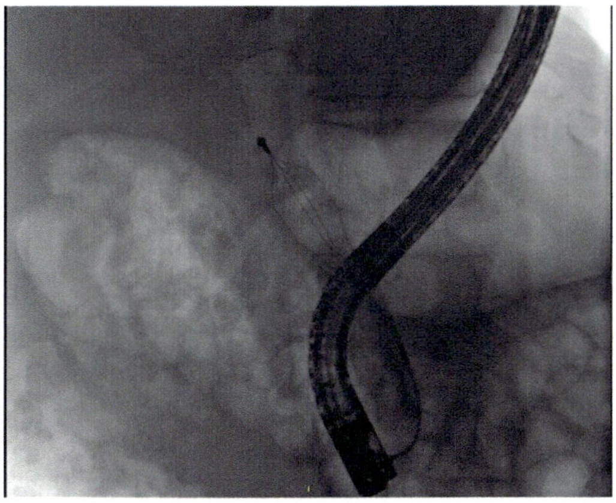

Fig. 26.5 Mechanical lithotripsy. The mechanical lithotripter can be passed into the common bile duct. The lithotripter basket is opened and the basket is used to ensnare large stones. After stones are ensnared, the basket is gradually closed until stones are crushed or fragmented

achieved, a plastic or covered-metal biliary stent should be placed to maintain biliary drainage until repeat ERCP is performed [47].

Interval cholecystectomy should be performed in the vast majority of patients following stone clearance, given the high rate (20%) of recurrent symptoms including cholecystitis, pancreatitis, and recurrent choledocholithiasis [48, 49].

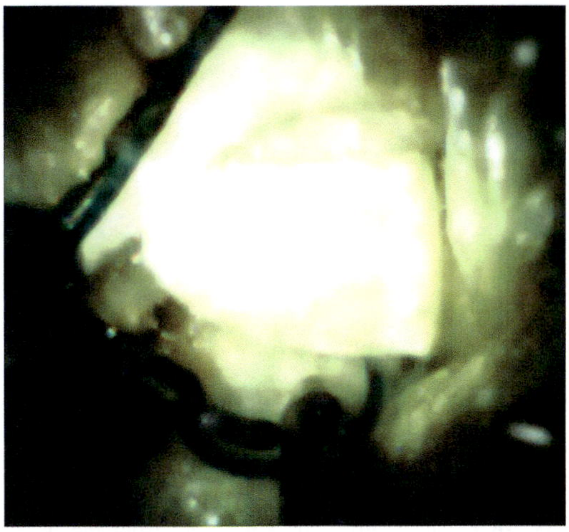

Fig. 26.6 Electrohydraulic lithotripsy. Cholangioscopic images demonstrating intraductal electrohydraulic lithotripsy to fracture a large common bile duct stones which was not amenable to retrieval using conventional methods. Surgical suture can be visualized which served as a nidus for stone formation

Cholangitis

Acute cholangitis, or infection in the bile duct, occurs when biliary obstruction results in cholestasis and infection (Fig. 26.7). This is most often secondary to a bile duct stone, but can also occur in the setting of malignancy, prior biliary instrumentation, biliary strictures secondary to surgery or chronic pancreatitis, or other infectious or auto-immune cholangiopathies [50]. Cholangitis classically presents with Charcot's triad [51], consisting of fever, right upper quadrant pain, and jaundice, or Reynold's pentad [52] (hypotension and altered mentation) if the patient is in shock. Historically, cholangitis carried a high mortality rate, particularly in the elderly [53]. In addition to antibiotics, timely biliary drainage is the cornerstone in management. Endoscopic transpapillary biliary drainage via ERCP is currently the standard of care, with success rates of >90–95% [54]. Reasons for failure of conventional ERCP include ampullary pathology (adenoma/carcinoma), periampullary diverticulum, gastric outlet or duodenal obstruction, or variant anatomy (e.g., Roux-ex-Y) [55]. When ERCP cannot be completed, alternative

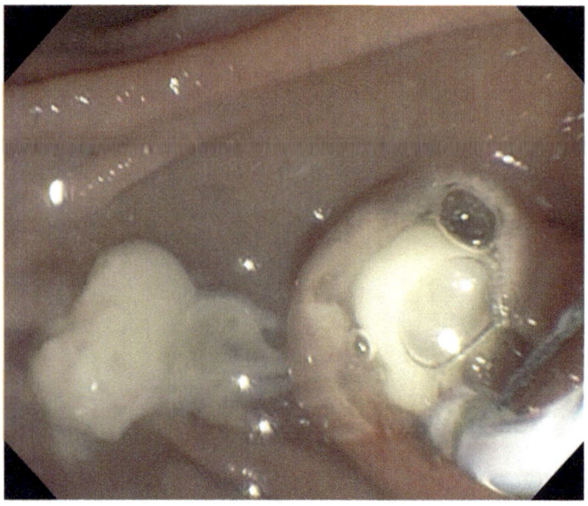

Fig. 26.7 Cholangitis. Pus emanating from the major papilla following endoscopic sphincterotomy

approaches include percutaneous transhepatic biliary drainage (PTBD), or EUS-guided biliary drainage [56].

Endoscopic Transpapillary Biliary Drainage

As noted above, endoscopic transpapillary biliary drainage is first line in the management of cholangitis [40]. ERCP performed within 48 h of presentation is associated with improved outcomes [57]. Patients with overt sepsis and frail, elderly patients who may decompensate quickly should undergo ERCP as soon as it is clinically safe to do so. The technical aspects of the procedure are identical to those used for choledocholithiasis. The primary goal is to establish biliary drainage. In patients with cholangitis secondary to choledocholithiasis, sphincterotomy and stone/sludge extraction are generally sufficient to provide adequate biliary drainage, with stent placement reserved for cases where the stone cannot be easily removed or the patient is too ill to undergo a prolonged procedure. Similarly, in patients with obstruction due to benign or malignant strictures, biliary stent placement with or without stricture dilation is generally needed to provide adequate drainage. The one exception to this approach is in patients with primary sclerosing cholangitis (PSC), whereby stent placement is avoided if possible, with focus on stricture dilation and stone removal to promote biliary drainage.

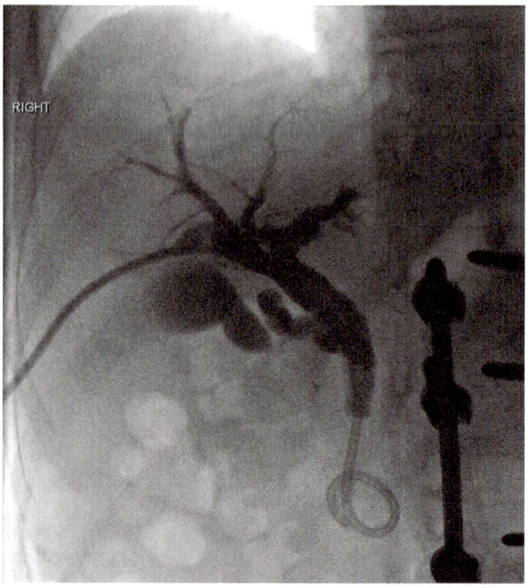

Fig. 26.8 Percutaneous transhepatic biliary drainage. A percutaneous cholangiogram obtained by contrast injection of an internal-external biliary drain

Percutaneous Transhepatic Biliary Drainage (PTBD)

Percutaneous bile duct access was first described in 1937 [58], and ultimately refined for routine clinical use in the 1980s with the advent of specially-designed needle catheters. The technique involves ultrasound-guided identification and percutaneous puncture of an intrahepatic bile duct using an 18–22-gauge needle. After confirming backflow of bile, a guidewire is advanced through the needle into the bile duct. Using fluoroscopic guidance, a 7–10 Fr catheter is advanced into the bile duct over the guidewire. If the guidewire can be passed into the duodenum, the catheter may provide both internal (into duodenal lumen) and external biliary drainage (into external bag) (Fig. 26.8). If the wire cannot reach the duodenum (e.g., obstructed by a stone or stricture), the catheter can be left in the bile duct, facilitating external drainage only.

PTBD has a high success rate (>90%) and can be done without general anesthesia. PTBD is often used to access to the biliary tree when endoscopic approaches are unsuccessful. Similar to percutaneous cholecystostomy, one major disadvantage is the need for an external catheter which may require frequent catheter exchanges and can be associated with catheter dislodgement, patient discomfort, and impaired quality of life [59]. Additional adverse events include sepsis (2.5%), bleeding (2.5%), inflammation/infection (1.2%—including abscess, peritonitis, cholecystitis, pancreatitis), and pneumothorax (0.5%) [60].

EUS-Guided Biliary Drainage

First described in 2001 by Giovannini et al. [61], endoscopic ultrasound-guided biliary drainage (EUS-BD) is a minimally invasive endoscopic option, increasingly offered as an alternative to PTBD for biliary decompression when conventional ERCP fails. In comparison with PTBD, a recent meta-analysis found that EUS-BD had better clinical success, fewer adverse events, and a lower rate of re-intervention [62]. EUS-BD has evolved over the last 20 years and encompasses three main techniques: EUS-guided biliary rendezvous (Fig. 26.9a–d), EUS-guided choledochoduodenostomy (extrahepatic bile duct drainage), and EUS-guided hepaticogastrostomy (intrahepatic bile duct drainage).

To perform EUS-guided biliary rendezvous (EUS-RV), the echoendoscope is advanced to either the duodenum to puncture the extrahepatic

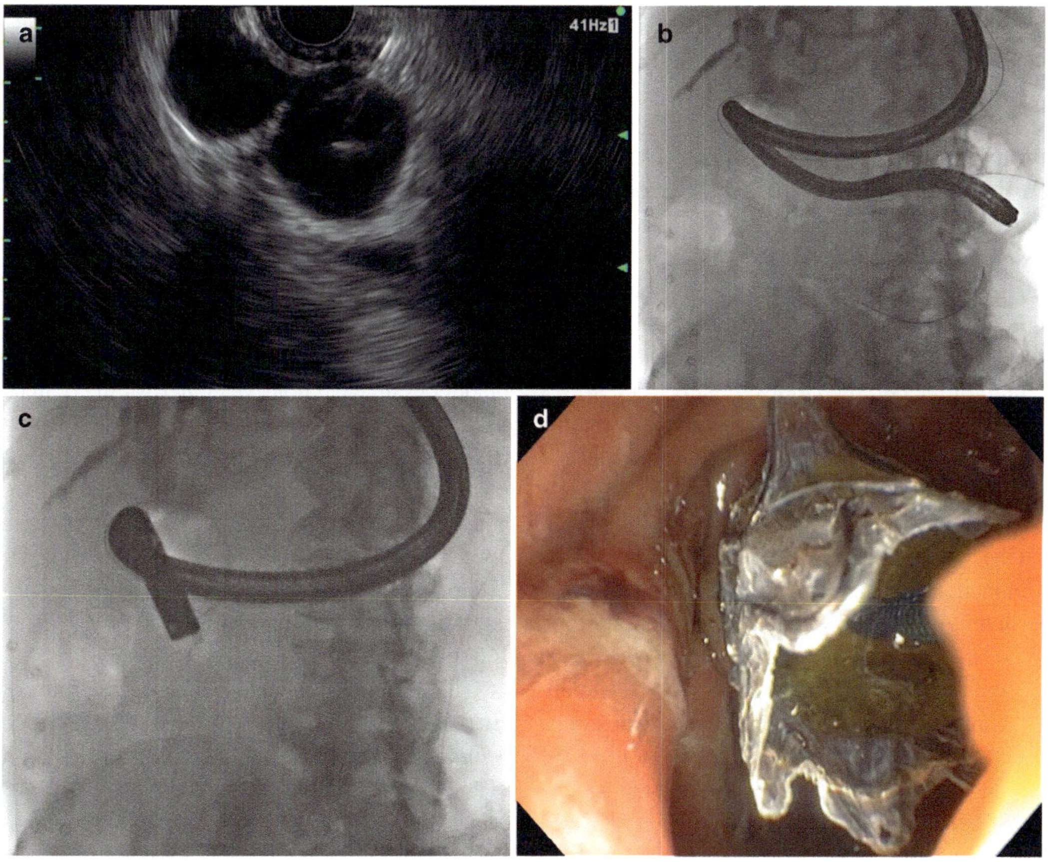

Fig. 26.9 EUS-guided biliary rendezvous procedure. (**a**) The bile duct is identified and punctured under EUS-guidance. Following access, a cholangiogram can be obtained and a guidewire is passed antegrade into the distal bile duct, through the major papilla and ultimately coiled in the duodenum. (**b**) The echoendoscope is exchanged for a duodenoscope. The duodenoscope is passed into the small bowel and the guidewire is located. (**c**) The guidewire is grasped and retrieved through the working channel of the duodenoscope allowing for conventional retrograde interventions. (**d**) Retrograde placement of a fully covered self-expandable metal stent across a benign distal bile duct stricture using the rendezvous technique

biliary duct, or the stomach to puncture a left intrahepatic bile duct. After confirmation of access (i.e., bile aspiration and contrast injection), a guidewire is passed through the EUS-FNA needle into the biliary system with the goal of traversing the ampulla and coiling in the duodenum. Following placement of the "rendezvous" guidewire, the echoendoscope is removed leaving the guidewire in place. A duodenoscope is then passed transorally in parallel to the guidewire and into position within the second portion of the duodenum. The bile duct may then be cannulated alongside the "rendezvous" guidewire, or the guidewire can be grasped and withdrawn through the working channel of the duodenoscope to allow for device/accessory passage over the grasped "rendezvous" guidewire [63].

For EUS-guided choledochoduodenostomy (EUS-CDS), the echoendoscope is positioned in the duodenal bulb and the CBD is punctured with an EUS-FNA needle. After confirmation of needle location, the tract between the duodenum and extrahepatic bile duct is dilated using mechanical dilation (i.e., rigid graduated dilating catheters, dilation balloon) or electrocautery (i.e., electrocautery enhanced LAMS, cystotome) or a combination of the two modalities. Finally, a FCSEMS or LAMS, depending on the chosen approach, is placed to create an anastomosis between the CBD and the duodenum.

For EUS-guided hepaticogastrostomy (EUS-HGS), the echoendoscope is positioned in the stomach to identify a left intrahepatic biliary radicle. An EUS-FNA needle is then used to puncture the bile duct, aspirate bile to confirm location, and inject contrast to obtain a cholangiogram. Similar to choledochoduodenostomy, the tract is dilated using a variety of devices, dependent on the endoscopist's preference. A FCSEMS is placed across the tract, generally not less than 8 cm in length, with the distal flange in the left hepatic duct and the proximal flange in the gastric lumen. Often a plastic double-pigtail stent may be placed to straighten the stent and prevent stent migration/separation of the tract. This EUS-guided approach allows for immediate or future antegrade therapies using conventional ERCP techniques (i.e., balloon dilation or FCSEMS placement across a distal bile duct stricture, stone fragmentation with lithotripsy devices followed by stone removal, etc.). Uncommonly, antegrade therapies may be performed without formal creation of a hepaticogastrostomy tract. This less common technique involves passage of a guidewire into the biliary system followed by over-the-guidewire tract dilation using a rigid graduated catheter or balloon dilator. Antegrade therapy, most commonly a FCSEMS across a distal bile duct stricture, can then be performed without creation of an anastomosis. This idea relies on the premise that bile will flow in the path of least resistance (i.e., through the bile duct stent) and not out the site of puncture/access [64]. The technical success rate for the EUS-antegrade approach (77%) is less than other EUS-guided biliary drainage (EUS-BD) techniques, owing to the difficulty of guidewire passage and stent delivery from an intrahepatic access site to traverse an area of obstruction [56].

Lastly, and less commonly, EUS-guided gallbladder drainage (cholecystoenterostomy) can be used to decompress the biliary system, assuming the cystic duct is patent and above the level of obstruction [65]. This approach is as described above for the non-surgical management of acute cholecystitis. When this technique is used for biliary drainage, it is often in the setting of malignant distal bile duct obstruction with failed ERCP [66].

The cumulative technical success rate of EUS-BD has been reported around 90–95%, with a clinical success rate of 90–95%, and adverse event rate of 15–23% [67, 68]. Adverse events include bleeding (4%), bile leak (4%), pneumoperitoneum (3%), stent migration (2.7%), and cholangitis (2.4%). In terms of comparing the EUS-BD methods, EUS-CDS and EUS-HGS have been found to have equal efficacy and safety, with nearly identical technical success rates [69]. These methods are generally superior to EUS-RV, which has an overall success rate of 80% and adverse event rate of 15% [63]. In the context of currently available literature, there is no optimal EUS-BD approach. Rather, the endoscopist must factor in the clinical circumstance and individual anatomy (e.g., level of obstruction, degree of duct dilation, surgical alteration) as well as the goals of the procedure when choosing the appropriate EUS-BD therapy [70].

Biliary Access in Surgically-Altered Anatomy

Surgically-altered gastrointestinal anatomy may result in anatomic changes that make endoscopic access to the biliary tree technically difficult or impossible. These include gastric resections (e.g., Billroth II gastrectomy), bypass procedures or weight loss operations (e.g., Roux-en-Y gastric bypass [RYGB], loop gastrojejunostomy, duodenal switch with biliopancreatic diversion), pancreatic resections (e.g., Whipple pancreaticoduodenectomy), or biliary drainage surgeries (e.g., Roux-en-Y hepaticojejunostomy or choledochojejunostomy). Depending on the length of the Roux limb in resection surgeries, a duodenoscope or forward-viewing endoscope may be able to reach the major papilla to allow for "conventional" ERCP. However, in patients with RYGB anatomy or a long Roux limb, this is usually not feasible. There are three major endoscopic approaches for biliary interventions in patients with surgically-altered anatomy when conventional accessories cannot be utilized: (1) device-assisted enteroscopy ERCP, (2) laparoscopic-assisted ERCP, and (3) EUS-directed transgastric ERCP.

Device-assisted or "deep" enteroscopy permits advancement of an endoscope deep into the small bowel by "telescoping" the small-bowel over an overtube to bring the target closer, rather than relying on forward propulsion [71]. Devices used in practice include the single-balloon enteroscope, double-balloon enteroscope, and spiral enteroscope. In the context of Roux-en-Y anatomy, the enteroscope must traverse the Roux limb and advance into the pancreaticobiliary limb in order to reach the biliary orifice, at which point ERCP can be performed. This approach has several limitations and has fallen out of favor at many institutions. First, the surgical anastomosis or major papilla may not be reachable. Second, the enteroscope—which is not designed for ERCP—is forward-viewing, lacks an elevator, and is more difficult to maneuver in the region of the papilla, all of which make biliary cannulation technically challenging. Furthermore, accessories for therapeutic interventions are limited because of the long length (200 cm) and small-diameter working channel of the enteroscopes. The success rate varies widely in the literature, with technical success rate ranging from 60–70% at best [72, 73].

Laparoscopic-assisted ERCP requires a surgeon to access the excluded gastric remnant laparoscopically followed by placement of a 15-mm laparoscopic port. The duodenoscope can then be passed through the port and into position for conventional ERCP. Following ERCP, surgical closure of the gastrostomy is performed; however, if repeat ERCP will be required (e.g., removal of stents, stone removal, etc.), a gastrostomy tube can be placed through the tract to maintain patency. Tract dilation may be needed prior to subsequent ERCP to allow scope passage. A major advantage of this approach is that it allows for concomitant cholecystectomy in the same operation. Very high rates of technical success, nearing 100%, have been reported [74]. The most significant limitation of the laparoscopic approach is the need to coordinate logistics between surgical and gastroenterological teams to perform a combined procedure [75].

Most recently, EUS-guided approaches have been described with equally high success rates. One method, EUS-directed transgastric ERCP (EDGE), involves the creation of a gastrogastrostomy between the gastric pouch and gastric remnant in patients with RYGB (Fig. 26.10a–d). To perform this procedure, the gastric remnant is located endosonographically from either the gastric pouch or the blind jejunal pouch of the Roux limb. A 19-gauge needle is used to puncture the gastric remnant, which is then filled with dilute contrast and a coloring agent. Following instillation of ~500 cc of dilute contrast, the gastric remnant is adequately distended and can serve as an endosonographic target. A LAMS is then deployed

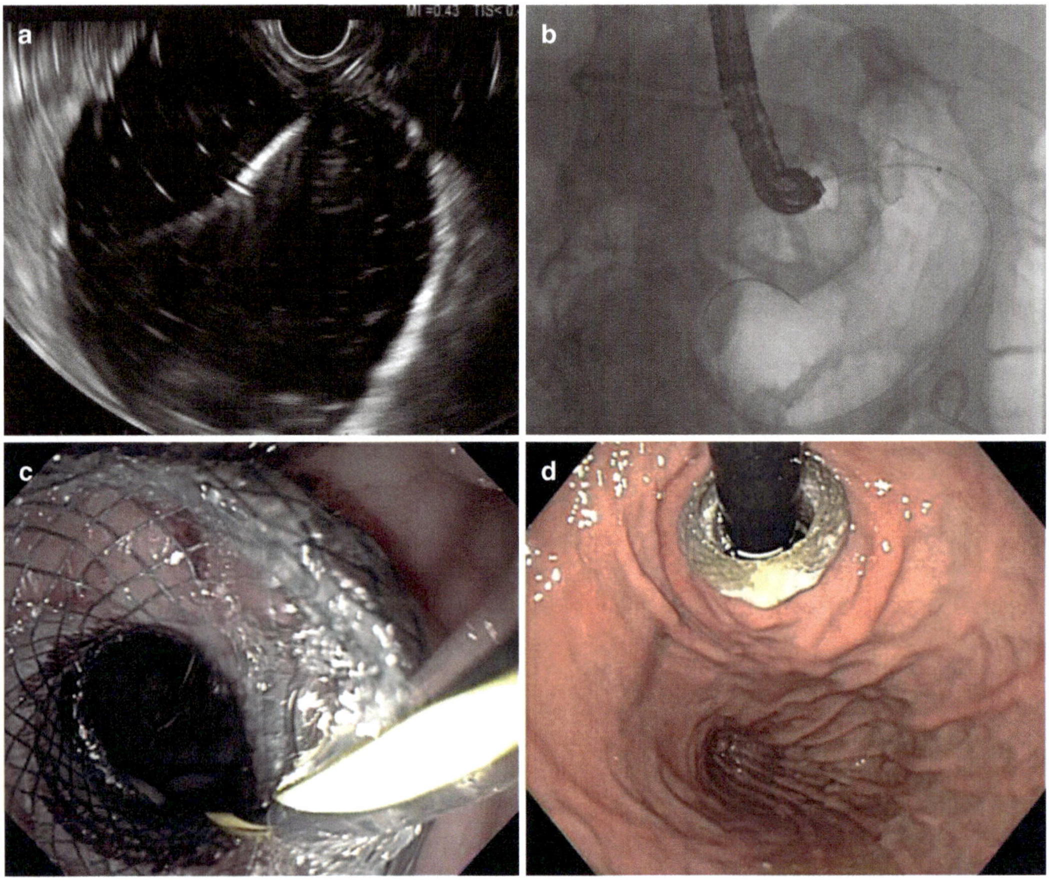

Fig. 26.10 EUS-direct transgastric ERCP (EDGE) procedure. (**a**) The excluded gastric remnant is identified endosonographically and is punctured using a 19-g FNA needle. Dilute contrast is instilled to distend the gastric remnant. (**b**) Fluoroscopic image immediately after deployment of the lumen-apposing metal stent creating the gastrogastric anastomosis. (**c**) Endoscopic confirmation of transgastric access following balloon dilation of the stent lumen. The mucosa of the gastric remnant can be visualized through the stent lumen after dilation. (**d**) Passage of the duodenoscope through the lumen-apposing metal stent to perform conventional ERCP

into the gastric remnant using a cautery-enhanced catheter, either over a guidewire or using a freehand technique, thereby creating a gastrogastric or jejunogastric anastomosis. Subsequently, the LAMS can then be balloon dilated to allow for passage of the duodenoscope into the gastric remnant to complete ERCP during the same session. Alternatively, in stable patients, ERCP can be deferred to a later date (i.e., minimum 2 weeks) to allow tract maturation. It should be noted that the single-session approach carries an increased risk of stent dislodgement during duodenoscope passage [76]. Once interventions are complete, the LAMS is removed at a subsequent procedure, and the tract can be closed via endoscopic suturing or placement of an over-the-scope clip, or left to close without endoscopic closure. Procedural success rates with EDGE are >95% [73, 77]. Serious adverse events occur rarely in expert hands, and include stent migration, perforation, bleeding, and chronic fistulization with risk of weight regain. EDGE is becoming the preferred procedure at centers with expertise in therapeutic EUS and ERCP, as it confers many advantages including high success rates, low rates of serious adverse events, cost-effectiveness, and the ability to use a standard duodenoscope and accessories [78–80].

An alternative EUS-guided approach is EUS-HGS, as described above. Therapeutic interventions can be performed in an antegrade fashion as necessary (i.e., stricture dilation and stent placement, stone removal, etc.). Similar to EDGE, interventions can be performed during the index procedure or in subsequent staged procedures. Recent studies have reported success rates over 90% with an acceptable adverse event rate [81, 82]; however, this approach is limited by the need for a sufficiently dilated intrahepatic duct and the availability of technical expertise.

Finally, percutaneous transhepatic biliary drainage (PTBD), as described above, is also an option; however, this approach requires an external drainage catheter and is associated with the limitations previously mentioned. Ultimately, the procedural approach depends on the clinical scenario and local expertise.

Section 2: Bile Leaks and Bile Duct Injury

Introduction

Bile duct injury (BDI) is a rare and dreaded adverse event of cholecystectomy, which is associated with significant morbidity and mortality. While the incidence of BDI has increased in the laparoscopic era, it remains low at approximately 0.5%, ranging in severity from minor bile leaks to complete bile duct transection [83, 84]. While the majority of BDIs can be treated with endoscopic interventions, some require surgical repair. Prompt recognition of BDI and involvement of a multidisciplinary team including hepatobiliary surgeons, interventional endoscopists, and interventional radiologists is essential to optimize outcomes [85]. In terms of endoscopic management, the most important factor is whether or not there is continuity of the injured bile duct with the CBD. While various classification schemata have been proposed to guide management decisions (Fig. 26.11a–c), the Strasberg system remains the most popular and widely used (Table 26.2) [86].

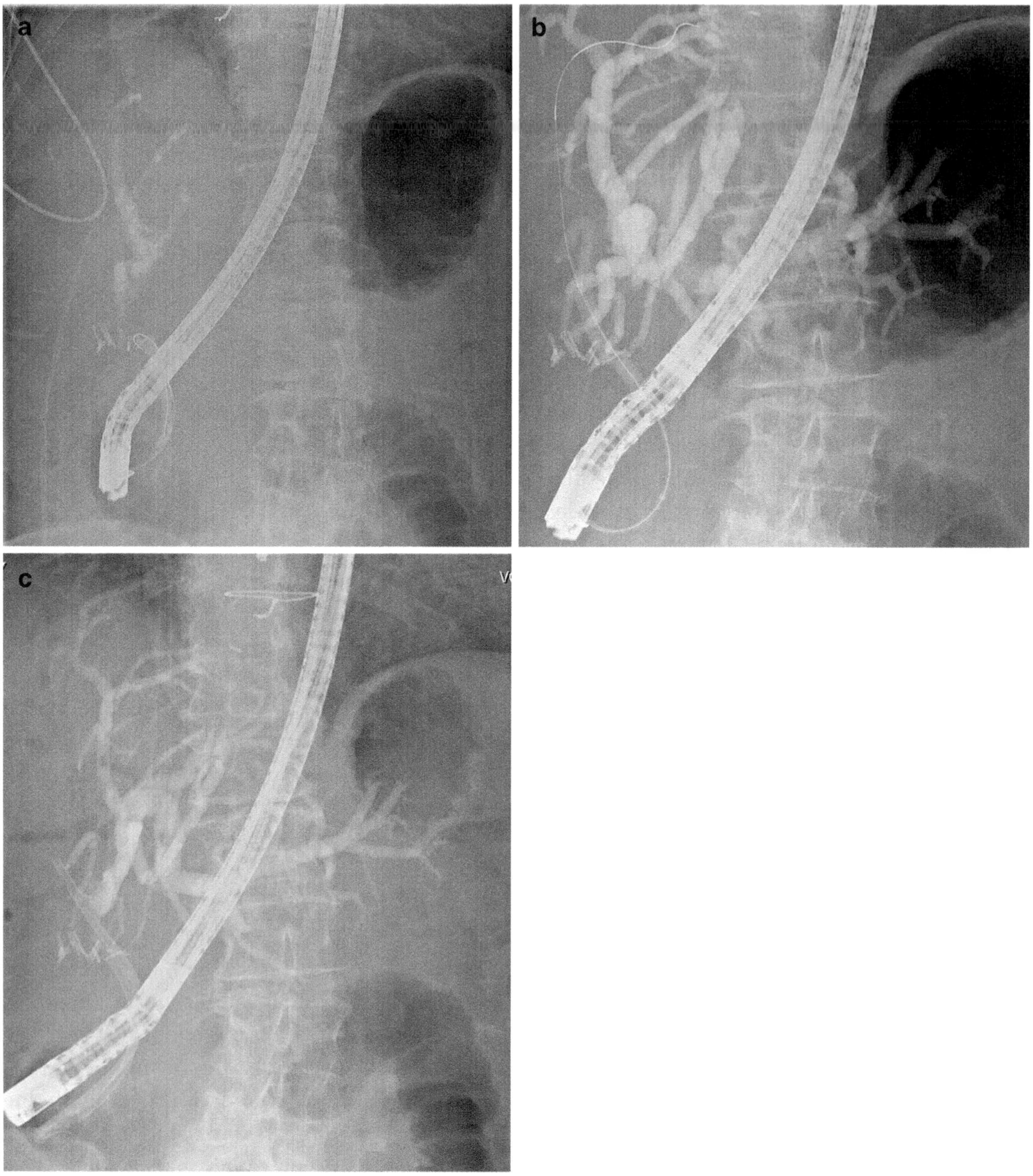

Fig. 26.11 Near-complete bile duct transection. (**a**) Cholangiography demonstrating near-complete clip transection of the common bile duct at the level of the cystic duct insertion. No contrast extravasation is seen and the common hepatic duct and intrahepatics opacify suggesting partial connection to the distal common bile duct. (**b**) Balloon dilation across the site of clip transection. (**c**) Placement of two plastic common bile duct stents to recanalize the bile duct thus promoting antegrade bile drainage and prevent the need for surgical intervention

Table 26.2 Strasberg classification of bile duct injury

Strasberg classification	Definition	Frequency	Treatment
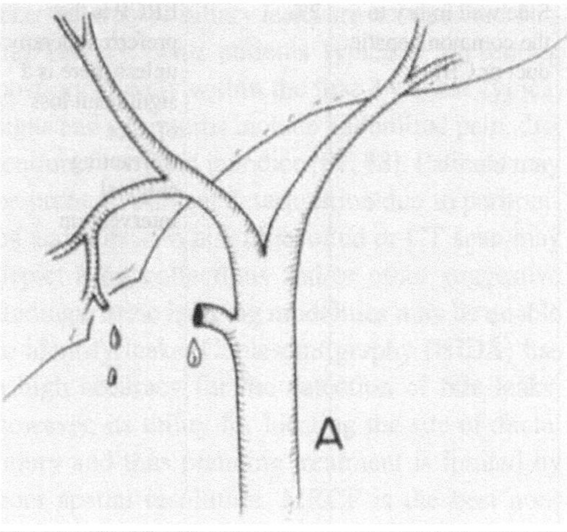	Leak from the cystic duct or duct of Luschka	45–85% 75% from cystic duct stump 10% from the ducts of Luschka	ERCP
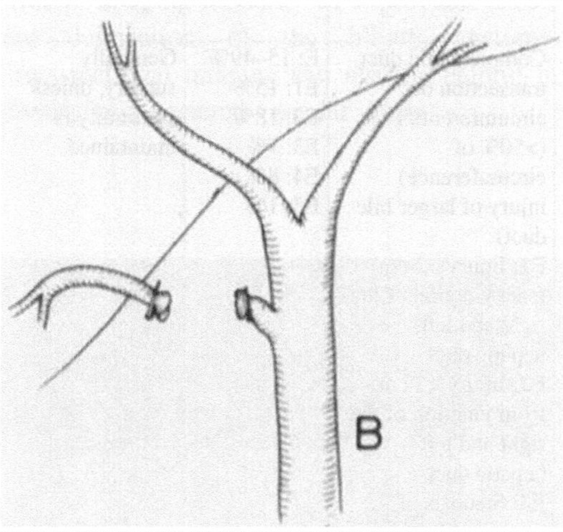	Ligated sectoral duct	1%	Communication with CBD branches: ERCP No communication with CBD branches: Surgery
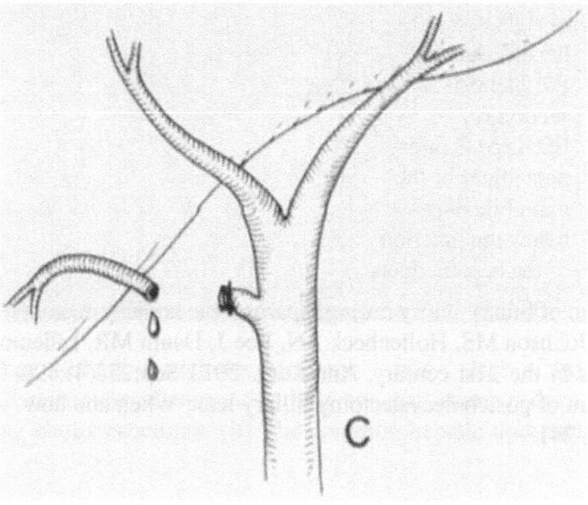	Leak from non-ligated sectoral duct	1%	Communication with CBD branches: ERCP No communication with CBD branches: Surgery

(continued)

placement alone (failure rate 4%) or combination therapy (failure rate 3%) were superior to sphincterotomy alone (failure rate 11%) [91].

In clinical practice, most endoscopists perform sphincterotomy with placement of a short (i.e., <7 cm) 10 Fr plastic stent. This approach can be applied to most bile leaks. In cases where there is a leak from a branch of the hepatic duct, placement of a longer and possibly smaller caliber stent which traverses the leak site should be considered. Placement of a FCSEMS should be considered for high-grade leaks or leaks secondary to large disruption of the CBD wall [92]. Data are limited regarding the optimal approach, and thus, the choice of endoscopic intervention is often made based on several factors, such as location and grade of the leak, presence of concomitant bile duct stones, and individualized patient considerations (i.e., use of antithrombotic agents, etc.).

Stents are left in place for approximately 4–6 weeks, at which point ERCP is repeated to remove the stent and determine if the leak has resolved. Of note, if a percutaneous drain was placed as part of management of the bile leak, the drain should be removed, or the output should be <10 mL/day, prior to biliary stent removal. In cases of refractory bile leak (i.e., persistent leak on cholangiography or persistent high output percutaneous drainage), rescue endoscopic options include the following: placement of a stent which bridges the leak site, placement of multiple plastic stents, or placement of a FCSEMS, with data suggesting that FCSEMS are superior [92–94].

In the setting of complete transection of the bile duct (Strasberg E), the treatment of choice has traditionally been surgical hepaticojejunostomy, given biliary discontinuity. However, in select cases, recanalization of the bile duct may be feasible with a percutaneous-endoscopic rendezvous procedure [95]. A recent retrospective review of 47 patients undergoing this rendezvous procedure found a primary success rate of 94%, with procedure-related adverse events occurring in 18% of patients, none of which were life-threatening. Rendezvous was the final successful treatment in 55% and served as a bridge to surgery in 30% [96].

Biloma

A bile leak may result in the formation of a biloma. While the majority of bilomas will resolve spontaneously, up to 20% will require drainage due to clinically significant symptoms such as abdominal pain, nausea, vomiting, gastric outlet obstruction, or abscess formation [86]. Percutaneous drainage remains the treatment of choice for most patients [97]; however, if the biloma is close to the gastric or duodenal wall, it may be drained via EUS-guided drainage [98].

Biliary Stricture

Post-operative injuries can result in biliary strictures, which often present much later than biliary leaks (median of 2 months). This delayed presentation is usually a result of ischemic injury with resultant fibrosis [99]. Patients typically present with signs of biliary obstruction, namely jaundice, cholestatic liver biochemistries, and biliary dilation on imaging.

Endoscopic treatment involves stricture dilation and serial placement of multiple plastic stents until stricture resolution (often over 12 months), with exchanges approximately every 3 months [100–102]. Alternatively, FCSEMS appear to have excellent efficacy and require less frequent exchanges (Fig. 26.13a, b) [91]. When using FCSEMS, the stent should be left in place

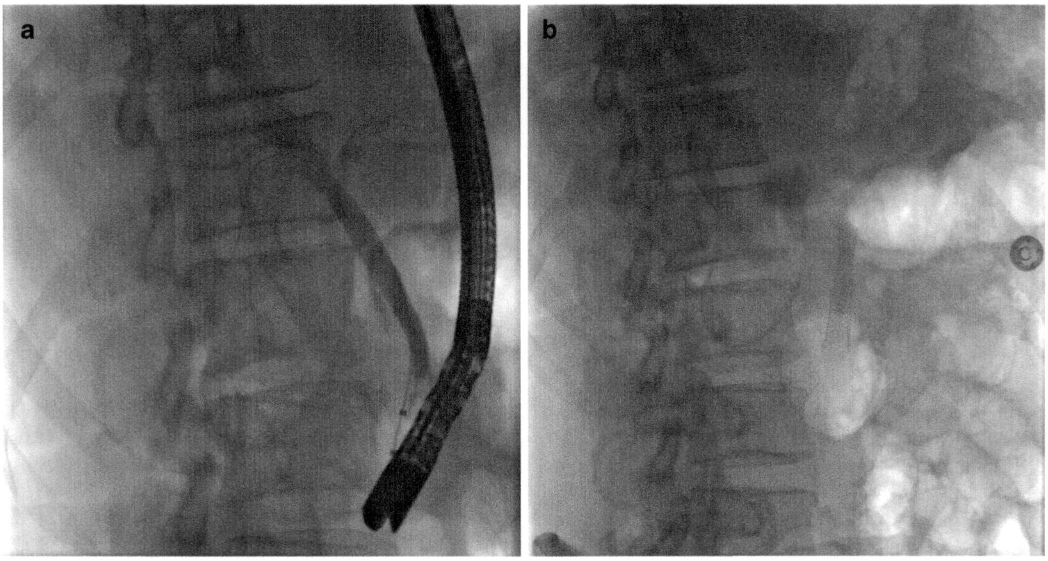

Fig. 26.13 Distal common bile duct stricture. (**a**) Cholangiogram images showing a refractory distal common bile duct stricture in the setting of chronic pancreatitis. (**b**) Placement of a fully covered self-expandable metal stent into the distal bile duct

for a minimum of 3 months to treat the stricture. In rare cases, biliary strictures refractory to endoscopic therapy may require surgical biliary bypass.

Conclusion

Non-operative interventions are valuable tools in the management of biliary diseases and bile duct injuries. In patients unfit for surgery, endoscopic and/or percutaneous procedures may serve as primary treatment modalities or as a bridge to future surgical intervention. Recent advances in endoscopic tools and techniques, particularly EUS-guided interventions, have greatly enhanced the armamentarium. The increasing complexity of patients and therapies alike underscore the importance of multidisciplinary and team-based care.

References

1. Kimura Y, Takada T, Strasberg SM, Pitt HA, Gouma DJ, Garden OJ, Büchler MW, Windsor JA, Mayumi T, Yoshida M, Miura F, Higuchi R, Gabata T, Hata J, Gomi H, Dervenis C, Lau WY, Belli G, Kim MH, Hilvano SC, Yamashita Y. TG13 current terminology, etiology, and epidemiology of acute cholangitis and cholecystitis. J Hepatobiliary Pancreat Sci. 2013;20(1):8–23.
2. Radder RW. Ultrasonically guided percutaneous catheter drainage for gallbladder empyema. Diagn Imaging. 1980;49:330–3.
3. Stanek A, Dohan A, Barkun J, et al. Percutaneous cholecystostomy: a simple bridge to surgery or an alternative option for the management of acute cholecystitis? Am J Surg. 2018;216(3):595–603.
4. Duszak R Jr, Behrman SW. National trends in percutaneous cholecystostomy between 1994 and 2009: perspectives from Medicare provider claims. J Am Coll Radiol. 2012;9:474–9.
5. Winbladh A, Gullstrand P, Svanvik J, Sandström P. Systematic review of cholecystostomy as a treat-

ment option in acute cholecystitis. HPB (Oxford). 2009;11(3):183–93.
6. Penas-Herrero I, de la Serna-Higuera C, Perez-Miranda M. Endoscopic ultrasound-guided gallbladder drainage for the management of acute cholecystitis (with video). J Hepatobiliary Pancreat Sci. 2015;22:35–43.
7. Alvino DML, Fong ZV, McCarthy CJ, et al. Long-term outcomes following percutaneous cholecystostomy tube placement for treatment of acute calculous cholecystitis. J Gastrointest Surg. 2017;21(5):761–9.
8. Loozen CS, van Santvoort HC, van Duijvendijk P, Besselink MGH, Gouma DJ, Nieuwenhuijzen GAP, et al. Laparoscopic cholecystectomy versus percutaneous catheter drainage for acute cholecystitis in high risk patients (CHOCOLATE): multicentre randomised clinical trial. BMJ. 2018;363:k3965.
9. Arvanitakis M. Endoscopic transpapillary gallbladder stent placement for high-risk patients with cholecystitis: an oldie but still a goodie. Gastrointest Endosc. 2020;92(3):645–7.
10. de Mestral C, Gomez D, Haas B, Zagorski B, Rotstein OD, Nathens AB. Cholecystostomy: a bridge to hospital discharge but not delayed cholecystectomy. J Trauma Acute Care Surg. 2013;74(1):175–80.
11. McKay A, Abulfaraj M, Lipschitz J. Short- and long-term outcomes following percutaneous cholecystostomy for acute cholecystitis in high-risk patients. Surg Endosc. 2012;26(5):1343–51.
12. Elmunzer BJ, Novelli PM, Taylor JR, Piraka CR, Shields JJ. Percutaneous cholecystostomy as a bridge to definitive endoscopic gallbladder stent placement. Clin Gastroenterol Hepatol. 2011;9:18–20.
13. Law R, Grimm IS, Stavas JM, Baron TH. Conversion of percutaneous cholecystostomy to internal transmural gallbladder drainage using an endoscopic ultrasound-guided, lumen-apposing metal stent. Clin Gastroenterol Hepatol. 2016;14(3):476–80.
14. Feretis CB, Manouras AJ, Apostolidis NS, Golematis BC. Endoscopic transpapillary drainage of gallbladder empyema. Gastrointest Endosc. 1990;36:523–5.
15. Itoi T, Kawakami H, Katanuma A, Irisawa A, Sofuni A, Itokawa F, et al. Endoscopic nasogallbladder tube or stent placement in acute cholecystitis: a preliminary prospective randomized trial in Japan (with videos). Gastrointest Endosc. 2015;81:111–8.
16. Ridtitid W, Piyachaturawat P, Teeratorn N, Angsuwatcharakon P, Kongkam P, Rerknimitr R. Single-operator peroral cholangioscopy cystic duct cannulation for transpapillary gallbladder stent placement in patients with acute cholecystitis at moderate to high surgical risk (with videos). Gastrointest Endosc. 2020;92(3):634–44.
17. Baron TH, Grimm IS, Swanstrom LL. Interventional approaches to gallbladder disease. N Engl J Med. 2015;373(4):357–65.
18. Lee TH, Park DH, Lee SS, et al. Outcomes of endoscopic transpapillary gallbladder stenting for symptomatic gallbladder diseases: a multicenter prospective follow-up study. Endoscopy. 2011;43(8):702–8.
19. Siegel J. Stone extraction, lithotripsy, stents and stones. In: Siegel J, editor. Endoscopic retrograde cholangiopancreatography. New York: Raven Press; 1991. p. 227–71.
20. Higa JT, Sahar N, Kozarek RA, et al. EUS-guided gallbladder drainage with a lumen-apposing metal stent versus endoscopic transpapillary gallbladder drainage for the treatment of acute cholecystitis (with videos). Gastrointest Endosc. 2019;90(3):483–92.
21. Sagami R, Hayasaka K, Ujihara T, et al. Endoscopic transpapillary gallbladder drainage for acute cholecystitis is feasible for patients receiving antithrombotic therapy. Dig Endosc. 2020; https://doi.org/10.1111/den.13650. [Published online ahead of print, 13 Feb 2020].
22. Schlenker C, Trotter JF, Shah RJ, et al. Endoscopic gallbladder stent placement for treatment of symptomatic cholelithiasis in patients with end-stage liver disease. Am J Gastroenterol. 2006;101(2):278–83.
23. Tujios SR, Rahnama-Moghadam S, Elmunzer JB, et al. Transpapillary gallbladder stents can stabilize or improve decompensated cirrhosis in patients awaiting liver transplantation. J Clin Gastroenterol. 2015;49(9):771–7.
24. Baron TH, Topazian MD. Endoscopic transduodenal drainage of the gallbladder: implications for endoluminal treatment of gallbladder disease. Gastrointest Endosc. 2007;65:735–7.
25. Law R, Baron TH. Endoscopic ultrasound-guided gallbladder drainage. Gastrointest Endosc Clin N Am. 2018;28(2):187–95.
26. Dollhopf M, Larghi A, Will U, et al. EUS-guided gallbladder drainage in patients with acute cholecystitis and high surgical risk using an electrocautery-enhanced lumen-apposing metal stent device. Gastrointest Endosc. 2017;86(4):636–43.
27. Walter D, Teoh AY, Itoi T, et al. EUS-guided gall bladder drainage with a lumen-apposing metal stent: a prospective long-term evaluation. Gut. 2016;65:6–8.
28. Anderloni A, Buda A, Vieceli F, Khashab MA, Hassan C, Repici A. Endoscopic ultrasound-guided transmural stenting for gallbladder drainage in high-risk patients with acute cholecystitis: a systematic review and pooled analysis. Surg Endosc. 2016;30(12):5200–8.
29. Teoh AYB. Outcomes and limitations in EUS-guided gallbladder drainage. Endosc Ultrasound. 2019;8(Suppl 1):S40–3.
30. Small AJ, Irani S. EUS-guided gallbladder drainage vs. percutaneous gallbladder drainage. Endosc Ultrasound. 2018;7(2):89–92.
31. Jang JW, Lee SS, Song TJ, et al. Endoscopic ultrasound-guided transmural and percutaneous transhepatic gallbladder drainage are comparable for acute cholecystitis. Gastroenterology. 2012;142:805–11.
32. Kedia P, Sharaiha RZ, Kumta NA, et al. Endoscopic gallbladder drainage compared with percutaneous drainage. Gastrointest Endosc. 2015;82(6):1031–6.
33. Teoh AYB, Kitano M, Itoi T, et al. Endosonography-guided gallbladder drainage versus percutaneous cholecystostomy in very high-risk surgical patients with

acute cholecystitis: an international randomised multicentre controlled superiority trial (DRAC 1). Gut. 2020;69(6):1085–91.
34. Oh D, Song TJ, Cho DH, et al. EUS-guided cholecystostomy versus endoscopic transpapillary cholecystostomy for acute cholecystitis in high-risk surgical patients. Gastrointest Endosc. 2019;89(2):289–98.
35. Mohan BP, Khan SR, Trakroo S, et al. Endoscopic ultrasound-guided gallbladder drainage, transpapillary drainage, or percutaneous drainage in high risk acute cholecystitis patients: a systematic review and comparative meta-analysis. Endoscopy. 2020;52:96–106.

Choledocholithiasis

36. Paumgartner G, Sauerbruch T. Gallstones: pathogenesis. Lancet. 1991;338:1117–21.
37. Frossard JL, Morel PM. Detection and management of bile duct stones. Gastrointest Endosc. 2010;72:808–16.
38. Chisholm PR, Patel AH, Law RJ, et al. Preoperative predictors of choledocholithiasis in patients presenting with acute calculous cholecystitis. Gastrointest Endosc. 2019;89(5):977–83.
39. ASGE Standards of Practice Committee, Buxbaum JL, Abbas Fehmi SM, et al. ASGE guideline on the role of endoscopy in the evaluation and management of choledocholithiasis. Gastrointest Endosc. 2019;89(6):1075–1105.e15.
40. ASGE Standards of Practice Committee, Chathadi KV, Chandrasekhara V, et al. The role of ERCP in benign diseases of the biliary tract. Gastrointest Endosc. 2015;81(4):795–803.
41. Baron TH, Harewood GC. Endoscopic balloon dilation of the biliary sphincter compared to endoscopic biliary sphincterotomy for removal of common bile duct stones during ERCP: a meta-analysis of randomized, controlled trials. Am J Gastroenterol. 2004;99:1455–60.
42. Kogure H, Kawahata S, Mukai T, et al. Multicenter randomized trial of endoscopic papillary large balloon dilation without sphincterotomy versus endoscopic sphincterotomy for removal of bile duct stones: MARVELOUS trial. Endoscopy. 2020;52:736–44.
43. Fujisawa T, Kagawa K, Hisatomi K, Kubota K, Nakajima A, Matsuhashi N. Is endoscopic papillary balloon dilatation really a risk factor for post-ERCP pancreatitis? World J Gastroenterol. 2016;22(26):5909–16.
44. Meine GC, Baron TH. Endoscopic papillary large-balloon dilation combined with endoscopic biliary sphincterotomy for the removal of bile duct stones (with video). Gastrointest Endosc. 2011;74(5):1119–5.
45. Leung JW, Tu R. Mechanical lithotripsy for large bile duct stones. Gastrointest Endosc. 2004;59:688–90.
46. Cecinato P, Fuccio L, Azzaroli F, et al. Extracorporeal shock wave lithotripsy for difficult common bile duct stones: a comparison between 2 different lithotripters in a large cohort of patients. Gastrointest Endosc. 2015;81(2):402–9.
47. Cerefice M, Sauer B, Javaid M, et al. Complex biliary stones: treatment with removable self-expandable metal stents: a new approach (with videos). Gastrointest Endosc. 2011;74:520–6.
48. Pereira-Lima JC, Jakobs R, Winter UH, et al. Long-term results (7 to 10 years) of endoscopic papillotomy for choledocholithiasis. Multivariate analysis of prognostic factors for the recurrence of biliary symptoms. Gastrointest Endosc. 1998;48:457–64.
49. Yi SY. Recurrence of biliary symptoms after endoscopic sphincterotomy for choledocholithiasis in patients with gallbladder stones. J Gastroenterol Hepatol. 2000;15:661–4.

Cholangitis

50. Gigot JF, Leese T, Dereme T, Coutinho J, Castaing D, Bismuth H. Acute cholangitis. Multivariate analysis of risk factors. Ann Surg. 1989;209(4):435–8.
51. Charcot JM. Leçons sur les maladies du foie, des voies biliaires et des reins faites à la Faculté de Médecine de Paris. Recueillies et publliées par Bourneville et Sevestre. Paris: Bureaux du Progrés Médical & Adrien Delahaye; 1877.
52. Reynolds BM, Dargan EL. Acute obstructive cholangitis: a distinct clinical syndrome. Ann Surg. 1959;150:299–303.
53. Kiriyama S, Kozaka K, Takada T, et al. Tokyo guidelines 2018: diagnostic criteria and severity grading of acute cholangitis (with videos). J Hepatobiliary Pancreat Sci. 2018;25(1):17–30.
54. Cote GA, Singh S, Bucksot LG, et al. Association between volume of endoscopic retrograde cholangiopancreatography at an academic medical center and use of pancreatobiliary therapy. Clin Gastroenterol Hepatol. 2012;10:920–4.
55. Puspok A, Lomoschitz F, Dejaco C, et al. Endoscopic ultrasound guided therapy of benign and malignant biliary obstruction: a case series. Am J Gastroenterol. 2005;100:1743–7.
56. Mukai S, Itoi T, Baron TH, et al. Indications and techniques of biliary drainage for acute cholangitis in updated Tokyo guidelines 2018. J Hepatobiliary Pancreat Sci. 2017;24:537–49.
57. Iqbal U, Khara HS, Hu Y, et al. Emergent versus urgent ERCP in acute cholangitis: a systematic review and meta-analysis. Gastrointest Endosc. 2020;91:753–60.
58. Huard P. Do-Xuan-Hop: La ponction transhépatique des canaux biliaries. Bull Soc Med Chir Indochine. 1937;15:1090–100.
59. Oh HC, Lee SK, Lee TY, et al. Analysis of percutaneous transhepatic cholangioscopy-related complications and the risk factors for those complications. Endoscopy. 2007;39:731–6.

60. Saad WE, Wallace MJ, Wojak JC, Kundu S, Cardella JF. Quality improvement guidelines for percutaneous transhepatic cholangiography, biliary drainage, and percutaneous cholecystostomy. J Vasc Interv Radiol. 2010;21(6):789–95.
61. Giovannini M, Moutardier V, Pesenti C, et al. Endoscopic ultrasound-guided bilioduodenal anastomosis: a new technique for biliary drainage. Endoscopy. 2001;33:898–900.
62. Sharaiha RZ, Khan MA, Kamal F, et al. Efficacy and safety of EUS-guided biliary drainage in comparison with percutaneous biliary drainage when ERCP fails: a systematic review and meta-analysis. Gastrointest Endosc. 2017;85(5):904–14.
63. Iwashita T, Yasuda I, Mukai T, et al. EUS-guided rendezvous for difficult biliary cannulation using a standardized algorithm: a multicenter prospective pilot study (with videos). Gastrointest Endosc. 2016;83(2):394–400.
64. Iwashita T, Doi S, Yasuda I. Endoscopic ultrasound-guided biliary drainage: a review. Clin J Gastroenterol. 2014;7(2):94–102. https://doi.org/10.1007/s12328-014-0467-5.
65. Imai H, Kitano M, Omoto S, et al. EUS-guided gallbladder drainage for rescue treatment of malignant distal biliary obstruction after unsuccessful ERCP. Gastrointest Endosc. 2016;84(1):147–51.
66. Issa D, Irani S, Law R, et al. Endoscopic ultrasound-guided gallbladder drainage as a rescue therapy for unresectable malignant biliary obstruction: a multicenter experience. Endoscopy. 2020; https://doi.org/10.1055/a-1259-0349.
67. Wang K, Zhu J, Xing L, Wang Y, Jin Z, Li Z. Assessment of efficacy and safety of EUS-guided biliary drainage: a systematic review. Gastrointest Endosc. 2016;83(6):1218–27.
68. Khan MA, Akbar A, Baron TH, et al. Endoscopic ultrasound-guided biliary drainage: a systematic review and meta-analysis. Dig Dis Sci. 2016;61(3):684–703.
69. Uemura RS, Khan MA, Otoch JP, Kahaleh M, Montero EF, Artifon ELA. EUS-guided choledochoduodenostomy versus hepaticogastrostomy: a systematic review and meta-analysis. J Clin Gastroenterol. 2018;52(2):123–30.
70. Canakis A, Baron TH. Relief of biliary obstruction: choosing between endoscopic ultrasound and endoscopic retrograde cholangiopancreatography. BMJ Open Gastroenterol. 2020;7:e000428.

Biliary Access in Surgically-Altered Anatomy

71. Shah RJ, Smolkin M, Yen R, et al. A multicenter, U.S. experience of single-balloon, double-balloon, and rotational overtube-assisted enteroscopy ERCP in patients with surgically altered pancreaticobiliary anatomy (with video). Gastrointest Endosc. 2013;77(4):593–600.
72. Skinner M, Popa D, Neumann H, Wilcox CM, Mönkemüller K. ERCP with the overtube-assisted enteroscopy technique: a systematic review. Endoscopy. 2014;46(7):560–72.
73. Bukhari M, Kowalski T, Nieto J, et al. An international, multicenter, comparative trial of EUS-guided gastrogastrostomy-assisted ERCP versus enteroscopy-assisted ERCP in patients with Roux-en-Y gastric bypass anatomy. Gastrointest Endosc. 2018;88(3):486–94.
74. Mohammad B, Richard MN, Pandit A, et al. Outcomes of laparoscopic-assisted ERCP in gastric bypass patients at a community hospital center. Surg Endosc. 2019; https://doi.org/10.1007/s00464-019-07310-y.
75. Schreiner MA, Chang L, Gluck M, et al. Laparoscopy-assisted versus balloon enteroscopy-assisted ERCP in bariatric post-Roux-en-Y gastric bypass patients. Gastrointest Endosc. 2012;75(4):748–56.
76. Krafft MR, Fang W, Nasr JY. Shortened-interval dual-session EDGE reduces the risk of LAMS dislodgement while facilitating timely ERCP. Dig Dis Sci. 2020; https://doi.org/10.1007/s10620-020-06551-5.
77. Kedia P, Tarnasky PR, Nieto J, et al. EUS-directed transgastric ERCP (EDGE) versus laparoscopy-assisted ERCP (LA-ERCP) for Roux-en-Y gastric bypass (RYGB) anatomy: a multicenter early comparative experience of clinical outcomes. J Clin Gastroenterol. 2019;53(4):304–8.
78. Forster E, Elmunzer BJ. Endoscopic retrograde cholangiopancreatography in patients with Roux-en-Y gastric bypass. Am J Gastroenterol. 2020;115(2):155–7.
79. James HJ, James TW, Wheeler SB, Spencer JC, Baron TH. Cost-effectiveness of endoscopic ultrasound-directed transgastric ERCP compared with device-assisted and laparoscopic-assisted ERCP in patients with Roux-en-Y anatomy. Endoscopy. 2019;51(11):1051–8.
80. Wang TJ, Thompson CC, Ryou M. Gastric access temporary for endoscopy (GATE): a proposed algorithm for EUS-directed transgastric ERCP in gastric bypass patients. Surg Endosc. 2019;33(6):2024–33.
81. James TW, Fan YC, Baron TH. EUS-guided hepaticoenterostomy as a portal to allow definitive antegrade treatment of benign biliary diseases in patients with surgically altered anatomy. Gastrointest Endosc. 2018;88(3):547–54.
82. Mukai S, Itoi T, Sofuni A, et al. EUS-guided antegrade intervention for benign biliary diseases in patients with surgically altered anatomy (with videos). Gastrointest Endosc. 2019;89(2):399–407.

Bile Leaks and Bile Duct Injury

83. Flum DR, Cheadle A, Prela C, Dellinger EP, Chan L. Bile duct injury during cholecystectomy and survival in medicare beneficiaries. JAMA. 2003;290(16):2168–73.
84. Fong ZV, Pitt HA, Strasberg SM, et al. Diminished survival in patients with bile leak and ductal injury:

management strategy and outcomes. J Am Coll Surg. 2018;226(4):568–76.
85. Perera MT, Silva MA, Hegab B, et al. Specialist early and immediate repair of post-laparoscopic cholecystectomy bile duct injuries is associated with an improved long-term outcome. Ann Surg. 2011;253(3):553–60.
86. Strasberg SM, Hertl M, Soper NJ. An analysis of the problem of biliary injury during laparoscopic cholecystectomy. J Am Coll Surg. 1995;180(1):101–25.
87. Bergman JJ, van den Brink GR, Rauws EA, et al. Treatment of bile duct lesions after laparoscopic cholecystectomy. Gut. 1996;38:141–7.
88. Sandha GS, Bourke MJ, Haber GB, Kortan PP. Endoscopic therapy for bile leak based on a new classification: results in 207 patients. Gastrointest Endosc. 2004;60(4):567–74.
89. Rustagi T, Aslanian HR. Endoscopic management of biliary leaks after laparoscopic cholecystectomy. J Clin Gastroenterol. 2014;48(8):674–8.
90. Bjorkman DJ, Carr-Locke DL, Lichtenstein DR, et al. Postsurgical bile leaks: endoscopic obliteration of the transpapillary pressure gradient is enough. Am J Gastroenterol. 1995;90(12):2128–33.
91. Vlaemynck K, Lahousse L, Vanlander A, et al. Endoscopic management of biliary leaks: a systematic review with meta-analysis. Endoscopy. 2019;51:1074–81.
92. Irani S, Baron TH, Law R, et al. Endoscopic treatment of nonstricture-related benign biliary diseases using covered self-expandable metal stents. Endoscopy. 2015;47(4):315–21.
93. Canena J, Liberato M, Meireles L, et al. A non-randomized study in consecutive patients with postcholecystectomy refractory biliary leaks who were managed endoscopically with the use of multiple plastic stents or fully covered self-expandable metal stents (with videos). Gastrointest Endosc. 2015;82:70–8.
94. Canena J, Horta D, Coimbra J, et al. Outcomes of endoscopic management of primary and refractory postcholecystectomy biliary leaks in a multicentre review of 178 patients. BMC Gastroenterol. 2015;15:105.
95. Sondhi AR, Pomerantz BJ, Kazanjian S, Nathan H, Law R. Recanalization of the bile duct by using percutaneous and endoscopic methods after iatrogenic injury. VideoGIE. 2020;5(7):308–10.
96. Schreuder AM, Booij KAC, de Reuver PR, et al. Percutaneous-endoscopic rendezvous procedure for the management of bile duct injuries after cholecystectomy: short- and long-term outcomes. Endoscopy. 2018;50(6):577–87.
97. Thompson CM, Saad NE, Quazi RR, Darcy MD, Picus DD, Menias CO. Management of iatrogenic bile duct injuries: role of the interventional radiologist. Radiographics. 2013;33(1):117–34.
98. Shami VM, Talreja JP, Mahajan A, Phillips MS, Yeaton P, Kahaleh M. EUS-guided drainage of bilomas: a new alternative? Gastrointest Endosc. 2008;67(1):136–40.
99. Zepeda-Gómez S, Baron TH. Benign biliary strictures: current endoscopic management. Nat Rev Gastroenterol Hepatol. 2011;8(10):573–81.
100. Costamagna G, Pandolfi M, Mutignani M, et al. Long-term results of endoscopic management of postoperative bile duct strictures with increasing numbers of stents. Gastrointest Endosc. 2001;54:162.
101. Draganov P, Hoffman B, Marsh W, Cotton P, Cunningham J. Long-term outcome in patients with benign biliary strictures treated endoscopically with multiple stents. Gastrointest Endosc. 2002;55(6):680–6.
102. Costamagna G, Tringali A, Mutignani M, et al. Endotherapy of postoperative biliary strictures with multiple stents: results after more than 10 years of follow-up. Gastrointest Endosc. 2010;72(3):551–7.

Acute Urologic Emergencies

27

Niels V. Johnsen and Hunter Wessells

Case Report

A 63-year-old man with a history of poorly controlled diabetes and coronary artery disease presents to the emergency room with a 2-day history of fevers, fatigue, and scrotal pain. Laboratory evaluation shows a marked leukocytosis with associated hyponatremia and lactic acidosis. Physical examination reveals significant edema and erythema of the scrotum with palpable crepitus and a 4-cm eschar on the inferior surface. The patient was hemodynamically stable and, thus, brought for cross-sectional imaging that revealed diffuse genital soft-tissue infection with associated subcutaneous emphysema. He was initiated on broad-spectrum antibiotics and brought urgently to the operating room for extensive tissue debridement of the scrotum, perineum, and gluteal regions. Following debridement, he required prolonged vasopressor support and ICU-level care until the entirety of infected and necrotic tissue was able to be fully debrided in two subsequent procedures. Long-term wound care and closure plans were then initiated.

Introduction

Acute surgical emergencies involving the genitourinary tract may arise from a multitude of factors. However, exclusive of traumatic injuries, these emergencies are most commonly due to infectious or obstructive etiologies. Specifically, while both urinary tract obstruction and infection alone can be problematic for patients, the combination of the two can be particularly life-threatening and immediate intervention is often required to achieve appropriate urinary drainage, source control, and targeted antimicrobial therapy. Furthermore, the genitalia are particularly at risk for necrotizing soft-tissue infections that require prompt evaluation, diagnosis, and aggressive surgical debridement to avoid significant morbidity or mortality. Herein, the evaluation, diagnosis, and management of patients with acute surgical emergencies related to the genitourinary system will be reviewed. For organiza-

N. V. Johnsen (✉)
Department of Urology, Vanderbilt University Medical Center, Nashville, TN, USA
e-mail: niels.v.johnsen@vumc.org

H. Wessells
Department of Urology, University of Washington School of Medicine, Seattle, WA, USA
e-mail: wessells@uw.edu

M. D. Zielinski, O. Guillamondegui (eds.), *The Acute Management of Surgical Disease*,
https://doi.org/10.1007/978-3-031-07881-1_27

tion purposes, disease processes will be presented by region of the genitourinary system affected.

Upper Urinary Tract

Upper Tract Obstruction

The upper urinary tract is comprised of paired kidneys and their accompanying drainage system: the renal pelvis and ureter. Obstruction of urinary drainage can be the result of intrinsic, extrinsic, or congenital causes and lead to the severe, paroxysmal pain associated with renal colic. The clinical presentation of upper urinary tract obstruction can be variable due to differences in the degree and chronicity of obstruction. The pain present in acute obstruction results from distension of the proximal segment of the obstructed system and is often referred to the flank, costovertebral angle, ipsilateral groin or lower quadrant, and/or scrotum. This pain is not improved by changes in positioning and is often accompanied by significant nausea and vomiting due to the concomitant passage of afferent nerve fibers from the renal pelvis and proximal ureter along the course of the vagus nerve. Conversely, long-standing chronic obstruction is often entirely asymptomatic in the absence of associated upstream infection.

Table 27.1 Primary differential diagnosis of acute flank pain

Urologic
Ureteral calculi
Urothelial malignancy
Ureteropelvic junction obstruction
Ureteral stricture
Extrinsic obstruction of ureter
Pyelonephritis
Renal/perinephric abscess
Clot obstruction
Polycystic kidney disease
Adrenal hemorrhage
Gastrointestinal
Cholecystitis
Appendicitis
Pancreatitis
Peptic ulcer disease
Diverticulitis
Inflammatory bowel disease
Volvulus
Gynecologic
Ectopic pregnancy
Ovarian torsion
Endometriosis
Vascular
Abdominal aortic aneurysm
Aortic dissection
Renal/iliac artery aneurysm
Renal vein thrombosis
Renal artery embolus

While the symptoms and history of renal colic are often pathognomonic for upper urinary tract obstruction, numerous other diseases involving other organ systems should be included in the initial differential diagnosis (Table 27.1). Gynecologic, gastrointestinal, adrenal, and vascular etiologies should be specifically considered and appropriately evaluated even in the presence of apparently straightforward renal colic. Disease processes such as ectopic pregnancy, diverticulitis, pancreatitis, appendicitis, and aortic dissection can all be mistaken for acute renal colic and thus be mismanaged if the diagnosis is not verified.

The most common etiology of renal colic in an otherwise healthy individual is obstruction due to urolithiasis, and this should be high on one's differential diagnosis list when evaluating the acute patient. Other common causes include upper tract urothelial cancer, congenital ureteropelvic junction obstruction, ureteral stricture, and extrinsic ureteral compression due to retroperitoneal tumors or retroperitoneal fibrosis.

Evaluation

Initial evaluation should include an in-depth history and physical examination. In particular, a history of prior urolithiasis is a significant predictor of recurrent stone formation, with first-time stone formers having an approximately 50% risk for recurrence in the subsequent 10 years [1]. Patients with histories of stones and prior stone procedures are also at risk for obstruction due to stricture formation within the ureter from prior ischemic injury, which can present with identical symptoms as an acute stone episode. Patients may also have other medical histories that put them at particular risk for stone formation. These include prior weight-loss surgeries, malignancy, and urinary or fecal diversion, as well medications such as protease inhibitors or the anti-epileptic topiramate [2–6].

Laboratory evaluation at initial presentation includes urinalysis, routine basic metabolic panel, and a complete blood count. One primary decision point in the initial evaluation of a patient with suspected upper urinary tract obstruction is the determination of concomitant infection. Patients with obstruction and infection are at significant risk for developing bacteremia and sepsis, and this should be considered a surgical emergency. Patients with unilateral renal obstruction in the absence of infection may be considered for urgent intervention if severely symptomatic with uncontrollable pain, nausea, or vomiting. However, patients with unilateral obstruction due a stone who can be symptomatically managed with oral medications and hydration can often be considered for delayed management and allowed time to pass the offending stone. Patients with bilateral renal obstruction or obstruction of a solitary kidney, however, require immediate intervention.

Historically, patients with suspicion for obstruction due to urolithiasis were imaged with plain film KUBs, and this practice has generally been retired in the United States in favor for more definitive evaluation methods. Renal ultrasound is often used as a preliminary modality for evaluating patients with suspected nephrolithiasis and has been shown in a large, multicenter randomized trial to decrease unnecessary computed tomography (CT) scan usage and limit unnecessary radiation exposure, without significantly impacting patient outcomes [7]. However, while ultrasounds may show evidence of hydronephrosis supporting a diagnosis of upper tract obstruction, this imaging modality has relatively poor sensitivity for identifying ureteral calculi as the obstructive etiology in particular, which may lead to delays in diagnosis and even to unnecessary further imaging [8]. Non-contrast abdominal CT scans are generally the most frequently used diagnostic imaging tool available, with reported sensitivities and specificities for detecting ureteral stones of 94–100% [9]. CT allows for identification and localization of multiple potential obstructive etiologies, as well as visualization of secondary findings such as forniceal rupture, edema, or perinephric stranding.

Management

Indications for acute surgical management for patients with upper urinary tract obstruction are based on symptoms and concern for infection. As previously stated, bilateral renal obstruction or any degree of obstruction in the presence of associated urinary tract infection or signs of systemic inflammatory response (SIRS) are indications for emergent intervention. Similarly, fever, anuria, obstruction of a transplanted or solitary kidney, or intractable pain and vomiting are all indications for intervention. The goals of urgent intervention are to relieve the obstruction, protect renal function, and facilitate drainage of infected urine. Also of importance is the obtaining of a urine sample from proximal to the obstruction to send for culture to ensure that targeted antibiotics can be provided.

There are two options for acute intervention for renal colic and upper urinary tract obstruction, with the primary goal of simply obtaining appropriate drainage and returning in a delayed fashion for definitive treatment of the obstruction. Cystoscopy and retrograde stent placement are the standard first-line management options and are appropriate in all but the most severely ill patients. While this procedure routinely involves a general anesthetic which may be associated with increased risk in some patients, some providers have recently advocated for performance of this procedure bedside in awake patients using just local anesthesia in order to minimize time delays of going to the operating room or potential risks associated with anesthesia [10]. These authors found that bedside placement was successful in 71% of patients and may serve a role in expediting decompression in certain patients.

In more severely ill patients, or in those in which retrograde attempts to place a stent are unsuccessful, referral to interventional radiology for a percutaneous nephrostomy tube is appropriate. Potential benefits of a percutaneous nephrostomy tube include expeditious drainage of the obstructed kidney and the ability to be placed under ultrasound or fluoroscopic guidance with only local anesthesia, thus avoiding the potential risks associated with a general anesthetic. However, unlike an indwelling ureteral stent which drains the kidney into the bladder, a nephrostomy tube requires an externalized drainage bag that the patient must carry and maintain until he or she obtains definitive treatment of the obstruction.

Special Considerations

Ureteropelvic Junction Obstruction

Ureteropelvic junction (UPJ) obstruction represents a unique form of urinary tract obstruction often triaged in the emergency department. This condition is often congenital and usually presents during infancy or childhood, but may progress undiagnosed into adulthood. Adult patients presenting with acute renal colic and imaging consistent with isolated UPJ obstruction in the absence of prior urologic instrumentation or procedures often have congenital UPJ obstructions that went undiagnosed during childhood. These patients frequently present with a syndrome of severe flank pain, nausea, and vomiting that is intermittent and often preceded by excessive fluid or diuretic intake. This syndrome, known as *Dietl's crisis*, is due to a rapid dilation of the renal pelvis with large volume diuresis, but an inability to rapidly excrete this fluid due to obstruction at the level of the junction to the proximal ureter. Contrary to many other etiologies of acute renal colic, patients with congenital UPJ obstruction often do not require immediate surgical intervention, as their pain often resolves as their hydration status equilibrates. However, for patients with intractable symptoms, either a nephrostomy tube or a ureteral stent may be used for management, although a nephrostomy tube is often preferred by urologists prior to eventual reconstruction.

Renal Colic in Pregnancy

One special scenario that warrants mention is renal colic in pregnancy, which is one of the top non-obstetric causes for hospital admission in pregnant women [11]. While relatively rare, this situation presents unique diagnostic and therapeutic difficulties that require special consideration. Pregnant women are at high risk for developing physiologic hydroureteronephrosis during pregnancy due to three primary causes: dextrorotation of the uterus causing ureteral compression, reduced ureteral peristalsis due to progesterone effects, and increased glomerular filtration leading to increased urine volumes [12]. As such, women presenting with acute flank pain should be evaluated for urolithiasis, but care should be taken to ensure that there is an identifiable obstructing offender, as these women often have physiologic hydroureteronephrosis that can ultrasonically or radiographically appear as acute obstruction.

In pregnant women with concern for acute renal colic, appropriate diagnosis and management are paramount, as renal colic has been associated with preterm rupture of membranes and preterm delivery [13]. Renal ultrasound has been considered the first-line diagnostic tool given the low cost and lack of radiation exposure to the fetus, but overall has low sensitivity in identifying ureteral calculi and interpretation can be influenced by the degree of physiologic upper urinary tract dilation present [14]. Magnetic resonance urography (MRU) has emerged as a highly touted second-line imaging modality due to the lack of ionizing radiation, with numerous studies failing to identify negative effects of MRU on developing fetuses [15, 16]. CT without contrast remains superior to MR in detection of ureteral calculi and remains the most definitive evaluation tool for renal colic in pregnant patients suspected of having urolithiasis. Nonetheless, CT is generally avoided in the first trimester and is only recommended in patients with unclear pathology and only after consultation between urology, obstetrics, and radiology to determine risks versus benefits for that particular patient.

Management of urinary tract obstruction in pregnant patients has other unique considerations.

For pregnant patients with urolithiasis and well-controlled symptoms, observation should be first-line management. Observation is often performed in conjunction with medical expulsive therapy, which consists of pharmacologic treatment with an oral alpha blocker such as tamsulosin to hasten stone passage. However, women should be counseled that although the use of alpha blockers in pregnancy has not been rigorously evaluated, initial studies suggest that they are safe [17]. For patients not appropriate for conservative management, initial management with either a ureteral stent or a nephrostomy tube, or immediate endoscopic treatment of offending stones in the absence of infection, is appropriate [18]. However, pregnant women are at high-risk for encrustation of both stents and nephrostomy tubes and may require frequent replacement throughout the course of pregnancy until treatment of the obstruction is undertaken. Thus, for stable women in their second trimester, once infection has been treated or ruled out, definitive ureteroscopic laser treatment of urolithiasis is recommended to limit risks of stent encrustation and to minimize multiple anesthetic trips to the operating room for stent exchanges.

Renal and Perinephric Abscesses

Renal abscesses, also sometimes referred to as renal carbuncles, are an uncommon secondary infection following acute pyelonephritis [19]. These lesions represent localized collections of purulent fluid confined to the renal parenchyma and are most commonly due to the same gram-negative bacteria often responsible for pyelonephritis [20]. Prior to the current widespread use of antibiotics, however, the majority of renal abscesses were due to hematogenous spread of gram-positive bacteria from non-urinary sources. While hematogenously spread abscesses are still occasionally encountered, these are most often identified in patients with a history of intravenous drug use and immunosuppression. Similarly, formation of a renal abscess in an otherwise immunologically intact individual is relatively rare, with 30–50% of cases occurring in patients with diabetes mellitus [19–21].

Perinephric abscesses differ from renal abscesses in that they are not completely contained to the renal parenchyma and often represent renal abscesses that have ruptured and spread within Gerota's fascia. As such, they have a similar etiology to renal abscesses and are most often due to ascending gram-negative bacteria, although they too can be due to hematogenous spread of gram-positives as well. Furthermore, both renal and perinephric abscesses are relatively uncommon in healthy and anatomically normal individuals and most often occur in patients with recent instrumentation, obstruction, or injury. These lesions can also be found in individuals with large staghorn renal calculi, vesicoureteral reflux, distal ureteral obstruction, or polycystic kidney disease [22].

Clinical presentation of renal or perinephric abscesses is generally indistinguishable from acute pyelonephritis, with flank pain, fever, chills, fatigue, and malaise. Large perinephric abscesses may cause upper quadrant pain or even present with associated empyema. However, many patients will present with a history of recent similar symptomatology with failure to improve despite appropriate antibiotics, as these lesions often progress from simple pyelonephritis. As such, clinical suspicion for a potential abscess should be high in any patient with persistent symptoms despite previous antibiotic treatment or a rapid recurrence of symptoms after treatment.

Evaluation

Laboratory evaluation will often show a leukocytosis; however, urinalysis and urine culture may in fact be negative, especially if the patient's predisposing pyelonephritis has previously been treated with antibiotics or if hematogenous spread is suspected. Blood cultures, on the other hand, may be positive in patients with possible hematogenous spread and should be obtained at presentation for any patient with SIRS or history concerning for intravenous drug use.

Patients with suspected renal or perinephric abscesses require imaging to determine the diagnosis as well as to guide management. Ultrasonography has a limited role, but may help

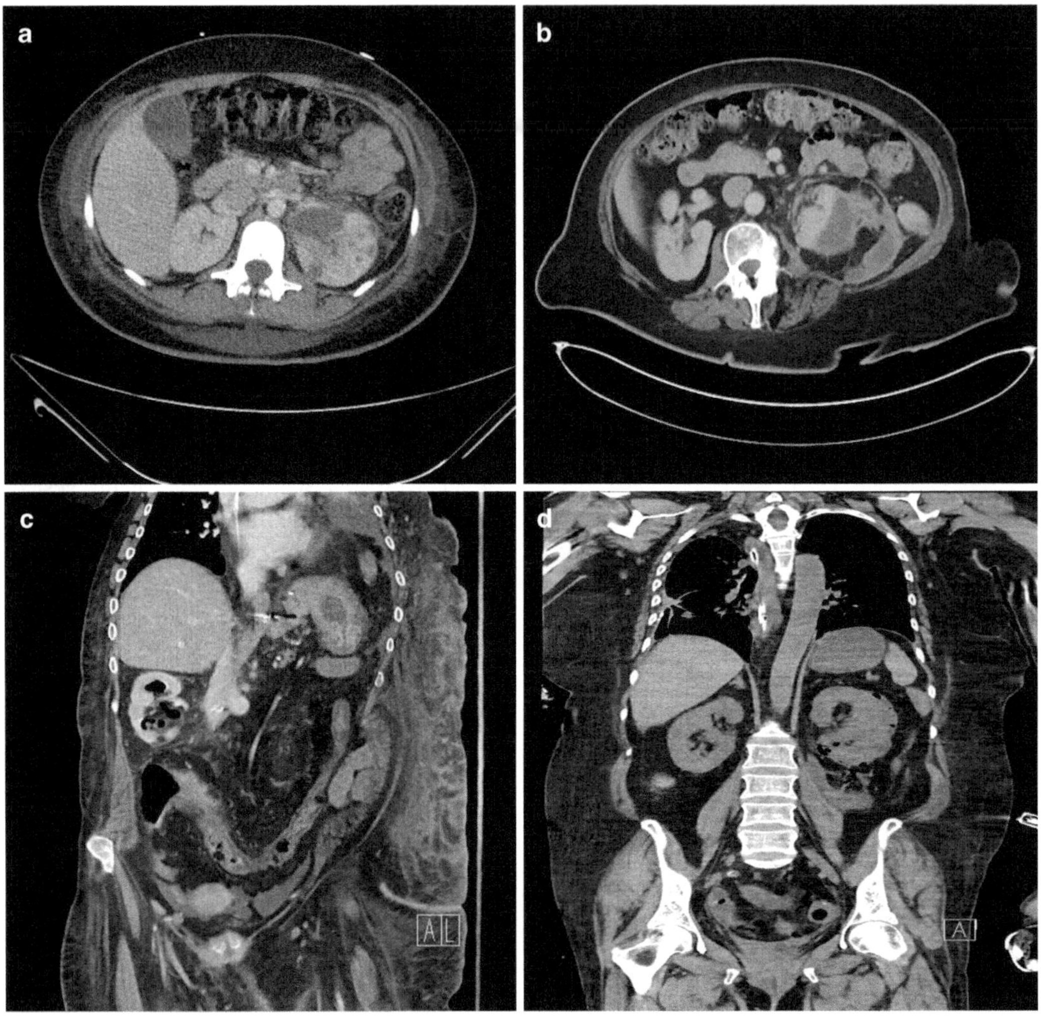

Fig. 27.1 CT images showing multifocal left renal abscess (**a**), left perinephric abscess with expansion into Gerota's fascia (**b**), right emphysematous pyelitis (**c**), and left emphysematous pyelonephritis (**d**)

identify a fluid-filled cavity in the renal cortex or perirenal space. Contrast-enhanced CT remains the gold standard for identifying and diagnosing renal and perinephric abscesses (Fig. 27.1). These images can definitively diagnose a rim-enhancing, low-density lesion on or around the kidney, as well as any evidence of locoregional invasion and involvement of surrounding structures including the psoas muscle. Also often identified with contrast-enhanced CT is lobar nephronia, a term utilized by radiologist to identify a hypodense region of the kidney suggestive of infection with possible progression to a renal abscess, but without liquefaction and rim enhancement.

Management

Management of patients with renal and perinephric abscesses depends on size and associated symptoms. All patients should be initiated on appropriate broad-spectrum antibiotics at presentation based on clinical suspicion. If a urinary source is suspected, gram-negative coverage is required. For patients at risk for hematogenous spread from intravenous drug use, gram-positive coverage including coverage for methicillin-resistant Staphylococcus with vancomycin is often required. Therapy should then be directed to the causative organism once culture data are available.

Determining the size of the lesion is vital, as abscesses larger than approximately 3–5 cm have been shown to respond poorly to intravenous antibiotics alone and require CT or ultrasound-guided percutaneous drainage [23–25]. Once appropriate source control is obtained, patients can generally be transitioned to culture-specific oral antibiotics for 2–4 weeks. In select cases, however, where severe anatomic abnormalities such as a nonfunctioning kidney or a large staghorn calculus are present, or where percutaneous drainage is either not possible or ineffective, open surgical debridement and possible nephrectomy may be warranted, although in contemporary series this has been infrequently reported [19]. Follow-up imaging is recommended in patients who fail to clinically progress, as well as to confirm that loculated collections have been completely drained prior to drain removal and cessation of antimicrobials.

Emphysematous Pyelonephritis

Emphysematous pyelonephritis represents a potentially life-threatening urologic emergency that requires prompt intervention. This disease process results from necrotizing infection of the renal parenchyma due to gas-forming bacterial infections and occurs almost exclusively in diabetic patients who have poor tissue perfusion and urinary obstruction [26–28]. The most common bacterial offenders include *E. coli*, *Klebsiella*, and *Proteus*, as well as *Clostridium*.

Evaluation

Patients present with clinical findings similar to both acute pyelonephritis and renal or perinephric abscesses with flank pain, fever, chills, and malaise. Diagnosis is confirmed by the use of CT that identifies the presence of air within the parenchyma of the kidney. This should not be confused with air within the collecting system (*emphysematous pyelitis*), which is a much less serious condition that can be treated as pyelonephritis with antibiotics alone (Fig. 27.1).

Management

Management consists of early initiation of broad-spectrum antibiotics, tight blood glucose control, and supportive care. Traditionally, this diagnosis has represented a true surgical emergency and has been treated with immediate open drainage and nephrectomy; however, more contemporary series have reported excellent management with antibiotics and percutaneous drainage alone [29–31]. A systematic review found that patients treated with antibiotics alone had a 50% mortality rate, while those treated with antibiotics plus nephrectomy had a 25% mortality rate and those treated with antibiotics plus percutaneous drainage a 13.5% mortality rate [31]. However, patients not treated with immediate nephrectomy should be carefully monitored and undergo surgical drainage and nephrectomy if the infection fails to resolve or patients fail to improve clinically. There are no standardized guidelines as to the duration of antibiotics, but treatment courses similar to those for percutaneously drained abscesses (2–4 weeks) have been regularly utilized.

Spontaneous Retroperitoneal Hematoma

Acute, nontraumatic spontaneous retroperitoneal hematoma (SRH) is a relatively rare entity and usually occurs secondary to either vascular rupture of an underlying pathologic lesion or a systemic coagulopathy. While patients often present with acute flank or truncal pain, many present in a delayed fashion in acute hemorrhagic shock due to significant blood loss into the retroperitoneal space [32]. As such, this entity has the potential for significant morbidity and even mortality if the diagnosis is missed or inappropriately managed.

Patients with known bleeding diathesis or those on anticoagulation are at particular increased risk for SRH. Prior reports have suggested that up to 6.6% of patients on heparin and 0.6% of patients on warfarin are at risk for SRH; however, up to 15% of patients in one series of SRH were on no form of anticoagulation [33–

be needed for follow-up management. Urinalysis and urine culture often cannot be obtained until retention has been relieved but are vital in further evaluation and management. While imaging is often not required if the initial diagnosis is clinically clear, pelvic ultrasound may be useful acutely to visualize a large, distended bladder. Follow-up imaging should, however, be considered in the diagnosis of the potential etiology of urinary retention and for consideration of long-term management strategies. This is especially true in patients in which urethral catheterization is not possible and percutaneous placement of a suprapubic catheter is required. Also, bladder ultrasound may show a large intravesical clot burden as the etiology of outlet obstruction, which may further guide treatment decisions. However, a simple ultrasonic bladder scanner that can quantify the volume of bladder contents is often sufficient to establish a diagnosis of AUR.

Management

Management of AUR involves prompt establishment of bladder drainage, most frequently through placement of a urethral catheter. In general, difficult catheterization in women is due to body habitus or sometimes a hypospadiac meatus within the vaginal canal that is difficult to visualize or access. Trendelenburg positioning and use of assistants to aid in retraction can help in exposure in the obese patient, while placement of a gloved fingertip inside the vagina can help guide the catheter into the meatus in women with hypospadias. Difficult catheterization in men can be due to a multitude of conditions but is most often due to the BPH or urethral stricture. Coudé catheters can help navigate the posterior urethra in men with BPH, while urologic consultation for cystoscopy, dilation, and Councill tip catheter placement over a guidewire may be needed in patients with urethral stricture disease. In any scenario, multiple attempts should be avoided and early urologic consultation obtained in order to prevent significant urethral trauma that may make catheter placement more difficult and potentially lead to later stricture formation.

Suprapubic catheterization may be required in situations where urethral catheter placement is not possible or not appropriate. This procedure can be performed with local anesthesia alone in the emergency department, although some patients and providers may prefer a general anesthetic if possible. Bedside, ultrasonography, as previously stated, can be useful in visualizing the location of the distended bladder and ensuring appropriate trajectory and depth of percutaneous trocar passage. Special note should be taken of any previous abdominal surgeries that may have disrupted the space of Retzius or of pelvic radiation that may have caused significant fibrosis. Patients should be placed in Trendelenburg position to encourage the bowels to move cephalad away from the bladder and a small punch suprapubic catheter can be placed approximately 2 fingerbreadths above the pubic symphysis. For patients with a history of pelvic surgery or other concerning findings on ultrasound, open suprapubic tube placement in the operating room may be preferred to avoid inadvertent injury to the bowel.

Once bladder drainage has occurred, urine should be sent for culture and antibiotics considered if an infectious etiology is suspected. Most importantly, patients with long-standing obstruction should be monitored for the development of *post-obstructive diuresis*. Post-obstructive diuresis has been variably defined in the literature, but in general refers to excess urine output (>3 L per 24 h) following relief of bilateral renal obstruction [45, 46]. While physiologic post-obstructive diuresis occurs as a normal result of long-term obstruction as the body attempts to regain fluid homeostasis, pathologic post-obstructive diuresis can cause significant dehydration and electrolyte abnormalities. Excessive urine output >200 mL/h following decompression should prompt providers to closely monitor the volume and electrolyte status of patients. Many patients can regulate their volume with sufficient oral fluid intake, but in some instances fluid replacement with intravenous fluids is required. Common practice is to replace urine losses with 0.45% normal saline at half the rate of urine output per hour until patients normalize and can maintain sufficient fluid intake orally.

Providers should not forget that once the acute process has been addressed, patients still require complete evaluation to identify the underlying pathologic process. While the long-term management of these underlying etiologies is beyond the scope of this text, special consideration should be given to patients in retention secondary to large clot burdens within the bladder that often requires aggressive bedside hand irrigation or cystoscopic clot evacuation in the operating room. Also, acute urinary retention may be a presenting symptom of a new neurologic lesion that requires prompt evaluation and treatment by specialists.

Scrotum

Fournier's Gangrene

Fournier's gangrene is a rapidly progressive necrotizing soft-tissue infection of the genitals and perineum. This represents a true life-threatening emergency with historical mortality rates reaching nearly 50%, although contemporary mortality appears to be closer to 5–20% [47–51]. Appropriate management requires prompt diagnosis, aggressive surgical debridement of involved tissues, intravenous antibiotics, and fluid resuscitation to stave off mortality.

While *Escherichia coli* is the most commonly isolated bacteria in patients with Fournier's gangrene, this disease process most often represents a synergistic polymicrobial infection. Other causative organisms commonly found include *Klebsiella*, enterococci, *Bacteroides*, *Clostridium*, *Pseudomonas*, and *streptococci* variants [52–54]. Fournier's gangrene is almost entirely limited to individuals with significant medical comorbidities, with up to 70% of patients having diabetes mellitus [55]. Other predisposing risk factors include immunosuppression, alcoholism, malignancy, obesity, and malnutrition [52, 55–60]. As such, patients with these comorbid conditions and recent histories of perirectal or perianal abscesses, urethral stricture disease with periurethral infection, scrotal abscesses, genital skin wounds, or epididymitis are particularly at risk for development of this necrotizing infection [52, 61].

As is true with other necrotizing soft-tissue infections, the pattern of spread of Fournier's gangrene is along the fascial planes of the genitals and perineum and can progress to the medial thighs, glutes, and anterior abdominal wall. In the genitals, infection spreads along Colles' and dartos fascial planes in particular often sparing the deeper structures unless advanced disease is present. Necrosis occurs as infection causes small vessel thrombosis leading to ischemia and, thus, further extension of the infection [62]. Notably, histologic studies have previously shown that the epidermis and superficial dermis are often spared from the necrotizing process, while the deeper soft-tissues show extensive vasculitis, thrombosis, and tissue necrosis [63].

Evaluation

Clinical presentation of patients with Fournier's gangrene is variable. Some patients present early prior to systemic signs of illness and before extensive visible tissue destruction, while others may present in septic shock and in immediate need for resuscitation and vasopressor support. However, in both cases, the urgency with which the patient requires antibiotics and surgical debridement are similar and intervention should not be delayed. Early presenters may have pain, erythema, and swelling of the involved scrotal or perineal tissues, while patients with more progressed disease will have signs of black or purple tissue discoloration, skin sloughing, and crepitus (Fig. 27.2). Patients capable of providing a history may report history of recent genital wounds, scrotal pain, rectal or urethral instrumentation, or perirectal drainage or pain.

Laboratory evaluation often shows a significant leukocytosis, as well as hyponatremia, elevated creatinine, and lactic acidosis [62, 64]. In patients with advanced disease with palpable crepitus and visible tissue necrosis, imaging is not required for diagnosis but may be useful in showing the extent of underlying soft-tissue involvement. However, in patients with visible cellulitis but who lack a definitive diagnosis, CT provides a high degree of specificity and sensitivity for diagnosis [65] and can guide surgical debridement. Pathognomonic of necrotizing soft-

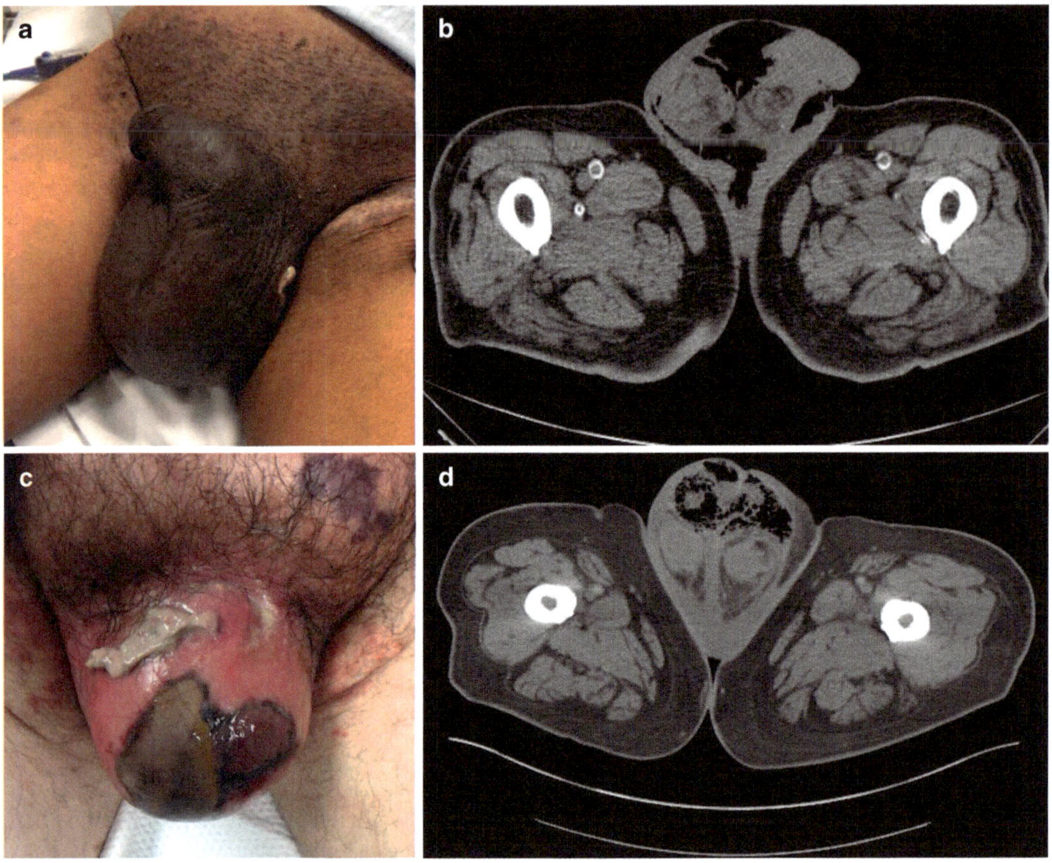

Fig. 27.2 Variable clinical presentations of Fournier's gangrene. Scrotal swelling and discomfort without overt skin necrosis (**a**), but diffuse soft-tissue emphysema (**b**). Frank necrosis and purulence (**c**) with similar CT findings of subcutaneous emphysema (**d**)

tissue infection is the presence of subcutaneous or deep tissue gas on CT imaging, which should prompt immediate surgical debridement.

Management

Initial management of patients with Fournier's gangrene involves early initiation of broad-spectrum antibiotics, intravenous fluid resuscitation, vasopressor support if needed, and emergent surgical debridement of infected and necrotic tissues. Blood cultures should be obtained prior to starting antibiotics as patients are at risk for bacteremia. Antibiotics should cover gram-positive, gram-negative, and anaerobic bacteria. Clindamycin, in particular, is recommended for the first 48 h after presentation as it has the added benefit of inhibiting the effects of potential *Clostridium* toxins.

Aggressive surgical debridement should be undertaken immediately to remove devitalized tissues and any signs of infection and should be performed until healthy bleeding tissues are encountered. Wound cultures should be sent to microbiology for culture in order to help tailor antibiotics. As a rule, repeat debridements are required every 24–48 h to ensure that all involved tissues have been removed and, as such, any attempts at wound closure or coverage should be delayed until patients have clinically improved and show no recurrent signs of soft-tissue infection. Although the skin and deep tissues of the penis and scrotum are regularly involved, the corpus spongiosum, corpora cavernosa, and the testicles tend to be spared given their independent blood supplies and separation along fascial planes. However, patients presenting with epididymo-orchitis as the inciting infection may require orchiectomy, while patients with periurethral abscesses from extravasation of infected urine due to distal urethral obstruction may have involvement of the corpus spongiosum and urethra.

Large wounds with perirectal involvement may require fecal diversion to aid in wound healing and minimize further wound contamination. Urethral catheterization is generally sufficient for urinary diversion, but suprapubic catheter placement may be required in patients with significant obesity or those with urethral involvement. We generally recommend wrapping denuded testicles in Xeroform or Vaseline gauze between initial debridements. Long-term management of the testicles depends on patient and surgeon preference and may consist of either creation of thigh pouches for skin coverage or scrotal reconstruction with meshed split-thickness skin grafts in a delayed fashion (Fig. 27.3).

It is our practice to stop antibiotics once patients have been completely debrided, are afe-

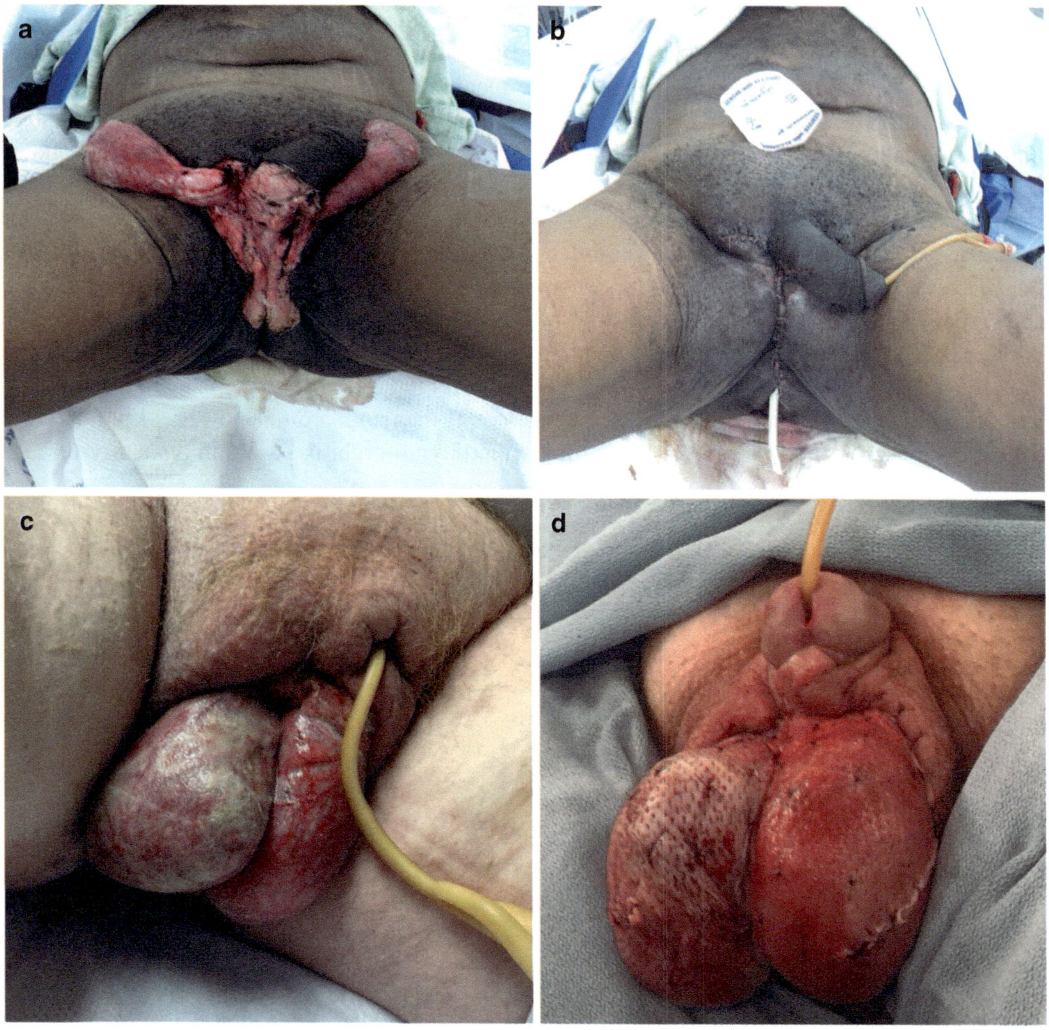

Fig. 27.3 Genital wound management following serial debridements for Fournier's gangrene. Exposed testicles (**a**) managed with bilateral thigh pouches and delayed primary wound closure of perineum (**b**). Separate patient with exposed testicles (**c**) managed with meshed split-thickness skin grafting (**d**)

brile, and show signs of clinical improvement with a down-trending leukocytosis and fever curve. Patients with bacteremia will require a longer duration of intravenous antibiotics based on the particular microbiology and recommendations from infectious disease specialists. Delayed primary wound closure is often able to be performed for the perineum as well as the scrotum, assuming at least 50% of the scrotal tissue has been spared. In patients with larger defects, meshed split-thickness grafts for scrotal reconstruction have excellent results.

Testicular Torsion

Any patient presenting with acute scrotal pain, tenderness and swelling requires prompt evaluation to rule out emergent etiologies. While the differential is broad, the most significant acute scrotal pathology that requires surgical intervention, aside from a necrotizing soft-tissue infection, is testicular torsion. Testicular torsion in adolescents and adults involves the twisting of the spermatic cord within the tunica vaginalis due to a congenital abnormality in how the testicle and epididymis are fixated within the scrotum called a *bell clapper deformity* (Fig. 27.4) [66]. While more common in adolescents, testicular torsion can occur in adults and may present in an intermittent fashion, where patients have intermittent twisting of the spermatic cord causing pain that spontaneously resolves without intervention.

Evaluation

Testicular torsion presents with acute onset, unilateral scrotal pain and is often associated with nausea and vomiting. Physical signs of testicular torsion include a firm, high-riding testicle with a horizontal lie and absence of the ipsilateral cremasteric reflex. While testicular torsion remains a clinical diagnosis and obtaining imaging in a patient with a high suspicion for torsion is not required, many patients will undergo scrotal ultrasonography prior to going to the operating room. Color Doppler ultrasound has been shown to have a sensitivity of approximately 90% and a specificity of 99% in diagnosing acute testicular torsion [67]. Diagnosis is confirmed by a lack of arterial blood flow within the parenchyma of the affected testicle.

There are a number of other diagnoses on the differential that must be considered when evaluating the acute scrotum, however. Epididymitis/epididymo-orchitis is an inflammatory disease

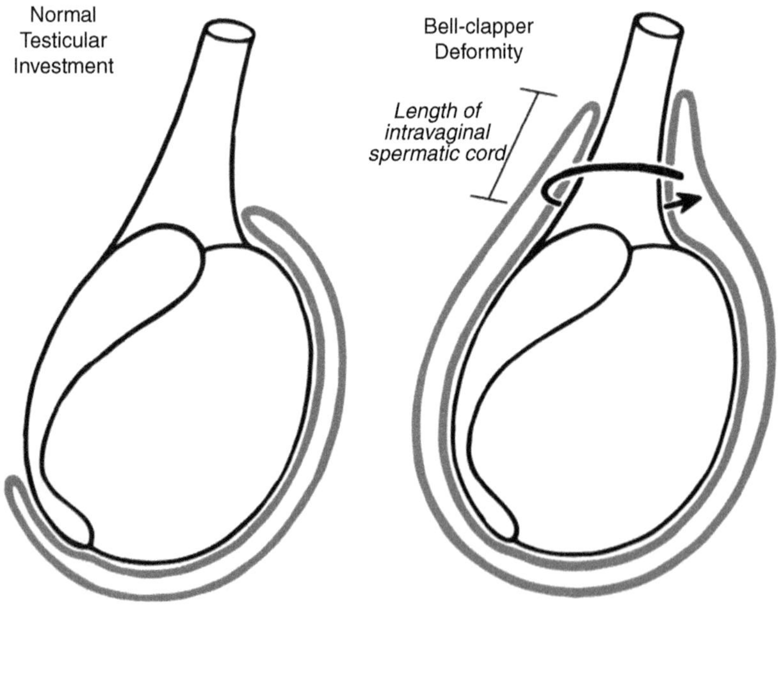

Fig. 27.4 Anatomic representation of bell clapper deformity leading to testicular torsion. (Adapted with permission from Taghavi K., et al., *The bell-clapper deformity of the testis: The definitive pathological anatomy*. J Ped Surg, 2020, E-pub ahead of print)

that can have both viral and bacterial etiologies, as well as noninfectious etiologies such as reflux of sterile urine into the epididymis. This diagnosis can clearly be distinguished for testicular torsion by the presence of hypervascularity of the involved testicle or epididymis of Doppler ultrasonography. While acute epididymo-orchitis rarely requires acute surgical intervention, failure of patients to clinically respond to intravenous antibiotics may prompt surgical exploration and orchiectomy. Torsion of a testicular or epididymal appendage can also present similarly, although some patients will present with the "blue dot sign," which is pathognomonic of torsion of the appendix testis or epididymis. Unlike testicular torsion, this is not a surgical emergency and supportive care is all that is warranted. Other disease processes such as hydroceles, varicoceles, spermatoceles, and testicular tumors can similarly be verified on ultrasonography, and although many do not warrant emergent surgical intervention, there is a risk for urgent or emergent intervention in some cases.

Management

Patients with confirmed or suspected testicular torsion should undergo immediate surgical intervention, and this should not be delayed by unnecessary radiographic evaluation in patients with clinical examination findings consistent with torsion. Previous work has shown that the likelihood of testicular salvage following testicular torsion declines precipitously with delays in surgical intervention, with 97% of testicles being salvaged if intervention occurs within 6 h [68]. However, testicular salvage rates decline to 80% at 7–12 h, 61% at 13–18 h, and 42% at 19–24 h. Manual detorsion may be performed as a temporizing maneuver, but should not preclude scrotal exploration. To perform manual detorsion, an "open book" approach should be taken where the testicle is rotated medial to lateral initially. Success will be noted if the patient has immediate relief of acute pain, but may only be successful in approximately 26% of cases [69]. If this is not successful, attempts to rotate lateral to medial may be attempted.

Surgical treatment involves exploration of the affected hemiscrotum and detorsion of the testicle. Once the spermatic cord has been untwisted and blood flow restored, the testicle should be wrapped in moist gauze and attention can be turned to the contralateral testicle. For this reason, the procedure is best performed through a single midline raphe incision to allow access to both testicles. The contralateral testicle should then be exposed and an orchiopexy performed, as the congenital malformation responsible for torsion of the affected side is believed to be present in both testicles. Orchiopexy is generally performed by direct suturing of the tunica albuginea of the testicle to the scrotal dartos in at least three points to minimize the risk of torsion. Attention is then turned back to the affected testicle. If pink and viable, a similar orchiopexy procedure is performed on that side. If the testicle fails to show signs of perfusion, viability may be assessed with an intraoperative Doppler of the spermatic cord or by incising the tunica albuginea of the testicle to assess for arterial bleeding. If the testicle is not perfused, scrotal orchiectomy is completed.

Penis

Priapism

Priapism is defined as a persistent erection unrelated to sexual stimulation that lasts for at least 4 h in duration [70]. While relatively rare, it is one of the more common urologic emergencies and often requires procedural intervention either in the emergency department or in the operating room. There are two types of priapism: *nonischemic priapism* and *ischemic priapism*. Nonischemic priapism is due to unregulated cavernous artery inflow and is most commonly due to acute trauma [71]. Ischemic priapism, however, is due to impaired venous outflow from the penis, which subsequently impairs arterial inflow and leads to hypoxia, cell death, and fibrosis within the corpora cavernosa [72]. There is also a variant of ischemic priapism known as *stuttering* or recurrent priapism, in which patients have intermittent ischemic priapism.

Ischemic priapism is much more common than nonischemic and is most often idiopathic. However, numerous associated etiologies of ischemic priapism have been identified. Medications such as trazodone, phosphodiesterase type-5 inhibitors, amphetamines, and cocaine have all been implicated in cases of ischemic priapism [73–75]. Spinal cord injuries and pelvic malignancies have similarly been associated. One of the more common causes of ischemic priapism, in pediatric populations in particular, is sickle cell disease [76]. While the pathology of sickle cell disease causing priapism is not entirely clear, it is believed that low pH and oxygen tensions present in the cavernosal tissues during erection may cause sickling of diseased erythrocytes that then block venous outflow, leading to ischemia.

Evaluation

Patients presenting with priapism will have a firm erection that usually only involves the corpora cavernosa, as the corpus spongiosum and glans are generally soft and not involved. Painful erections are more likely in ischemic priapism, while nonischemic priapism is less frequently associated with pain. Patients should be queried on recent medication or illicit drug use, recent perineal or penile trauma, and history of prior priapism episodes. Special concern should be taken to evaluate for history of sickle cell disease or other hematologic disorders that could be contributing causes. While priapism itself requires acute management, patients should be simultaneously evaluated and managed for underlying causes as well.

Once a diagnosis of priapism has been made, it is vital to determine if it is ischemic or nonischemic in nature. Nonischemic priapism is not a surgical emergency and can most often be managed with observation alone. For patients who do not resolve spontaneously and remain erect, angiographic embolization may be attempted as an outpatient. Ischemic priapism, however, requires prompt surgical intervention, as the duration of ischemic priapism is directly related to the likelihood of long-term erectile dysfunction. Previous work has shown that resolution of priapism within 24 h results in approximately 92% of men regaining baseline erectile function, while only 22% of those that persisted greater than 7 days did [77]. Furthermore, conservative management of ischemic priapism without intervention was associated with just 31% of patients maintaining potency from the same study.

There are two primary methods for differentiating ischemic from nonischemic priapism: penile Doppler ultrasound and corporal blood gas measurement. In either test, the goal of evaluation is determination of the presence or absence of maintained cavernosal arterial blood flow. Documentation of cavernosal artery flow on Doppler ultrasound confirms the absence of ischemic priapism. Corporal aspiration of blood in ischemic priapism often reveals dark, hypoxic blood, while the oxygenated blood in nonischemic priapism is bright red. Blood gas measurements in ischemic priapism, furthermore, will typically show hypoxia ($P_{O2} < 30$ mmHg), hypercarbia ($P_{CO2} > 60$ mmHg), and acidosis (pH < 7.25) [70].

Management

As previously stated, nonischemic priapism does not require immediate intervention and may be observed. However, patients with ischemic priapism require urgent intervention, as oral medications have failed to show clinical efficacy. Initial management involves aspiration of old, ischemic blood from the corpora, often with concomitant administration of intracavernous phenylephrine. The use of 100–500 μg/mL of phenylephrine every 3–5 min for 1 h has been recommended and patients should be closely monitored for adverse side effects including hypertension, palpitations, and reflex bradycardia. Patients who fail to respond to aspiration and injection of sympathomimetic mediations should then be considered for surgical decompression. Successful treatment will be identified by detumescence and resolution of pain. However, patients are at risk of early recurrence and should be monitored following treatment prior to discharge to home.

There are a number of surgical options for patients who fail to respond to lesser invasive treatments. Historically, the goal has been to create a surgical shunt between the corpora cavernosa with either the corpus spongiosum or the venous system in order to divert blood away from the engorged penis and allow restoration of arterial blood blow. A corporoglanular shunt should be the initial surgical procedure performed given its ease and low likelihood of complication. The most commonly performed corporoglanular shunt procedures include the *Winter's shunt*, where a large-bore biopsy needle is passed through the glans into the tip of the corpora cavernosa, and the *Ebbehoj* or T-shunt, where a scalpel blade is inserted through the glans into the distal tip of the corpora cavernosa [78, 79]. However, the most effective corporoglanular shunt is the *Al-Ghorab* shunt, where a small 2-cm horizontal incision is made on the dorsum of the glans to expose the engorged tips of the corpora cavernosa. The tips are then excised to create a shunt to the corpus spongiosum [80]. This procedure is often coupled with corporal dilation through the excised corporal tips to aid in evacuation and decompression of the corpora [81].

Proximal shunts have also been reported but are less commonly employed contemporarily. These include the *Quackels* shunt, where a proximal shunt is created by anastomosing the corpus spongiosum to the cavernosa, and the *Grayhack* shunt, where the saphenous vein is anastomosed to the corpora cavernosa [82, 83]. A newer approach to management of recurrent ischemic priapism has employed performing simple decompression of the corpora cavernosa via a penoscrotal skin incision [84]. In this approach, shunting is not performed, and priapism is treated like a penile compartment syndrome, in which after decompression the corpora are then closed. Early reports suggest excellent results that may change the paradigm for management of recurrent ischemic priapism in patients in whom distal shunting has failed.

Prostate

Prostatitis and Prostate Abscess

Much like renal and perinephric abscesses that may form following acute pyelonephritis, prostatic abscesses often arise following acute bacterial prostatitis. Patients at risk for acute bacterial prostatitis include patients with prior history of urinary tract infection, urethral instrumentation, prostate biopsy, or immunosuppressive states including diabetes mellitus, HIV, and chronic kidney disease [85–87]. The most common causative organisms are gram-negative bacteria and include *E. coli*, *Proteus*, *Klebsiella*, and *Pseudomonas* species [88, 89]. However, up to a quarter of men will have gram-positive infections due to hematogenous spread [90].

Evaluation

Presenting symptoms of prostatic abscess and prostatitis are often quite similar, and the diagnoses are often only distinguishable by cross-sectional imaging. Patients most often report lower urinary tract symptoms such as dysuria, urinary urgency, sensation of incomplete bladder emptying, and perineal pain, but also often present with fevers, chills, and low back pain as well [90]. Other generalized symptoms such as malaise and myalgias may be present. Physical examination often reveals a painful, irregular, and boggy prostate gland on digital rectal examination, although aggressive digital prostatic examinations are not recommended due to the potential to induce bacteremia [91]. Laboratory evaluation should include urinalysis with urine culture to identify causative organisms, while a complete blood count and blood cultures may be indicated based on clinical presentation. Ensuring that patients are not in urinary retention via ultrasound is also vital during initial evaluation. Patients in retention have traditionally been managed with suprapubic catheter placement due to concerns related to inducing bacteremia with passage of a urethral catheter; however, this dogma has been shifting toward acceptance of urethral catheterization when indicated due to lack of clear evidence that this worsens patient outcomes [92].

Management

Initial management involves initiation of appropriate antimicrobial agents based on urine culture data. Early empiric antibiotic selection should

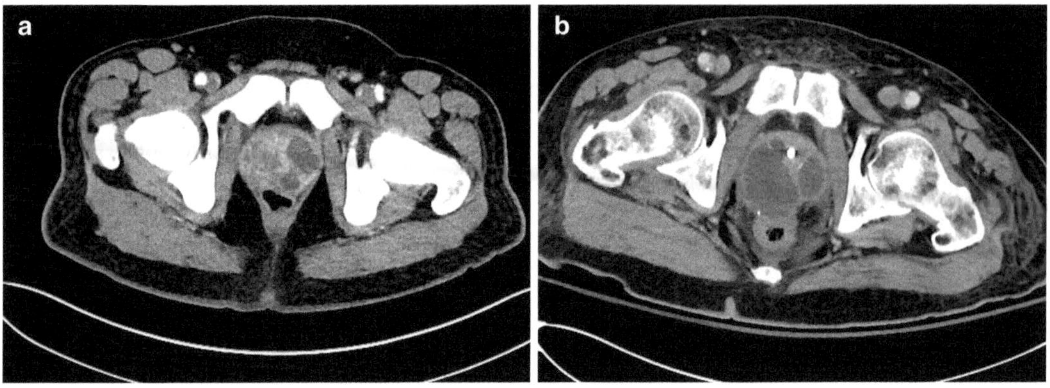

Fig. 27.5 CT imaging showing large, multifocal prostatic abscesses in two patients (**a** and **b**), both treated with transurethral unroofing

cover likely causative organisms, primarily gram-negative bacteria, unless patients are at risk for gram-positive hematogenously spread infections. Fluoroquinolones and trimethoprim-sulfamethoxazole have shown to have excellent prostatic tissue penetration and are often chosen as first-line therapies for the majority of patients until culture data are available to more appropriately guide antibiotic choices. Men younger than 35 who are sexually active should also be considered for coverage of *N. gonorrhea* and *C. trachomatis* due to possible sexually transmitted infection as the cause of prostatitis [93].

While the incidence is low, patients who fail to clinically improve despite appropriate antimicrobial treatment should be specifically evaluated for development of a prostatic abscess. Cross-sectional imaging with contrasted CT serves as the optimal imaging modality for diagnosis of prostatic abscesses with the highest specificity and sensitivity (Fig. 27.5). Transrectal ultrasonography may also be useful, but is less commonly used in the initial diagnostic phase today. CT showing a non-enhancing fluid collection within the prostatic parenchyma, possibly with septations or rim enhancement, is diagnostic.

Traditionally, patients with small abscesses <1 cm in size have been managed with culture-specific antibiotics and follow-up imaging alone, as these smaller lesions often respond without surgical intervention [94]. However, more recent work has suggested that patients with abscesses up to 2 cm in size may also do well with antibiotic therapy alone [95]. Patients with larger lesions, or those who are severely ill or immunocompromised, often require drainage. Multiple different approaches have been reported in the literature, all with high rates of success. Transrectal ultrasound-guided drainage, percutaneous transperineal drainage, and transurethral unroofing utilizing a resectoscope are all viable options. Larger, multiloculated abscesses are often best served by transurethral unroofing, while smaller solitary abscesses are generally well managed with drainage procedures. For patients treated with drainage procedures, follow-up imaging should be performed to ensure abscess resolution. Patients treated with transurethral procedures generally keep a urethral catheter in place for 1 week and are monitored for clinical signs of improvement.

References

1. Uribarri J, Oh MS, Carroll HJ. The first kidney stone. Ann Intern Med. 1989;111(12):1006–9.
2. Kuo RL, et al. Topiramate-induced nephrolithiasis. J Endourol. 2002;16(4):229–31.
3. Maalouf NM, et al. Nephrolithiasis in topiramate users. Urol Res. 2011;39(4):303–7.
4. Gentle DL, et al. Protease inhibitor-induced urolithiasis. Urology. 1997;50(4):508–11.
5. Matlaga BR, et al. Effect of gastric bypass surgery on kidney stone disease. J Urol. 2009;181(6):2573–7.
6. Cruz DN, Huot SJ. Metabolic complications of urinary diversions: an overview. Am J Med. 1997;102(5):477–84.

7. Smith-Bindman R, et al. Ultrasonography versus computed tomography for suspected nephrolithiasis. N Engl J Med. 2014;371(12):1100–10.
8. Ray AA, et al. Limitations to ultrasound in the detection and measurement of urinary tract calculi. Urology. 2010;76(2):295–300.
9. Miller OF, Kane CJ. Unenhanced helical computed tomography in the evaluation of acute flank pain. Curr Opin Urol. 2000;10(2):123–9.
10. Nourparvar P, et al. Safety and efficacy of ureteral stent placement at the bedside using local anesthesia. J Urol. 2016;195(6):1886–90.
11. Semins MJ, Matlaga BR. Management of urolithiasis in pregnancy. Int J Women's Health. 2013;5:599–604.
12. Blanco LT, et al. Renal colic during pregnancy: diagnostic and therapeutic aspects. Literature review. Cent European J Urol. 2017;70(1):93–100.
13. Lewis DF, et al. Urolithiasis in pregnancy. Diagnosis, management and pregnancy outcome. J Reprod Med. 2003;48(1):28–32.
14. Andreoiu M, MacMahon R. Renal colic in pregnancy: lithiasis or physiological hydronephrosis? Urology. 2009;74(4):757–61.
15. Expert Panel on MR Safety, et al. ACR guidance document on MR safe practices: 2013. J Magn Reson Imaging. 2013;37(3):501–30.
16. Ray JG, et al. Association between MRI exposure during pregnancy and fetal and childhood outcomes. JAMA. 2016;316(9):952–61.
17. Bailey G, et al. Perinatal outcomes with tamsulosin therapy for symptomatic urolithiasis. J Urol. 2016;195(1):99–103.
18. Assimos D, et al. Surgical management of stones: American Urological Association/Endourological Society Guideline, part II. J Urol. 2016;196(4):1161–9.
19. Coelho RF, et al. Renal and perinephric abscesses: analysis of 65 consecutive cases. World J Surg. 2007;31(2):431–6.
20. Dielubanza EJ, Mazur DJ, Schaeffer AJ. Management of non-catheter-associated complicated urinary tract infection. Infect Dis Clin N Am. 2014;28(1):121–34.
21. Gardiner RA, Gwynne RA, Roberts SA. Perinephric abscess. BJU Int. 2011;107(Suppl 3):20–3.
22. Dembry LM, Andriole VT. Renal and perirenal abscesses. Infect Dis Clin N Am. 1997;11(3):663–80.
23. Dalla Palma L, Pozzi-Mucelli F, Ene V. Medical treatment of renal and perirenal abscesses: CT evaluation. Clin Radiol. 1999;54(12):792–7.
24. Siegel JF, Smith A, Moldwin R. Minimally invasive treatment of renal abscess. J Urol. 1996;155(1):52–5.
25. Fowler JE Jr, Perkins T. Presentation, diagnosis and treatment of renal abscesses: 1972-1988. J Urol. 1994;151(4):847–51.
26. Huang JJ, Tseng CC. Emphysematous pyelonephritis: clinicoradiological classification, management, prognosis, and pathogenesis. Arch Intern Med. 2000;160(6):797–805.
27. Mokabberi R, Ravakhah K. Emphysematous urinary tract infections: diagnosis, treatment and survival (case review series). Am J Med Sci. 2007;333(2):111–6.
28. Ubee SS, McGlynn L, Fordham M. Emphysematous pyelonephritis. BJU Int. 2011;107(9):1474–8.
29. Chen MT, et al. Percutaneous drainage in the treatment of emphysematous pyelonephritis: 10-year experience. J Urol. 1997;157(5):1569–73.
30. Mydlo JH, Maybee GJ, Ali-Khan MM. Percutaneous drainage and/or nephrectomy in the treatment of emphysematous pyelonephritis. Urol Int. 2003;70(3):147–50.
31. Somani BK, et al. Is percutaneous drainage the new gold standard in the management of emphysematous pyelonephritis? Evidence from a systematic review. J Urol. 2008;179(5):1844–9.
32. Kasotakis G. Retroperitoneal and rectus sheath hematomas. Surg Clin North Am. 2014;94(1):71–6.
33. Mant MJ, et al. Haemorrhagic complications of heparin therapy. Lancet. 1977;1(8022):1133–5.
34. Sagel SS, et al. Detection of retroperitoneal hemorrhage by computed tomography. AJR Am J Roentgenol. 1977;129(3):403–7.
35. Baekgaard JS, et al. Spontaneous retroperitoneal and rectus sheath hemorrhage-management, risk factors and outcomes. World J Surg. 2019;43(8):1890–7.
36. Sunga KL, et al. Spontaneous retroperitoneal hematoma: etiology, characteristics, management, and outcome. J Emerg Med. 2012;43(2):e157–61.
37. McDougal WS, Kursh ED, Persky L. Spontaneous rupture of the kidney with perirenal hematoma. J Urol. 1975;114(2):181–4.
38. Zhang JQ, Fielding JR, Zou KH. Etiology of spontaneous perirenal hemorrhage: a meta-analysis. J Urol. 2002;167(4):1593–6.
39. Nguyen HT, et al. Acute retroperitoneal hemorrhage due to transitional cell carcinoma of the renal pelvis. J Urol. 1995;153(1):140–1.
40. Heyns CF, Rossouw DJ. Spontaneous rupture of adult Wilms' tumor. Cancer. 1989;64(1):173–7.
41. Aragona F, et al. Sarcomatous carcinoma of the kidney presenting as spontaneous retroperitoneal hemorrhage. Report of a case with immunocytochemical study. Eur Urol. 1988;14(5):417–21.
42. Oesterling JE, et al. The management of renal angiomyolipoma. J Urol. 1986;135(6):1121–4.
43. Sahu KK, et al. Clinical spectrum, risk factors, management and outcome of patients with retroperitoneal hematoma: a retrospective analysis of 3-year experience. Expert Rev Hematol. 2020;13(5):545–55.
44. Ekici Y, et al. Treatment approaches for spontaneous retroperitoneal bleeding. Int Surg. 2009;94(2):171–5.
45. Halbgewachs C, Domes T. Postobstructive diuresis: pay close attention to urinary retention. Can Fam Physician. 2015;61(2):137–42.
46. Leinum LR, Berthelsen C, Azawi N. Post-obstructive diuresis; underlying causes and hospitalization. Scand J Urol. 2020;54(3):253–7.
47. Furr J, et al. Contemporary trends in the inpatient management of Fournier's gangrene: predictors of length of stay and mortality based on population-based sample. Urology. 2017;102:79–84.

48. Osbun N, et al. Low-volume vs high-volume centers and management of Fournier's gangrene in Washington state. J Am Coll Surg. 2017;224(3):270–275.e1.
49. Sorensen MD, et al. Fournier's gangrene: population based epidemiology and outcomes. J Urol. 2009;181(5):2120–6.
50. Yim SU, et al. Neutrophil to lymphocyte and platelet to lymphocyte ratios are more effective than the Fournier's gangrene severity index for predicting poor prognosis in Fournier's gangrene. Surg Infect (Larchmt). 2016;17(2):217–23.
51. Radcliffe RS, Khan MA. Mortality associated with Fournier's gangrene remains unchanged over 25 years. BJU Int. 2020;125(4):610–6.
52. Eke N. Fournier's gangrene: a review of 1726 cases. Br J Surg. 2000;87(6):718–28.
53. Baskin LS, et al. Necrotising soft tissue infections of the perineum and genitalia. Bacteriology, treatment and risk assessment. Br J Urol. 1990;65(5):524–9.
54. Basoglu M, et al. Management of Fournier's gangrene: review of 45 cases. Surg Today. 2007;37(7):558–63.
55. Morpurgo E, Galandiuk S. Fournier's gangrene. Surg Clin North Am. 2002;82(6):1213–24.
56. Clayton MD, et al. Causes, presentation and survival of fifty-seven patients with necrotizing fasciitis of the male genitalia. Surg Gynecol Obstet. 1990;170(1):49–55.
57. Dahm P, et al. Outcome analysis in patients with primary necrotizing fasciitis of the male genitalia. Urology. 2000;56(1):31–5; discussion 35–6.
58. Elem B, Ranjan P. Impact of immunodeficiency virus (HIV) on Fournier's gangrene: observations in Zambia. Ann R Coll Surg Engl. 1995;77(4):283–6.
59. Norton KS, et al. Management of Fournier's gangrene: an eleven year retrospective analysis of early recognition, diagnosis, and treatment. Am Surg. 2002;68(8):709–13.
60. Smith GL, Bunker CB, Dinneen MD. Fournier's gangrene. Br J Urol. 1998;81(3):347–55.
61. Corman JM, Moody JA, Aronson WJ. Fournier's gangrene in a modern surgical setting: improved survival with aggressive management. BJU Int. 1999;84(1):85–8.
62. Paty R, Smith AD. Gangrene and Fournier's gangrene. Urol Clin North Am. 1992;19(1):149–62.
63. Stamenkovic I, Lew PD. Early recognition of potentially fatal necrotizing fasciitis. The use of frozen-section biopsy. N Engl J Med. 1984;310(26):1689–93.
64. Anaya DA, et al. Predicting death in necrotizing soft tissue infections: a clinical score. Surg Infect (Larchmt). 2009;10(6):517–22.
65. Levenson RB, Singh AK, Novelline RA. Fournier gangrene: role of imaging. Radiographics. 2008;28(2):519–28.
66. Taghavi K, et al. The bell-clapper deformity of the testis: the definitive pathological anatomy. J Pediatr Surg. 2020; https://doi.org/10.1016/j.jpedsurg.2020.06.023.
67. Baker LA, et al. An analysis of clinical outcomes using color doppler testicular ultrasound for testicular torsion. Pediatrics. 2000;105(3 Pt 1):604–7.
68. Mellick LB, et al. A systematic review of testicle survival time after a torsion event. Pediatr Emerg Care. 2019;35(12):821–5.
69. Vasconcelos-Castro S, et al. Manual detorsion in testicular torsion: 5 years of experience at a single center. J Pediatr Surg. 2020;55:2728–31.
70. Montague DK, et al. American urological association guideline on the management of priapism. J Urol. 2003;170(4 Pt 1):1318–24.
71. Hakim LS, et al. Evolving concepts in the diagnosis and treatment of arterial high flow priapism. J Urol. 1996;155(2):541–8.
72. Spycher MA, Hauri D. The ultrastructure of the erectile tissue in priapism. J Urol. 1986;135(1):142–7.
73. Carson CC 3rd, Mino RD. Priapism associated with trazodone therapy. J Urol. 1988;139(2):369–70.
74. Eiland LS, Bell EA, Erramouspe J. Priapism associated with the use of stimulant medications and atomoxetine for attention-deficit/hyperactivity disorder in children. Ann Pharmacother. 2014;48(10):1350–5.
75. Munarriz R, et al. Cocaine and ephedrine-induced priapism: case reports and investigation of potential adrenergic mechanisms. Urology. 2003;62(1):187–92.
76. Fowler JE Jr, et al. Priapism associated with the sickle cell hemoglobinopathies: prevalence, natural history and sequelae. J Urol. 1991;145(1):65–8.
77. Kulmala RV, Lehtonen TA, Tammela TL. Preservation of potency after treatment for priapism. Scand J Urol Nephrol. 1996;30(4):313–6.
78. Brant WO, et al. T-shaped shunt and intracavernous tunneling for prolonged ischemic priapism. J Urol. 2009;181(4):1699–705.
79. Ebbehoj J. A new operation for priapism. Scand J Plast Reconstr Surg. 1974;8(3):241–2.
80. Muller A. al-Ghorab shunt for priapism. J Sex Med. 2016;13(8):1279–84.
81. Burnett AL, Pierorazio PM. Corporal "snake" maneuver: corporoglanular shunt surgical modification for ischemic priapism. J Sex Med. 2009;6(4):1171–6.
82. Quackels R. [Treatment of a case of priapism by cavernospongious anastomosis]. Acta Urol Belg. 1964;32:5–13.
83. Wendel EF, Grayhack JT. Corpora cavernosa-glans penis shunt for priapism. Surg Gynecol Obstet. 1981;153(4):586–8.
84. Fuchs JS, et al. Penoscrotal decompression-promising new treatment paradigm for refractory ischemic priapism. J Sex Med. 2018;15(5):797–802.
85. Breyer BN, et al. HIV status is an independent risk factor for reporting lower urinary tract symptoms. J Urol. 2011;185(5):1710–5.
86. Mosharafa AA, et al. Rising incidence of acute prostatitis following prostate biopsy: fluoroquinolone resistance and exposure is a significant risk factor. Urology. 2011;78(3):511–4.

87. Wyndaele JJ. Complications of intermittent catheterization: their prevention and treatment. Spinal Cord. 2002;40(10):536–41.
88. Cornia PB, Takahashi TA, Lipsky BA. The microbiology of bacteriuria in men: a 5-year study at a Veterans' Affairs hospital. Diagn Microbiol Infect Dis. 2006;56(1):25–30.
89. Roberts RO, et al. A review of clinical and pathological prostatitis syndromes. Urology. 1997;49(6):809–21.
90. Ackerman AL, Parameshwar PS, Anger JT. Diagnosis and treatment of patients with prostatic abscess in the post-antibiotic era. Int J Urol. 2018;25(2):103–10.
91. Krieger JN. Prostatitis syndromes: pathophysiology, differential diagnosis, and treatment. Sex Transm Dis. 1984;11(2):100–12.
92. Pfau A. Prostatitis. A continuing enigma. Urol Clin North Am. 1986;13(4):695–715.
93. Brede CM, Shoskes DA. The etiology and management of acute prostatitis. Nat Rev Urol. 2011;8(4):207–12.
94. Ludwig M, et al. Diagnosis and therapeutic management of 18 patients with prostatic abscess. Urology. 1999;53(2):340–5.
95. Lee DS, et al. Acute bacterial prostatitis and abscess formation. BMC Urol. 2016;16(1):38.

28 Acute Gynecologic Emergencies

Elise Bardawil and Eric Strand

Case Presentation

A 32-year-old female, gravid 2, para 2, presents to the emergency department with the sudden onset of right lower quadrant pain, nausea, and vomiting. The patient reports no significant prior medical or surgical history. She was in her normal state of health until the onset of sharp, colicky pain that started ~18 h prior to presentation. On physical examination, the patient's temperature is 99.1 °F, pulse 110 bpm, and BP 118/64. Her abdomen is tender in the RLQ with moderate guarding. Laboratory evaluation reveals a Hgb of 11.2 g/dL and a WBC of 13.2 k/mm^3. A urine pregnancy test is negative. A CT scan performed reveals a complex right lower quadrant mass without clear visualization of the appendix, interpreted as suspicious for appendiceal rupture and/or abscess.

As the general surgeon on call, you are consulted and take the patient to the operating room for a laparoscopic evaluation. At the time of surgery, you discover a 7 cm torsed right ovary with a bluish hue. The appendix is visualized and appears normal.

E. Bardawil
Division of Minimally Invasive Gynecologic Surgery, Department of Obstetrics and Gynecology, Washington University School of Medicine, St. Louis, MO, USA
e-mail: e.bardawil@wustl.edu

E. Strand (✉)
Division of General Obstetrics and Gynecology, Department of Obstetrics and Gynecology, Washington University School of Medicine, St. Louis, MO, USA
e-mail: eastrand@wustl.edu

M. D. Zielinski, O. Guillamondegui (eds.), *The Acute Management of Surgical Disease*, https://doi.org/10.1007/978-3-031-07881-1_28

Introduction

Although uncommon, the general surgeon may encounter situations in which knowledge regarding the management of common OB/GYN diagnoses would be valuable. In this chapter, we describe some of these common diagnoses, reviewing clinical presentations, relevant anatomy, and directed surgical (or nonsurgical) management.

Adnexal Torsion

Symptoms and Causes

As this case presentation has illustrated, the presenting symptom of adnexal torsion is the abrupt onset of unilateral lower quadrant pain which is often associated with nausea and vomiting. Torsion is a common gynecologic emergency accounting for 2.7% of emergent gynecologic surgical cases [1]. Adnexal torsion occurs when the blood supply to the ovary gets twisted and compromised. This is most frequently caused by an ovarian cyst which causes the ovary to become enlarged. Less frequently paratubal cysts may cause torsion of the ovary or even of the fallopian tube. Usually, the ovary twists around both of its ligamentous supports, the infundibulopelvic ligament and the utero-ovarian ligament. As a result, there is continued partial influx of arterial blood and a marked decreased egress of the compressed venous blood flow. This causes the ovary to become edematous and enlarged, distending the ovarian capsule. If left untreated, the tissue becomes necrotic and ultimately causes peritonitis.

Relevant Pelvic Anatomy

Ovarian torsion is a surgical emergency. In order to discuss surgical management options, it is worth reviewing the relevant pelvic anatomy. The major blood supply to the ovary is supplied by the ovarian artery, which is a branch of the descending aorta (Fig. 28.1). The ovarian artery and vein travel across the pelvic brim in the infundibulopelvic ligament, also called the sus-

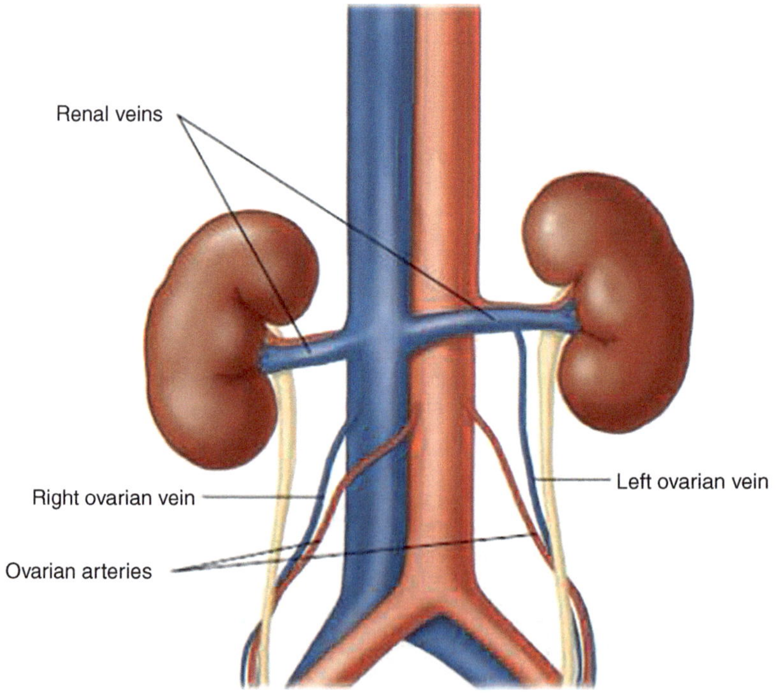

Fig. 28.1 Ovarian vasculature. (*Reproduced with permission from Falcone, Tommaso, et al. Operative Techniques in Gynecologic Surgery: Gynecology. Philadelphia: Wolters Kluwer, 2017. Copyright @2017 Wolters Kluwer*)

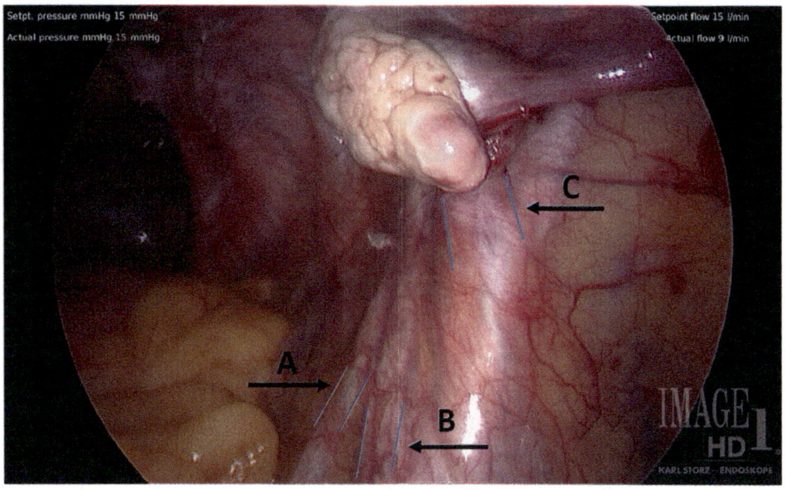

Fig. 28.2 Surgical photo of right pelvic brim, illustrating the proximity of the ureter to the right infundibulopelvic ligament (a: internal iliac artery; b: ureter; c: infundibulopelvic ligament)

pensory ligament of the ovary. The suspensory ligament attaches the ovary to the pelvic sidewall, while the utero-ovarian ligament attaches the ovary to the uterus. A branch of the uterine artery also supplies blood to the ovary through the utero-ovarian ligament. The mesosalpinx is the portion of the broad ligament that connects the ovary to the fallopian tube. The fallopian tube extends from the cornua of the uterus and runs superior and anterior to the ovary.

It is also important to recognize the path of the ureter in the female pelvis as it relates to ovarian anatomy, as it can easily be injured during adnexal surgery (Fig. 28.2b). The ureter courses across the bifurcation of the common iliac from lateral to medial as it crosses the pelvic brim. Anatomic studies have shown that the mean distance between the ureter and infundibulopelvic ligaments is 2.2 cm on the right (range 0.5–3.5 cm) and 2.6 cm on the left (range 1.0–4.5 cm) [2]. Given this close proximity, it is important to identify the ureter before ligating and transecting that ligament to avoid a ureteral injury.

Surgical Management

The first step in surgical management of adnexal torsion is to reestablish normal anatomy. This usually involves untwisting the ovary multiple times. If an ovary has been torsed for multiple hours, it may appear black. When it is untwisted, it should start to return to a normal color. Numerous studies in pediatric adolescent gynecology illustrate that detorsed ovaries remain functional the vast majority of the time [3]. The trend in gynecology is toward conservative management by leaving the ovaries in place, either with or without an ovarian cystectomy.

If the ovary is detorsed and appears viable, it is reasonable to end the case, leaving the ovary, and the likely cyst behind. When adnexal pathology was present, Adiyemi-Fowode et al. found the rate of recurrent ovarian torsion to be 2–12%. They discuss a higher rate of repeat torsion in girls without adnexal pathology [3]. If there is an identifiable ovarian cyst, another treatment option is to proceed with an ovarian cystectomy in order to decrease the likelihood of recurrent torsion.

Abdominal Ovarian Cystectomy

To perform an abdominal ovarian cystectomy, the ovary must be visualized. The patient should be placed in slight Trendelenburg. A retractor may be necessary, and the bowel may need to be packed away. An abdominal ovarian cystectomy is performed by grasping the ovary. The infundibulopelvic ligament and utero-ovarian ligament should be identified. The outermost layer, the ovarian cortex, should be carefully incised with a scalpel or cautery to the level of the cyst wall. The incision should be located where the cyst is taut, distal from both of the ovary's suspending ligaments. A knife handle is then used to shell out the cyst from the surrounding ovarian cortex. The cyst wall can be grasped with Allis clamps to aid in the dissection. It is important to remove the cyst wall completely to prevent recurrence. To achieve hemostasis, the ovarian cortex can then be sutured together using a fine absorbable suture, such as 3-0 polyglactin, in a continuous fashion. If the ovary is hemostatic after the cystectomy, suturing is not required. Pathologic examination of the cyst wall should be performed to determine whether the cyst was benign or malignant, the potential risk of recurrence, and if future medical management might be indicated (as with an endometrioma). Future follow-up can be arranged with the patient's gynecologist.

Laparoscopic Ovarian Cystectomy

A laparoscopic ovarian cystectomy is performed in a similar manner. The patient is placed in Trendelenburg so that the bowel falls into the upper abdomen and the pelvic organs can be identified. The ovary is identified and often brought out from posterior cul-de-sac behind the uterus. The infundibulopelvic ligament and utero-ovarian ligament are identified. The ovary is stabilized with a bowel grasper or atraumatic grasper. An incision is made in the cortex of the ovary using an advanced energy device like a harmonic scalpel or a monopolar device like the monopolar scissors. It is more difficult to make an incision in the ovarian cortex without rupturing the cyst laparoscopically. If the cyst is kept intact, the ovarian cortex is grasped, and a second instrument gently, and often bluntly, peels the cyst wall away. Sometimes, sharp dissection is needed to cut away tissue attaching the cyst wall to the ovary. If the cyst is ruptured, the same technique is used to separate the cyst wall from the cortex. It is important to keep track of which instrument is grasping the ovarian cortex and which is holding onto the cyst wall, especially after a cyst rupture, as the color and texture of the ovarian cortex and cyst wall are very similar. Consistent identification of the cyst wall ensures this tissue is dissected and removed (and not ovarian cortex).

Sometimes, the ovarian bed bleeds after a cystectomy. Hemostasis may be achieved using a bipolar device. If this is unsuccessful, a 2-0 or 3-0 barbed suture can be used to close the ovarian defect. This usually establishes hemostasis.

Once the cyst is resected, it should be placed into a specimen retrieval bag. When the bag is removed, specimen extraction may be limited by the fascia. If the cyst is intact, it can be ruptured and the fluid should be drained using wall suction. The cyst can then be removed using Kocher clamps to grasp it. If the cyst does not deliver easily through the laparoscopic incision, the incision can be widened, or the cyst morcellated. If there is concern for an ovarian malignancy, it is important to ensure the specimen's removal is contained within the specimen retrieval bag, so that malignant cells are not spread throughout the pelvis.

Abdominal Oophorectomy

If the ovary is detorsed and remains hemorrhagic and necrotic, then the treatment becomes an oophorectomy. An oophorectomy is accomplished by cutting off the blood supply to the ovary by transecting the infundibulopelvic ligament and the utero-ovarian ligament. The ovary is then removed from the mesosalpinx. In an abdominal oophorectomy, the ovary is identified. In order to see the uterus and ovary, the patient should be placed in Trendelenburg and the bowel should be packed away. Once again, this may require a retractor. The ovary is then grasped and tented upward. The peritoneum lateral to the infundibulopelvic ligament is grasped with blunt pickups and incised, opening up the retroperitoneum. The ureter is located retroperitoneally coursing along the medial leaf of the broad ligament. Blunt dissection is performed until the ureter is identified. A hole is made in the broad ligament between the infundibulopelvic ligament and ureter. A large clamp, like a Kelly clamp or Haney clamp, is placed through this hole from lateral to medial, clamping the infundibulopelvic ligament. A second clamp should be placed distally. The tissue between the two clamps is cut. A free tie is used to secure the pedicle. A transfixion suture is then placed between the free tie and the clamp. The infundibulopelvic ligament is now secure.

A second window is then made between the fallopian tube and utero-ovarian ligament in order to isolate the utero-ovarian ligament. Again, two clamps are placed on this pedicle. The tissue between the clamps is cut. A free tie, followed by a transfixion suture, is placed on the pedicle. When the ligaments are both transected, the mesosalpinx can be severed using cautery. It is not necessary to remove the fallopian tube as it can still play a role in fertility, even when the ipsilateral ovary has been removed.

Laparoscopic Oophorectomy

The steps for an oophorectomy laparoscopically are the same except that an advanced bipolar device is used for every step. The patient is placed in steep Trendelenburg. The ovary is identified, and peritoneum is incised lateral to the infundibulopelvic ligament. The infundibulopelvic ligament is grasped with a blunt grasper and tented toward the opposite sidewall. Blunt dissection is used to open the retroperitoneum to identify the ureter. A hole is made in the retroperitoneum between the ureter and the infundibulopelvic ligament. This hole can be made bluntly using an instrument with a sharper tip like a Maryland or by using an advanced hemostatic device. When the infundibulopelvic ligament is isolated, the pedicle is coagulated and transected using an advanced hemostatic device. The hemostatic device is placed through the opening made in the peritoneum. It is important to coagulate, or triple burn, the pedicle so that when it is transected and retracts, it does not bleed.

The utero-ovarian ligament should then be identified. It should be coagulated and transected using an advanced hemostatic device. Avoidance of the uterine artery running laterally up the uterus is necessary as it can bleed briskly. When this vessel is secure, an advanced hemostatic device should then be used to remove the ovary from the mesosalpinx. Small vessels run within the mesosalpinx, so it is easier to use energy when cutting through this tissue than performing this step without energy.

Oophoropexy

The risk of a repeat ovarian torsion may be decreased by performing a suspending procedure—the oophoropexy. This involves either shortening the utero-ovarian ligament or suturing the ovary to a structure like the utero-sacral ligament with a permanent suture. The gynecology data are unclear regarding the risks and benefits of this procedure, and it is usually reserved for patients who have repeat ovarian torsions. In a review of ovarian torsion in the pediatric literature, there was no evidence to support oophoropexy after a single episode of ovarian torsion. In this setting, a fixation procedure did not eliminate the possibility of future torsion events and also demonstrated that the oophoropexy may negatively affect future fertility for the patient due to altering the ovarian anatomy and blood supply [4]. As a general surgeon, it is unlikely that you would perform this procedure in the acute setting.

Hemorrhagic Ovarian Cysts: Symptoms and Management

The presenting symptom of a ruptured hemorrhagic cyst is the acute onset of severe unilateral pelvic pain with imaging demonstrating blood or free fluid in the pelvis. This presentation can mimic that of a patient with a ruptured ectopic pregnancy. Since a ruptured ectopic pregnancy is another common cause of an adnexal mass with free fluid in the pelvis, the workup for a patient with these symptoms should always include a pregnancy test. Most patients with a ruptured hemorrhagic cyst are managed nonoperatively with observation and pain medication in the acute setting. Infrequently, patients with a hemorrhagic cyst will need a transfusion due to blood loss from the cyst. Even in this situation, the bleeding from the ovary usually resolves on its own. In the outpatient setting, patients are often initiated on oral contraceptives in order to suppress future ovarian cyst formation.

Uncommonly, patients who present with hemorrhagic cysts may have unstable vital signs. This occurs because the ovaries have a dual blood supply and can bleed quickly into the peritoneal cavity. Patients may also present with peritoneal signs. The decision to operate should be based on the patient's full clinical picture and if the patient can be stabilized medically (typically with blood product replacement). If the patient remains unstable despite resuscitation, surgical management should aim at clearing the pelvis of any blood or clot so that the site of bleeding can be identified. If any ongoing bleeding is found, it should be rendered hemostatic. Either advanced bipolar devices or suturing may be used. If this is unsuccessful, an ovarian cystectomy or oophorectomy should be performed as described previously. Commonly, no obvious site of bleeding can be identified during these procedures as the ovarian bleeding if often self-limited.

Vulvar Abscess/Necrotizing Fasciitis

Vulvar abscesses are a common gynecologic problem. Most represent polymicrobial infections, often arising in the hair-bearing areas of the labia majora (an exception, the Bartholin's gland abscess, should be managed by a gynecologic specialist and will not be addressed here). Although the exact incidence of vulvar abscess is unknown, there are a number of risk factors associated with their development, including diabetes mellitus, obesity, shaving or waxing of the pubic hair, and pregnancy [5].

Anatomic Considerations

The skin of the vulva contains a number of glands that carry the potential for infection. Holocrine sebaceous glands are associated with the hair shafts of the labia majora. Apocrine sweat glands are also located lateral to the vaginal introitus and the anus—these glands may become chronically infected in circumstances such as hidradenitis suppurativa and may require surgical debridement.

The subcutaneous tissue underlying the labia majora consists of lobules of fat interlaced with fine connective tissue septae. This fatty tissue is quite similar to that encountered in the anterior abdominal wall. Beneath this layer is a more fibrinous, membranous layer (also known as Colles fascia). This layer is similar to Scarpa's fascia of the abdominal wall. Notably, this membranous layer attaches laterally to the ischiopubic rami and posteriorly to the perineal membrane. It does not, however, have an anterior attachment to the pubic rami. Thus, infections or hematomas of the vulva may spread to the anterior abdominal wall (and, similarly, infections or hematomas from the anterior abdominal wall may spread to the perineum) [6].

Surgical Management

The initial management of small vulvar abscesses (<2 cm) can be conservative in nature—application of warm compresses 3–4 times a day will often lead to spontaneous drainage of the abscess. Antibiotics may be added if the lesion does not resolve after 1–2 days. A broad-spectrum agent including coverage for methicillin-resistant *Staphylococcus aureus* (MRSA) should be selected (trimethoprim–sulfamethoxazole or doxycycline are common choices).

Abscesses over 2 cm in size generally should be incised and drained. This may be accomplished in the office setting, although larger abscesses should be drained in the operating room under general anesthesia to facilitate patient comfort. The area should be prepped, and a local anesthetic should be injected at both the incision site and around the base of the abscess. Usually, the drainage incision should be made in the anterior–posterior axis of the vulva; this maximizes exposure and assists with healing as there will be less tension on the incision. The incision should be large enough to facilitate complete debridement of the abscess. During drainage, an aerobic and anaerobic culture should be obtained. After drainage, the abscess cavity should be irrigated and packed with a saline-soaked gauze. Most commonly, this dressing is changed daily, allowing healing of the abscess cavity by secondary intention. However, for larger abscess cavities, a wound vacuum may be used. Although the data supporting continued antibiotic use after surgical drainage are unclear, most experts recommend continued antibiotics for patients at high risk for failure or recurrence, including:

- Diabetes
- Abscess size >5 cm
- Infection extending into the abdominal wall/extensive cellulitis
- High likelihood of MRSA infection [7]

Necrotizing Fasciitis

Although rare, necrotizing fasciitis can result from vulvar infections. Diabetic patients are at particular risk [5]. As with other anatomic regions, symptoms will often include fever, perceived pain out of proportion to physical examination findings, and possible hemodynamic instability.

Vulvar necrotizing fasciitis represents a surgical emergency. The patient's clinical status should be optimized with intravenous fluids and/or vasopressor support. Central venous access and placement of a urinary catheter to monitor urine output are also indicated. Blood cultures should be obtained and broad-spectrum antimicrobial therapy initiated. Informed consent for surgical debridement should be obtained, ensuring to review both the potential need for extensive debridement as well as the prolonged postoperative course of wound healing.

In the OR, the patient should be placed in the lithotomy position to facilitate exposure. As the area of necrosis may extend beyond what was initially expected, the surgeon should be prepared to debride extensively until normal, healthy, bleeding tissue is encountered. Given the anatomic considerations of the vulvar fascia mentioned previously, necrotizing fasciitis of the vulva may extend to the lower abdomen, requiring extensive vulvar and abdominal debridement (Fig. 28.3).

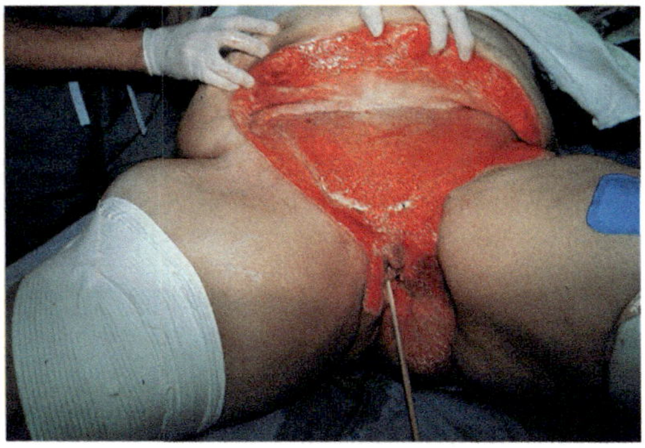

Fig. 28.3 Wide surgical excision of a diabetic patient with necrotizing fasciitis of the left vulva; photograph taken on approximately hospital day 28, when closure was performed. (*Reproduced with permission from Sweet RL, Gibbs RS. Atlas of Infectious Diseases of the Female Genital Tract. Philadelphia: Lippincott Williams & Wilkins, 2005. Copyright ©2005 Lippincott Williams & Wilkins*)

Postoperative care is similar to other cases of necrotizing fasciitis, focused on repeated debridement (if needed), antibiotic administration, pan management, and wound care. A variety of antimicrobial dressings may be employed (dilute Dakin's solution, silver-impregnated dressings) and negative pressure wound therapies may also be utilized—to either facilitate granulation tissue formation in anticipation of future skin grafts or as a mechanism for final wound closure. Although the anatomy of the vulva may present challenges in securing a reliable seal, the use of various fillers and adhesive agents will usually allow for the successful use of this technology.

Cesarean Delivery

Cesarean delivery is the most common surgical procedure performed in the United States, representing approximately 1.3 million cases annually [8]. Roughly one-third of all deliveries are currently performed via cesarean [8]. Although there are a number of acceptable indications (Table 28.1), the most common include repeat cesarean delivery, arrest of dilation or descent, and nonreassuring fetal status during labor.

Table 28.1 Indications for cesarean delivery

Indications for planned cesarean delivery:
• Elective cesarean after prior cesarean delivery
• Prior classical cesarean incision
• Prior full-thickness myomectomy
• Fetal malpresentation
• Placenta previa or abnormal placentation
• Obstructive genital tract mass (e.g., cervical cancer)
• Significant birth trauma in a prior vaginal delivery
• Fetal macrosomia
Indications for unplanned cesarean delivery:
• Arrest of cervical dilation
• Arrest of fetal descent
• Nonreassuring fetal status/abnormal fetal heart rate
• Failed operative vaginal delivery

Preoperative Preparation

As with any surgical procedure, informed consent should be obtained. The major risks of cesarean delivery include bleeding, postoperative pain, infection (either endometritis or wound infection), damage to other abdominal organs such as the bladder or intestines, and the potential need for future cesarean deliveries. As cesarean deliveries are often pursued when a safe vaginal delivery cannot be accomplished, these risks are seen as acceptable in the majority of cases.

As cesarean delivery is associated with an increased risk of infection compared to vaginal delivery, antibiotic prophylaxis is indicated. Most commonly, cefazolin 2 g IV as a single dose is utilized, with consideration of 3 g in patients with a weight >120 kg. For patients in labor or with ruptured membranes, the addition of azithromycin 500 mg IV has been shown to decrease infectious morbidity and should be considered standard of care [9]. For penicillin-allergic patients, a combination of gentamycin and clindamycin may be used.

Procedure/Surgical Anatomy

Cesarean deliveries are most commonly performed through a low transverse Pfannenstiel incision, although a vertical incision or a transverse muscle-splitting incision such as the Maylard may be used in certain circumstances. The Pfannenstiel incision allows for improved cosmesis, lower levels of postoperative pain, and a decreased incidence of incisional hernias compared with vertical incisions [10]. At the level of the Pfannenstiel incision, the abdominal wall fascia lies completely anterior to the rectus muscles. Typically, the fascia will be incised transversely and dissected from the underlying rectus muscles, exposing the peritoneum in the midline. This peritoneum may then be entered either bluntly or sharply at the surgeon's discretion. The peritoneal incision should be extended, with attention paid to the inferior margin and the location of the bladder.

Once the peritoneal cavity is entered, retractors are placed to expose the lower uterine segment and retract the bladder inferiorly. Ideally, the uterine incision should be placed transversely across the lower uterine segment, typically ~1 cm above the vesicouterine peritoneum. Under most circumstances, dissecting the bladder inferiorly is not required. However, adhesions from a prior cesarean delivery may result in cephalad scarring of the bladder to the lower uterine segment—in this case, the vesicouterine peritoneum should be incised and the bladder dissected inferiorly to allow access to the lower uterine segment. The low transverse incision typically provides enough space for atraumatic delivery of the fetus and also has several advantages, including limiting blood loss, allowing easy reapproximation, and decreasing the risk of uterine rupture in subsequent pregnancies [11]. A vertical or "classical" incision extending cephalad into the upper muscular portion of the uterus may be needed under certain circumstances including:

- A underdeveloped, narrow lower uterine segment (often seen in severely preterm deliveries)
- A densely adherent bladder
- Lower uterine segment pathology (e.g., uterine fibroid) preventing access to the lower uterine segment
- When significant manipulation is anticipated for delivery, including extreme macrosomia or fetal malpresentation
- Postmortem delivery

Classical incisions can lead to heavier bleeding from the myometrium as well as an increased risk of extension of the incision into the bladder or cervix. These incisions also carry a higher risk of uterine rupture in subsequent pregnancies. Given these reasons, the vast majority of cesareans utilize a low transverse incision.

Once the uterine cavity is entered, the incision can be extended bluntly in a cephalad/caudad direction (the transverse nature of the uterine muscle fibers will result in the incision naturally extending transversely instead of vertically). For a classical incision, bandage scissors will be required to sharply extend the incision vertically into the muscular upper segment. Once the incision is extended, the fetal vertex can be delivered by flexing the fetal head, bringing it to the level of the hysterotomy and applying fundal pressure. After the fetus is delivered and the umbilical cord is clamped, the uterus should be massaged to allow spontaneous delivery of the placenta.

The uterus may be exteriorized at this point to facilitate exposure. The uterine incision may be closed in a single or double layer; either is considered acceptable. Single-layer closures are associated with a lower operative time and less blood loss; double-layer closures are believed to decrease the risk of a subsequent uterine rupture, but overall the evidence is unclear [11]. Classical incisions will always require more than one layer to approximate the thicker upper uterus and ensure hemostasis. A 0 or No. 1 synthetic delayed absorbable suture such as polyglactin or polyglecaprone is a common choice. After replacing the uterus into the abdominal cavity, the remainder of the abdominal wall closure (peritoneum, fascia, subcutaneous space, and skin) may be closed via standard closure techniques. If the subcutaneous depth is >2 cm, data clearly support closure to minimize postoperative wound complications [12].

Management of Postpartum Hemorrhage

One of the most likely complications of cesarean delivery is postpartum hemorrhage. Given the uterine artery blood flow of ~500–600 cc/min at term, the risk of massive hemorrhage is substantial. Postdelivery hemostasis is primarily achieved by myometrial contraction, which compresses the blood vessels previously supplying the placental bed. Uterine atony, or a suboptimal contraction of the uterine myometrium, represents the most common cause of postpartum hemorrhage.

When brisk bleeding due to uterine atony is encountered, the problem may be approached medically or surgically. Nonsurgical approaches are usually attempted initially, including the following interventions aimed at increasing uterine tone:

- Brisk manual massage of the uterine fundus
- IV oxytocin infusion (typically 40 units/1 L normal saline infused at a rate of up to 500 cc/h)
- IM methylergonovine (0.2 mg; contraindicated in patients with hypertension); may be repeated every 2–4 h
- IM carboprost tromethamine (250 mcg; contraindicated in patients with asthma); may be repeated every 15–90 min
- Misoprostol (400 μg sublingual or 800 μg rectal)

If the above measures do not resolve the atony, the antifibrinolytic tranexamic acid (1 g IV over 20 min) may be administered.

Should medical therapy not resolve the hemorrhage, ligation of the uterine arteries may reduce bleeding by decreasing perfusion pressure to the uterus. Knowledge of pelvic anatomy is critical as the ureter lies just lateral to the uterine arteries. Typically, a 0-polyglycolic acid suture on a CT-1 needle will be passed through the lateral lower uterine segment as close to cervix as possible and then passed through the broad ligament lateral to the uterine arteries. The sutures can be placed and tied bilaterally, if needed.

References

1. Rock JA, et al. Te Linde's operative gynecology. Philadelphia: Lippincott Williams & Wilkins; 2015.
2. Nezhat CH, Nezhat F, Brill AI, Nezhat C. Normal variations of abdominal and pelvic anatomy evaluated at laparoscopy. Obstet Gynecol. 1999;94(2):238–42.

3. Adeyemi-Fowode O, McCracken KA, Todd NJ. Adnexal torsion. J Pediatr Adolesc Gynecol. 2018;31(4):333–8.
4. Dasgupta R, Renaud E, Goldin AB, et al. Ovarian torsion in pediatric and adolescent patients: a systematic review. J Pediatr Surg. 2018;53(7):1387–91.
5. Kilpatrick CC, Alagkiozidis I, Orejuela FJ, Chohan L, Hollier LM. Factors complicating surgical management of the vulvar abscess. J Reprod Med. 2010;55(3–4):139.
6. Corton MM, DeLancey JL. Surgical anatomy of the female pelvis. In: Handa VL, Van Le L, editors. Te Linde's operative gynecology. 12th ed. Philadelphia: Lippincott Williams & Wilkins; 2020. p. 3–42.
7. Liu C, et al. Clinical practice guidelines by the infectious diseases society of America for the treatment of methicillin-resistant Staphylococcus aureus infections in adults and children. Clin Infect Dis. 2011;52(3):e18. Epub 2011 Jan 4.
8. Hamilton BE, Martin JA, Osterman MJ. Births: Preliminary Data for 2015. Natl Vital Stat Rep. 2016;65(3):1–15. PMID: 27309256.
9. Tita AT, Szychowski JM, Boggess K, et al. Adjunctive azithromycin prophylaxis for cesarean delivery. N Engl J Med. 2016;375(13):1231–41.
10. Dahlke JD, Mendez-Figueroa H, Rouse DJ, Berghella V, Baxter JK, Chauhan SP. Evidence-based surgery for cesarean delivery: an updated systemic review. Am J Obstet Gynecol. 2013;209(4):294–306. Epub 2013 Mar 1.
11. Di Spiezio SA, Saccone G, McCurdy R, Bujold E, Bifulco G, Berghella V. Risk of cesarean scar defect following single- vs double-layer uterine closure: systematic review and meta-analysis of randomized controlled trials. Ultrasound Obstet Gynecol. 2017;50(5):578. Epub 2017 Oct 9.
12. Chelmow D, Rodriguez EJ, Sabatini MM. Suture closure of subcutaneous fat and wound disruption after cesarean delivery: a meta-analysis. Obstet Gynecol. 2004;103(5 Pt 1):974–80.

Ruptured Abdominal Aortic Aneurysm

29

Anna N. Romagnoli and Joseph J. DuBose

Case Report

You are called to see a patient in the emergency room presenting with abdominal pain and hypertension. The patient is a 61-year-old male with a history of hypertension and an abdominal aortic aneurysm for which he was being followed by vascular surgery. His last ultrasound measurement of the aneurysm was 3.8 cm in maximal diameter 2 years prior, and he has neglected to follow up with his vascular surgeon since. He has no surgical history. He complains of tearing low back and abdominal pain and is diaphoretic with a blood pressure of 88/45. On examination, he has a palpable pulsatile mass in the infraumbilical region that is tender, but does not have frank peritonitis. He responds to fluid resuscitation, with an increase in blood pressure to 95/52, and receives a subsequent contrast-enhanced CT examination demonstrating contained rupture of a 5.2 cm infrarenal abdominal aortic aneurysm.

Introduction

While the prevalence of abdominal aortic aneurysm has been declining in the past decades [1], the progression of the disease process to rupture continues to be associated with a greater than 80% mortality rate in all comers and a >40% mortality rate in those who survive to operation [2]. Aortic aneurysms are more common in men than in women. They have the highest incidence in the ninth decade of life. Age and genetic predisposition, including connective tissue disorders, are nonmodifiable risk factors associated with their development. Modifiable risk factors include atherosclerotic disease, hypertension, hypercholesterolemia, inflammation, and smoking [1]. The relationship between cigarette smoking, matrix metalloproteinases, and aneurysmal degeneration has been well described and is implicated in both initial development and expansion of abdominal aortic aneurysms [3].

Risk of aneurysm rupture is directly correlated to aneurysmal diameter. As explained by the law of Laplace, as the radius of the aneurysm sac increases, the wall tension increases, thereby increasing the risk of rupture [4]. Estimated annual risk of rupture for abdominal aortic aneurysms increases dramatically as diameter increases (Table 29.1) [5], with rupture risk sur-

A. N. Romagnoli
Division of Vascular and Endovascular Surgery, Massachusetts General Hospital, Boston, MA, USA
e-mail: aromagnoli@mgh.harvard.edu

J. J. DuBose (✉)
Division of Trauma and Critical Care, R Adams Cowley Shock Trauma Center, University of Maryland Medical Center, Baltimore, MD, USA
e-mail: joseph.dubose@umm.edu

M. D. Zielinski, O. Guillamondegui (eds.), *The Acute Management of Surgical Disease*,
https://doi.org/10.1007/978-3-031-07881-1_29

Table 29.1 Annual rupture risk of abdominal aortic aneurysms (AAA) based on diameter [5]

AAA diameter (cm)	Annual risk of rupture (%)
<4	0
4–5	0.5–5
5–6	3–15
6–7	10–20
7–8	20–40
>8	30–50

passing general operative risk of elective repair at >5 cm. Elective repair in otherwise healthy patients is recommended with fusiform aneurysms with diameter >5.4 cm and for all saccular aneurysms [6].

In the setting of elective aortic aneurysm repair, endovascular aneurysm repair (EVAR) has been demonstrated to be associated with a marked reduction in 30-day mortality in comparison with open repair [7–9]; however, there is conflicting data in the literature regarding its benefit in ruptured abdominal aortic aneurysms. Three notable multicenter randomized controlled trials have evaluated the topic. The Amsterdam Acute Aneurysm Trial (n = 116) showed no significant difference in death/severe complications; however, it did demonstrate decreased blood product transfusion, ICU admission, and ventilator dependence [10]. The Endovasculaire ou Chirurgie dans les Aneurysmes aorto-iliaques Rompus (ECAR) trial (n = 107) failed to show a mortality benefit at 30 days or 1 year; however, ruptured endovascular aneurysm repair (REVAR) was associated with a lower complication rate [11]. The largest randomized controlled trial on the topic to date is the Immediate Management of Patients with Rupture: Open versus Endovascular Repair (IMPROVE) trial (n = 623). No difference in 30-day mortality between the two repair modalities was detected in all comers; however, a subgroup analysis did demonstrate a survival benefit in women. Additionally, patients undergoing REVAR were more likely to be discharged home [12]. While there was no difference in mortality at 1 year [13], the 3-year follow-up analysis of the IMPROVE study was notable for a survival advantage, improved quality of life, and reduced cost in the REVAR group [14].

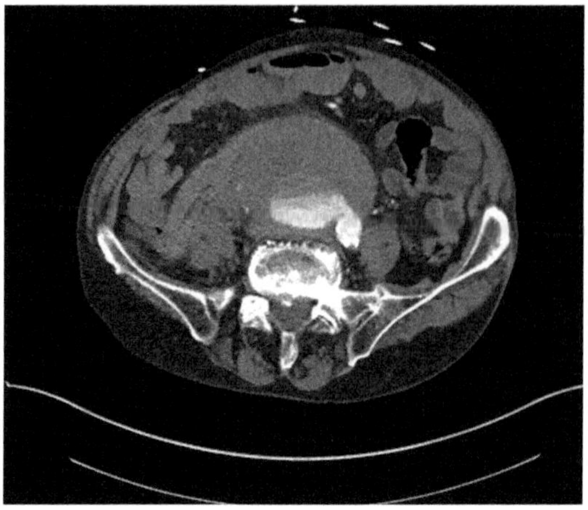

Fig. 29.1 Computed tomographic angiography (CTA) demonstrating ruptured abdominal aortic aneurysm

Diagnosis

Hypotension and abdominal pain in a patient with a known abdominal aortic aneurysm should be considered a rupture until proven otherwise. However, patients with a contained or early rupture may have a more subtle presentation including abdominal or back pain with other signs of systemic illness. A palpable abdominal mass may be appreciated on examination, but can be obscured by body habitus. Hypotension on presentation is a worrisome finding, which increases mortality in the setting of aneurysmal rupture. Definitive diagnosis is achieved by computed tomographic angiography (CTA—contrast-enhanced CT), which will both reveal the diagnosis and delineate pertinent anatomy for subsequent treatment (Fig. 29.1).

Initial Management

Large-bore IV access should be rapidly obtained. Laboratory tests include blood typing and cross-matching. While no randomized controlled trials comparing hypotensive to normotensive resuscitation in the setting of ruptured abdominal aortic aneurysm have been performed [15], animal studies suggest that hypotensive resuscitation may be beneficial [16]. Resuscitation to a systolic blood pressure between 70 and 90 mmHg (hypotensive resuscitation) as long as the patient has intact mentation is recommended by the Society of Vascular Surgery (SVS) [6] (Fig. 29.2). Caution should be taken, however, when extrapolating the widely accepted principles of damage control resuscitation in trauma [17, 18] to this patient population. Unlike the trauma population, patients with ruptured abdominal aortic aneurysms are older and likely have concomitant cerebrovascular and cardiovascular disease. The effect of prolonged hypotension in the setting of aortic rupture

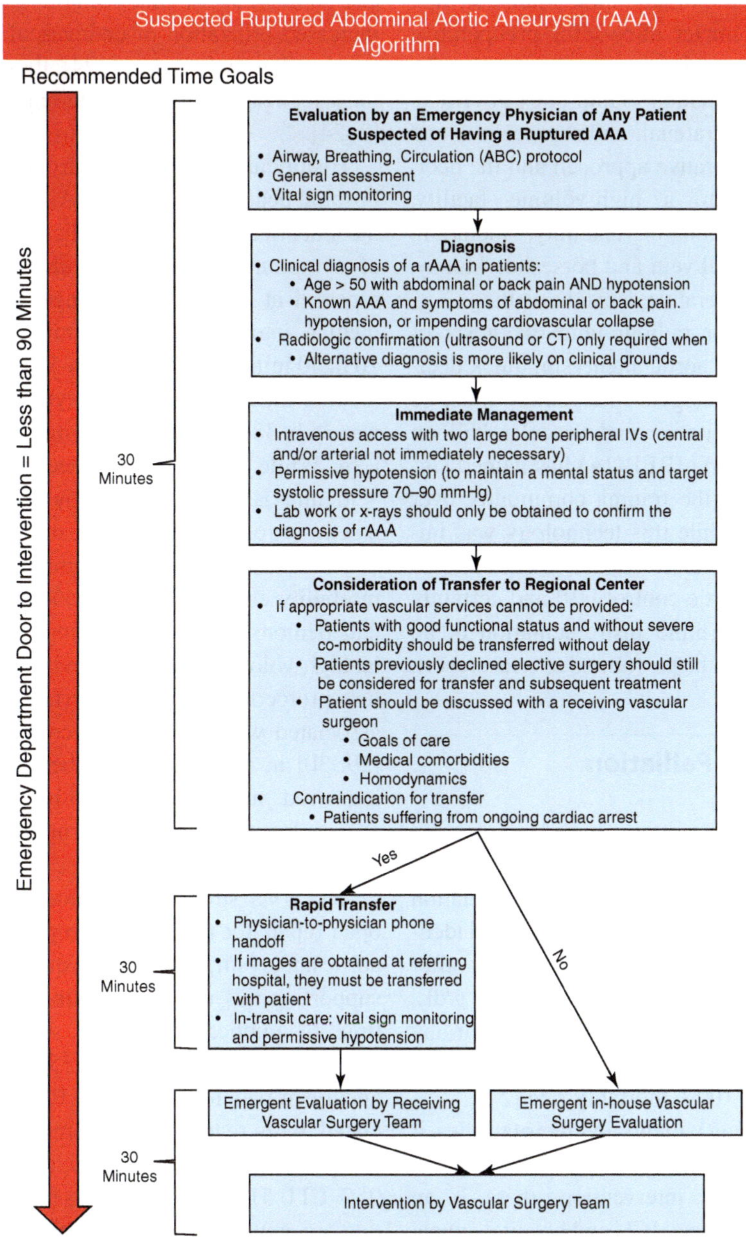

Fig. 29.2 Algorithm for management of suspected rAAA [6]

on cerebral, coronary, and spinal cord perfusion in this patient population has not been well studied.

Every effort should be maintained to obtain a preoperative CTA. This allows for assessment of anatomic suitability for endovascular repair and planning for both endovascular and open surgical repairs. The assessment of aneurysm neck length and angulation, proximal aortic diameter, and access vessel diameter allows for preoperative endograft selection. Prior to open repair, the identification of potential clamp sites is critical (i.e., infrarenal, suprarenal, and supraceliac) and may impact the operative approach and the decision to transfer to a high-volume facility. Additional evaluation of anatomy, including retro-aortic left renal vein and horseshoe kidney, may also inform operative decision making.

Upon clinical or radiographic diagnosis of ruptured abdominal aortic aneurysm, quick decision making and emergent intervention must be undertaken. Resuscitative endovascular balloon occlusion of the aorta (REBOA) has gained significant traction in the trauma community over the past decade. While this technology was initially coopted from endovascular maneuvers to obtain proximal aortic control [19] and certainly can be life-saving, blind instrumentation of an injured aorta should be performed as a last resort.

Intervention vs Palliation

A number of scoring systems have been devised to quantify chances of survival; however, most have not demonstrated consistent correlation with outcome [20]. One simplified scale did identify the following predictors of mortality after open repair: age >76 years, creatinine >2.0 g/dL, pH <7.2, and blood pressure <70 mmHg at any time. When all four are present, open repair is associated with a 100% mortality rate [21].

When counseling patients and their families, it is critical that they understand that if they survive the initial operative intervention, there is an almost certain prolonged ICU and hospital course to follow, which may include tracheostomy, dependence on enteral feeds, temporary or permanent dialysis, or paralysis.

Stabilization and Transfer

Institutions with an established protocol for management of patients with rAAA have demonstrated a reduction in mortality [22, 23], with one study demonstrating a 30-day mortality reduction from 57.8% to 35.3% [23]. Analysis of trends and outcomes in the United States reveals increased utilization of endovascular repair and improved mortality rate [1, 24]; these benefits are most realized in high-volume teaching facilities [2, 24].

Historically, mean time from admission to hospital death from ruptured AAA is 8 h [25]. In the modern era, however, median time from onset of symptoms to hospital admission has been reported at 2 h, 30 min (range 44 min–36 h), median interval between admission and death 10 h, 40 min (range 1 h–143 h 55 min), while the median time from onset of symptoms to death was 16 h, 38 min (range 2 h 6 min–146 h 50 min) [26]. While a goal door-to-intervention time of ≤90 min is recommended by the SVS [6], a recent retrospective review suggests that this benchmark does not have significant impact on morbidity and mortality [27]. Although there is data demonstrating lower perioperative mortality in high-volume institutions with in-place "rupture protocols" [23, 28], interfacility transfer is associated with an overall increase in mortality [29, 30] in some studies. Other studies suggest improved mortality rate with a regionalized approach to management of ruptured abdominal aortic aneurysms [23, 31].

The SVS strongly recommends EVAR over open repair for treatment of ruptured abdominal aortic aneurysm; however, the quality of evidence supporting this recommendation was low at the time of publication [6]. A subsequent meta-analysis which included 267,259 ruptured aortic aneurysm patients found that REVAR was associated with reduced perioperative mortality in comparison to open surgical repair (OR 0.54, 95% CI 0.51–0.57, $p < 0.001$) [32]. Many facilities are not equipped with personnel or equipment to perform EVAR at all or in the setting of a ruptured AAA. If preoperative CTA demonstrates a pararenal or paravisceral aneurysm, unless the operating surgeon is familiar with supraceliac clamping and visceral reconstruction, expeditious transfer is necessary. Because of the potential mortality benefit associated with transfer to high-volume facilities, the probable mortality and known morbidity benefit of REVAR, as well as the often relatively long window between symptom onset and mortality, the risks and benefits of transfer should be considered in all patients presenting with rAAA.

Endotracheal intubation should be undertaken thoughtfully and with caution. Resuscitation should be initiated prior to intubation, particularly for those patients presenting with significant hypotension. It is prudent to prepare for decompensation at the time of intubation by prepping the abdomen for immediate surgical entry or by being prepared to counter the anticipated loss of vasomotor tone with the utilization of an endovascular balloon. Via femoral access with the patient yet awake, the balloon can be positioned under fluoroscopic guidance above the aneurysmal rupture in amenable patients.

For open repair, the use of a suction-based cell saver collection system is prudent. Planning in this fashion will permit autotransfusion of shed blood within the abdominal cavity. Enteric contamination is uncommon in simple ruptured abdominal aneurysms, affording the utilization of this blood in subsequent resuscitation.

Operative Management

Regardless of operative management strategies, proximal aortic control must be obtained expeditiously. Indications for aortic occlusion balloon placement include cardiac arrest, hemodynamic instability, and anatomic limitations preventing expeditious repair [23, 33]. While endovascular balloon occlusion of the aorta has been shown to reduce intraoperative mortality, it has not been shown to improve other outcomes [34]. Similarly, open aortic cross-clamping has traditionally been associated with improved hemorrhage control and remains a critical maneuver of open repair—but has not been well studied.

In the setting of elective open and endovascular aneurysm repair, systemic anticoagulation is routinely administered. When managing a ruptured AAA, the decision to anticoagulate should be made on a case-by-case basis based on the patient's intrinsic coagulation status, as determined by traditional laboratories, thromboelastography, or clinical evidence of coagulopathy.

Endovascular Repair

For elective EVAR, general exclusion criteria include aortic neck diameter ≤32 mm, neck length ≤15 mm, circumferential calcifications, thrombus >40%, >60° aortic neck angulation, and access vessel diameter <6.5 mm [23]. There are now a number of devices on the market which can safely be used with fewer anatomic exclusions. Comprehensive review of available devices and their limitations, however, is beyond the scope of this chapter. In the setting of a ruptured aneurysm, it is not uncommon for the operating vascular surgeon to perform off-IFU REVAR. However, off-IFU REVAR has been reported at the abstract level to be associated with a higher mortality rate than on-IFU REVAR. When compared to OSR patients with supraceliac clamp, off-IFU REVAR was associated with improved mortality rate. This was not observed when off-IFU REVAR was compared with OSR with infrarenal or suprarenal clamps [35].

Open Surgical Repair

Unless the operating surgeon routinely performs aortic surgery via a thoracoabdominal incision in the lateral position, a transperitoneal supine approach is recommended (Fig. 29.3). If an infrarenal or immediately suprarenal clamp site is feasible, after performing a generous midline laparotomy the transverse colon should be reflected superiorly and the small bowel packed off to the right. The ligament of Treitz is sharply taken down, allowing for the entirety of the small bowel to be packed into the right side of the abdo-

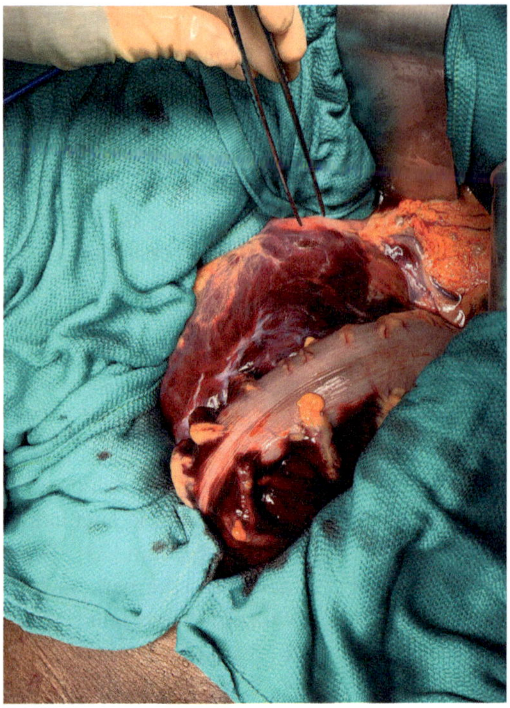

Fig. 29.3 Ruptured abdominal aortic aneurysm (rAAA) at operation, exposed via peritoneal approach

men. The aneurysm neck should be identified by palpation, and the peritoneum is sharply divided. The dissection should be carried out posteriorly on both sides of the aorta until the vertebral bodies are palpable. Circumferential mobilization of the aorta is not necessary and can result in the avulsion of hidden lumbar arteries. A large aortic clamp should be placed with the handle directed cephalad.

For heavily calcified aortas, an infrarenal or immediately suprarenal clamp may not coapt the aortic walls adequately enough to provide hemostasis. In this setting, supraceliac aortic control should be attempted, as this region of the aorta is generally spared from calcific disease. After midline laparotomy and division of the falciform ligament, the left lobe of the liver is retracted to the patient's right, allowing the gastrohepatic ligament is being divided. The stomach and distal esophagus are retracted to the left. To clamp the aorta at this location, the right crus of the diaphragm must be divided; a clamp can then be passed taking care to not injure posterior branches of the vagus nerve. If suprarenal or supraceliac control is initially obtained, it is critical to move the clamp to an infrarenal location as soon as is feasible to limit warm ischemia time to the viscera and kidneys.

After proximal control has been obtained, attention should be turned to obtaining distal control. Common iliac arteries should be dissected and clamped. Again, circumferential dissection is unnecessary and may result in iatrogenic injury to the iliac veins which will result in torrential hemorrhage. If the calcium burden of these vessels precludes occlusive clamping, Pruitt occlusion balloons can be passed under direct vision to provide distal control.

After satisfactory clamp application, the aneurysm sac is opened from below the cross-clamp to a centimeter or two above the iliac bifurcation. Unless the rupture involves one of the iliac arteries, bifurcate grafts should be avoided in the emergent setting. The aneurysm sac is tee-d off at its cephalad and caudad extents. Mural thrombus and other debris are then scooped out of the sac to permit clear visualization of any bleeding lumbar vessels. These should be suture ligated with figure-of-eight 2-0 or 3-0 silk suture; visualization may be aided by placing a self-retaining retractor within the aneurysm sac. An appropriately sized Dacron graft is brought onto the field; the proximal anastomosis is performed using 3-0 or 4-0 polypropylene suture. The inlay technique described by Creech in 1966 is still widely employed today, whereby the proximal aspect of the posterior wall of the aneurysm sac is incorporated into the suture line [36]. Once the proximal anastomosis is complete, the graft is clamped distally, and the proximal suture line is checked for hemostasis. Repair stitches are placed as needed. The graft is then trimmed to size, and the distal anastomosis is then performed in similar fashion.

Diminished back bleeding from the iliac arteries should prompt the operating surgeon to consider the potential for embolization of intra-aortic debris or formation of thrombus during clamping. Fogarty embolectomy should be performed until all clot or debris is removed and robust back bleeding occurs, followed by an additional pass of the balloon catheter.

The graft should be forward and back flsuhed with any trapped air evacuated prior to completing the distal anastomosis. Before perfusion is restored to the lower extremities, the anesthesia team must be notified, as the washout of ischemic byproducts from aortic cross-clamping can have significant effects on hemodynamics, up to and including cardiac arrest.

Consideration should be given to reimplanting the inferior mesenteric artery (IMA) into the distal aortic graft, utilizing a carrel patch. If robust back bleeding is observed from the orifice of the IMA indicating adequate collateral flow through the arc of Riolan and superior rectal arteries, the IMA can be ligated. However, in the setting of postoperative hypotension and vasopressor use, the left colon may be at risk for ischemia in spite of intraoperative observation of intact collateral flow.

Once hemostasis has again been verified, the aneurysm sac is closed using running 2-0 vicryl suture. The aorta should then be reperitonealized or covered with omentum to mitigate the risk of future development of an aortoenteric fistula.

Consideration should be given to open abdominal management/damage control laparotomy in the same fashion as applied to traumatic operations. As such, hypothermia, acidosis, or the presence of clinical or laboratory documented coagulopathy should be considered prudent markers for the utility of temporary damage control laparotomy with or without a suction assisted dressing. Return to the operating room for re-exploration and closure should then occur only after this "deadly triad" has been corrected through thoughtful resuscitation.

Prior to leaving the operating room, the distal lower extremities should be assessed for adequate blood flow via pulse or hand-held Doppler examination. If there is a discrepancy in, distal embolization of thrombus or debris should be presumed. Open cutdown and fogarty embolectomy should then be performed. If there was a prolonged interruption of flow to the lower extremities, or clinical examination is concerning for compartment syndrome, compartment pressures should be checked, or fasciotomies empirically performed.

Postoperative Complications

If the patient survives the operation, they can expect to move on to a prolonged critical care phase. Open surgical repair following ruptured AAA is associated with a longer ICU length of stay and a higher rate of major complications (respiratory, cardiac, cerebrovascular, renal failure, lower limb ischemia) [37].

Abdominal Compartment Syndrome

Abdominal compartment syndrome represents the extreme of the intra-abdominal hypertension spectrum and occurs when sustained elevations in the intra-abdominal pressure (IAP) result in new end-organ dysfunction. IAP should be measured via the bladder after a maximal instillation of 25 mL sterile saline, at end expiration, with muscles relaxed and transducer at the mid-axillary line. In critically ill adults, normal IAP is 5–7 mmHg. Intra-abdominal hypertension is defined by a sustained or repeated pathological elevation in IAP $\geq$12 mmHg. Abdominal compartment syndrome (ACS) is defined as a sustained IAP >20 mmHg, with or without abdominal perfusion pressure <60 mmHg (mean arterial pressure—IAP), accompanied with new organ dysfunction or failure [38].

ACS occurs following ruptured abdominal aortic aneurysm repair in 4–34% of patients [39–43], mortality rate of those with ACS ranges from 30% to 70% [39, 41, 43]. A recent review of the Swedish Vascular Registry demonstrated high mortality following abdominal aortic aneurysm repair. Three pathophysiological findings were identified at decompressive laparotomy: bowel ischemia (21%), bleeding (29%), and edema (50%). Poor outcomes were associated with longer suprarenal clamp and greater volume of transfused blood products. On multivariate analysis, however, the only independent predictor for development of abdominal compartment syndrome was age [39]. Duration of IAP $\geq$20 mmHg was an independent predictor for renal replacement therapy. Abdominal compartment syndrome following ruptured abdominal aortic aneurysm repair and abdominal compartment syndrome secondary to bleeding were negative predictors for survival [39]. The standard of care for treatment of ACS is decompressive laparotomy. Timing of decompressive laparotomy after ruptured abdominal aortic aneurysm repair has not been studied; however, extrapolation from the trauma literature suggests that earlier decompression is associated with improved survival [44, 45].

In addition to the abovementioned etiologies for abdominal compartment syndrome, patients who have undergone REVAR are also at risk for continued hemodynamically significant endoleak. Type II endoleaks (persistent perfusion of the aneurysm sac via collateral vessels, most commonly lumbar arteries or the IMA) may result in continued pressurization of the aneurysm sac in spite of excluding its major in-flow and out-flow vessels. This potentially places the patient with a contained rupture at continued risk for free rupture. In the setting of an aneurysm sac that has already ruptured, continued bleeding through the lumbar vessels or the IMA into the peritoneal space may contribute to ongoing hemodynamic instability and development of ACS. This potential risk is reflected in the lower threshold to perform decompressive laparotomy following REVAR in comparison to patients who had undergone open repair for ruptured abdominal aortic aneurysm (median 2.8 vs 30.8 h, $p < 0.001$) [39].

Acute Renal Failure

Acute renal failure (ARF) following ruptured abdominal aortic aneurysm repair is associated with high mortality rates [46–48] and is an independent predictor for in-hospital mortality [49, 50]. The incidence of postoperative ARF in survivors of ruptured abdominal aortic aneurysms is 20–34% [46, 51]. The development of postoperative ARF is multifactorial, with age, pre-existing renal disease, hypotension, contrast administration, and aortic cross-clamping contributing [52]. REVAR eliminates the need for prolonged aortic occlusion and can be done under local anesthetic which mitigates any hypotension associated with induction of general anesthesia and may be the reason it has a lower rate of postoperative ARF (6.9% vs 13.5% $p < 0.001$) [53] and long-term hemodialysis [50].

Colonic Ischemia

Colonic ischemia occurs in 6–44% of survivors of ruptured abdominal aortic aneurysm [10, 12, 54]. The patency of the IMA is likely complicit in development of ischemic colitis; however, treatment or nontreatment of the IMA at time of operation was not associated with development of colonic ischemia. Preoperative shock, greater intraoperative blood loss [54], and high postoperative vasopressor requirement [55] were associated with the development of colonic ischemia. In one small study, most patients with postoperative bowel ischemia had chronically occluded IMAs and therefore would not have been candidates for reimplantation [54]. In the absence of a frankly bloody bowel movement, colonic ischemia can be challenging to diagnose in the perioperative period. Flexible sigmoidoscopy has been demonstrated to be a valuable tool in this setting [55].

Other

Spinal cord infarction is a rare complication (<1%) of ruptured abdominal aortic aneurysm repair and occurs with equal incidence after both open and endovascular intervention [10, 56]. In the modern era, postoperative respiratory failure and myocardial infarction are independent predictor for mortality in survivors of ruptured AAA, but neither has an increased incidence following OSR compared with REVAR [50].

Case Conclusion

The patient was rapidly delivered to the operating room, where he underwent placement of an aortic occlusive balloon in the proximal abdominal aorta to facilitate intubation and open exposure of the aneurysm. The aneurysm then underwent repair utilizing a Dacron interposition graft to repair his infrarenal aorta. The graft was covered with retroperitoneum, and the abdomen was left open in a damage control fashion. The next day, the patient underwent re-exploration and abdominal closure. After 2 days in the intensive care unit and 6 days of hospitalization, he was discharged to home.

References

1. Mureebe L, Egorova N, Giacovelli JK, Gelijns A, Kent KC, McKinsey JF. National trends in the repair of ruptured abdominal aortic aneurysms. J Vasc Surg. 2008;48(5):1101–7.
2. Karthikesalingam A, Holt PJ, Vidal-Diez A, Ozdemir BA, Poloniecki JD, Hinchliffe RJ, et al. Mortality from ruptured abdominal aortic aneurysms: clinical lessons from a comparison of outcomes in England and the USA. Lancet. 2014;383(9921):963–9.
3. Li Z-Z, Dai Q-Y. Pathogenesis of abdominal aortic aneurysms: role of nicotine and nicotinic acetylcholine receptors. Mediat Inflamm. 2012;2012:103120.
4. Hall AJ, Busse EF, McCarville DJ, Burgess JJ. Aortic wall tension as a predictive factor for abdominal aortic aneurysm rupture: improving the selection of patients for abdominal aortic aneurysm repair. Ann Vasc Surg. 2000;14(2):152–7.
5. Brewster DC, Cronenwett JL, Hallett JW Jr, Johnston KW, Krupski WC, Matsumura JS. Guidelines for the treatment of abdominal aortic aneurysms. Report of a subcommittee of the Joint Council of the American Association for Vascular Surgery and Society for Vascular Surgery. J Vasc Surg. 2003;37(5):1106–17.
6. Chaikof EL, Dalman RL, Eskandari MK, Jackson BM, Lee WA, Mansour MA, et al. The Society for Vascular Surgery practice guidelines on the care of patients with an abdominal aortic aneurysm. J Vasc Surg. 2018;67(1):2–77.e2.
7. Schermerhorn ML, O'Malley AJ, Jhaveri A, Cotterill P, Pomposelli F, Landon BE. Endovascular vs. open repair of abdominal aortic aneurysms in the Medicare population. N Engl J Med. 2008;358(5):464–74.
8. Greenhalgh RM, Brown LC, Kwong GP, Powell JT, Thompson SG, EVAR Trial Participants. Comparison of endovascular aneurysm repair with open repair in patients with abdominal aortic aneurysm (EVAR trial 1), 30-day operative mortality results: randomised controlled trial. Lancet. 2004;364(9437):843–8.
9. Prinssen M, Verhoeven EL, Buth J, Cuypers PW, van Sambeek MR, Balm R, et al. A randomized trial comparing conventional and endovascular repair of abdominal aortic aneurysms. N Engl J Med. 2004;351(16):1607–18.
10. Reimerink JJ, Hoornweg LL, Vahl AC, Wisselink W, van den Broek TA, Legemate DA, et al. Endovascular repair versus open repair of ruptured abdominal aortic aneurysms: a multicenter randomized controlled trial. Ann Surg. 2013;258(2):248–56.
11. Desgranges P, Kobeiter H, Katsahian S, Bouffi M, Gouny P, Favre JP, et al. Editor's choice—ECAR (Endovasculaire ou Chirurgie dans les Anévrysmes aorto-iliaques Rompus): a French randomized controlled trial of endovascular versus open surgical repair of ruptured aorto-iliac aneurysms. Eur J Vasc Endovasc Surg. 2015;50(3):303–10.
12. Powell JT, Sweeting MJ, Thompson MM, Ashleigh R, Bell R, Gomes M, et al. Endovascular or open repair strategy for ruptured abdominal aortic aneurysm: 30 day outcomes from IMPROVE randomised trial. BMJ. 2014;348:f7661.
13. IMPROVE Trial Investigators. Endovascular strategy or open repair for ruptured abdominal aortic aneurysm: one-year outcomes from the IMPROVE randomized trial. Eur Heart J. 2015;36(31):2061–9.
14. IMPROVE Trial Investigators. Comparative clinical effectiveness and cost effectiveness of endovascular strategy v open repair for ruptured abdominal aortic aneurysm: three year results of the IMPROVE randomised trial. BMJ. 2017;359:j4859.
15. Moreno DH, Cacione DG, Baptista-Silva JC. Controlled hypotension versus normotensive resuscitation strategy for people with ruptured abdominal aortic aneurysm. Cochrane Database Syst Rev. 2018;6(6):CD011664.
16. Roberts K, Revell M, Youssef H, Bradbury AW, Adam DJ. Hypotensive resuscitation in patients with ruptured abdominal aortic aneurysm. Eur J Vasc Endovasc Surg. 2006;31(4):339–44.
17. Cannon JW, Khan MA, Raja AS, Cohen MJ, Como JJ, Cotton BA, et al. Damage control resuscitation in patients with severe traumatic hemorrhage: a practice management guideline from the Eastern Association for the Surgery of Trauma. J Trauma Acute Care Surg. 2017;82(3):605–17.
18. Roberts DJ, Ball CG, Feliciano DV, Moore EE, Ivatury RR, Lucas CE, et al. History of the innovation of damage control for management of trauma patients: 1902-2016. Ann Surg. 2017;265(5):1034–44.
19. Romagnoli A, Brenner M. Principles of REBOA. In: Horer T, DuBose J, Rasmussen T, White J, editors. Endovascular resuscitation and trauma management, Hot topics in acute care surgery and trauma. Cham: Springer; 2020.
20. Tambyraja AL, Murie JA, Chalmers RT. Prediction of outcome after abdominal aortic aneurysm rupture. J Vasc Surg. 2008;47(1):222–30.
21. Garland BT, Danaher PJ, Desikan S, Tran NT, Quiroga E, Singh N, et al. Preoperative risk score for the prediction of mortality after repair of ruptured abdominal aortic aneurysms. J Vasc Surg. 2018;68(4):991–7.

22. Mehta M, Taggert J, Darling RC 3rd, Chang BB, Kreienberg PB, Paty PS, et al. Establishing a protocol for endovascular treatment of ruptured abdominal aortic aneurysms: outcomes of a prospective analysis. J Vasc Surg. 2006;44(1):1–8; discussion 8.
23. Starnes BW, Quiroga E, Hutter C, Tran NT, Hatsukami T, Meissner M, et al. Management of ruptured abdominal aortic aneurysm in the endovascular era. J Vasc Surg. 2010;51(1):9–17; discussion 17–8.
24. Lesperance K, Andersen C, Singh N, Starnes B, Martin MJ. Expanding use of emergency endovascular repair for ruptured abdominal aortic aneurysms: disparities in outcomes from a nationwide perspective. J Vasc Surg. 2008;47(6):1165–70; discussion 70–1.
25. Walker EM, Hopkinson BR, Makin GS. Unoperated abdominal aortic aneurysm: presentation and natural history. Ann R Coll Surg Engl. 1983;65(5):311–3.
26. Lloyd GM, Bown MJ, Norwood MG, Deb R, Fishwick G, Bell PR, et al. Feasibility of preoperative computer tomography in patients with ruptured abdominal aortic aneurysm: a time-to-death study in patients without operation. J Vasc Surg. 2004;39(4):788–91.
27. Davis FM, Sutzko DC, Smith ME, Gallagher K, Henke PK, Osborne N. Variation in hospital door-to-intervention time for ruptured AAAs and its association with outcomes. Ann Vasc Surg. 2020;62:83–91.
28. Moore R, Nutley M, Cina CS, Motamedi M, Faris P, Abuznadah W. Improved survival after introduction of an emergency endovascular therapy protocol for ruptured abdominal aortic aneurysms. J Vasc Surg. 2007;45(3):443–50.
29. Mell MW, Wang NE, Morrison DE, Hernandez-Boussard T. Interfacility transfer and mortality for patients with ruptured abdominal aortic aneurysm. J Vasc Surg. 2014;60(3):553–7.
30. Brattheim BJ, Eikemo TA, Altreuther M, Landmark AD, Faxvaag A. Regional disparities in incidence, handling and outcomes of patients with symptomatic and ruptured abdominal aortic aneurysms in Norway. Eur J Vasc Endovasc Surg. 2012;44(3):267–72.
31. van Beek SC, Reimerink JJ, Vahl AC, Wisselink W, Reekers JA, van Geloven N, et al. Effect of regional cooperation on outcomes from ruptured abdominal aortic aneurysm. Br J Surg. 2014;101(7):794–801.
32. Kontopodis N, Galanakis N, Antoniou SA, Tsetis D, Ioannou CV, Veith FJ, et al. Meta-analysis and meta-regression analysis of outcomes of endovascular and open repair for ruptured abdominal aortic aneurysm. Eur J Vasc Endovasc Surg. 2020;59(3):399–410.
33. Malina M, Holst J. Balloon control for ruptured AAAs: when and when not to use? J Cardiovasc Surg (Torino). 2014;55(2):161–7.
34. Raux M, Marzelle J, Kobeiter H, Dhonneur G, Allaire E, Cochennec F, et al. Endovascular balloon occlusion is associated with reduced intraoperative mortality of unstable patients with ruptured abdominal aortic aneurysm but fails to improve other outcomes. J Vasc Surg. 2015;61(2):304–8.
35. Zarkowsky DS, Ramirez JL, Holscher CM, Goodney PP, Malas MB, Iannuzzi JC, et al. Ruptured AAA patients treated with EVAR off-IFU demonstrate lower in-hospital survival than those with on-IFU repair. Ann Vasc Surg. 2020;63:13–4.
36. Creech O Jr. Endo-aneurysmorrhaphy and treatment of aortic aneurysm. Ann Surg. 1966;164(6):935–46.
37. von Meijenfeldt GC, Ultee KH, Eefting D, Hoeks SE, ten Raa S, Rouwet EV, et al. Differences in mortality, risk factors, and complications after open and endovascular repair of ruptured abdominal aortic aneurysms. Eur J Vasc Endovasc Surg. 2014;47(5):479–86.
38. Malbrain ML, Cheatham ML, Kirkpatrick A, Sugrue M, Parr M, De Waele J, et al. Results from the international conference of experts on intra-abdominal hypertension and abdominal compartment syndrome. I. Definitions. Intensive Care Med. 2006;32(11):1722–32.
39. Ersryd S, Djavani Gidlund K, Wanhainen A, Smith L, Björck M. Editor's choice—abdominal compartment syndrome after surgery for abdominal aortic aneurysm: subgroups, risk factors, and outcome. Eur J Vasc Endovasc Surg. 2019;58(5):671–9.
40. De Waele JJ, Kimball E, Malbrain M, Nesbitt I, Cohen J, Kaloiani V, et al. Decompressive laparotomy for abdominal compartment syndrome. Br J Surg. 2016;103(6):709–15.
41. Karkos CD, Menexes GC, Patelis N, Kalogirou TE, Giagtzidis IT, Harkin DW. A systematic review and meta-analysis of abdominal compartment syndrome after endovascular repair of ruptured abdominal aortic aneurysms. J Vasc Surg. 2014;59(3):829–42.
42. Fietsam R Jr, Villalba M, Glover JL, Clark K. Intra-abdominal compartment syndrome as a complication of ruptured abdominal aortic aneurysm repair. Am Surg. 1989;55(6):396–402.
43. Ersryd S, Djavani-Gidlund K, Wanhainen A, Björck M. Editor's choice—abdominal compartment syndrome after surgery for abdominal aortic aneurysm: a Nationwide population based study. Eur J Vasc Endovasc Surg. 2016;52(2):158–65.
44. Balogh Z, McKinley BA, Holcomb JB, Miller CC, Cocanour CS, Kozar RA, et al. Both primary and secondary abdominal compartment syndrome can be predicted early and are harbingers of multiple organ failure. J Trauma. 2003;54(5):848–59; discussion 59–61.
45. Maxwell RA, Fabian TC, Croce MA, Davis KA. Secondary abdominal compartment syndrome: an underappreciated manifestation of severe hemorrhagic shock. J Trauma. 1999;47(6):995–9.
46. Sarac TP, Bannazadeh M, Rowan AF, Bena J, Srivastava S, Eagleton M, et al. Comparative predictors of mortality for endovascular and open repair of ruptured infrarenal abdominal aortic aneurysms. Ann Vasc Surg. 2011;25(4):461–8.
47. Gordon AC, Pryn S, Collin J, Gray DW, Hands L, Garrard C. Outcome in patients who require renal support after surgery for ruptured abdominal aortic aneurysm. Br J Surg. 1994;81(6):836–8.

48. Nasim A, Sayers RD, Thompson MM, Healey PA, Bell PR. Trends in abdominal aortic aneurysms: a 13 year review. Eur J Vasc Endovasc Surg. 1995;9(2):239–43.
49. Antonopoulos CN, Kakisis JD, Andrikopoulos V, Dervisis K, Georgopoulos S, Giannoukas A, et al. Predictors affecting in-hospital mortality of ruptured abdominal aortic aneurysms: a Greek multicenter study. Ann Vasc Surg. 2014;28(6):1384–90.
50. Acher C, Acher CW, Castello Ramirez MC, Wynn M. Operative mortality and morbidity in ruptured abdominal aortic aneurysms in the endovascular age. Ann Vasc Surg. 2020;66:70–6.
51. Giles KA, Hamdan AD, Pomposelli FB, Wyers MC, Dahlberg SE, Schermerhorn ML. Population-based outcomes following endovascular and open repair of ruptured abdominal aortic aneurysms. J Endovasc Ther. 2009;16(5):554–64.
52. Cherr GS, Hansen KJ. Renal complications with aortic surgery. Semin Vasc Surg. 2001;14(4):245–54.
53. Aziz F, Azab A, Schaefer E, Reed AB. Endovascular repair of ruptured abdominal aortic aneurysm is associated with lower incidence of post-operative acute renal failure. Ann Vasc Surg. 2016;35:147–55.
54. Piotrowski JJ, Ripepi AJ, Yuhas JP, Alexander JJ, Brandt CP. Colonic ischemia: the Achilles heel of ruptured aortic aneurysm repair. Am Surg. 1996;62(7):557–60; discussion 60–1.
55. Jalalzadeh H, van Schaik TG, Duin JJ, Indrakusuma R, van Beek SC, Vahl AC, et al. The value of sigmoidoscopy to detect colonic ischaemia after ruptured abdominal aortic aneurysm repair. Eur J Vasc Endovasc Surg. 2019;57(2):229–37.
56. Gialdini G, Parikh NS, Chatterjee A, Lerario MP, Kamel H, Schneider DB, et al. Rates of spinal cord infarction after repair of aortic aneurysm or dissection. Stroke. 2017;48(8):2073–7.

Management of Esophageal Perforation

30

Nabeel H. Gul, Valerie X. Du, and Shawn S. Groth

Case Report

A 55-year-old man presented to the emergency department with sudden onset of excruciating chest pain and dyspnea after a bout of forceful vomiting. Upon presentation, he was tachycardiac, tachypneic, afebrile, and had normal blood pressure. EKG and troponin were normal. Laboratory investigation revealed leukocytosis and mild elevation of creatinine. Chest X-ray showed a large left-sided pleural effusion. CT scan of the chest revealed large loculated left pleural effusion, lung collapse, and pneumomediastinum. He was resuscitated with fluids and broad-spectrum antibiotics were initiated. A large-bore chest tube was placed and drained turbid appearing fluid with food particles. A diagnosis of Boerhaave syndrome was suspected and the patient was taken to the operating room for intervention.

Overview

Esophageal perforations fall on a spectrum of severity, from clinically inconsequential microperforations on one end to septic shock from large uncontrolled perforations surrounded by devitalized tissue on the other end. Esophageal perforations are associated with significant morbidity and mortality rates, particularly if there are signs of sepsis on presentation. Indeed, though a systematic review of the literature noted a mortality rate of 13.3%, mortality rates over 30% have been reported [1]. Importantly, experienced centers have reported mortality rates of 5–10%, highlighting the importance of understanding the nuances of managing these patients.

Although esophago-cutaneous fistula secondary to rupture was mentioned in the Smith Papyrus from 2500 BC [2], the first case of spontaneous esophageal rupture was reported by Herman Boerhaave in 1724. After consuming a gluttonous meal,[1] Baron Jan Gerrit van Wassenaer heer van Rosenberg, the Grand Admiral of the Dutch Fleet, tried to induce emesis after drinking

N. H. Gul
Division of Thoracic Surgery, Michael E. DeBakey Department of Surgery, Baylor College of Medicine/Texas Heart Institute, Houston, TX, USA

V. X. Du · S. S. Groth (✉)
Division of Thoracic Surgery, Michael E. DeBakey Department of Surgery, Baylor College of Medicine, Houston, TX, USA
e-mail: Shawn.Groth@bcm.edu

[1] "At the last meal on the day he took sick he ate veal soup with fragrant herbs; he took a little white cabbage boiled with sheep; spinach; and calf sweetbreads lightly roasted (or fried); a little duck, the thigh and breast; two larks; a bit of apple compote and bread; and ended his meal with dessert consisting of pears, grapes, and sweetmeats. With his meal he drank a little beer, and a little wine from Moselle."

M. D. Zielinski, O. Guillamondegui (eds.), *The Acute Management of Surgical Disease*,
https://doi.org/10.1007/978-3-031-07881-1_30

several cups of *Carduus Benedictus* (a thistle used for various medicinal purposes including indigestion) forcefully vomited, perforated his esophagus, and "*suddenly gave forth a horrifying cry*" [3]. During the ensuing 16 h before the Admiral died of septic shock, Hermann Boerhaave carefully scribed the clinical course.

The dramatic description of the Admiral's condition by Boerhaave as "*the most atrocious malady*" which "*cannot be remedied by any assistance of the medical profession*", resonated fear among many physicians for centuries. Indeed, for two centuries, esophageal perforation was left for an autopsy before evaluation [4]. It was not until 1947 that Norman Barrett in London and O.T. Clagett at Mayo Clinic independently reported the first cases of timely diagnosis and successful repair [5, 6]. Other reports of successful intervention led to primary repair becoming the standard of care for the majority of the twentieth century. In 1965, Mengold and Klassen first reported the "non-operative" management of esophageal perforations [7]. With the evolution of minimally invasive surgery and interventional endoscopy, there is a growing array of options for managing esophageal perforations. What began as a paradigm of early surgical intervention has evolved into a multi-disciplinary hybrid approach [8].

Etiology

Today, the most common cause of esophageal perforation is an iatrogenic injury during diagnostic or therapeutic interventions, accounting for nearly 60% of all perforations [9]. The risk of iatrogenic perforation is predicated on the type of endoscope and the therapeutic intent of the endoscopic intervention. Indeed, there is a higher risk of perforation with rigid endoscopy (0.11%), as compared with flexible endoscopy (0.03%). Furthermore, as compared with diagnostic endoscopy, the risk of perforation is higher for therapeutic interventions such as dilation, stenting, sclerotherapy, and endoscopic resection of lesions.

The area at greatest risk of perforation is the Killian's triangle, a weakness in the posterior wall of the pharynx between the cricopharyngeal and thyropharyngeal muscles, followed by the distal esophagus just proximal to the gastroesophageal junction and the mid-esophagus, where the aortic arch and the left main stem bronchus impinge on the esophagus. Intraoperative injury to the esophagus can also occur during paraesophageal surgery. Such injuries have been reported with fundoplication and hiatal hernia repair, vagotomy, tracheostomy, lung transplantation, pneumonectomy, thoracic aortic aneurysm repair, and cervical spine surgery [10–13].

Though it has received much attention, Boerhaave's syndrome accounts for only 10–15% of all esophageal perforations. These spontaneous esophageal perforations are barogenic—the result of a sudden increase in the intra-esophageal pressure and simultaneous failure of the upper esophageal sphincter to relax. Though forceful vomiting is a common cause, spontaneous rupture can also result from childbirth, coughing, or weightlifting [14]. It results in a longitudinal tear that mostly occurs in the distal third of the esophagus, typically 1–8 cm in length [15]. The majority of these perforations in the distal esophagus communicates with the left pleural cavity but can communicate with the right pleural space, highlighting the importance of accurate pre-interventional diagnostic evaluation.

Foreign body ingestion is a less common cause of esophageal perforation; although, most foreign bodies that reach the gastrointestinal tract will pass spontaneously. Bones are the most common foreign body ingestion. While fishbones are the most common foreign body ingested in Asia, chicken bones are the most common foreign body ingestion in the West. The pharynx is the most common location where foreign bodies become lodged and cause perforation. While most can be removed endoscopically; the risk of perforation is rare and the reported incidence is 0.001% [16].

Traumatic injuries to the esophagus are rare and account for less than 1% of all trauma injuries. The most common mechanism is penetrating injury. The thoracic esophagus is deeply seated in the chest cavity and well protected by the rib cage, making it exceedingly rare to have an isolated esophageal injury. Typically such patients also have rib fractures and a pneumothorax. The cervical esophagus, however, lies in the neck and is susceptible to penetrating injuries. Mortality and morbidity are likely results of injuries to other major structures. In a retrospective analysis of 641 patients with esophageal trauma, it was found that the largest risk of mortality with esophageal trauma was a high injury severity score [17].

Other less common etiologies include caustic ingestions, esophageal cancer, transesophageal echocardiography, or perforation from surrounding infection, especially in immunocompromised patients.

The etiology has a significant impact on the outcome. Spontaneous esophageal perforations carry the greatest mortality rate of 36% (0–72%), likely due to a delay in diagnosis because the presenting symptoms are often confused with other diagnoses. In contrast, iatrogenic perforations are often diagnosed during the procedure, can be managed expeditiously, and have a reported mortality of 19% (7–33%). Traumatic perforations are typically limited to the cervical esophagus, which is contained by the fascial planes in the neck and carries a mortality of 7% (0–33%) [18–30].

Clinical Presentation

The clinical presentation of esophageal perforation differs depending on the etiology, location of the injury, time interval since perforation, and the degree of contamination. Common symptoms include chest pain, dysphagia, dyspnea, fever, chills, neck, or abdominal pain. These symptoms may be mild if the presentation is early or perforation is contained within the mediastinum. Often, presenting symptoms following cervical esophageal perforation is less severe, because such perforations are contained within the fascial planes of the neck. In contrast, perforation of the thoracic esophagus may result in mediastinal and pleural space contamination, which initiates an intense cytokine-mediated reaction that leads to fluid sequestration, hypotension, and sepsis.

Pain is a common presenting symptom. Pain from posterior mediastinal contamination is often localized in the epigastric region with radiation to the infra-scapular region. Pleural contamination can result in pleuritic chest pain on the affected side. Intraperitoneal contamination may be accompanied by acute abdominal signs. During the initial evaluation, it is important to obtain a focused history on pre-existing symptoms of gastroesophageal reflux disease, dysphagia, weight loss, prior esophageal surgeries, and intervention, since it may influence the treatment modality.

Physical examination may reveal fever, tachycardia, hypotension, tachypnea, crepitus, and edema of the chest or neck. Hamman sign, a crunching, rasping sound heard over the precordium synchronous with cardiac rhythm, due to emphysema of the mediastinum can be found in nearly half of the patients [31]. Subcutaneous emphysema is detected by the physical examination in 60% of patients after cervical perforation and 40% after thoracic perforation [20].

Diagnosis

The initial symptoms are vague, and perforation of the esophagus is usually not at the top of the differential diagnosis in patients presenting with chest pain. The timely diagnosis of perforation is crucial in mitigating the deleterious effects of mediastinal and pleural contamination. Therefore, it is imperative to have high suspicion.

Radiological studies are paramount to diagnose esophageal perforation. A quick and inexpensive chest X-ray may reveal pleural effusion, hydro-pneumothorax, pneumomediastinum, mediastinal widening, pneumoperitoneum, or subcutaneous emphysema. However, it is important to understand that a normal chest X-ray does not reliably rule out perforation, particularly early in the disease process or with contained perforations. Some of the findings such as pleural effusion and widening of the esophagus might require several hours to appear [32].

A contrast esophagram is the gold standard for diagnosing esophageal perforations. It has the advantages of assessing esophageal anatomy and underlying pathology (i.e., strictures, masses, and hiatal hernias), identifying the location (and side) of the perforation, and evaluating the extent of the contamination. The study is performed using water-soluble, iodinated contrast (e.g., diatrizoate sodium-diatrizoate meglumine solution; Gastrografin®). Gastrografin® is rapidly absorbed and safer than barium, which can potentially exacerbate the inflammatory response to mediastinal, pleural, or abdominal contamination. Of note, the patient must be alert and cooperative to safely complete a contrast esophagram. Gastrografin, if aspirated, can cause severe chemical pneumonitis. In an intubated patient, the study can be performed by instilling the contrast via a naso-esophageal tube or through the working channel of a flexible esophagoscope under fluoroscopy. Despite the advantages of water-soluble contrast, barium has a high viscosity, has better mucosal adherence, and hence offers greater anatomic detail. Consequently, if there is a high index of suspicion of esophageal perforation, a negative water-soluble contrast study should be followed by an esophagram with thin barium to increase the sensitivity of the test. Indeed, the false-negative rate for water-soluble contrast esophagograms (22–50%) is higher than barium esophagograms (10–12%) [20].

Contrast esophagography has inherent limitations in an emergent setting, including the availability of experienced radiology staff, the ability of the patient to cooperate, and potentially the time needed to obtain the appropriate views. As an alternative, computed tomography (CT) avoids many of these limitations. CT scan can typically detect pneumomediastinum, mediastinal abscesses, pleural effusions, and esophago-pleural fistulas. In a recent large retrospective analysis conducted in an emergency department setting, CT was associated with a higher sensitivity for diagnosing esophageal perforation (100%), as compared to contrast esophagograms (77%). However, due to the high false-positive rates with the CT scan, the authors recommended following up a positive CT scan with an esophagram to confirm the diagnosis, when possible [33].

Fiberoptic esophagoscopy provides the added benefit of directly visualizing the degree of mucosal injury and identifying underlying pathology, such as strictures, diverticula, or malignancy. In traumatic esophageal perforation, esophagoscopy is associated with a sensitivity of 100% and a specificity of 83% [34]. Concern has been raised about the safety of esophagoscopy in the setting of non-traumatic perforations as insufflation could create a tension pneumothorax, worsen pneumoperitoneum, or convert a small or partial-thickness perforation to a larger defect. However, in experienced hands with careful attention to detail, flexible esophagoscopy can be performed safely and provides invaluable information for guiding treatment.

Each diagnostic modality has inherent risks, benefits, and limitations. The application of each study must be carefully weighed in the appropriate clinical circumstances. These diagnostic modalities are not mutually exclusive; rather, they are complementary. Finding the location of the perforation and the extent of contamination is critical information for treatment planning.

Treatment

Initial Management

Like all severe illnesses, the basic tenants of critical care—source control, resuscitation according to oxygen transport criteria, and metabolic support—provide a framework for managing patients with esophageal perforation [35]. Furthermore, a mindful, proactive approach is necessary to mitigate the risk of morbidity and mortality from esophageal perforation. Once the diagnosis is suspected, antimicrobials to cover gram positives, gram negatives, anaerobes, and fungus should be given during the initial evaluation and within 1 h of triage for both sepsis and septic shock [36]. Anti-fungal treatment is especially important for patients on proton pump inhibitors, which are known to increase the fungal colonization in the stomach [37]. If a large pleural effusion or hydro-pneumothorax is present, a tube thoracostomy provides temporary control of pleural contamination while the patient is stabilized, assessed, and triaged to treatment.

Due to the controversy in the proper management of this condition, Luketich and colleagues proposed the Pittsburgh Perforation Severity Score (PSS), to provide a framework for making treatment decisions based on 10 clinical variables at the time of presentation. The score was based on 119 cases of esophageal perforations treated at the University of Pittsburgh Medical Center [38]. The pre-existing conditions and clinical variables at the time of presentation are assigned points (range 1–3) for a possible total score of 18. Points are given according to the following scale: 1 = age >75 years, tachycardia (>100 bpm), leukocytosis (>10,000 white blood cells/mL), or pleural effusion (on chest radiograph, computed tomography, or barium swallow); 2 = fever (>38.5 °C), non-contained leak (on barium swallow or computed tomography), respiratory compromise (respiratory rate >30, increasing oxygen requirement, or need of mechanical ventilation), or time to diagnosis >24 h; and 3 = presence of cancer or hypotension. It has been shown that the PSS may be a useful tool to stratify patients into low, intermediate, and high-risk groups [39, 40]. However, the PSS was devised from retrospective studies, and its value in treatment allocation remains debatable [41].

Primary Repair

Primary repair remains the gold standard for the definitive treatment of esophageal perforation.

Traditional "Open" Approach

The location of the perforation dictates the approach. While cervical esophageal perforations are typically performed via a left neck incision and mid-thoracic perforations are often best approached through the right chest, a distal esophageal perforation is usually approached through the left chest, classically via a muscle-sparing thoracotomy through the left seventh intercostal space. Upon entering the chest, the pleural space is lavaged clear and, if needed, a decortication is performed.

If the location of the perforation is not immediately apparent, on-table endoscopy is a helpful adjunct. A longitudinal myotomy is performed overlying the perforation to expose the full extent of the mucosal injury. Often, the degree of mucosal injury is greater than what is initially appreciated by examining the area of full-thickness injury. Necrotic, devitalized tissue should be debrided. At this point, the surgeon must ascertain whether the esophagus can be repaired (or at least spared). If not, an esophagectomy is required.

Once the extent of the mucosal injury is fully exposed and the devitalized tissue has been debrided, the repair is performed in two layers. The inner layer (mucosa and submucosa) is closed with absorbable suture and the outer layer (muscularis propria) is closed with non-absorbable suture. Importantly, the repair should be performed over a Bougie (i.e., 40–48 French) both to mitigate the risk of stricturing and to relieve any distal obstruction (e.g., an esophageal stricture) [42]. For patients with untreated esophageal outflow obstruction (i.e., achalasia), a contralateral esophageal myotomy should be performed and carried 2 cm onto the stomach. Despite meticulous closure, the esophageal leak is a common complication. Consequently, the suture line should be buttressed with a vascularized pedicle of intercostal muscle, serratus anterior, latissimus dorsi, pleura, or pericardial fat pad to reduce the rate of fistula formation. Nonetheless, leaks are a common (15–50%), even with tissue reinforcement [38, 43]. Consequently, we recommend leaving a small drain (i.e., #10 Jackson-Pratt) adjacent to the repair for chronic fistula management.

For distal esophageal perforations, a gastrostomy (or gastro-jejunostomy) is placed for chronic gastric decompression and a feeding jejunostomy is placed for nutritional support. For proximal perforations in the absence of a hiatal hernia or chronic symptoms of reflux, a gastrostomy alone may be sufficient. Depending on the stability of the patient and the length of operative time for the primary repair, the gastrostomy and jejunostomy may be placed on a separate day.

Minimally Invasive Approach

The safety, feasibility, and advantages of standard video-assisted thoracoscopic surgery (VATS) and laparoscopy and robot-assisted approaches for elective transthoracic procedures are well-documented [44]. However, most of the literature regarding the utilization of minimally invasive approaches for esophageal perforation is limited to case reports and small case series. Most of the reported cases describe the treatment of Boerhaave perforation and repair of perforation caused by pneumatic dilation in achalasia [45–50]. Patients in these series were stable, had minimal contamination, and were diagnosed early after the injury. The same principles of open repair apply to minimally invasive approaches: (1) perform a longitudinal myotomy to expose the full extent of the injury; (2) repair the esophagus in two layers over a Bougie; (3) reinforce the repair with vascularized tissue; (4) leave a drain for chronic fistula management.

Timing of Repair

Esophageal perforations should be managed as expeditiously as possible. Unfortunately, patients with esophageal perforation often have a delayed presentation. An older (now outdated) dogma of managing esophageal perforations is to avoid attempts at repair for perforations more than 24 h old, due to concern of an inordinate risk of failure of the repair [51]. Instead, some advocated drainage alone, esophagectomy (with or without reconstruction), or esophageal diversion for those patients with a delayed presentation. Grillo and Wilkins were among the first to challenge this surgical dogma and recommended repair whenever possible, regardless of the time interval between injury and intervention [52].

With increasing experience, additional reports of primary repair of perforations more than 24 h old have documented the safety and feasibility of repair in this subset of patients to avoid the morbidity associated with resection or diversion and the need for a second reconstructive operation [9]. A number of patients who undergo diversion are never able to undergo reconstruction. Though morbidity and mortality rates are higher among those patients who have a delayed presentation, what is likely more important than timing is the clinical status of the patient, underlying esophageal pathology, and the quality of the tissue that is injured.

Outcomes of Primary Repair

In a seminal paper, Dr. Orringer and colleagues reported their series of 22 patients who were treated at their institution over 17 years (1976–1993). They noted an 80% successful closure rate and a remarkably low (5%) 30-day mortality rate [53]. Since then, numerous other investigators have reported the safety and efficacy of primary repair including a 3–30% mortality rate, a 40–65% complication rate (depending on the severity of sepsis upon presentation), and a 15–30% leak rate [34, 54–58]. After primary repair, 20% of patients require (unplanned) re-intervention. Therefore, it is inaccurate to presume that primary repair is a "one-and-done" procedure, as compared to interventional techniques which frequently require repeat interventions.

Dr. Orringer and colleagues also evaluated long-term functional outcomes of primary repair. In their series of 25 patients who underwent primary repair over a nearly 20-year period (1977–1995) with a mean follow-up of 3.7 years, 40% required at least 1 dilatation. At a mean of 21 months after the primary repair, 5 of the 10 patients who required dilation ultimately underwent esophagectomy due to a recalcitrant peptic stricture. In the total cohort, 90% of patients were subjectively satisfied with their swallowing function afterward. The 10% of patients that were dissatisfied all had peptic strictures [59]. Despite the limitations of this study, select patients who have a perforation in the setting of a severe peptic stricture may be best served by esophagectomy.

Esophagectomy

Esophagectomy is usually reserved for patients whose esophagus is not salvageable because of underlying esophageal pathology (e.g., esophageal cancer, end-stage achalasia, and recalcitrant peptic and caustic strictures) or poor tissue quality. The approach (transthoracic vs transhiatal) and technique (minimally invasive vs. open) is dictated by the nature and location of the injury and by the experience of the surgeon. Contaminated pleural and mediastinal spaces should be washed out, debrided/decorticated, and drained. Not surprisingly, the mortality rate from esophagectomy is higher in the emergent, as compared with the elective setting. In one literature review (1990–2003), 129 patients underwent esophagectomy for esophageal perforation, a mean mortality rate of 17% (range, 0–43%) was noted among the reported series [9].

One-Staged Reconstruction

For hemodynamically stable patients, esophagectomy and primary reconstruction is a safe treatment plan [25]. One-staged reconstruction can potentially avoid the need for a second operation but requires careful selection of patients. The feared complication of anastomotic leak after an emergent reconstruction has led some surgeons to prefer deferring reconstruction to a later stage.

Bipolar Exclusion and Delayed Reconstruction

For hemodynamically unstable patients who require esophagectomy, reconstruction should be delayed. As an alternative, some surgeons have advocated for proximal and distal diversion without esophagectomy and leaving reconstruction after recovery. Proximal diversion can be performed via an end cervical esophagostomy or placement of an esophageal T-tube and loop cervical esophagostomy. The need for the second operation and the technical challenges in restoring gastrointestinal continuity at a later stage have made this option less desirable. Furthermore, if the esophagus is left in situ, a mucocele will ensue unless the mucosa is resected. We also find a loop esophagostomy often problematic since it tends to retract into the wound, even with an external bolster.

Consequently, for patients who require esophagectomy but are not candidates for reconstruction, we recommend end cervical esophagostomy. Typically, 20–25 cm (approximately the level of the azygous arch) of the remnant esophagus will remain viable. The remnant esophagus should be brought through the sternocleidomastoid and under the skin over the clavicle and out the left chest wall. The chest wall provides a more rigid structure for the application of an ostomy bag and is more comfortable for patients than an ostomy bag overlying the left neck.

"Non-operative" Hybrid Treatment

In 1965, Manigold and Klassen reported their experience with "non-operative" management of esophageal perforations. Their approach entailed interventional endoscopy, drainage of all collections, intravenous antibiotics, and parenteral or enteric nutritional support [7]. Since then, with advancements in interventional endoscopy, there has been a paradigm shift in the utilization of endoscopic techniques for managing esophageal perforations from 37% in 1994 to 80% in 2009 [8]. Of note, the term "non-operative" management is somewhat of a misnomer since intervention (including the potential need for pleural drainage and decortication) is a cornerstone of this treatment approach. This approach has been applied to patients at all time intervals from perforation and provides the benefit of combining the diagnostic and treatment capabilities of advanced endoscopy. Currently available endoscopic strategies include esophageal stenting, endoluminal suturing (OverStitch™, Apollo Endosurgery, Inc., Austin, TX), through-the-scope (TTS) clips, over-the-scope clips (OTSC® System, Ovesco Endoscopy, Cary, NC), and endoscopic vacuum therapy (endoVAC).

Several investigators have published criteria to identify patients who are candidates for this approach [60]:

- Early diagnosis (or delayed diagnosis of a contained leak)
- Contained in neck or mediastinum (not abdomen or pleural space)
- Not traversing neoplastic tissue
- No distal obstruction
- No signs of sepsis
- Experienced thoracic surgeon available

Endoluminal Stenting

Self-expanding metal stents (SEMS) offer many advantages as a minimally invasive treatment for esophageal perforations. Initially, early metal stents were used for only palliative procedures of malignant strictures, but the addition of synthetic polymer coatings has broadened its applications and decreased rates of complications (e.g., tissue in-growth) after placement.

Pre-procedural assessment includes radio-opaque markers placed to indicate proximal and distal boundaries of the planned stent placement. While the procedure can be performed without fluoroscopy by placing the endoscope adjacent to the stent and deploying the stent under endoscopic visualization, we prefer the use of fluoroscopy under general anesthesia. The diameter and length of the chosen stent are dictated by the anatomy of the esophagus and the location of the perforation. In general, stent positioning at the upper esophageal sphincter is poorly tolerated by patients. Though unavoidable at times, stenting across the gastroesophageal junction increases the risk of gastroesophageal reflux and aspiration. Stent migration is a common complication of covered stents, occurring in 8–40% of patients [61–71]. This risk can be mitigated by fixing the stent in place with clips or suture.

Care must be taken when deploying the stent. While it is relatively easy to reposition a stent that was placed slightly too distal to the desired location, it is generally not possible to advance a fully deployed stent that was initially positioned too proximal to the desired location. A chest X-ray is obtained after the procedure to establish a baseline for assessing any future stent migration. To minimize the risk of stent erosion/perforation and to assess for healing, we recommend removing the stent and re-evaluating the perforation every 2–4 weeks.

Due to the rarity of esophageal perforations and differences in training and treatment biases between practitioners who manage these patients, there will never be a randomized controlled trial comparing stenting and primary repair. Nonetheless, multiple observational studies have demonstrated comparable morbidity (including leak) and mortality rates of esophageal stenting and primary repair in appropriately selected patients [8]. Freeman and colleagues used the Premiere database (2009–2012) and propensity-matched 30 patients who underwent primary repair and 30 who underwent stenting for iatrogenic perforation. They found that stenting was associated with a shorter intensive care unit and total hospital length of stay, earlier initiation of oral intake, reduced morbidity, lower likelihood of discharging to a long-term acute care hospital, lower total hospital costs, and no difference in leak rates, the need for re-intervention, or mortality [72].

Endoscopic Clipping

Endoscopic clipping in acute esophageal perforations is ideally undertaken for smaller lacerations with healthy tissue margins, such as iatrogenic perforations. Initially used for post-operative anastomotic leaks, its applications have broadened to spontaneous and iatrogenic perforations and for fistulas after transluminal endoscopic surgeries [73]. Of note, endoscopic clipping has a higher success rate (69.1%) as a primary intervention rather than a salvage intervention after previously failed management attempts (46.9%) as the tissue quality becomes less amenable to clipping [74]. Perforations are characterized radiographically before endoluminal therapy to allow identification of the location and appropriate clip size. Through-the-scope (TTS) clips are ideal for smaller perforations (<1 cm) surrounded by healthy tissue. The newer over-the-scope clips (OTSC System) can also be used for larger perforations. The clip size is chosen based on the margins of healthy tissue surrounding the pathologic portion to allow proper adhesion and seal after application. Suction is applied to the perforation to gather tissue through the distal scope for the approximation of margins and control. The jaws of the clips are closed, inspected for correct placement, and deployed. Successful closure can be determined as complete closure without leakage 24 h after contrast esophagogram or water-soluble contrast X-ray.

The efficacy of clipping is limited by the size of perforation and the dimension of available clips currently available OTSC diameters are 6, 11, 12, and 14 mm while TTS clips typically have a wingspan of 9–16-mm. Though success rates for OTSC for managing esophageal perforations approach 85%, these are best reserved by perforations 10-mm or less in size [75]. Though longer perforations can be managed with a series of TTS clips (or endoscopic suturing), such perforations have a higher risk of treatment failure with endoscopic clips. In addition to size, perforations with minimal inflammation and perforations that are acute (rather than chronic fistulas) are other factors favorable for endoscopic clipping [73].

Endoluminal Vacuum-Assisted Closure

Endoluminal vacuum-assisted closure (also known as endoVAC or EVAC) devices were first used to treat rectal anastomotic leaks. Its application has since expanded to other defects in the gastrointestinal tract, including esophageal leaks and perforations. Though a prefabricated device is not available in the United States, it can be readily constructed using a standard black VAC sponge, suture, and nasogastric (NG) tube. Negative pressure applied through the NG tube (typically 175 mmHg) allows for relief of edema and removal of infectious secretions, gradually closing the lesion. CT or contrast esophagogram can be performed after the first endoscopic placement to confirm correct placement and exclude pneumothorax or other abscesses requiring external drainage [76]. Importantly, surgical or interventional radiology drains next to the perforation will compete with the endoVAC system and should be removed as soon as possible. We recommend sponge exchange every 3–5 days, with successful therapy indicated by shrinkage of the mediastinal cavity and development of healthy granulation tissue. The longer the sponge is left in place, the more likely esophageal secretions will overwhelm the capacity of the VAC foam and suction (and therefore efficacy) is impaired. Many groups have reported success rates for endoVAC treatment ranging from 88% concurrently with surgical and endoscopic therapies as well as 73.3% with endoVAC alone [77, 78]. Though success rates over 90% for esophageal leaks and perforations have been reported, typically patients require 3–4 weeks of (inpatient) therapy to achieve closure [79].

Indications for the inclusion of endoVAC therapy include poor surgical candidacy for extensive surgery, contained perforations with paraesophageal abscesses, or failure of other aforementioned therapies. Common complications include stricture secondary to granulation tissue development, requiring additional dilation repairs. Due to the risk of fistula formation, endoVACs should not be placed when there is no tissue between the perforation and airways or aorta.

Nutritional Management: Enteral vs. Parenteral

Determinants of nutritional management during repair and hospitalization can be assessed based on the individual patient's condition and the surgeon's judgment. For more conservative repairs with anticipated oral feedings 2–3 weeks after the repair, peripheral access to total parenteral nutrition (TPN) can be sufficient, though we prefer enteric nutritional support for all patients whenever possible. However, long-term feeding methods are required in the management of complex cases such as intra-pleural leaks and complicated esophageal repairs. Enteral nutrition with a pharyngostomy, gastrostomy, or jejunostomy avoids the catheter-related complications associated with TPN and maintains the health of the intestinal microbiome [80]. Consideration of the extent of esophageal damage, additional mediastinal com-

stapled anastomosis. J Thorac Cardiovasc Surg. 2000;119(2):277–88.
43. Pasricha PJ, Fleischer DE, Kalloo AN. Endoscopic perforations of the upper digestive tract; a review of their pathogenesis, prevention and management. Gastroenterology. 1994;106:787–802.
44. Gul NH, Hennon M. Advances in video-assisted thoracoscopic surgery. Indian J Thorac Cardiovasc Surg. 2018;34:36–9. https://doi.org/10.1007/s12055-017-0590-2.
45. Nguyen NT, Follette DM, Roberts PF, et al. Thoracoscopic management of postoperative esophageal leak. J Thorac Cardiovasc Surg. 2001;121:391–2.
46. Scott HJ, Rosin RD. Thoracoscopic repair of a transmural rupture of the oesophagus. J R Soc Med. 1995;88:414–5.
47. Landen S, El Nakadi I. Minimally-invasive approach to Boerhaave's syndrome: a pilot study of three cases. Surg Endosc. 2002;16:1354–7.
48. Vaidya S, Prabhudessai S, Jhawar N, et al. Boerhaave's syndrome: thoracolaparoscopic approach. J Minim Access Surg. 2010;6:76–9. https://doi.org/10.4103/0972-9941.68585.
49. Cho JS, Kim YD, Kim JW, et al. Thoracoscopic primary esophageal repair in patients with Boerhaave's syndrome. Ann Thorac Surg. 2011;91:1552–5. https://doi.org/10.1016/j.athoracsur.2011.01.082.
50. Elliott JA, Buckley L, Albagir M, et al. Minimally invasive surgical management of spontaneous esophageal perforation (Boerhaave's syndrome). Surg Endosc. 2019;33:3494–502. https://doi.org/10.1007/s00464-019-06863-2.
51. Wang N, Razzouk AJ, Safavi A, et al. Delayed primary repair of intrathoracic esophageal perforation: is it safe? J Thorac Cardiovasc Surg. 1996;111:114–21.
52. Grillo HC, Wilkins EW Jr. Esophageal repair following late diagnosis of intrathoracic perforation. Ann Thorac Surg. 1975;20(4):387–99.
53. Whyte RI, Iannettoni MD, Orringer MB. Intrathoracic esophageal perforation. The merit of primary repair. J Thorac Cardiovasc Surg. 1995;109(1):140–4; discussion 144–6. https://doi.org/10.1016/S0022-5223(95)70429-9.
54. Felmly LM, Kwon H, Denlinger CE, Klapper JA. Esophageal perforation: a common clinical problem with many different management options. Am Surg. 2017;83(8):911–7.
55. Ohri SK, Liakakos TA, Pathi V, Townsend ER, Fountain SW. Primary repair of iatrogenic thoracic esophageal perforation and Boerhaave's syndrome. Ann Thorac Surg. 1993;55(3):603–6. https://doi.org/10.1016/0003-4975(93)90261-f.
56. Jougon J, Mc Bride T, Delcambre F, Minniti A, Velly JF. Primary esophageal repair for Boerhaave's syndrome whatever the free interval between perforation and treatment. Eur J Cardiothorac Surg. 2004;25(4):475–9. https://doi.org/10.1016/j.ejcts.2003.12.029.
57. Wright CD, Mathisen DJ, Wain JC, Moncure AC, Hilgenberg AD, Grillo HC. Reinforced primary repair of thoracic esophageal perforation. Ann Thorac Surg. 1995;60(2):245–8; discussion 248–9. https://doi.org/10.1016/0003-4975(95)00377-w.
58. Lawrence DR, Ohri SK, Moxon RE, Townsend ER, Fountain SW. Primary esophageal repair for Boerhaave's syndrome. Ann Thorac Surg. 1999;67(3):818–20. https://doi.org/10.1016/s0003-4975(99)00043-0.
59. Iannettoni MD, Vlessis AA, Whyte RI, Orringer MB. Functional outcome after surgical treatment of esophageal perforation. Ann Thorac Surg. 1997;64(6):1606–9; discussion 1609–10. https://doi.org/10.1016/s0003-4975(97)01090-4.
60. Altorjay A, Kiss J, Vörös A, Bohák A. Nonoperative management of esophageal perforations. Is it justified? Ann Surg. 1997;225(4):415–21. https://doi.org/10.1097/00000658-199704000-00011.
61. Blackmon SH, Santora R, Schwarz P, Barroso A, Dunkin BJ. Utility of removable esophageal covered self-expanding metal stents for leak and fistula management. Ann Thorac Surg. 2010;89(3):931–6; discussion 936–7. https://doi.org/10.1016/j.athoracsur.2009.10.061.
62. Van Halsema EE, van Hooft JE. Clinical outcomes of self-expandable stent placement for benign esophageal diseases: a pooled analysis of the literature. World J Gastrointest Endosc. 2015;7(2):135–53. https://doi.org/10.4253/wjge.v7.i2.135.
63. Ott C, Ratiu N, Endlicher E, et al. Self-expanding Polyflex plastic stents in esophageal disease: various indications, complications, and outcomes. Surg Endosc. 2007;21:889–96.
64. Wang MQ, Sze DY, Wang ZP, Wang ZQ, Gao YA, Dake MD. Delayed complications after esophageal stent placement for treatment of malignant esophageal obstruction and esophagorespiratory fistulas. J Vasc Interv Radiol. 2001;12:465–74.
65. Eubanks S, Edwards CA, Fearing NM, et al. Use of endoscopic stents to treat anastomotic complications after bariatric surgery. J Am Coll Surg. 2008;206:935–8.
66. Fiorni A, Fleischer D, Valero J, Israeli E, Wengrower D, Goldin E. Self-expandable metal coil stents in the treatment of benign esophageal strictures refractory to conventional therapy: a case series. Gastrointest Endosc. 2000;52:259–62.
67. Radecke K, Gerken G, Treichel U. Impact of self-expanding plastic esophageal stent on various esophageal stenosis, fistulas and leakages: a single-center experience in 39 patients. Gastrointest Endosc. 2005;61:812–8.
68. Shin JH, Song HY, Ko GY, Lim JO, Yoon HK, Sung KB. Esophagorespiratory fistula: long-term results of palliative treatment with covered expandable metallic stents in 61 patients. Radiology. 2004;232:252–9.
69. Adam A, Ellul J, Watkinson A, et al. Palliation of inoperable esophageal carcinoma: a prospective randomized trial of laser therapy and stent placement. Radiology. 1997;202:344–8.

70. Sabharwal T, Hamady MS, Chui S, Atkinson S, Mason R, Adam A. A randomised prospective comparison of the Flamingo Wallstent and Ultraflex stent for palliation of dysphagia associated with lower third oesophageal carcinoma. Gut. 2003;52:922–6.
71. So H, Ahn JY, Han S, Jung K, Na HK, Lee JH, Jeong KW, Kim DH, Choi KD, Song HJ, Lee GH, Jung HY. Efficacy and safety of fully covered self-expanding metal stents for malignant esophageal obstruction. Dig Dis Sci. 2018;63(1):234–41. https://doi.org/10.1007/s10620-017-4839-9. Epub 2017 Nov 17.
72. Freeman RK, Herrera A, Ascioti AJ, Dake M, Mahidhara RS. A propensity-matched comparison of cost and outcomes after esophageal stent placement or primary surgical repair for iatrogenic esophageal perforation. J Thorac Cardiovasc Surg. 2015;149(6):1550–5. https://doi.org/10.1016/j.jtcvs.2015.01.066. Epub 2015 Feb 11.
73. Watkins JR, Farivar AS. Endoluminal therapies for esophageal perforations and leaks. Thorac Surg Clin. 2018;28(4):541–54. https://doi.org/10.1016/j.thorsurg.2018.07.002.
74. Haito-Chavez Y, et al. International multicenter experience with an over-the-scope clipping device for endoscopic management of GI defects (with video). Gastrointest Endosc. 2014;80(4):610–22.
75. Kobara H, Mori H, Nishiyama N, Fujihara S, Okano K, Suzuki Y, Masaki T. Over-the-scope clip system: a review of 1517 cases over 9 years. J Gastroenterol Hepatol. 2019;34(1):22–30. https://doi.org/10.1111/jgh.14402. Epub 2018 Aug 16.
76. Heits N, Stapel L, Reichert B, Schafmayer C, Schniewind B, Becker T, Hampe J, Egberts JH. Endoscopic endoluminal vacuum therapy in esophageal perforation. Ann Thorac Surg. 2014;97(3):1029–35. https://doi.org/10.1016/j.athoracsur.2013.11.014. Epub 2014 Jan 18.
77. Manfredi MA, Clark SJ, Staffa SJ, Ngo PD, Smithers CJ, Hamilton TE, Jennings RW. Endoscopic esophageal vacuum therapy: a novel therapy for esophageal perforations in pediatric patients. J Pediatr Gastroenterol Nutr. 2018;67(6):706–12. https://doi.org/10.1097/MPG.0000000000002073.
78. Jung CFM, Müller-Dornieden A, Gaedcke J, Kunsch S, Gromski MA, Biggemann L, Seif Amir Hosseini A, Ghadimi M, Ellenrieder V, Wedi E. Impact of endoscopic vacuum therapy with low negative pressure for esophageal perforations and postoperative anastomotic esophageal leaks. Digestion. 2020;11:1–11. https://doi.org/10.1159/000506101. Epub ahead of print.
79. Leeds SG, Mencio M, Ontiveros E, Ward MA. Endoluminal vacuum therapy: how I do it. J Gastrointest Surg. 2019;23(5):1037–43. https://doi.org/10.1007/s11605-018-04082-z. Epub 2019 Jan 22.
80. Moron R, Galvez J, Colmenero M, Anderson P, Cabeza J, Rodriguez-Cabezas ME. The importance of the microbiome in critically ill patients: role of nutrition. Nutrients. 2019;11(12):3002. https://doi.org/10.3390/nu11123002.
81. Ong GKB, Freeman RK. Endoscopic management of esophageal leaks. J Thorac Dis. 2017;9(Suppl 2):S135–45. https://doi.org/10.21037/jtd.2017.03.100.

Introduction to Acute Upper Gastrointestinal Hemorrhage

31

Caroline Park and Michael Cripps

Case 1

A 45-year-old male presented with hematemesis and melena. Symptoms began earlier this morning with melena; he most recently developed hematemesis in the emergency room. His past medical history is significant for an open right inguinal hernia repair, moderate alcohol consumption of 2–6 beers per night, and occasional ibuprofen for back pain. On exam, the patient appears anxious, is tachycardic to 120 s, blood pressure is 140/110, respiratory rate of 20 breaths/min, with an O_2 saturation of 96% on room air. There is no evidence of scleral icterus, palmar erythema, or abdominal wall varices. His abdomen is obese and non-tender without evidence of ascites or palpable liver or splenomegaly. Digital rectal exam reveals melena without masses or hemorrhoidal disease. His point of care hemoglobin is 11 mg/dL. Two large-bore IVs were placed, and a type and cross was sent. A nasogastric tube was placed, revealing bright-red blood. At this time, his blood pressure drops to 80/58 with an increase in tachycardia to 140. Given the persistent tachycardia, narrowed pulse pressure, and hypotension, the patient received two units of packed red blood cells with an appropriate improvement in vital signs. He was transferred to the surgical intensive care unit where he received two additional units over the next 12 h, for a total 4 units within 24 h. Viscoelastic testing was sent at the time, demonstrating coagulopathy and need for fresh frozen plasma. GI consultation was obtained, and the patient was prepared for upper gastrointestinal endoscopy with a single dose of erythromycin. At endoscopy, he was found to have a large ulcer, Forrest 2a with a visible vessel; this was treated with epinephrine injection and clipping with adequate hemostasis. He went on to recover in the SICU while remaining on proton-pump inhibitor therapy without further signs of hemorrhage.

C. Park (✉)
Division of Burn, Trauma and Acute Care Surgery, Department of Surgery, University of Texas Southwestern Medical Center at Dallas, Dallas, TX, USA

Biomedical Engineering, Graduate School of Biomedical Sciences, University of Texas Southwestern Medical Center, Dallas, TX, USA
e-mail: Caroline.Park@UTSouthwestern.edu

M. Cripps
Division of Burn, Trauma and Acute Care Surgery, Department of Surgery, Parkland Memorial Hospital, University of Texas Southwestern Medical Center at Dallas, Dallas, TX, USA
e-mail: Michael.Cripps@CUAnschutz.edu

M. D. Zielinski, O. Guillamondegui (eds.), *The Acute Management of Surgical Disease*,
https://doi.org/10.1007/978-3-031-07881-1_31

Early Management

Once the diagnosis of UGIH is suspected, it is paramount to stabilize and resuscitate, focusing on protecting the airway and establishing large-bore IV access. Patients should be connected to continuous cardiac monitoring and pulse oximetry, and an airway established if required. Crystalloid boluses [24] can be the initial form of volume resuscitation, but should soon be followed with blood products and activation of massive transfusion protocol if the patient presents with hemorrhagic shock [25]. Early identification and resuscitation can mitigate the increased risk of mortality and cardiovascular complication [26].

While establishing IV access, it is critical to send a type and cross-match in additional to a full panel of laboratory studies, including CBC, full chemistry panel, lactate, liver function tests, bilirubin, prothrombin/partial thromboplastin/INR and viscoelastic testing such as rotational thromboelastometry (ROTEM) or thromboelastography (TEG), whichever one is available to help guide resuscitation. A point of care hemoglobin is useful in obtaining a baseline but should not help direct the provider in transfusion if the patient is actively hemorrhaging.

Serial hemoglobin, lactate, and coagulation studies, which could include ROTEM, TEG, or PT/PTT/INR, should be drawn during active resuscitation to help guide transfusions. ROTEM and TEG are preferred blood analyses to address the coagulopathy associated with massive bleeding and can help target transfusions to prevent ongoing non-surgical hemorrhage [27]. In the setting of acute blood loss, vitamin K antagonists (VKA), direct oral anticoagulants (DOACs), and antiplatelets should be held with appropriate reversal of the first two. Vitamin K antagonists can be reversed with prothrombin complex concentrate, fresh frozen plasma, and vitamin K, with respective increase in time to efficacy of reversal [24]. These agents are not as effective in reversing DOACs, which generally have a shorter half-life and will require time to eliminate by clearance.

Restrictive Versus Liberal Transfusion

Similar to other studies on transfusion strategies and risk of mortality, a restrictive transfusion strategy in patients with non-massive, non-variceal UGIH is recommended (target Hb 7–9 g/dL) to a liberal threshold of Hb 9–11 g/dL with improved survival and reduced re-bleeding rates [28, 29]. However, in massive UGIH, massive transfusion protocol should be activated with a focus on restoring circulatory volume until hemorrhage is controlled and the patient is stabilized. Transfusion targets may shift to higher hemoglobin levels in patients with other significant liver, cardiac [30], and pulmonary comorbidities.

Breathing and Securing the Airway

Oftentimes during active hematemesis, patients will prefer to sit upright, which is a critical step in avoiding aspiration. If the patient is actively vomiting blood, and the airway is not protected, a nasogastric tube should be inserted and the patient intubated. If airway protection in a patient with hematemesis is required, endotracheal intubation should be performed ideally with a rapid sequence intubation strategy. This includes nasogastric decompression to avoid aspiration and enough initial resuscitation to avoid cardiovascular collapse on induction. While cardiopulmonary complications may occur after endoscopy, prophylactic endotracheal intubation for UGIH may not necessarily increase these complications [31]. However, pre-induction resuscitation may help mitigate the cardiovascular collapse [32] and aspiration that may occur with sedation and paralysis [33].

Nasogastric Decompression

Nasogastric decompression and lavage can be utilized to evaluate for UGIH, but the studies are mixed depending on the severity of the bleeding. In patients without hematemesis, the sensitivity is poor [34]. Sensitivity of nasogastric lavage in defining an upper versus lower GIH can be as low as 44% but with high specificity of 95%. However, in patients with severe UGIH, including hematemesis, the sensitivity and specificity are improved to 77% and 76% respectively [35, 36]. Another critical role of nasogastric decompression is also to reduce the risk of aspiration of blood, particularly if airway control is necessary for endoscopy. Although providers may hesitate to place a nasogastric tube in patients with known varices or variceal bleeds, this is a critical step in potential diagnosis and in decreasing aspiration risk.

In the setting of suspected or known variceal bleeding, achieving early tamponade of these engorged varices can temporize the massive bleeding that can occur secondary to longstanding portal hypertension.

The three most commonly used balloon devices include (1) Sengstaken-Blakemore, (2) Minnesota, and (3) Linton-Nachlas tubes. However, these balloon devices are temporary measures for hemorrhage control by compression of these varices along the gastric wall, GE-junction and esophagus and carry risks of perforation, additional bleeding, and/or necrosis of the tissues. Balloon tamponade can be employed while the patient undergoes active resuscitation, correction of coagulopathy, and provides time to transition to definitive measures.

Obtaining a History and Physical Exam

After initial stabilization, a thorough history and physical examination should be performed to evaluate for risk factors for UGIH, including non-variceal and variceal, the latter which is most often seen in patients with advanced cirrhosis. Patients with advanced cirrhosis may present with jaundice, encephalopathy, fluid-wave secondary to ascites, and less common, abdominal wall varices.

Risk factors for non-variceal UGIH (NVUGIH) include peptic ulcer disease (NSAID, *H. pylori*), recent abdominal trauma (including liver and pancreas), history of malignancy, and use of anticoagulation medication. Variceal UGIH is commonly associated with advanced cirrhosis with subsequent portal hypertension, but other less common etiologies include splenic vein thrombosis with associated gastric varices.

Table 31.3 Glasgow-Blatchford Score: risk of intervention and re-bleeding

	Points
Systolic blood pressure, mmHg	
100–109	1
90–99	2
<90	3
Blood urea nitrogen, mmol/L	
6.5–7.9	2
8.0–9.9	3
10.0–24.9	4
≥25.0	6
Hemoglobin for men, g/dL	
12.0–12.9	1
10.0–11.9	3
<10.0	6
Hemoglobin for women, g/dL	
10.0–11.9	1
<10.0	6
Other risk variables	
Pulse ≥100	1
Melena	1
Syncope	2
Hepatic disease	2
Cardiac failure	2

Assessing Risk of Re-bleeding, Intervention, and Mortality

Several risk-scoring systems exist to stratify risk of bleeding, need for endoscopic intervention, need for acute level of care, and mortality. However, the most commonly referenced scoring systems include the Glasgow-Blatchford Score (GBS) to predict re-bleeding and need for intervention [37], and the Rockall score for risk of mortality from UGIH [38] (Tables 31.3 and 31.4).

Initial Diagnosis

Early diagnosis and control of UGIH are essential to mitigate morbidity and mortality. As outlined above, nasogastric tube placement should be

Table 31.4 Rockall Scoring System to predict mortality from UGIH. Maximum additive score prior to diagnosis = 7, maximum additive score following diagnosis = 11

	Score			
Variable	0	1	2	3
Age	<60 years	60–79 years	≥80 years	
Shock	SBP ≥100, pulse <100	SBP ≥100, pulse ≥100	SBP <100	
Comorbidity	No major comorbidity		Cardiac failure, ischemic heart disease, major comorbidity	Renal failure, liver failure, disseminated malignancy
Diagnosis	Mallory-Weiss tear, no lesion identified, and no signs of recent hemorrhage	All other diagnoses	Malignancy upper GI tract	
Major signs of recent hemorrhage	None or dark spot only			Blood in upper GI tract, adherent clot, visible or spurting vessel

inserted as a first-line diagnostic approach in patients with UGIH. It is also important to incorporate knowledge of the patient's history (e.g., anticoagulants), recent sleeve-gastrectomy, and prior history of GI bleed and interventions to narrow the differential and exclude lower gastrointestinal hemorrhage. Up to 60% of GI bleeds are related to previously known lesion [39], thus a thorough history and review of recent interventions can help expedite diagnosis and source control.

Medical Management

After hemodynamic stabilization and reversal of coagulopathy, there are other medical, pharmacologic therapies that should be implemented to reduce the need for intervention and alleviate symptoms.

Acid-Reduction

Acid-reduction therapies should be implemented early, especially for stress-ulcer gastritis, gastric and duodenal or marginal ulcers where acid exposure propagates ulceration and bleeding [40]. Two main therapies exist, including histamine-2 receptor blockers and proton-pump inhibitors, although the latter has demonstrated improved outcomes and reduced incidence in bleeding [41].

After bleeding cessation, twice daily high-dose IV or PO (in patients that can tolerate) has been shown to be as effective as continuous infusion [42, 43]. However, in the immediate setting for UGIH, high-dose PPI with 80 mg IV bolus followed by an 8 mg infusion/hr. can help accelerate the resolution of signs of bleeding and the need for endoscopic intervention [44, 45].

Pro-kinetics

Pro-kinetic agents as metoclopramide and odansetron help with motility of blood products and alleviating symptoms of nausea. Dose of 10 mg IV of metoclopramide prior to induction may also help reduce the risk of aspiration and help empty the stomach prior to endoscopy [46, 47]. However, erythromycin in a single dose of 250 mg IV infused 30–120 min prior to endoscopy may have the same result and has also been associated with decreased rates of repeat endoscopy, transfusions, and length of stay [48, 49].

Antibiotic and Other Therapies

Lastly, patients with advanced cirrhosis should be initiated on antibiotics, specifically a third-generation generation cephalosporin (such as ceftriaxone) for prophylaxis of spontaneous bacterial peritonitis. Recent data suggests the benefit of empiric antibiotic prophylaxis is more pronounced for Child's B and C cirrhosis [50]. Many of these patients are generally borderline hypotensive while on beta-blockers (propranolol), diuretics (spironolactone) or cathartics (rifaximin, lactulose), and require vasopressor support. Vasopressin remains a first-line choice in this population as it is more selective on the splanchnic system for its vasoconstrictive effects [51]. Beta-blockers such as nadolol or propranolol are important for medical maintenance but should be avoided in the resuscitation phase [52, 53].

Diagnostic (and Therapeutic) Modalities

The first-line diagnostic modality for UGIH has been endoscopy for the past few decades, with many therapeutic additions [54]. Endoscopy remains the gold standard and is a quality indicator [55] given its diagnostic and potentially therapeutic potential and should be performed within 24 h or earlier (<12 h) for patients presenting with an acute UGIH with signs of hemodynamic instability. However, computed tomography angiography (CTA) and angiogram can play essential roles in the diagnosis of bleed that cannot be localized or is not amenable to endoscopy.

Endoscopy

The use of endoscopy blossomed in the 1980s and since then has evolved with new over the scope techniques, including clipping, banding, thermal and argon-plasma coagulation, and other techniques and topicals for hemostasis.

The timing of endoscopy very early (<12 h), early (<24 h), or delayed (>24 h) is dictated by the patient's hemodynamic stability and failure of medical management with active resuscitation and contraindication to cessation of anticoagulation [24]. Early endoscopy can decrease the length of stay, and potentially decrease the risk of re-bleeding, and the need for surgery [56].

Assessing the risk of re-bleeding is important as it impacts decision-making (therapeutic techniques) and consideration of a second-look endoscopy and characterization of low- or high-risk lesion. The Forrest classification is most commonly used to characterize ulcers from low risk to high risk of bleeding (Table 31.5, Fig. 31.2).

Endoscopic Techniques

Endoscopic techniques for non-variceal UGIH include injection, thermal, mechanical, and topical sprays. Endoscopic injection typically consists of epinephrine with good success [59]. Thermal treatments include monopolar and argon-plasma coagulation [60] (Fig. 31.3). Mechanical treatments include clipping [61] and banding [62]. Lastly, hemostatic spray [63] and glues have been implemented in conjunction with clipping, injection, and thermal treatments with recent success in hemostasis, particularly with areas of diffuse bleeding.

For bleeding in the small bowel distal to the ligament of Treitz, typically angiodysplasia and arterio-venous malformations, double-balloon enteroscopy may be useful to examine the entire small bowel [64].

Table 31.5 Forrest classification of ulcer disease

Grade	Endoscopic characteristics	Risk of re-bleeding (%)
I	Active hemorrhage	
Ia	Spurting	60–100
Ib	Oozing	25
II	Signs of recent hemorrhage	
IIa	Visible vessel	50
IIb	Adherent clot	30
IIc	Hematin-covered flat spot	<10
III	No hemorrhage—clean ulcer bed	<3

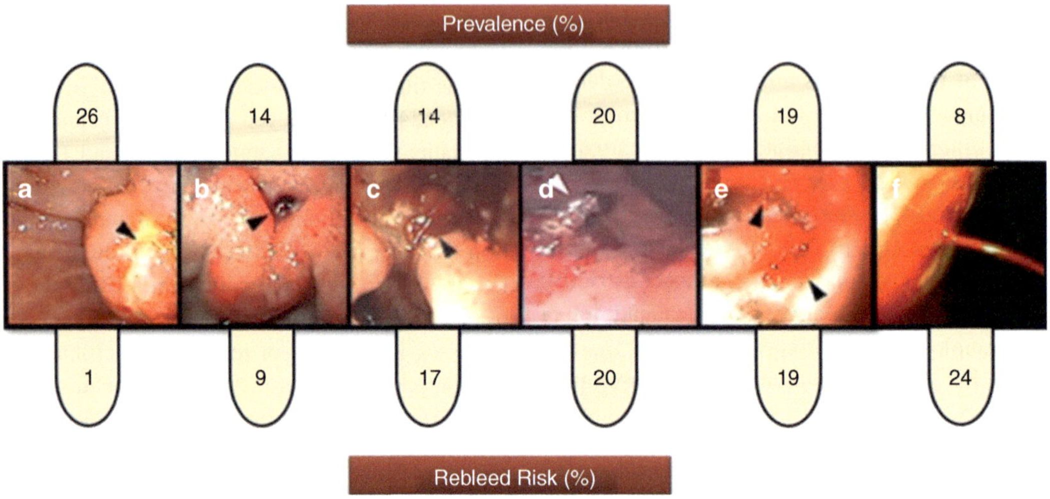

Fig. 31.2 Forrest classification of PUD with prevalences and post-endotherapy re-bleed risks based on data from Guglielmi et al. [57]. (**a**) Forrest 3: Clean base, (**b**) Forrest 2c: Flat pigmented spot, (**c**) Forrest 2b: Adherent clot, (**d**) Forrest 2a: Visible vessel, (**e**) Forrest 1b: Oozing vessel, (**f**) Forrest 1a: Spurting vessel. (Courtesy of Keith Siau, MD, Department of Gastroenterology, Russell's Hall Hospital, Dudley [58])

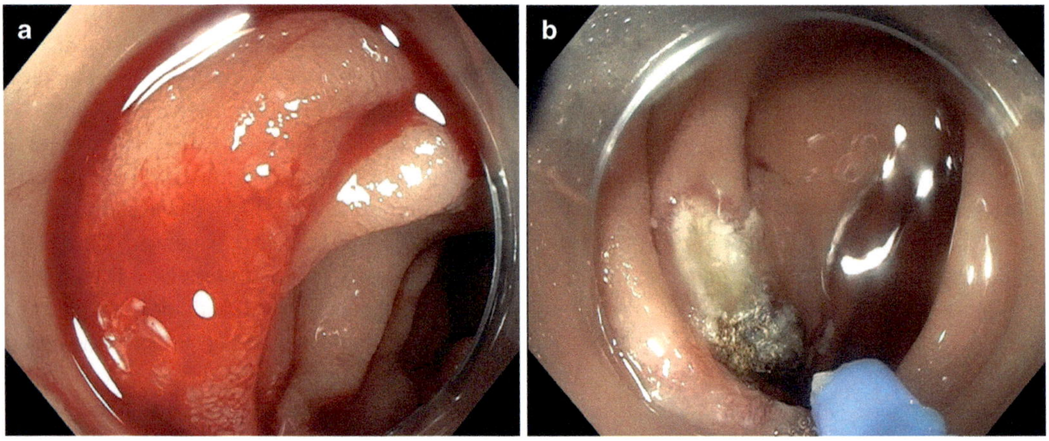

Fig. 31.3 (**a**, **b**) AV malformation before and after argon plasma coagulation. (Courtesy of Anna Tavakkoli, MD, MSc, Division of Digestive and Liver Diseases, University of Texas Southwestern Medical Center)

Computed Tomography Angiography (CTA)

When endoscopy cannot be performed, or cannot localize bleeding secondary to patient anatomy (such as a Roux-en-Y gastric bypass), CTA can be performed to more precisely localize bleeding. This modality is especially useful for bleeding within the small bowel that may be less accessible with standard endoscopy. In one study, the overall location-based accuracy, sensitivity and specificity for the detection of GI bleeding by 64-row CTA was 98.8% and 95.0% respectively [65]. Limitations include contrast exposure, and the inability to provide simultaneous therapeutic options. However, it has been shown to be accurate, and cost-effective in the diagnosis of acute UGIH [66] as it can guide interventional radiologists to the likely source of bleeding during an angiogram, minimize contrast and radiation exposure, and decrease time to hemorrhage control.

Percutaneous: Endovascular Techniques

Interventional radiology techniques, including endovascular techniques, have exponentially increased in utility and application since the 1980s, when its use played a pivotal role in the treatment of hemobilia after major liver trauma [67]. Trans-catheter arterial embolization (TAE) can play a significant role in the identification and treatment of UGIH but should be considered generally after appropriate resuscitation and endoscopic attempts have failed.

Since the 1980s, the application and diversity of endovascular techniques have increased dramatically to include bleeding duodenal ulcers [68], arterial hemorrhage from pancreatic pseudocysts [69], and bleeding from hypervascular malignancies [70]. Within this armamentarium includes coils, plugs with gelfoam [71], local instillation of heparin to provoke bleeding and of vasopressin to create vasoconstriction [72].

Lastly, the creation of intra-hepatic portosystemic shunts has replaced a classically morbid operation of selective shunting for patients with advanced cirrhosis. This percutaneous technique, the trans-jugular intrahepatic portosystemic shunt (TIPS), requires access to the hepatic vein and creation of a shunt between the portal and hepatic veins. This procedure can reduce portal venous pressure by 10–15 mmHg and subsequently decrease in bleeding from engorged esophago-gastric varices [73]. Patients who otherwise fail TIPS may require devascularization either open with splenectomy (Sugiura procedure) or laparoscopically [74, 75].

Nuclear-Medicine Studies

The role of nuclear medicine studies is limited in the diagnosis of UGIH, as its utility is best in occult bleeding with rates as low as 0.1 mL/min [76]. Heparin administration can provoke bleeding to aid in localization using tagged RBC studies [77]. However, compared to endoscopy, angiogram, or surgery, the sensitivity of localization is quite low [78] and is not recommended in the setting of UGIH.

Capsule Endoscopy

Capsule endoscopy (CE) retains a limited role in the diagnosis of UGIH. It historically has been a more effective method in evaluating occult GI bleed, particularly in the small bowel with a high positive predictive value of 95.5% and negative predictive value of 100% [79]. However, in the setting of UGIH, CE can facilitate patient triage, identify gross blood, and prompt earlier endoscopy, but should not be considered a substitute for endoscopy [80] (Fig. 31.4).

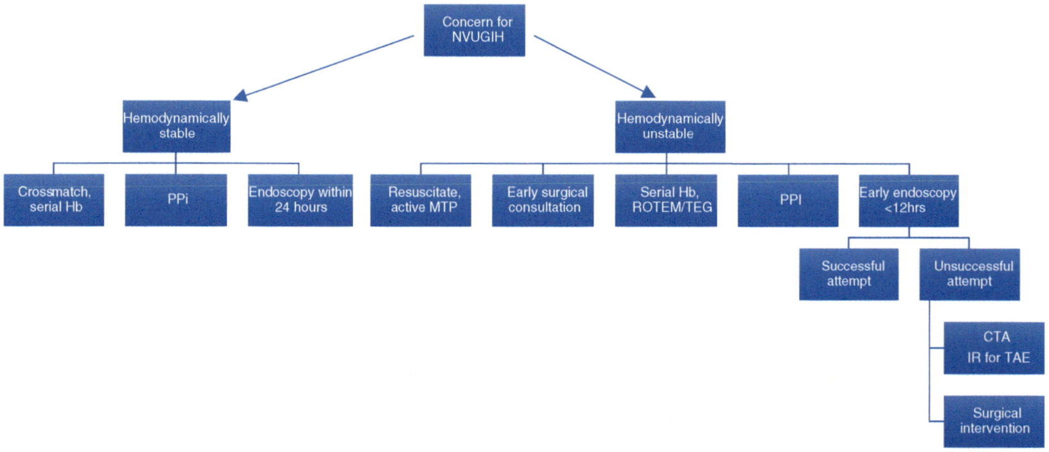

Fig. 31.4 Approach to non-variceal upper gastrointestinal hemorrhage. *NVUGIH* non-variceal upper gastrointestinal hemorrhage, *PPi* proton-pump inhibitor, *Hb* hemoglobin, *ROTEM* rotational thromboelastometry, *TEG* thromboelastography, *IR* interventional radiology, *CTA* computed tomography angiography, *TAE* trans-catheter arterial embolization

Key Points

- Resuscitate and address coagulopathy
- Early endoscopy for patients with hemodynamic instability
- Risk-stratify the patient based on clinical factors, ulcer appearance
- Continue medical management post-endoscopic intervention with PPI, transfusions
- Consider other diagnostic adjuncts—CTA or percutaneous angiography with difficult anatomy or failed endoscopy

Specific Considerations for Surgical Management

With the advent of acid-reduction therapies, and the availability of advanced endoscopy and interventional percutaneous, surgical intervention for acute UGIH is increasingly rare and limited to patients with refractory bleeding not amenable to the above strategies. We discuss a few scenarios with an emphasis on additional work-up and surgical approach.

Scenario:
47F with history of *H. pylori* and NSAID use presenting with a bleeding peptic ulcer; patient has failed two endoscopic attempts at epinephrine and injection of an actively bleeding, large ulcer. Patient is undergoing active resuscitation but is becoming coagulopathic. Percutaneous attempt with embolization of the left gastric artery is moderately successful. Patient however continues to require blood transfusions in the next 24 h.

Patients with refractory bleeding are those that may be pre-disposed to bleeding (cannot come off anticoagulation, uremia from renal disease) or with large ulcers and may require surgical intervention.

Prior to surgery:

1. Secure access: the patient should have confirmed, secure IV access and active type and cross-match.
2. Localize bleed: most of these patients have undergone an attempt at an endoscopy, CTA, or percutaneous angiography with localization of the bleed, which is critical in triaging an upper versus lower GIH.

Case #1: Bleeding Gastric Ulcer

Other adjuncts or equipment to consider:

- Concomitant endoscopy may be helpful in localizing the bleed to perform a limited wedge resection.

Approach:
Minimally invasive or open approach may be used depending on the comfort level of the surgeon.

Depending on the ulcer location, such as the greater curvature or anterior stomach, a limited wedge resection might be sufficient.

However, large ulcers near the lesser curvature or antrum may be more appropriate for antrectomy with Billroth I or II anastomosis. If the patient is stable, truncal vagotomy should be performed, especially if the patient has failed medical therapy with ant-acid reduction in the past. Small ulcers near the GE junction may be approached with an anterior gastrotomy with biopsy and oversewing; if the ulcer is large, a Csendes procedure may be necessary.

For juxta-cardial or more posterior ulcers that are not amenable to wedge resection and/or if endoscopy is not available for localization, an anterior gastrotomy can be performed to visualize the posterior wall and oversew bleeding vessels [81]. This approach is less appropriate for large, cratered ulcers or tumors that should be resected.

Case #2: Bleeding Duodenal Ulcer

Other adjuncts or equipment to consider:

- Potential choledochoscope or Fogarty catheter to thread in common bile duct if near gastroduodenal artery.
- Resuscitative endovascular balloon occlusion of the aorta has been implemented in case reports for stabilization purposes [82].

Approach:
Minimally invasive or open approach can be performed based on surgeon-comfort level.

Bleeding duodenal ulcers are often posterior with involvement of the gastroduodenal artery (GDA). It is imperative to palpate or doppler the GDA and localize in relation to the proper hepatic artery to avoid inadvertent ischemia to the liver.

Kocherize the duodenum after taking down the hepatic flexure. Create a longitudinal incision from the distal stomach across the pylorus and place stay sutures on the posterior and anterior aspects of the incision. The GDA typically traverses north to south (12 o'clock, and 6 o'clock) under the ulcer, which can individually be controlled with three independent stitches using PDS. There should be a superior and inferior U-stitches to control the GDA and a medial stitch to control the transverse pancreatic branches that are typically at 3 o'clock underneath the ulcer.

The common bile duct (CBD) is located lateral to the GDA, so caution must be taken when placing the superior and inferior stitches, as to not injure the CBD. If there is any concern for proximity to the common bile duct, a Fogarty catheter or choledochoscope should be threaded into the CBD from the cystic duct or cystic-CBD junction and palpated during this suture ligation.

The incision should then be closed transversely via Heineke-Mikulicz pyloroplasty and a truncal vagotomy performed if the patient has a history of failed medical management.

Case #3: Aorto-Enteric Fistula

Scenario:
65Y male patient with history of hypertension, prior open abdominal aortic aneurysm repair with Dacron graft presenting with hematemesis and syncope. He is tachycardic and hypotensive to 90/60 but mentating with mild mid-epigastric abdominal pain. Two large-bore IVs are placed and two units of packed red blood cells transfused. Given his history, a CTA is obtained, and demonstrates air around his graft concerning for aorto-enteric fistula (Fig. 31.5).

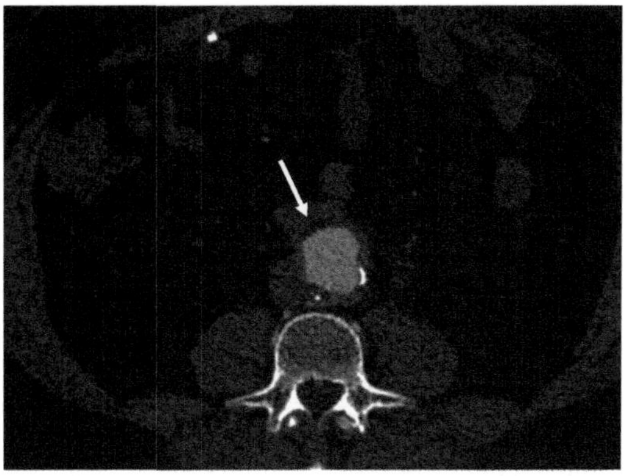

Fig. 31.5 Air outside of and proximal to aorto-bifemoral graft. (Courtesy of Fatemeh Malekpour, MD; Department of Vascular Surgery, University of Texas Southwestern Medical Center)

Patients with prior aortic intervention, particularly open aortic bypass (aorto-bifemoral, abdominal aortic aneurysm) are at risk for developing this potentially fatal complication [83]. Aorto-enteric fistula is a result of graft inflammation, most commonly at the proximal anastomosis between the third and fourth portions of the duodenum.

A thorough history and physical is critical to excluding this diagnosis as soon as possible in patients with UGIH. Patients may present with the classic "sentinel bleed" with large volume hematemesis or melena, which may cease and then propagate into massive hemorrhage. Endoscopy may demonstrate a large ulceration of the third portion of the duodenum [84]. CTA is often performed initially given the patient's history of aortic instrumentation and may show extravasation into the duodenum, although air around the graft is a more common radiologic finding in more stable patients that can undergo CTA.

Other adjuncts or equipment to consider:

- Endovascular balloon occlusion.

Approach:
Major tenets to this operation include: (1) obtain hemorrhage control, (2) ligate and protect the

proximal aortic stump, (3) washout and control of enteric contents, and (4) extra-anatomic bypass or replacement.

A generous laparotomy incision is created and right medial visceral rotation is performed to expose the second and third portion of the duodenum. Proximal aortic control should be obtained, endovascular technique is recommended, and a side-biting clamp placed on the aorta proximal to the fistula as the para-aortic tissues tend to be friable. The fistula is then taken down, and the graft removed in its entirety. The remaining aortic cuff is ligated and covered with an omental flap, if available. The wound bed is washed out and irrigated thoroughly and the enteric portion of the fistula—typically the third portion of the duodenum, requires excision and bypass (Fig. 31.6).

Options include primary repair, patch repair, and fistula-takedown with resection and primary anastomosis. Primary and patch repair with omentum or serosal patch are unlikely to heal given a chronic inflammatory state. Therefore, duodenojejunostomy may be required. The bed should be widely drained and distal feeding access obtained.

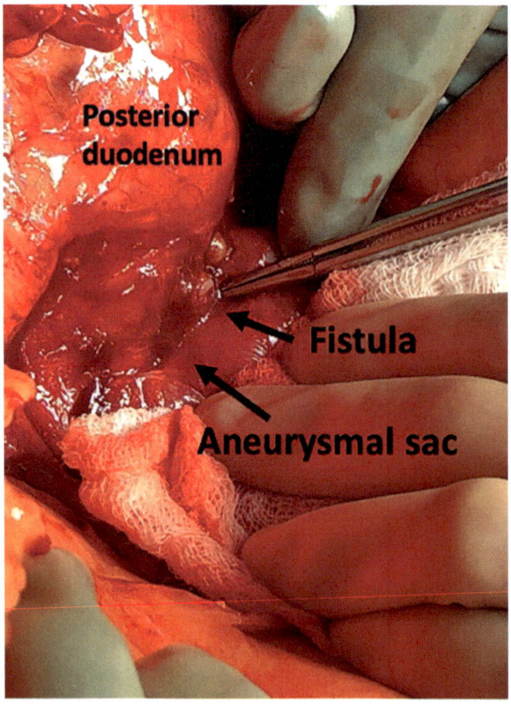

Fig. 31.6 Intra-operative findings of aorto-enteric fistula. (Courtesy of Fatemeh Malekpour, MD; Department of Vascular Surgery, University of Texas Southwestern Medical Center)

A critical step is restoring aortic continuity, which typically consists of extra-anatomic bypass (axillo-bifemoral) in a more controlled situation or rifampin-soaked graft placement in-situ. There are more recent explorations in endovascular replacement in this setting, but have not been widely studied, and have been typically employed for palliative purposes [84].

Key Points

- Establish access early and resuscitate
- Early endoscopy for patients with hemodynamic instability
- Localize bleed with endoscopy for suspected PUD
- Pursue interventional percutaneous embolization after failed endoscopy
- Localize bleed with CTA for suspected aorto-enteric fistula
- Consider other adjuncts in the operating room, including on-table endoscopy, choledochoscopy, or Fogarty catheter to identify the common bile duct, endovascular occlusion of the aorta

Take-Home Points

- Upper gastrointestinal hemorrhage remains a morbid condition with associated complications, prolonged length of stay, and utilization of resources. Early diagnosis, resuscitation, and hemorrhage control are critical to mitigating these complications.
- A thorough history, including medical, surgical history, and medications, is essential to triaging an upper versus lower GIH with decreased time to appropriate intervention.
- Endoscopy is the standard of care in diagnosis and should be performed early in patients with hemodynamic instability.
- Repeat endoscopy may be utilized in patients with high-risk lesions, however other diagnos-

tic and therapeutic modalities, such as CTA or percutaneous angiography, should be considered early in the algorithm.

- Indications for surgery include failure of the above modalities, hemodynamic instability, or ongoing transfusions.

References

1. van Leerdam ME. Epidemiology of acute upper gastrointestinal bleeding. Best Pract Res Clin Gastroenterol. 2008;22(2):209–24.
2. Hearnshaw SA, et al. Acute upper gastrointestinal bleeding in the UK: patient characteristics, diagnoses and outcomes in the 2007 UK audit. Gut. 2011;60(10):1327–35.
3. Roberts SE, Button LA, Williams JG. Prognosis following upper gastrointestinal bleeding. PLoS One. 2012;7(12):e49507.
4. Saltzman JR, et al. A simple risk score accurately predicts in-hospital mortality, length of stay, and cost in acute upper GI bleeding. Gastrointest Endosc. 2011;74(6):1215–24.
5. Cook DJ, et al. The attributable mortality and length of intensive care unit stay of clinically important gastrointestinal bleeding in critically ill patients. Crit Care. 2001;5(6):368–75.
6. Adler DG, et al. ASGE guideline: the role of endoscopy in acute non-variceal upper-GI hemorrhage. Gastrointest Endosc. 2004;60(4):497–504.
7. Lau JY, et al. Challenges in the management of acute peptic ulcer bleeding. Lancet. 2013;381(9882):2033–43.
8. Larson G, et al. Upper gastrointestinal bleeding: predictors of outcome. Surgery. 1986;100(4):765–73.
9. al-Assi MT, et al. Ulcer site and complications: relation to Helicobacter pylori infection and NSAID use. Endoscopy. 1996;28(2):229–33.
10. Rockall TA, et al. Variation in outcome after acute upper gastrointestinal haemorrhage. The National Audit of Acute Upper Gastrointestinal Haemorrhage. Lancet. 1995;346(8971):346–50.
11. Strodel WE, et al. Intraoperative fiberoptic endoscopy. Am Surg. 1984;50(6):340–4.
12. Bharucha AE, Gostout CJ, Balm RK. Clinical and endoscopic risk factors in the Mallory-Weiss syndrome. Am J Gastroenterol. 1997;92(5):805–8.
13. Johnson DC, et al. Gastric lipomas: a rare cause of massive upper gastrointestinal bleeding. Am J Gastroenterol. 1981;75(4):299–301.
14. Sharon P, Stalnikovicz R, Rachmilewitz D. Endoscopic diagnosis of duodenal neoplasms causing upper gastrointestinal bleeding. J Clin Gastroenterol. 1982;4(1):35–8.
15. Savides TJ, et al. Severe upper gastrointestinal tumor bleeding: endoscopic findings, treatment, and outcome. Endoscopy. 1996;28(2):244–8.
16. Camus M, et al. Severe upper gastrointestinal hemorrhage from linear gastric ulcers in large hiatal hernias: a large prospective case series of Cameron ulcers. Endoscopy. 2013;45(5):397–400.
17. Gray DM, et al. Cameron lesions in patients with hiatal hernias: prevalence, presentation, and treatment outcome. Dis Esophagus. 2015;28(5):448–52.
18. Kruger R, et al. Diffuse vascular ectasia of the gastric antrum. Am J Gastroenterol. 1987;82(5):421–6.
19. Novitsky YW, et al. Watermelon stomach: pathophysiology, diagnosis, and management. J Gastrointest Surg. 2003;7(5):652–61.
20. Lambert CJ Jr, Williamson JW. Splenic artery aneurysm. A rare cause of upper gastrointestinal bleeding. Am Surg. 1990;56(9):543–5.
21. Aboujaoude M, et al. Pseudoaneurysm of the proper hepatic artery with duodenal fistula appearing as a late complication of blunt abdominal trauma. J Trauma. 1996;40(1):123–5.
22. Yeh TS, et al. Massive extra-enteric gastrointestinal hemorrhage secondary to splanchnic artery aneurysms. Hepato-Gastroenterology. 1997;44(16):1152–6.
23. Saeed M, et al. Bleeding following endoscopic sphincterotomy: angiographic management by transcatheter embolization. Gastrointest Endosc. 1989;35(4):300–3.
24. Gralnek IM, et al. Diagnosis and management of non-variceal upper gastrointestinal hemorrhage: European Society of Gastrointestinal Endoscopy (ESGE) guideline. Endoscopy. 2015;47(10):a1–46.
25. Feinman M, Haut ER. Upper gastrointestinal bleeding. Surg Clin North Am. 2014;94(1):43–53.
26. Baradarian R, et al. Early intensive resuscitation of patients with upper gastrointestinal bleeding decreases mortality. Am J Gastroenterol. 2004;99(4):619–22.
27. Kumar M, et al. Thromboelastography-guided blood component use in patients with cirrhosis with nonvariceal bleeding: a randomized controlled trial. Hepatology. 2020;71(1):235–46.
28. Marik PE, Corwin HL. Efficacy of red blood cell transfusion in the critically ill: a systematic review of the literature. Crit Care Med. 2008;36(9):2667–74.
29. Villanueva C, et al. Transfusion strategies for acute upper gastrointestinal bleeding. N Engl J Med. 2013;368(1):11–21.
30. Barkun AN, et al. Management of nonvariceal upper gastrointestinal bleeding: guideline recommendations from the International Consensus Group. Ann Intern Med. 2019;171(11):805–22.
31. Rehman A, et al. Prophylactic endotracheal intubation in critically ill patients undergoing endoscopy for upper GI hemorrhage. Gastrointest Endosc. 2009;69(7):e55–9.
32. Hayat U, et al. Association of prophylactic endotracheal intubation in critically ill patients with upper

GI bleeding and cardiopulmonary unplanned events. Gastrointest Endosc. 2017;86(3):500–509.e1.
33. Rudolph SJ, Landsverk BK, Freeman ML. Endotracheal intubation for airway protection during endoscopy for severe upper GI hemorrhage. Gastrointest Endosc. 2003;57(1):58–61.
34. Palamidessi N, et al. Nasogastric aspiration and lavage in emergency department patients with hematochezia or melena without hematemesis. Acad Emerg Med. 2010;17(2):126–32.
35. Srygley FD, et al. Does this patient have a severe upper gastrointestinal bleed? JAMA. 2012;307(10):1072–9.
36. Aljebreen AM, Fallone CA, Barkun AN. Nasogastric aspirate predicts high-risk endoscopic lesions in patients with acute upper-GI bleeding. Gastrointest Endosc. 2004;59(2):172–8.
37. Blatchford O, Murray WR, Blatchford M. A risk score to predict need for treatment for upper-gastrointestinal haemorrhage. Lancet. 2000;356(9238):1318–21.
38. Rockall TA, et al. Risk assessment after acute upper gastrointestinal haemorrhage. Gut. 1996;38(3):316–21.
39. McGuirk TD, Coyle WJ. Upper gastrointestinal tract bleeding. Emerg Med Clin North Am. 1996;14(3):523–45.
40. Fennerty MB. Pathophysiology of the upper gastrointestinal tract in the critically ill patient: rationale for the therapeutic benefits of acid suppression. Crit Care Med. 2002;30(6 Suppl):S351–5.
41. Conrad SA, et al. Randomized, double-blind comparison of immediate-release omeprazole oral suspension versus intravenous cimetidine for the prevention of upper gastrointestinal bleeding in critically ill patients. Crit Care Med. 2005;33(4):760–5.
42. Sachar H, Vaidya K, Laine L. Intermittent vs continuous proton pump inhibitor therapy for high-risk bleeding ulcers: a systematic review and meta-analysis. JAMA Intern Med. 2014;174(11):1755–62.
43. Javid G, et al. Comparison of p.o. or i.v. proton pump inhibitors on 72-h intragastric pH in bleeding peptic ulcer. J Gastroenterol Hepatol. 2009;24(7):1236–43.
44. Lau JY, et al. Omeprazole before endoscopy in patients with gastrointestinal bleeding. N Engl J Med. 2007;356(16):1631–40.
45. Lin HJ. Pre-endoscopic PPI therapy reduces recurrent adverse outcomes in acute non-variceal upper gastrointestinal bleeding. Aliment Pharmacol Ther. 2007;25(3):343–4; author reply 344–5.
46. Coffin B, et al. Erythromycin improves the quality of EGD in patients with acute upper GI bleeding: a randomized controlled study. Gastrointest Endosc. 2002;56(2):174–9.
47. Frossard JL, et al. Erythromycin intravenous bolus infusion in acute upper gastrointestinal bleeding: a randomized, controlled, double-blind trial. Gastroenterology. 2002;123(1):17–23.
48. Winstead NS, Wilcox CM. Erythromycin prior to endoscopy for acute upper gastrointestinal haemorrhage: a cost-effectiveness analysis. Aliment Pharmacol Ther. 2007;26(10):1371–7.
49. Bai Y, Guo JF, Li ZS. Meta-analysis: erythromycin before endoscopy for acute upper gastrointestinal bleeding. Aliment Pharmacol Ther. 2011;34(2):166–71.
50. Chang TS, et al. Limited effects of antibiotic prophylaxis in patients with Child-Pugh class A/B cirrhosis and upper gastrointestinal bleeding. PLoS One. 2020;15(2):e0229101.
51. Hussey KP. Vasopressin therapy for upper gastrointestinal tract hemorrhage. Has its efficacy been proven? Arch Intern Med. 1985;145(7):1263–7.
52. Pascal JP, Cales P. Propranolol in the prevention of first upper gastrointestinal tract hemorrhage in patients with cirrhosis of the liver and esophageal varices. N Engl J Med. 1987;317(14):856–61.
53. Kiire CF. Controlled trial of propranolol to prevent recurrent variceal bleeding in patients with non-cirrhotic portal fibrosis. BMJ. 1989;298(6684):1363–5.
54. Webb WA, et al. Endoscopic evaluation of 125 cases of upper gastrointestinal bleeding. Ann Surg. 1981;193(5):624–7.
55. Kanwal F, et al. Measuring quality of care in patients with nonvariceal upper gastrointestinal hemorrhage: development of an explicit quality indicator set. Am J Gastroenterol. 2010;105(8):1710–8.
56. Cooper GS, et al. Early endoscopy in upper gastrointestinal hemorrhage: associations with recurrent bleeding, surgery, and length of hospital stay. Gastrointest Endosc. 1999;49(2):145–52.
57. Guglielmi A, et al. Risk assessment and prediction of rebleeding in bleeding gastroduodenal ulcer. Endoscopy. 2002;34(10):778–86.
58. Siau K, et al. Management of acute upper gastrointestinal bleeding: an update for the general physician. J R Coll Physicians Edinb. 2017;47(3):218–30.
59. Chung SC, et al. Endoscopic injection of adrenaline for actively bleeding ulcers: a randomised trial. Br Med J (Clin Res Ed). 1988;296(6637):1631–3.
60. Kanai M, et al. Efficacy of argon plasma coagulation in nonvariceal upper gastrointestinal bleeding. Endoscopy. 2004;36(12):1085–8.
61. Ljubicic N, et al. Endoclips vs large or small-volume epinephrine in peptic ulcer recurrent bleeding. World J Gastroenterol. 2012;18(18):2219–24.
62. Misra SP, et al. Endoscopic band ligation as salvage therapy in patients with bleeding peptic ulcers not responding to injection therapy. Endoscopy. 2005;37(7):626–9.
63. Prei JC, et al. EndoClot polysaccharide hemostatic system in nonvariceal gastrointestinal bleeding: results of a prospective multicenter observational pilot study. J Clin Gastroenterol. 2016;50(10):e95–e100.
64. Manabe N, et al. Double-balloon enteroscopy in patients with GI bleeding of obscure origin. Gastrointest Endosc. 2006;64(1):135–40.
65. Ren JZ, et al. Lower gastrointestinal bleeding: role of 64-row computed tomographic angiography in diagnosis and therapeutic planning. World J Gastroenterol. 2015;21(13):4030–7.

66. Wu LM, et al. Usefulness of CT angiography in diagnosing acute gastrointestinal bleeding: a meta-analysis. World J Gastroenterol. 2010;16(31):3957–63.
67. Shenoy SS, Bergsland J, Cerra FB. Arterial embolization for traumatic hemobilia with hepato-portal fistula. Cardiovasc Intervent Radiol. 1981;4(3):206–8.
68. Abdel-Aal AK, et al. Embolization of bleeding duodenal ulcer using Amplatzer vascular plug II and hydrogel coils: case report. Vasc Endovasc Surg. 2011;45(3):307–10.
69. Adams DB, Zellner JL, Anderson MC. Arterial hemorrhage complicating pancreatic pseudocysts: role of angiography. J Surg Res. 1993;54(2):150–6.
70. Keller FS, et al. Percutaneous angiographic embolization: a procedure of increasing usefulness: review of a decade of experience. Am J Surg. 1981;142(1):5–13.
71. Yoon W, et al. Acute small bowel hemorrhage in three patients with end-stage renal disease: diagnosis and management by angiographic intervention. Cardiovasc Intervent Radiol. 2002;25(2):133–6.
72. Dempsey DT, et al. Angiography in poor-risk patients with massive nonvariceal upper gastrointestinal bleeding. Am J Surg. 1990;159(3):282–6.
73. Colapinto RF, et al. Formation of intrahepatic portosystemic shunts using a balloon dilatation catheter: preliminary clinical experience. AJR Am J Roentgenol. 1983;140(4):709–14.
74. Kitano S, et al. Laparoscopy-assisted devascularization of the lower esophagus and upper stomach in the management of gastric varices. Endoscopy. 1994;26(5):470–3.
75. Zilberstein B, et al. Video laparoscopy for the treatment of bleeding esophageal varices. Surg Laparosc Endosc. 1997;7(3):185–91.
76. Winzelberg GG, et al. Scintigraphic detection of gastrointestinal bleeding: a review of current methods. Am J Gastroenterol. 1983;78(6):324–7.
77. Chaudhuri TK, Brantly M. Heparin as a pharmacologic intervention to induce positive scintiscan in occult gastrointestinal bleeding. Clin Nucl Med. 1984;9(4):187–8.
78. Voeller GR, Bunch G, Britt LG. Use of technetium-labeled red blood cell scintigraphy in the detection and management of gastrointestinal hemorrhage. Surgery. 1991;110(4):799–804.
79. Delvaux M, Fassler I, Gay G. Clinical usefulness of the endoscopic video capsule as the initial intestinal investigation in patients with obscure digestive bleeding: validation of a diagnostic strategy based on the patient outcome after 12 months. Endoscopy. 2004;36(12):1067–73.
80. Gralnek IM, et al. Capsule endoscopy in acute upper gastrointestinal hemorrhage: a prospective cohort study. Endoscopy. 2013;45(1):12–9.
81. Camprodon RA, Al-Ghnaniem R, Camprodon R. Transgastric surgery for posterior juxtacardial ulcers: a minimal and safe approach. Arch Surg. 2003;138(7):757–61, discovery 762.
82. Samlowski E, et al. Catastrophic bleeding from gastroduodenal artery after whipple procedure managed with resuscitative endovascular balloon occlusion of the aorta. ACG Case Rep J. 2019;6(11):e00283.
83. Moulton S, Adams M, Johansen K. Aortoenteric fistula. A 7 year urban experience. Am J Surg. 1986;151(5):607–11.
84. Song Y, et al. Diagnosis and management of primary aortoenteric fistulas—experience learned from eighteen patients. Surgery. 2008;143(1):43–50.

32 Acute Lower Gastrointestinal Hemorrhage

Amelia Walling Maiga and Bradley M. Dennis

Case Scenario

A 65-year-old male presents with hematochezia. Symptoms began 1 week ago and have been intermittent. Earlier today he became lightheaded and nauseated, prompting his presentation to the emergency room.

Past medical history is pertinent for coronary artery disease and peripheral vascular disease. Past surgical history is pertinent for CABG 5 years ago. Social history is noted for a 30 pack-year smoking history. He takes metoprolol, aspirin, and Plavix.

On exam, patient appears anxious, HR 80s, BP 110/50, RR 22, and O_2 saturations are normal without oxygen. Orthostatics are notable for a drop in the BP to 90/48. Abdomen is obese and non-tender without evidence of ascites or palpable liver or splenomegaly. Digital rectal exams reveal hematochezia without masses or hemorrhoidal disease.

Point of care hemoglobin is 6.8 mg/dL.

Introduction

Acute lower gastrointestinal hemorrhage (LGIH) comprises bleeding originating distal to the ligament of Treitz, including the small bowel, colon, and anorectum. Approximately 20–24% of all major episodes of gastrointestinal hemorrhage are lower [1–3]. The clinical presentation of LGIH ranges from occult melena to intermittent hematochezia to massive bleeding [4]. LGIH is a common challenge encountered by acute care surgeons. Identification and management of the bleeding often necessitates a multidisciplinary approach with the involvement of gastroenterologists, interventional radiologists, surgeons, and intensivists.

A. W. Maiga
Division of Trauma and Surgical Critical Care, Department of Surgery, Vanderbilt University Medical Center, Nashville, TN, USA
e-mail: amelia.w.maiga@vumc.org

B. M. Dennis (✉)
LifeFlight Air Medical Program, Division of Trauma and Surgical Critical Care, Department of Surgery, Vanderbilt University Medical Center, Nashville, TN, USA
e-mail: bradley.m.dennis@vumc.org

M. D. Zielinski, O. Guillamondegui (eds.), *The Acute Management of Surgical Disease*,
https://doi.org/10.1007/978-3-031-07881-1_32

Incidence, Morbidity and Mortality, and Risk Factors.

The annual incidence of LGIH is 0.03% among adults, causing 30,000 deaths and 300,000 hospitalizations in the United States [1, 5]. Most deaths among patients with LGIH are not directly attributable to hemorrhage but rather to underlying comorbidities or nosocomial conditions [6]. LGIH is more common in men and increases in frequency with older age, particularly over 60 years [7].

Identifying the etiology of a LGIH can be particularly challenging due to the intermittent nature of blood loss and broad differential diagnosis. Patient age and history can help guide the differential diagnosis of undifferentiated LGIH. Younger patients are more likely to bleed from small bowel tumors, inflammatory bowel disease, and anatomic abnormalities such as Meckel's diverticulum and Dieulafoy lesions. Patients over age 40 most commonly bleed from angiodysplasias, neoplasms, and diverticulosis [8]. Use of nonsteroidal anti-inflammatory drugs (NSAIDs) is associated with diverticular bleeding [9]. Among patients already hospitalized in the ICU, ischemic colitis and acute hemorrhagic rectal ulcers are most common [10].

Anticoagulants and antiplatelet agents commonly unmask or exacerbate LGIH. Acute coronary syndrome (ACS) deserves special mention because these patients are frequently on antiplatelet agents and may develop LGIH requiring involvement of the acute care surgeon [11–13]. Bleeding is most common in patients with ACS over age 70, and ischemic colitis is the most common etiology of LGIH in this population [14, 15]. Among high-risk cardiac patients, troponin levels and an ECG should be obtained to rule out a silent MI in the setting of a LGIH [16].

Causes of Lower Gastrointestinal Hemorrhage

- **Diverticulosis** causes 20–55% of LGIH and is characterized by acute, painless hematochezia that ranges from indolent to massive [16]. Diverticular bleeding most commonly originates from right-sided diverticula due to rupture of the vasa recta of the marginal artery at the dome of the diverticulum or at the antimesenteric margin [17]. Although most diverticular bleeds are self-limited, up to 25% require intervention. Semi-elective surgical resection is usually offered after a second diverticular bleeding episode because once a second episode has occurred, the risk that a third will follow exceeds 50% [7].
- **Angiodysplasias** are responsible for 3–40% of LGIH and include vascular ectasias, arteriovenous malformations (AVMs), and angiomas due to degeneration of submucosal venules [18–21]. They are particularly common in the elderly and among patients with renal failure and aortic stenosis [22, 23]. Lesions are most common in the cecum and right colon, but they can cause intermittent, recurrent bleeding in any area of the small bowel or colon [24]. Multiple lesions are common. Angiodysplasias are often the diagnosis of exclusion for occult LGIH, particularly in the absence of diverticulosis. AVM bleeding will stop spontaneously in 85–90% of cases but recurs in 25–85%.
- **Colitis** is another frequent cause of LGIH, particularly among hospitalized patients [10, 25]. Colitis can be ischemic, inflammatory, or infectious.
  - ***Ischemic colitis*** causes transient bleeding due to a temporary, reversible reduction in small-vessel mesenteric blood flow, classically occurring in "low-flow" states and affecting the watershed areas of the colon, namely the splenic flexure and the rectosigmoid junction. Ischemic colitis is diagnosed as dusky mucosa on colonoscopy. Ischemic colitis rarely causes massive bleeding.
  - ***Inflammatory colitis*** includes inflammatory bowel disease (IBD), ulcerative colitis, and Crohn's disease. Bleeding can occur with either disease but is more common with Crohn's disease [26]. Clinical or family history usually suggests this diagnosis.
  - ***Infectious colitis*** in the immunocompetent patient is most commonly attributable to *Clostridium difficile* infection.
- **Anorectal** sources of LGIH account for 2–11% of acute severe hematochezia [5, 7, 27]. Hemorrhoids are common. Acute hemor-

rhagic rectal ulcer syndrome (AHRUS), while infrequent overall, is a relatively common cause of LGIH in the ICU [10]. AHRUS is characterized by massive, painless hematochezia in elderly bedridden patients with severe comorbidities [28, 29]. The pathophysiology is thought to be a stress-related mucosal injury. The ulcers appear endoscopically as single or multiple round Dieulafoy-like lesions in the lower rectum.

- **Neoplasm** is an uncommon cause of LGIH, and the associated bleeding tends to be insidious rather than massive. However, any patient with a family history of colorectal cancer or not up to date on colorectal screening merits a complete colonoscopy to exclude a neoplasm as the cause for LGIH [16, 30].
- **Dieulafoy lesions** can also affect the small intestine and colon and should also be included in the differential diagnosis of LGIH. In particular, stercocal ulceration from the pressure of solid stools in the colon can cause rupture of submucosal arterioles and precipitate unpredictable, massive bleeding [31, 32].
- **Recent interventions** can also cause LGIH, particularly polypectomies [33]. Post-polypectomy bleeding comprises 2–5% of LGIH and is the most likely cause of bleeding in the patient with a history of a recent colonoscopy and polypectomy. Most cases resolve without intervention, but these are most amenable to endoscopic intervention.
- **Other** less common etiologies include Meckel's diverticula in patients under 30 years, NSAID-induced coagulopathy, radiation proctitis in those with a history of pelvic radiation, CMV ulcers in the immunosuppressed population, and aortoenteric fistulae in patients with a history of aortic aneurysm repair.

Early Management

The management of an acute LGIH includes initial stabilization, bleeding localization, and site-specific interventions. Initial stabilization of acute LGIH mirrors that of acute UGIH – prioritization of the patient's airway, breathing, and circulation, including ensuring adequate IV access, blood product resuscitation, and correction of any coagulopathies. Of note, it may take up to 24 h for the hematocrit to equilibrate and accurately reflect blood loss.

Treatment options for LGIH include medical, endoscopic, angiographic, and surgical. The majority of cases of LGIH (>80%) respond to conservative management and/or stop spontaneously. Approximately 20% will require intervention and 5% will require surgery.

A careful and directed history and physical examination will guide localization and subsequent management. Faster passage of blood through the GI tract (i.e., less than 5 h) classically presents with hematochezia, whereas blood present in the GI tract for >20 h almost always presents as melena [34]. Guaiac and other fecal occult blood tests are rarely relevant for the massive LGIH patient population for which acute care surgeons are typically involved.

History should review any associated symptoms (i.e., abdominal pain, changes in bowel habits, weight loss, dizziness, other evidence of shock), previous surgeries and radiation, prior bleeding episodes, medications, and known coagulopathies. A careful physical exam includes a full set of vital signs, orthostatics, focused cardiopulmonary exam, complete abdominal exam, assessment for signs of liver disease, surgical scars, and a rectal exam. Standard laboratory tests should be sent including a complete blood count, complete metabolic panel, coagulation studies, and type and cross-match.

Rule Out Upper GIB and Anorectal Etiology

Early placement of an NGT and gastric washout is critical to identify the 10–15% of patients with an UGIH presenting instead with acute LGIH [35, 36]. Of note, approximately 20% of cases of UGIH may not yield bloody NGT output due to a duodenal source, and upper endoscopy is needed to rule out an UGIH in the case of non-bilious aspirate. Please refer to the first part of this chapter for further workup of UGIH.

After excluding an UGI source, bedside visual rectal and digital rectal exam is essential to rule out obvious anorectal causes of bleeding and confirm the color and quantity of the bleeding. Anoscopy or rigid sigmoidoscopy should be used as needed to supplement the rectal exam. Importantly, identification of an anorectal lesion does not obviate the need for proximal endoscopic evaluation in the context of ongoing hemorrhage.

Medical Management

In contrast to UGIH, medications do not play a key role in the management of LGIH, aside from IBD-directed therapies. Hormonal therapy with estrogen/progesterone compounds can be attempted as part of medical management of LGIH attributed to angiodysplasia, but recent reports suggest these are ineffective [37, 38].

Endoscopic Management

In a hemodynamically stable LGIH patient, colonoscopy should be the first intervention of choice [29, 39] (Fig. 32.1). Colonoscopy is important for diagnosing and potentially treating hemorrhagic pathologies, but also for localizing pathologies not amenable to endoscopic treatment. Localization of bleeding allows for more directed surgical therapy. Colonoscopy is consistently the most accurate methodology of diagnosing the cause of a LGIH, with a diagnostic yield above 75% in large studies [35, 40–44]. It can be performed on unprepped bowel with variable accuracy, but works best after a thorough bowel preparation, ideally within 24 h of the LGIH. Stigmata of bleeding are rarely identified on examinations delayed beyond 24 h in the absence of ongoing hemorrhage.

Diagnostic colonoscopy has a complication rate of 0.3–0.5%, and endoscopic interventions raise that to an acceptable 1.3% [45–47]. Bedside colonoscopy can be even safely performed in most patients with UGIH in the ICU [10].

Diverticuli are often visualized, particularly in most patients over age 50, but it is hard to definitely identify them as responsible for the hemorrhage (Fig. 32.2). Angiodysplasias may appear as flat, red lesions 2–10 mm in size, sometimes accompanied by a feeding vessel.

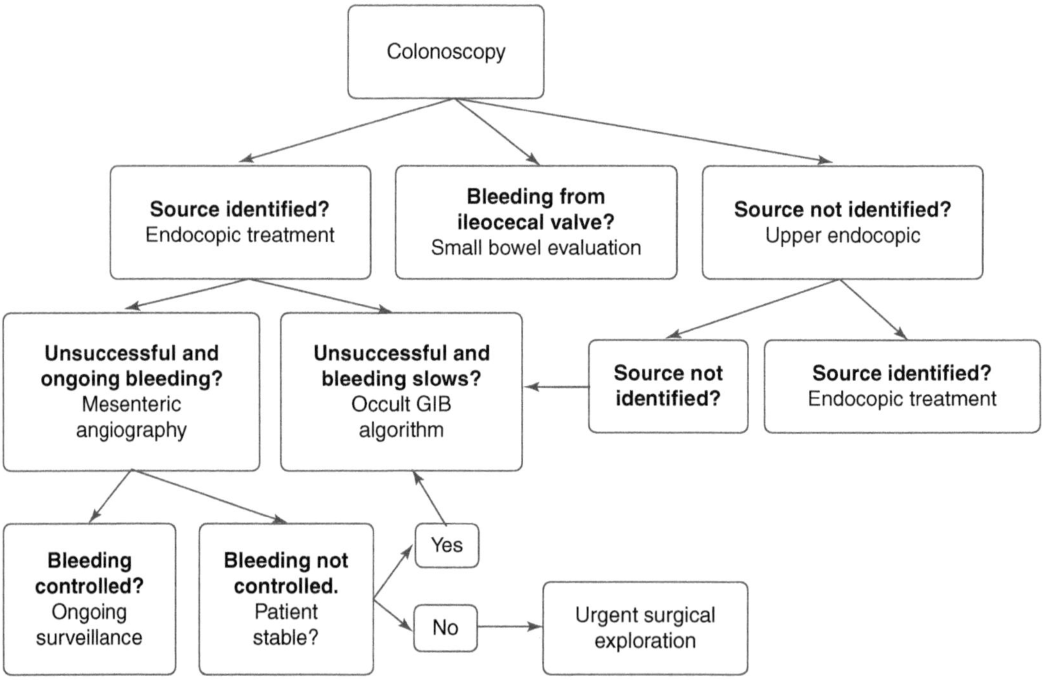

Fig. 32.1 Approach to the hemodynamically stable LGIH

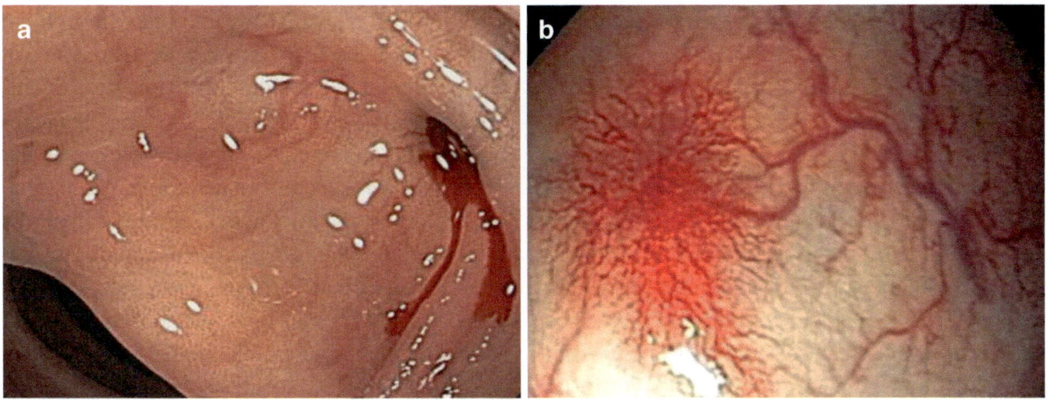

Fig. 32.2 Diverticula with active bleeding (**a**) and arteriovenous malformation (**b**)

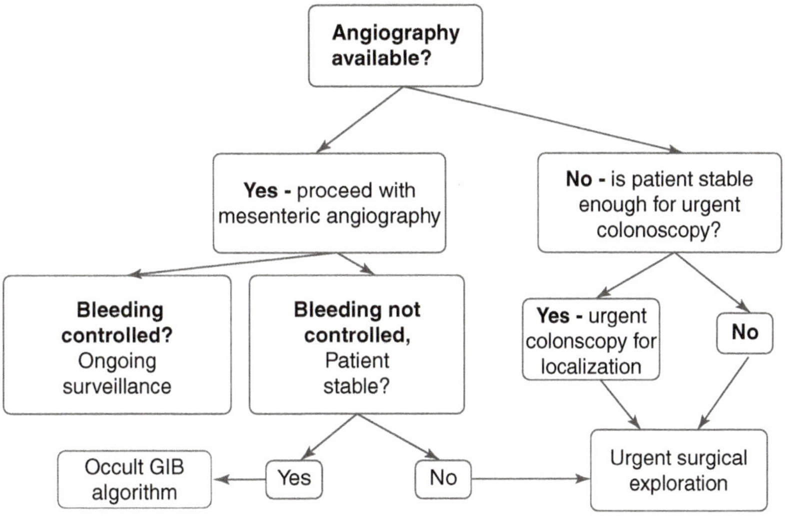

Fig. 32.3 Approach to the hemodynamically unstable LGIH

However, angiodysplasias detected during colonoscopy for LGIH should not automatically be assumed to be the source of bleeding unless there is active bleeding or stigmata of recent bleeding such as adherent clot, which is rare.

If the LGIH source is identified on colonoscopy, endoscopic treatment may be attempted.

Endoscopic interventions may include epinephrine injection, cautery, and hemoclips. However, in contrast to upper endoscopy, colonoscopy is often only diagnostic for LGIH.

If the entire colon is adequately inspected and no source of bleeding found, the terminal ileum should be intubated. Fresh blood in the terminal ileum reflects a small bowel source of the LGIH. If a bleeding source is not found, additional workup should be pursued to identify the bleeding before any attempt at operative management, including upper endoscopy and angiogram/CTA.

In a hemodynamically unstable patient, the diagnostic and therapeutic yield of an urgent colonoscopy is limited. Angiodysplasias are difficult to visualize in unstable patients with mesenteric vascular constriction. A timely middle-of-the-night unprepped colonoscopy is only helpful in select situations—e.g., when interventional radiology capabilities are unavailable and the patient is stable enough to undergo an attempt at localization prior to urgent surgical resection (Fig. 32.3).

Angiography

For the persistent LGIH that fails to respond to conservative management, mesenteric angiography is the next procedure of choice. Angiography has the added benefit of being potentially therapeutic as well as diagnostic. In some centers, cross-sectional imaging in the form of a CTA is routinely obtained prior to angiography to visualize bleeding (at least 0.3 cc/min) and help direct site-specific interventional radiology (IR) treatments. However, a pre-procedural CTA is not mandatory.

Angiography was first reported for the treatment of LGIH in the 1970s. Angiography successfully localizes the bleeding in 40–86% of patients with LGIH [47–49]. Of note, bleeding must be at least 0.5 cc/min in order to be detected on angiography [45]. Rapid, profuse bleeding is most easily identified. In one study, a systolic blood pressure <90 mmHg and the need for at least 5 units of blood had an 85% positive predictive value for bleeding localization [50].

Extravasation can be arrested with coil or gelfoam embolization with single-digit complication rates in the short-term [51]. Rates of downstream bowel ischemia initially ranged from 10% to 20%, but the routine use of superselective angioembolization has improved clinical success rates while lowering the risk of both ischemia and rebleeding [52–56]. Superselective embolization is an effective rescue treatment modality after failed endoscopic management. It has also almost entirely replaced catheter-directed vasoconstrictive therapy, thus avoiding the potential deleterious systemic effects of vasopressin administration. Other complications of angiography include access site complications, contrast reactions, and embolism from dislodged thrombus [57].

If embolization is not possible but a bleeding vessel is localized as contrast extravasation on angiography, the area should be marked to aid in intraoperative identification and segmental resection. Methylene blue can either be injected into the bleeding vessel while the patient is in the IR suite, or the superselective catheter can be left in place for the surgery. In the operating room, injecting 0.5 mL of methylene blue through the catheter will help to localize the segment for resection while avoiding diffusion of the dye throughout the operative field. Leaving the embolization catheter in place can also facilitate urgent operations for ischemia related to coil placement. Depending on the thickness of the mesentery, the coils can be difficult to palpate in some patients.

Some controversy exists regarding whether massive LGIH with hemodynamic compromise should be treated first with angiography, surgery, or colonoscopy. Colonoscopy in the unstable, unprepped, actively bleeding patient is rarely beneficial [1, 45]. Our preference is to proceed with urgent angiography before colonoscopy in this patient population, with or without CT angiography to define extravasation. Patients should only be sent for non-therapeutic localization studies if they are hemodynamically stable.

Approach to the Occult LGIH

Approximately 5% of patients will fall into the category of having an *occult* or *obscure GI bleeding*, defined as ongoing or recurrent bleeding without source on upper and lower endoscopy [58–60]. Repeat endoscopy may occasionally identify the source not seen on first examination [61, 62].

The small intestine is the "great unknown" for LGIH, responsible for one-third of all cases of LGIH yet arguably the majority of the diagnostic headaches [35, 47, 63, 64]. Various options exist to evaluate the small bowel endoscopically and radiographically. Cross-sectional imaging is most useful for identifying masses that may or may not be responsible for the bleeding. This includes standard contrasted CT, CT angiography (CTA), and CT enterography (CTE). CTA is occasionally useful in identifying colonic angiodysplasias [65].

CTE is a multiphase CT with both IV and oral contrast after patients have fasted for 4 h. Interpretation of these studies can be challenging, as 2-mm slices in both axial and coronal planes covering the entire abdomen and pelvis repeated for all three phases generate 1500–2500 images to review. CTE also involves significant patient radiation dose (approximately 35–40 mSv), which is most relevant in younger adults with an occult LGIH.

Options to evaluate the small intestine endoscopically include push enteroscopy, double-balloon endoscopy (DBE), capsule endoscopy, and intraoperative endoscopy. Intraoperative endoscopy is a messy, frustrating endeavor best only undertaken when other localization options have been unsuccessful. The lack of retroperitoneal attachments of the small attachments renders endoscopic navigation uniquely challenging. Push enteroscopy allows evaluation of anywhere from 60 to 160 cm of the proximal jejunum, depending on whether an overtube is used to prevent looping in the stomach [66]. Depending on the indication and technique used, diagnostic yield from push enteroscopy ranges from 13% to 78% [67].

DBE is technically challenging but, in theory, permits evaluation of the entire small bowel [68, 69]. DBE involves a specialized enteroscope with an overtube and two inflatable balloons. Once the distal end of the endoscope is reached, the overtube balloon is inflated, and the overtube and endoscope are gently withdrawn, causes pleating of the small intestine over the overtube/endoscope assembly. The endoscope balloon is then deflated, the endoscope is advanced further, and the entire process is repeated. While the goal is to reach the ileocecal valve, a retrograde approach may be necessary to do so.

Capsule endoscopy is a low-risk, well-tolerated diagnostic procedure that may aid in localizing a bleeding small bowel lesion, particularly if it is actively bleeding [70, 71]. Entrapment is an infrequent problem, and often occurs at the site of pathology, essentially marking it for segmental resection [72]. Clinical guidelines vary in their support for the use of capsule endoscopy due to low-quality data [73, 74].

Radionuclide studies, including ^{99m}Tc-labeled sulfur colloid scans and ^{99m}Tc-labeled tagged red blood cell scans, are noninvasive tests that may help detect slower active bleeding (0.1 cc/min) [75, 76]. These modalities may be over-represented in the literature and rarely provide clinically relevant localization. Of concern, radionuclide results are frequently either non-diagnostic or may result in a high proportion of incorrect segmental resections [77–81]. Anatomically selective colon resections for LGIB should never be performed based on localization obtained through radionuclide scanning alone. In the pediatric population, a Meckel's scan is still a useful, highly sensitive adjunct [81, 82].

Provocative Angiography

For experienced centers, provocative mesenteric angiography is an option if the initial angiography and other localization studies all fail to localize a recurrent bleed. Provocative angiography should only be attempted at specialized centers and with the close cooperation of a surgical team to ensure prompt operative management of uncontrolled bleeding [83]. It successfully identifies the source of LGIH about 33% of the time [84]. Protocols vary by institution but often involve a stacked approach. For example, a bolus of systemic heparin is first given (e.g., 5000 units IV followed by an infusion of 1000 units per hour). Next, 100 mcg of nitroglycerin is infused in the mesenteric vessel of interest followed by tissue plasminogen activator (tPA) in 5–10 mg increments until the desired effect is achieved. Typically, the SMA injected first, then the IMA, and finally the celiac trunk if provocation in the first two vessels is negative. As with non-provocative angiography, if extravasation is visualized but bleeding is not controlled, the catheter can be left in place in the vessel until management in the operating room.

Surgical Management

While only necessary in approximately 5% of patients with LGIH, surgical management plays an important role. Surgical resection should be reserved for bleeding lesions that are persistent or unable to be controlled with endoscopic or catheter-based interventions. Surgery equates to either a targeted or blind resection. Preoperative localization with the workup described above is ideal (e.g., colonoscopic tattoo, angiographic methylene blue injection, or positive Meckel's scan) as it facilitates a segmental resection of the affected area. In stable patients, open or laparoscopic approaches are both acceptable. Segmental resection with primary anastomosis is often feasible in patients who are stable and have localized, discrete bleeds. For more extensive bleeding etiologies, like ischemic colitis or inflammatory colitis, resection and anastomosis may not be advisable.

Unfortunately, the bleeding source is not always clearly identified preoperatively. Surgical exploration is occasionally necessary for patients with hemodynamic instability and persistent hemorrhage that has precluded further diagnostic workup [85]. Open exploration and resection should be performed for patients with unstable LGIH or unlocalized LGIH. As a general rule, blind segmental resections are ill-advised as they are associated with rebleeding rates as high as 75% and mortality as high as 50% [86, 87]. Few situations are more frustrating than an occult LGIH that cannot be localized intraoperatively. Exploration includes a thorough running of the entire small and large bowel to rule out any palpable lesions. Options in this scenario include intraoperative endoscopy with its limitations, a subtotal colectomy, and a temporizing or diagnostic ileostomy. While none of these are appealing, the least bad option in an unstable patient is a "blind" subtotal colectomy with end ileostomy. This procedure is associated with a ~4% rebleeding rate and mortality ranging from 20% to 50% [88].

Key Points

- Establish access early and resuscitate.
- Localize and stop bleed with colonoscopy followed by angiography.
- Occult GIB can be localized with a combination of cross-sectional imaging, endoscopic, and nuclear medicine techniques.
- Subtotal colectomy with end ileostomy is the procedure of choice in an unstable patient with an unlocalized LGIH.

Conclusion

- Most acute LGIH is self-limited. Only 20% require intervention and only 5% require surgery.
- Rule out an upper gastrointestinal source of an acute LGIH and obvious anorectal source early.
- Colonoscopy should be performed first except in cases of hemodynamic instability.
- Angiography is both diagnostic and therapeutic and should be performed early in cases of hemodynamic instability.
- Practically speaking, colonoscopy, angiography, and capsule endoscopy are most likely to assist in bleeding localization.
- Occult LGIH can occasionally be localized using push or double-balloon endoscopy, nuclear medicine scans, and in select cases, provocative angiography.
- Do not operate blindly if at all possible. Subtotal colectomy is the resection of choice with uncontrolled bleeding that cannot be further localized.

References

1. Peura DA, Lanza FL, Gostout CJ, Foutch PG. The American College of Gastroenterology Bleeding Registry: preliminary findings. Am J Gastroenterol. 1997;92(6):924–8.
2. Gostout C. Acute lower GI bleeding. In: Brandt L, editor. Current medicine clinical practice of gastroenterology. Philadelphia, PA: Churchill Livingstone; 1998. p. 651–62.
3. Zuccaro G. Management of the adult patient with acute lower gastrointestinal bleeding. American College of Gastroenterology. Practice Parameters Committee. Am J Gastroenterol. 1998;93(8):1202–8.
4. Proctor DD. Critical issues in digestive diseases. Clin Chest Med. 2003;24(4):623–32.
5. Bramley PN, Masson JW, McKnight G, Herd K, Fraser A, Park K, et al. The role of an open-access bleeding unit in the management of colonic haemorrhage. A 2-year prospective study. Scand J Gastroenterol. 1996;31(8):764–9.
6. Feinman M, Haut ER. Lower gastrointestinal bleeding. Surg Clin N Am. 2014;94(1):55–63.
7. Longstreth GF. Epidemiology and outcome of patients hospitalized with acute lower gastrointestinal hemor-

rhage: a population-based study. Am J Gastroenterol. 1997;92(3):419–24.
8. Mujica VR, Barkin JS. Occult gastrointestinal bleeding. General overview and approach. Gastrointest Endosc Clin N Am. 1996;6(4):833–45.
9. Laine L, Connors LG, Reicin A, Hawkey CJ, Burgos-Vargas R, Schnitzer TJ, et al. Serious lower gastrointestinal clinical events with nonselective NSAID or coxib use. Gastroenterology. 2003;124(2):288–92.
10. Lin CC, Lee YC, Lee H, Lin JT, Ho WC, Chen TH, et al. Bedside colonoscopy for critically ill patients with acute lower gastrointestinal bleeding. Intensive Care Med. 2005;31(5):743–6.
11. Bhatti N, Amoateng-Adjepong Y, Qamar A, Manthous CA. Myocardial infarction in critically ill patients presenting with gastrointestinal hemorrhage: retrospective analysis of risks and outcomes. Chest. 1998;114(4):1137–42.
12. Bellotto F, Fagiuoli S, Pavei A, Gregory SA, Cati A, Silverj E, et al. Anemia and ischemia: myocardial injury in patients with gastrointestinal bleeding. Am J Med. 2005;118(5):548–51.
13. Cappell MS. A study of the syndrome of simultaneous acute upper gastrointestinal bleeding and myocardial infarction in 36 patients. Am J Gastroenterol. 1995;90(9):1444–9.
14. Cappell MS. Gastrointestinal bleeding associated with myocardial infarction. Gastroenterol Clin N Am. 2000;29(2):423–44, vi.
15. Cappell MS. Risks versus benefits of flexible sigmoidoscopy after myocardial infarction: an analysis of 78 patients at three medical centers. Am J Med. 2004;116(10):707–10.
16. Foutch PG. Diverticular bleeding: are nonsteroidal anti-inflammatory drugs risk factors for hemorrhage and can colonoscopy predict outcome for patients? Am J Gastroenterol. 1995;90(10):1779–84.
17. Meyers MA, Alonso DR, Baer JW. Pathogenesis of massively bleeding colonic diverticulosis: new observations. AJR Am J Roentgenol. 1976;127(6):901–8.
18. Boley SJ, Brandt LJ. Vascular ectasias of the colon—1986. Dig Dis Sci. 1986;31(9 Suppl):26S–42S.
19. Boley SJ, DiBiase A, Brandt LJ, Sammartano RJ. Lower intestinal bleeding in the elderly. Am J Surg. 1979;137(1):57–64.
20. Welch CE, Athanasoulis CA, Galdabini JJ. Hemorrhage from the large bowel with special reference to angiodysplasia and diverticular disease. World J Surg. 1978;2(1):73–83.
21. Rogers BH. Endoscopic diagnosis and therapy of mucosal vascular abnormalities of the gastrointestinal tract occurring in elderly patients and associated with cardiac, vascular, and pulmonary disease. Gastrointest Endosc. 1980;26(4):134–8.
22. Marcuard SP, Weinstock JV. Gastrointestinal angiodysplasia in renal failure. J Clin Gastroenterol. 1988;10(5):482–4.
23. Imperiale TF, Ransohoff DF. Aortic stenosis, idiopathic gastrointestinal bleeding, and angiodysplasia: is there an association? A methodologic critique of the literature. Gastroenterology. 1988;95(6):1670–6.
24. Höchter W, Weingart J, Kühner W, Frimberger E, Ottenjann R. Angiodysplasia in the colon and rectum. Endoscopic morphology, localisation and frequency. Endoscopy. 1985;17(5):182–5.
25. Newman JR, Cooper MA. Lower gastrointestinal bleeding and ischemic colitis. Can J Gastroenterol. 2002;16(9):597–600.
26. Pardi DS, Loftus EV, Tremaine WJ, Sandborn WJ, Alexander GL, Balm RK, et al. Acute major gastrointestinal hemorrhage in inflammatory bowel disease. Gastrointest Endosc. 1999;49(2):153–7.
27. Vernava AM, Moore BA, Longo WE, Johnson FE. Lower gastrointestinal bleeding. Dis Colon Rectum. 1997;40(7):846–58.
28. Takeuchi K, Tsuzuki Y, Ando T, Sekihara M, Hara T, Ohno Y, et al. Clinical characteristics of acute hemorrhagic rectal ulcer. J Clin Gastroenterol. 2001;33(3):226–8.
29. Hung HY, Changchien CR, You JF, Chen JS, Chiang JM, Yeh CY, et al. Massive hematochezia from acute hemorrhagic rectal ulcer in patients with severe comorbid illness: rapid control of bleeding by per anal suturing of bleeder using anoretractor. Dis Colon Rectum. 2006;49(2):238–43.
30. Bjarnason I, Hayllar J, MacPherson AJ, Russell AS. Side effects of nonsteroidal anti-inflammatory drugs on the small and large intestine in humans. Gastroenterology. 1993;104(6):1832–47.
31. Franko E, Chardavoyne R, Wise L. Massive rectal bleeding from a Dieulafoy's type ulcer of the rectum: a review of this unusual disease. Am J Gastroenterol. 1991;86(10):1545–7.
32. Abdulian JD, Santoro MJ, Chen YK, Collen MJ. Dieulafoy-like lesion of the rectum presenting with exsanguinating hemorrhage: successful endoscopic sclerotherapy. Am J Gastroenterol. 1993;88(11):1939–41.
33. Suzuki S, Chino A, Kishihara T, Uragami N, Tamegai Y, Suganuma T, et al. Risk factors for bleeding after endoscopic submucosal dissection of colorectal neoplasms. World J Gastroenterol. 2014;20(7):1839–45.
34. Strate LL. Lower GI bleeding: epidemiology and diagnosis. Gastroenterol Clin N Am. 2005;34(4):643–64.
35. Jensen DM, Machicado GA. Diagnosis and treatment of severe hematochezia. The role of urgent colonoscopy after purge. Gastroenterology. 1988;95(6):1569–74.
36. Laine L, Shah A. Randomized trial of urgent vs. elective colonoscopy in patients hospitalized with lower GI bleeding. Am J Gastroenterol. 2010;105(12):2636–41; quiz 42.
37. van Cutsem E, Rutgeerts P, Vantrappen G. Treatment of bleeding gastrointestinal vascular malformations with oestrogen-progesterone. Lancet. 1990;335(8695):953–5.
38. Barkin JS, Ross BS. Medical therapy for chronic gastrointestinal bleeding of obscure origin. Am J Gastroenterol. 1998;93(8):1250–4.

39. Strate LL, Gralnek IM. ACG clinical guideline: management of patients with acute lower gastrointestinal bleeding. Am J Gastroenterol. 2016;111(5):755.
40. Tada M, Shimizu S, Kawai K. Emergency colonoscopy for the diagnosis of lower intestinal bleeding. Gastroenterol Jpn. 1991;26(Suppl 3):121–4.
41. Vellacott KD. Early endoscopy for acute lower gastrointestinal haemorrhage. Ann R Coll Surg Engl. 1986;68(5):243–4.
42. Green BT, Rockey DC, Portwood G, Tarnasky PR, Guarisco S, Branch MS, et al. Urgent colonoscopy for evaluation and management of acute lower gastrointestinal hemorrhage: a randomized controlled trial. Am J Gastroenterol. 2005;100(11):2395–402.
43. Rockey DC. Lower gastrointestinal bleeding. Gastroenterology. 2006;130(1):165–71.
44. Strate LL, Naumann CR. The role of colonoscopy and radiological procedures in the management of acute lower intestinal bleeding. Clin Gastroenterol Hepatol. 2010;8(4):333–43; quiz e44.
45. Zuckerman GR, Prakash C. Acute lower intestinal bleeding: part I: clinical presentation and diagnosis. Gastrointest Endosc. 1998;48(6):606–17.
46. Edelman DA, Sugawa C. Lower gastrointestinal bleeding: a review. Surg Endosc. 2007;21(4):514–20.
47. Leitman IM, Paull DE, Shires GT. Evaluation and management of massive lower gastrointestinal hemorrhage. Ann Surg. 1989;209(2):175–80.
48. Browder W, Cerise EJ, Litwin MS. Impact of emergency angiography in massive lower gastrointestinal bleeding. Ann Surg. 1986;204(5):530–6.
49. Britt LG, Warren L, Moore OF. Selective management of lower gastrointestinal bleeding. Am Surg. 1983;49(3):121–5.
50. Pennoyer WP, Vignati PV, Cohen JL. Mesenteric angiography for lower gastrointestinal hemorrhage: are there predictors for a positive study? Dis Colon Rectum. 1997;40(9):1014–8.
51. Miller M, Smith TP. Angiographic diagnosis and endovascular management of nonvariceal gastrointestinal hemorrhage. Gastroenterol Clin N Am. 2005;34(4):735–52.
52. Rosenkrantz H, Bookstein JJ, Rosen RJ, Goff WB, Healy JF. Postembolic colonic infarction. Radiology. 1982;142(1):47–51.
53. Guy GE, Shetty PC, Sharma RP, Burke MW, Burke TH. Acute lower gastrointestinal hemorrhage: treatment by superselective embolization with polyvinyl alcohol particles. AJR Am J Roentgenol. 1992;159(3):521–6.
54. Funaki B. Endovascular intervention for the treatment of acute arterial gastrointestinal hemorrhage. Gastroenterol Clin N Am. 2002;31(3):701–13.
55. Gordon RL, Ahl KL, Kerlan RK, Wilson MW, LaBerge JM, Sandhu JS, et al. Selective arterial embolization for the control of lower gastrointestinal bleeding. Am J Surg. 1997;174(1):24–8.
56. Luchtefeld MA, Senagore AJ, Szomstein M, Fedeson B, Van Erp J, Rupp S. Evaluation of transarterial embolization for lower gastrointestinal bleeding. Dis Colon Rectum. 2000;43(4):532–4.
57. Egglin TK, O'Moore PV, Feinstein AR, Waltman AC. Complications of peripheral arteriography: a new system to identify patients at increased risk. J Vasc Surg. 1995;22(6):787–94.
58. Spiller RC, Parkins RA. Recurrent gastrointestinal bleeding of obscure origin: report of 17 cases and a guide to logical management. Br J Surg. 1983;70(8):489–93.
59. Thompson JN, Salem RR, Hemingway AP, Rees HC, Hodgson HJ, Wood CB, et al. Specialist investigation of obscure gastrointestinal bleeding. Gut. 1987;28(1):47–51.
60. Raju GS, Gerson L, Das A, Lewis B, Association AG. American Gastroenterological Association (AGA) Institute technical review on obscure gastrointestinal bleeding. Gastroenterology. 2007;133(5):1697–717.
61. Zaman A, Katon RM. Push enteroscopy for obscure gastrointestinal bleeding yields a high incidence of proximal lesions within reach of a standard endoscope. Gastrointest Endosc. 1998;47(5):372–6.
62. Descamps C, Schmit A, Van Gossum A. "Missed" upper gastrointestinal tract lesions may explain "occult" bleeding. Endoscopy. 1999;31(6):452–5.
63. Farrands PA, Taylor I. Management of acute lower gastrointestinal haemorrhage in a surgical unit over a 4-year period. J R Soc Med. 1987;80(2):79–82.
64. Wagner HE, Stain SC, Gilg M, Gertsch P. Systematic assessment of massive bleeding of the lower part of the gastrointestinal tract. Surg Gynecol Obstet. 1992;175(5):445–9.
65. Junquera F, Quiroga S, Saperas E, Pérez-Lafuente M, Videla S, Alvarez-Castells A, et al. Accuracy of helical computed tomographic angiography for the diagnosis of colonic angiodysplasia. Gastroenterology. 2000;119(2):293–9.
66. Taylor AC, Chen RY, Desmond PV. Use of an overtube for enteroscopy—does it increase depth of insertion? A prospective study of enteroscopy with and without an overtube. Endoscopy. 2001;33(3):227–30.
67. Lin S, Branch MS, Shetzline M. The importance of indication in the diagnostic value of push enteroscopy. Endoscopy. 2003;35(4):315–21.
68. Yamamoto H, Kita H, Sunada K, Hayashi Y, Sato H, Yano T, et al. Clinical outcomes of double-balloon endoscopy for the diagnosis and treatment of small-intestinal diseases. Clin Gastroenterol Hepatol. 2004;2(11):1010–6.
69. May A, Nachbar L, Ell C. Double-balloon enteroscopy (push-and-pull enteroscopy) of the small bowel: feasibility and diagnostic and therapeutic yield in patients with suspected small bowel disease. Gastrointest Endosc. 2005;62(1):62–70.
70. Hartmann D, Schmidt H, Bolz G, Schilling D, Kinzel F, Eickhoff A, et al. A prospective two-center study comparing wireless capsule endoscopy with intraoperative enteroscopy in patients with obscure GI bleeding. Gastrointest Endosc. 2005;61(7):826–32.

71. Adler DG, Knipschield M, Gostout C. A prospective comparison of capsule endoscopy and push enteroscopy in patients with GI bleeding of obscure origin. Gastrointest Endosc. 2004;59(4):492–8.
72. Carey EJ, Fleischer DE. Investigation of the small bowel in gastrointestinal bleeding—enteroscopy and capsule endoscopy. Gastroenterol Clin N Am. 2005;34(4):719–34.
73. Gerson LB, Fidler JL, Cave DR, Leighton JA. ACG clinical guideline: diagnosis and management of small bowel bleeding. Am J Gastroenterol. 2015;110(9):1265–87; quiz 88.
74. Pennazio M, Spada C, Eliakim R, Keuchel M, May A, Mulder CJ, et al. Small-bowel capsule endoscopy and device-assisted enteroscopy for diagnosis and treatment of small-bowel disorders: European Society of Gastrointestinal Endoscopy (ESGE) clinical guideline. Endoscopy. 2015;47(4):352–76.
75. Awais M, Haq TU, Rehman A, Zaman MU, Haider Z, Khattak YJ, et al. Accuracy of 99mTechnetium-labeled RBC scintigraphy and MDCT with gastrointestinal bleed protocol for detection and localization of source of acute lower gastrointestinal bleeding. J Clin Gastroenterol. 2016;50(9):754–60.
76. Currie GM, Kiat H, Wheat JM. Scintigraphic evaluation of acute lower gastrointestinal hemorrhage: current status and future directions. J Clin Gastroenterol. 2011;45(2):92–9.
77. Hunter JM, Pezim ME. Limited value of technetium 99m-labeled red cell scintigraphy in localization of lower gastrointestinal bleeding. Am J Surg. 1990;159(5):504–6.
78. Levy R, Barto W, Gani J. Retrospective study of the utility of nuclear scintigraphic-labelled red cell scanning for lower gastrointestinal bleeding. ANZ J Surg. 2003;73(4):205–9.
79. Rantis PC, Harford FJ, Wagner RH, Henkin RE. Technetium-labelled red blood cell scintigraphy: is it useful in acute lower gastrointestinal bleeding? Int J Color Dis. 1995;10(4):210–5.
80. Garofalo TE, Abdu RA. Accuracy and efficacy of nuclear scintigraphy for the detection of gastrointestinal bleeding. Arch Surg. 1997;132(2):196–9.
81. Kong MS, Chen CY, Tzen KY, Huang MJ, Wang KL, Lin JN. Technetium-99m pertechnetate scan for ectopic gastric mucosa in children with gastrointestinal bleeding. J Formos Med Assoc. 1993;92(8):717–20.
82. Sfakianakis GN, Conway JJ. Detection of ectopic gastric mucosa in Meckel's diverticulum and in other aberrations by scintigraphy: II. Indications and methods—a 10-year experience. J Nucl Med. 1981;22(8):732–8.
83. Lin S, Rockey DC. Obscure gastrointestinal bleeding. Gastroenterol Clin N Am. 2005;34(4):679–98.
84. Kim CY, Suhocki PV, Miller MJ, Khan M, Janus G, Smith TP. Provocative mesenteric angiography for lower gastrointestinal hemorrhage: results from a single-institution study. J Vasc Interv Radiol. 2010;21(4):477–83.
85. Marion Y, Lebreton G, Le Pennec V, Hourna E, Viennot S, Alves A. The management of lower gastrointestinal bleeding. J Visc Surg. 2014;151(3):191–201.
86. McGuire HH, Haynes BW. Massive hemorrhage for diverticulosis of the colon: guidelines for therapy based on bleeding patterns observed in fifty cases. Ann Surg. 1972;175(6):847–55.
87. Parkes BM, Obeid FN, Sorensen VJ, Horst HM, Fath JJ. The management of massive lower gastrointestinal bleeding. Am Surg. 1993;59(10):676–8.
88. Setya V, Singer JA, Minken SL. Subtotal colectomy as a last resort for unrelenting, unlocalized, lower gastrointestinal hemorrhage: experience with 12 cases. Am Surg. 1992;58(5):295–9.

Emergency Surgery as a Team Sport

33

Alison A. Smith and Donald Jenkins

Emergency General Surgery Team Dynamics Case Report

A 68-year-old man with multiple co-morbid medical conditions presents to the Emergency Department complaining of abdominal pain for 1 day duration. A clerk immediately notifies the nurse of the patient's arrival. The patient is triaged by a nurse who quickly realizes that the patient is in critical condition. The medical technician records the patient's vital signs, medications, medical history, and contact information in an expeditious manner. She alerts the Emergency Medicine physician who promptly examines the patient, orders laboratory work, and other appropriate diagnostic tests. He then consults the Emergency General surgeon on call after discovering pneumoperitoneum on an X-ray.

After written informed consent and an in-depth discussion with the patient and his family, the patient completes the pre-operative process, and he is brought without delay to the operating room for an exploratory laparotomy. Prior to the case start, the surgeon discussed the operative plan with the operating room (OR) team in detail and ensures that all necessary equipment is present using the Emergency General Surgery (EGS) checklist. The team prepares for any potential pitfalls during the case and confirms that extra equipment is readily available. The surgical team regularly participates in simulation scenarios specific for emergent cases and is familiar with the EGS checklist.

At the start of the case, the surgeon leads the OR team through the standardized timeout prior to initiation of the procedure. All team members actively engage during the timeout. During the case, the OR nurse provides regular updates to the family. The surgeon and Anesthesia team discuss the progression of the case, and how the patient is tolerating anesthesia. The patient is extubated at the conclusion of the case. While being moved to the stretcher, he goes into cardiac arrest. The surgeon serves as the team leader for the code and assigns roles to each team member. The anesthesiologist quickly secures the airway and begins to bag the patient. The circulator nurse is the recorder while the nurse anesthetist administers medication. The scrub tech performs chest compressions alternating with another scrub tech. Return of spontaneous circulation is obtained, and the patient is transported to the (ICU). The surgeon leads a dynamic de-briefing with the operating room team to discuss areas in which the team performed well and where

A. A. Smith (✉)
Division of Trauma/Critical Care/Acute Care, Clinical Surgery, Department of Surgery, Louisiana State University, New Orleans, LA, USA

D. Jenkins
Department of Surgery, University of Texas Health Sciences Center San Antonio, San Antonio, TX, USA
e-mail: JenkinsD4@uthscsa.edu

M. D. Zielinski, O. Guillamondegui (eds.), *The Acute Management of Surgical Disease*,
https://doi.org/10.1007/978-3-031-07881-1_33

improvements could be made. All team members actively participate and freely voice any concerns. The suggested areas for improvement are relayed to the hospital's Quality Improvement Task Force.

While in the ICU, the attending surgeon rounds on the patient daily with a multi-disciplinary team comprised of ICU nurses, nutrition, pharmacy, case management, and physical/occupational therapy. A comprehensive daily plan is developed with all of the team's input. On post-operative day 5, the patient is transferred to an inpatient rehabilitation center. The patient's case data and outcomes are recorded into the hospital's EGS registry.

Background on Emergency General Surgery

Emergency general surgery (EGS) represents a rapidly expanding field of surgical disease. Although EGS was initially recognized as a surgical subspecialty in the early 2000s, it encompasses a wide variety of surgical diagnoses which were first formally defined in 2013 [1–3]. In the past decade, there has been an estimated increase in EGS cases by almost 30% [4]. Despite this vast experience, the population of EGS remains challenging to treat with on-going poor outcomes. EGS patients have an estimated eight-fold increase in mortality and 50% risk of post-operative complications compared to their elective surgery counterparts [5–7]. These patients also have higher rates of medical errors [8]. Some potential sources of the disparate outcomes for EGS patients likely stem from a sicker patient population at baseline with multiple pre-existing and often untreated co-morbid conditions. The sub-optimal circumstances revolving around the nature of EGS operative procedures due to limited time for patient and OR team preparation often lead to high-stress situations and lack of coordination that compound the likelihood of post-operative complications and medical errors [3].

The current costs associated with EGS are staggering with an estimated increase of greater than 40% anticipated over the next four decades [1]. This tremendous projected rise in EGS patients will likely place additional hindrances on an already strained healthcare system in the United States. Given the significant and growing burden of EGS on the medical infrastructure, an important goal in the near future should be to optimize the surgical and ancillary care teams for these high-risk patients.

An Introduction to Teamwork

A team is two or more individuals working together to achieve a shared goal through task-specific competencies, specialized work roles, shared resources, and communication in order to coordinate and adapt to a changing situation [9]. The multi-disciplinary approach is defined as a team-based structure that includes different levels of medical personnel (i.e., physicians, nurses, nursing assistants, technicians) collaborating together for the patient's plan of care [10]. In the field of medicine, this strategy was first pioneered through the development of tumor boards which bring together multiple medical specialties to discuss the patient's plan of care. The concept has expanded to include multi-disciplinary teams for daily patient care rounds [11, 12]. The goal of this approach is to break down conventional communication barriers between medical specialties and to encourage open dialogue among team members in order to improve safety, patient satisfaction, and to decrease hospital length of stay [10]. This structure has been shown to improve patient outcomes and provider efficency [10, 13]. For the trauma patient population, the standardization of trauma centers across the United States helped to improve outcomes and to provide a standard of care [14–16]. However, a similar strategy has not yet been instituted for the EGS patient population [1, 2, 4]. In order to combat the challenges associated with the lack of a consistent definition of EGS and its complex patient population, a team-based, multi-disciplinary approach could address particular areas of short-comings in this surgical subspecialty.

The Benefits of Team Sports

Team play is a unique attribute of the human species [17]. While evidence of humans engaging in sporting events can be traced back to pre-historic times, the exact period for the evolution of team sports remains unclear [18]. Through team sports, teammates work to develop cooperative relations in order to achieve common goals through complex relations and interactions that surpass the sum of individual performances [19]. In a study by Pluhar and colleagues, the importance of team sports was highlighted by the observation that athletes who participated in team sports had less anxiety and depression than individual athletes [20].

Team Dynamics

A growing area in sports science is the study of performance analysis and team dynamics [21, 22]. Observing the interpersonal interactions in performance analysis of team sports, which is based on the relationship between perception and action, is essential to understand how a team functions [23]. The individual team members face physical and social constraints that must be overcome with synergy for the team to collectively achieve the performance goals [24]. In addition, an analysis of how the individual team members interact with the environment helps to evaluate which circumstances result in success or failure [23].

The American Heart Association (AHA) identified and defined important elements of team dynamics. These elements are now incorporated into training as a part of AHA certification, and they are important to review in order to help improve team dynamics [25]. First, closed-loop communication is required to verify vital information that is conveyed between team members and to confirm the completion of tasks. Constructive intervention involves critiquing poor performance without criticizing [26]. Clear messages are essential to adequate team member communication, and it is necessary to provide additional clarification to the team as needed. Next, it is important for team members to have clear roles in order to ensure that the best care is provided to the patient by the most appropriate person. Understanding one's limitations is critical for knowing when to ask for help. Knowledge sharing is key to obtaining the most comprehensive assessment of a situation. Mutual respect is essential to provide positive feedback and a professional environment. Finally, re-evaluation and summarizing a situation can assist with reviewing essential information and developing a scientific-driven plan going forward.

Failure of the Team

What leads to a breakdown and subsequent failure of the team? First, team cohesiveness is essential for advancing team-related schemas and developing a collective sense of confidence amongst team members [27]. Mutual respect among team members serves as the foundation for success and subsequently the first step towards failure if respect is lacking [26]. The team will also falter if there is a lack of assertive communication. All team members regardless of position should feel empowered to voice concerns and not be fearful of the potential repercussions.

Wergin and colleagues investigated specific factors that led to collapse of the team [28, 29]. The investigators determined that it was a complex cascade of events that resulted in team collapse and not the summation of individual failures [29]. The major triggers identified were: emotional contagion, decreased performance contagion, lack of accountability, limited communication, and blaming other players for mistakes [29]. It has also been emphasized that team members should be questioned about their mistakes outside of the public arena. One framework to follow when addressing team member shortcomings is Pendleton's rules [30]. The team member should first be asked about his/her individual strengths, which is then followed by the leader stating the team member's strengths. Specific areas for improvement or how the situation could have been handled differently should be discussed. Suggestions for improvement with the team leader are also worth addressing [31].

When extrapolating the concepts of the team to surgery, it has been suggested that greater success will happen when the surgeon focuses on the team's welfare ahead of the individual surgeon's needs [26]. Further, the Joint Commission on Accreditation of Healthcare Organizations (JCAHO) identified communication breakdown of the team in the OR as a leading cause for sentinel events and medical errors [32]. Given this philosophy, it is important to review examples from the medical literature when the concepts of team sports have been applied in the medical community and how these principles could be applied to improve EGS outcomes.

Why Medicine Is a Team Sport

Given the far-reaching impacts of healthcare, the mitigation of medical errors and optimal patient safety should be viewed as a public health issue [33, 34]. There has been a major culture shift within the structure of hospitals to improve quality and standardize the delivery of care. Part of this revolution was ignited by the publication of a report in 1999 by the Institutes of Medicine titled, "To Err is Human: Building a Better Health System" [34]. The fallout from this groundbreaking report resulted in interest from many different stakeholders to overhaul to the existing system.

Teamwork has been a significant force in the movement to improve the delivery of healthcare. The hierarchical structures of medicine are being replaced with the creation of multi-disciplinary teams with representatives from all levels of healthcare workers that function together. Hospitals with team-based structures demonstrate improved staff satisfaction [35] and lower reported rates of burnout [36]. Further, dysfunctional team dynamics is linked to worsening the associated healthcare workers' attitudes and personal trauma when preventable patient errors occur [37]. Following reports of poor patient outcomes, the Department of Veterans Affairs (VA) system underwent a renaissance to improve the quality of care delivered across its system through the creation of the National Center for Patient Safety (NCPS) [38]. The basic tenets of the program focus on a nonpunitive approach to reporting unsafe behavior and an analysis of the system when errors occur to determine where the issues happened. The success of this program has been demonstrated in a significant improvement of outcomes at VA hospitals and the spread of this program to the private sector. In 1994, the VA also developed the National VA Surgical Quality Improvement Program (NSQIP) program to specifically address improvement in peri-operative care [39, 40]. As a result, the program led to a reduction in 30-day post-operative morbidity and mortality [40].

The Role of Team Sports and the Medical Trainee

The rigorous process of acceptance into medical school does not reward team-behavior but rather individual achievements [41]. However, efforts are being undertaken to incorporate team training into medical school curriculums [42–45]. A study by Chole and investigators found that the most successful otolaryngology residents had an established history of excelling in team sports [46]. In this study of 46 individuals, resident performance was not found to be linked to medical school grades, letters of recommendation, or standardized test scores. An investigation by Spitzer et al. showed that orthopedic residents with a history of participation in varsity sports were more likely to be selected as chief residents [47]. As the selection criteria for medical students and residents continues to evolve, it is likely that the ability of a trainee to participate effectively in teamwork should be considered.

Surgery as a Team Sport

The complex dynamics of the interactions between multiple levels of healthcare workers, and high-stake consequences when these relationships fail results in the surgical field as the prime battleground for teamwork. Preventable medical errors in the operating room (OR) are linked to a lack of communication and a failure of team leadership [48–50]. Accordingly, it is imperative to review the various components of the surgical team that are necessary to achieve success.

The Surgeon Athlete

The surgeon has traditionally been viewed as the "captain of the ship" in the OR [51, 52]. While surgeons are largely still regarded as the leader of the OR, it is important to recognize that the surgeon must learn to effectively lead the OR team and recognize the value of team members. To help improve performance, the training of a surgeon can thus be likened to the training of an elite athlete [53]. The rigors of surgical training can be improved if an approach for training athletes is undertaken, including one-on-one coaching, video-based review of performance, and development of tailored training programs targeting individual weaknesses [53, 54].

The Surgical Coach

Similar to professional athletes, surgeon and author, Dr. Atul Gawande, suggested that surgeons can improve technical performance by enlisting the help of a surgical coach [55]. The concept of coaching has drawn increased interest not only in the OR to improve technical skills, but also spread to varying aspects of the surgical profession, including one-on-one mentorship and strengthening of personal relationships [56–58]. There are two types of coaches: peer and expert. Peer coaching can involve video review of surgeon performance with directed critiques and coaching [58–60]. Several professional coaching organizations comprised of experts in coaching tactics specifically designed for surgeons have been created [61]. As team-based concepts in medicine continue to grow, it is likely that the idea of healthcare professional coaches will also continue to expand.

Team Work in the Operating Room

Given the complex dynamics that involve multiple levels of medical providers working together closely in the OR, this location has been identified as the most error-prone [62]. A team-based approach in the OR has thus been demonstrated to impact patient care and quality outcomes [63]. However, the OR team will fail if there is a lack of stability and the existing hierarchy overrides the team's ability to function [64]. Several studies found discrepancies between the surgeon's perception of the situation compared to other members of the OR team. In a simulation-based scenario of the OR, majority of surgeons reported that their most significant personal weakness is communication skills. OR nurses and anesthesiologists reported a need to work on improving self-assertiveness [65]. A survey conducted by Makary and colleagues found disparate responses between surgeons and OR nurses regarding the team's performance with nurses more often perceiving interactions as poor while surgeons were more likely to rate these same situations in a more favorable manner [66]. Further, a study by Mills and colleagues, which surveyed 384 OR staff across 6 Veteran's Affairs Hospital, found that nurses and anesthesiologists were more critical of team performance in the OR compared to surgeon's perception of the situation [67]. These studies highlight the importance of open communication and de-briefing with the OR team to understand all team member's perceptions.

Surgeon arrogance, which manifests as an unwillingness to solicit or respond to input from other team members, is a main cause of conflict among OR team members [68]. As a result, feedback or suggestions from team members could be perceived as questioning the surgeon's knowledge and authority. It remains important to train surgeons how to respond to team members' input with respect but without restricting the surgeon's need for autonomy [69].

The Surgeon's Playbook

In many professional sports, a playbook containing team strategies is utilized to help coordinate the team's plan [70]. Similarly, a surgeon's playbook should be developed in order to outline a plan for success in the OR. Important elements of this playbook include: clearly defined roles for OR team members, simulation practice scenarios, and pre-specified OR checklists. In 2008, the

World Health Organization (WHO) safety checklist was introduced as a tool to identify preventable errors prior to the start of the surgery [71]. Surgical checklists serve to improve team communication through reviewing protocols, goals, and encouraging case-specific discussion [72–74]. Checklists can also include charting of preoperative medications and post-operative instructions. An investigation led by Haynes and colleagues reported that the use of a surgical checklist was associated with a significant reduction in mortality, preventing 50% of deaths within 30 days of surgery [75]. Singer et al. found that surgeon engagement was needed to ensure the success of safety checklists [73]. Integrating checklists to improve teamwork requires team members to view the checklist as a trigger for discussion and not simply as a means to "check a box" [76, 77].

Structured Teamwork Training and Simulations

Highly functional teams demonstrate the best performance outcomes [78]. The airline industry has demonstrated that simulation training can improve human errors [79]. Therefore, routine structured training of team members is required. First, teamwork in the OR can be improved through several interventions focused on improving communication. OR team members should feel empowered to raise concerns without fear of the potential consequences. This type of communication has been termed "appropriate assertion" [49]. Other important elements of team communication include: critical language to identify certain phrases which will convey concern among team members, situational awareness of the "big picture," and debriefing [49]. Wolf and colleagues analyzed the implementation of 4863 standardized medical team trainings (MTT) [80]. MTT was an intensive 1 day training for the OR team that focused on a standardized briefing/debriefing/perioperative routine. This training resulted in improved OR function, including decreased case start time delays.

Clear expectations for every team member and institutional processes for error reporting should be established. Disruptive behavior from any team member should be immediately addressed and not tolerated. Multi-disciplinary morbidity and mortality conferences should be established with input from all involved healthcare workers, including OR nurses [41]. Support from leadership should enforce the principles of teamwork.

As a result of the recommendations from the Institute of Medicine report on medical errors, the Department of Defense and Agency for Healthcare Research and Quality (AHRQ) developed a systematic approach to facilitate training, Team Strategies and Tools to Enhance Performance and Patient Safety (TeamSTEPPS™) [34, 81]. The program is based on four core principles: communication, leadership, mutual support, and situation monitoring and provides healthcare teams with tools and strategies to succeed as a team [82, 83]. Since the introduction of TeamSTEPPS™, several studies have reported successful outcomes. It has been shown to increase on-time OR case starts, decrease OR case length, ameliorate issues with availability of OR equipment, help with turnover time, enhance team members' attitudes, and improve patient safety [83–86]. Mayer and colleagues described the implementation of the training program for staff in pediatric and surgical ICUs. Post-training evaluation 1 year after the training revealed continued improved communication between team members, increased time spent by staff at rapid response events, and lower nosocomial infections [87]. Despite the documented success of TeamSTEPPS™ in improving performance, several studies have demonstrated the culture deterioration of team skills learned during the course [88, 89]. The need for skill "refreshers" of TeamSTEPPS™ training has been proposed as a way to keep the team functional [89]. However, the optimal method to promote a sustainable culture of teamwork remains ill defined. Some fields of surgery demonstrated successful outcomes when applying these concepts to address specific areas.

Teamwork and Trauma Surgery

Advanced Trauma Life Support (ATLS) was first introduced in 1979 and has served as the worldwide standard for the initial assessment of the trauma patient [90]. ATLS focuses on the core principles of teamwork and subsequent programs such as the Rural Trauma Team Development Course (RTTDC) were developed to further integrate all players involved in the initial trauma patient encounter at critical access hospitals [91, 92]. The Trauma Evaluation and Management (TEAM) was adapted from ATLS to provide a structure for medical students to receive formalized training on the multi-disciplinary principles of trauma [93]. TeamSTEPPS™ has also been implemented for the trauma team to improve teamwork skills and efficiency in the trauma bay [94]. Another effort to improve team trauma resuscitation is the development of a specific Trauma care checklist by the WHO [95]. Finally, Dutton and colleagues described a multi-disciplinary approach to trauma rounds which included the Trauma fellow and senior staff, an orthopedic surgeon, the hospital bed manager, discharge planner, nursing staff, physical, occupational, and speech therapists. This approach was found to decrease patient length of stay through improved communication among multiple disciplines [12].

Teamwork and Cardiac Surgery

The body of literature on the importance of teamwork in cardiac surgery is extensive. The intensity and intricacies of running cardiopulmonary bypass (CPB) lend itself to fostering a culture of teamwork [96]. Since the inception of CPB in 1953, this technology thrives on closed-loop communication between team members and sharp attention to detail [96]. Given the high-risk nature of cardiac surgeries, the role of team interactions is important to help improve outcomes and meet the necessary quality metrics [11, 97–101]. A landmark study performed by the AHA in 2013 recommended that team training of all OR staff be incorporated into the cardiac OR [99]. A study by Hollingsworth and colleagues demonstrated that patients undergoing coronary artery bypass grafting (CABG) have improved outcomes including lower 60-day mortality rates if their surgery was performed at an institution with well-established teamwork [101]. Dahl et al. described the incorporation of TeamSTEPPS™ training of all cardiac OR team members to improve teamwork [102]. The progress of this initiative will be assessed using a pre and post questionnaire.

Teamwork and ECMO Programs

The increasing utilization of ECMO at many hospitals has also demonstrated the importance of a multi-disciplinary team approach to develop ECMO programs [103, 104]. ECMO programs require complex coordination of multiple levels of healthcare providers including physicians, nurses, perfusionists, and other support staff to work together to treat the most critically ill patients. Furthermore, the success of ECMO transport teams has re-enforced the importance of coordinated team efforts that can navigate multiple hospital systems in order to care for these patients [105–108]. Mayer and colleagues reported decreased time for placing patients on ECMO after the initiation of the TeamSTEPPS™ program for team members [87].

Teamwork and Orthopedic Surgery

Due to the nature of orthopedic surgery, the comparisons between this field and team sports are natural. Previous studies have identified a lack of teamwork as contributing to adverse events within the field of orthopedics [109, 110]. Caprari and colleagues identified four specific areas for improvement in orthopedic teams including: improve daily rounds by reducing cognitive overload and promoting confidence, collaboration by building empathy, connect the patient with the professional team, and support changes by fostering learning [111].

Several initiatives have been undertaken within the Orthopedic surgery community to help promote teamwork and improve outcomes. First, the American Academy of Orthopedic Surgeons made a commitment to integrate TeamSTEPPS™ into orthopedic surgery to improve teamwork and patient safety [112]. Lee et al. described the application of the TeamSTEPPS™ program to 24 orthopedic surgical teams with reinforcement in the form of lectures with videos on leadership skills, an online self-paced learning program on communication skills for nursing staff, a summary on leadership skills e-mailed to surgical staff, and a 1-h perioperative grand rounds. Nursing staff demonstrated improved leadership and communication skills whereas surgical staff showed enhanced leadership [82]. Another initiative by LeBlanc and colleagues to formulate a checklist specific for orthopedic patients has been investigated to help improve patient hand-offs [113]. Finally, patient-reported outcome measures (PROMs) are being developed in a multi-disciplinary fashion targeted to the needs of the orthopedic surgery population. The goal of PROMs is to improve efficiency and patient compliance [114].

Teamwork and Colorectal Surgery

The field of colorectal surgery has been a forerunner in leading efforts to develop multidisciplinary pathways for improving peri-operative care of patients. The Enhanced Recovery After Surgery (ERAS) largely took shape from advances in colorectal surgery [115–117]. ERAS has resulted in decreased hospital length of stay and associated costs [118]. In addition, a multi-disciplinary team at Mayo Clinic was pioneered to design a specific colorectal surgical site infection (SSI) reduction bundle. This strategy was utilized across all phases of patient care and frequent feedback was provided to the team members involved in the program. Cima and colleagues reported that this bundle resulted in a sustained reduction in SSIs [119].

The other area for improvement using a multidisciplinary approach has been the development of ileostomy pathways. The crux of these programs focuses on coordinated efforts between physicians, nurses, wound care nurses, nurse practitioners, and social workers to educate patients using a standardized program [120]. In addition, checklists, phone calls, and home visits are utilized to help increase patient compliance [121, 122]. Since the inception of these programs, there has been decreased hospital readmissions and dehydration secondary to high ileostomy output [120, 123–125]. Higher patient satisfaction and decreased hospital costs have also been reported [121].

Team Sports and Emergency Surgery: What Is the Future?

Given the vast experience with improving surgical outcomes in the fields of elective and trauma surgery, it remains important to review how these lessons could be applied to create a structured framework that will advance the burgeoning field of EGS. Based upon these experiences, both positive and negative, from previous studies in other surgical disciplines, the field of EGS can advance when the principles of teamwork serve as the foundation for improved patient outcomes and satisfaction. Several of these specific targets will be reviewed.

Structured de-briefing is an essential component to improving teamwork in the OR. A study by Ahmed and colleagues interviewed 33 surgeons, anesthesiologists, and OR nurses from the United States, United Kingdom, and Australia to identify key elements to debriefing. The themes identified included: appropriate approach, establishing a learning environment, learner engagement, managing learner reaction, reflection, analysis, diagnosis, and application to clinical practice [126]. These areas could serve as the starting framework to develop standardized debriefing tools for EGS specific-situations. Leadership must affirm that routine briefings and debriefings occur as part of the OR culture [77].

Another potential area to improve EGS is the development of a surgeon's playbook specific for this area. Important items to include in this playbook include a standardized WHO timeout, an OR checklist, and specified briefings directed to the needs and challenges of this field. Similar to the progress in other surgical fields, it is important to develop specific evidence-based materials to meet the demands of EGS. These materials are particularly invaluable for EGS as a result of the 24 h a day/7 days a week nature of this specialty, team members may not routinely work together. Additionally, the development of an EGS registry will help to support future research efforts and quality improvement initiatives.

Surgical education will be a large part of the success or failure of EGS evolving into a team sport in the future. As EGS fellowships become more common and formalized, the concepts of teamwork and opportunities to improve upon skills need to be incorporated into the education of trainees. One tool which could help to facilitate structured de-briefing sessions for EGS operative cases is the use of video-based learning. This strategy has proven to be successful for improving trauma resuscitations [127–131] and also for the structured training of surgical residents [132–136].

Several areas of team-dynamics in healthcare have un-answered questions which will require a thoughtful approach as this area develops within the sub-specialty of EGS. The optimal strategy for monitoring team dynamics and the frequency needed to refresh team skills needs to be addressed. Another area of potential teamwork breakdown that is particularly troublesome for EGS is patient handoffs [48, 137]. This form of communication is high-risk across all medical specialties but given the emergent and constant workflow of this surgical sub-specialty, this is a topic of particular interest. Possible solutions to this challenge include the development and implementation of structured hand-off tools [138] and standardized training of medical providers in communication techniques. To address these potential weaknesses, a rigorous multi-institutional research network must be built to provide a standardized and peer-reviewed process. Finally, the integration of patient participation into improving the OR team structure needs to be a consideration to achieve the best outcomes for patient safety and satisfaction.

Conclusion

As the field of EGS matures into a more structured field of surgery, the potential to create an evidence-based, quality-driven, and patient-centered standard of care remains plausible. Similar to the evolution of trauma surgery as a standardized surgical specialty many decades ago, EGS lies in a unique position to be steered into new but familiar territory. Transposing valuable lessons and scientific evidence on team dynamics and the multi-disciplinary approach from more mature surgical fields remains within reach and can shape the future of EGS to stand as an example of improvement in clinical and quality outcomes.Author Disclosures and Conflicts of InterestThe authors have no financial disclosures or conflicts of interest to disclose.

Funding Sources None.

References

1. Havens JM, Neiman PU, Campbell BL, Croce MA, Spain DA, Napolitano LM. The future of emergency general surgery. Ann Surg. 2019;270(2):221–2.
2. Shafi S, Aboutanos MB, Agarwal S Jr, et al. Emergency general surgery: definition and estimated burden of disease. J Trauma Acute Care Surg. 2013;74(4):1092–7.
3. Becher RD, Davis KA, Rotondo MF, Coimbra R. Ongoing evolution of emergency general surgery as a surgical subspecialty. J Am Coll Surg. 2018;226(2):194–200.
4. Gale SC, Shafi S, Dombrovskiy VY, Arumugam D, Crystal JS. The public health burden of emergency general surgery in the United States: a 10-year analysis of the Nationwide Inpatient Sample—2001 to 2010. J Trauma Acute Care Surg. 2014;77(2):202–8.
5. Lyu HG, Najjar P, Havens JM. Past, present, and future of emergency general surgery in the USA. Acute Med Surg. 2018;5(2):119–22.
6. Havens JM, Peetz AB, Do WS, et al. The excess morbidity and mortality of emergency general surgery. J Trauma Acute Care Surg. 2015;78(2):306–11.
7. Ingraham AM, Cohen ME, Raval MV, Ko CY, Nathens AB. Comparison of hospital performance in emergency versus elective general surgery operations at 198 hospitals. J Am Coll Surg. 2011;212(1):20–28 e21.

8. Gawande AA, Studdert DM, Orav EJ, Brennan TA, Zinner MJ. Risk factors for retained instruments and sponges after surgery. N Engl J Med. 2003;348(3):229–35.
9. Brannick MPC. An overview of team performance measurement. Mahwah: Lawrence Erlbaum Associates; 1997.
10. Epstein N. Multidisciplinary in-hospital teams improve patient outcomes: a review. Surg Neurol Int. 2014;5:S295–303.
11. Crawford TC, Conte JV, Sanchez JA. Team-based care: the changing face of cardiothoracic surgery. Surg Clin North Am. 2017;97(4):801–10.
12. Dutton RP, Cooper C, Jones A, Leone S, Kramer ME, Scalea TM. Daily multidisciplinary rounds shorten length of stay for trauma patients. J Trauma. 2003;55(5):913–9.
13. O'Mahony S, Mazur E, Charney P, Wang Y, Fine J. Use of multidisciplinary rounds to simultaneously improve quality outcomes, enhance resident education, and shorten length of stay. J Gen Intern Med. 2007;22(8):1073–9.
14. Miller PR. Defining burden and severity of disease for emergency general surgery. Trauma Surg Acute Care Open. 2017;2(1):e000089.
15. American College of Surgeons. Committee on Trauma. Resources for optimal care of the injured patient. 2014. https://www.facs.org/quality-programs/trauma/tqp/center-programs/vrc/resources. Accessed 18 Sept 2020.
16. Mackersie RC. History of trauma field triage development and the American College of Surgeons criteria. Prehosp Emerg Care. 2006;10(3):287–94.
17. Kniffin KM, Scalise SM. Toward a natural history of team sports. Hum Nat. 2018;29(3):211–8.
18. Capelo H. Symbols from the sky: heavenly messages from the depths of prehistory may be encoded on the walls of caves throughout Europe. 2010. https://web.archive.org/web/20120508010237/http://seedmagazine.com/content/article/symbols_from_the_sky/. Accessed 15 Sept 2020.
19. Duarte R, Araujo D, Correia V, Davids K, Marques P, Richardson MJ. Competing together: assessing the dynamics of team-team and player-team synchrony in professional association football. Hum Mov Sci. 2013;32(4):555–66.
20. Pluhar E, McCracken C, Griffith KL, Christino MA, Sugimoto D, Meehan WP 3rd. Team sport athletes may be less likely to suffer anxiety or depression than individual sport athletes. J Sports Sci Med. 2019;18(3):490–6.
21. Ramos J, Lopes RJ, Araujo D. What's next in complex networks? Capturing the concept of attacking play in invasive team sports. Sports Med. 2018;48(1):17–28.
22. Lord F, Pyne DB, Welvaert M, Mara JK. Methods of performance analysis in team invasion sports: a systematic review. J Sports Sci. 2020;38(20):2338–49.
23. Correia V, Araujo D, Vilar L, Davids K. From recording discrete actions to studying continuous goal-directed behaviours in team sports. J Sports Sci. 2013;31(5):546–53.
24. Araujo D, Davids K. Team synergies in sport: theory and measures. Front Psychol. 2016;7:1449.
25. American Heart Association. Team dynamics debriefing tool. 2016. https://ahainstructornetwork.americanheart.org/idc/groups/ahaecc-public/@wcm/@ecc/documents/downloadable/ucm_488325.pdf. Accessed 15 Sept 2020.
26. Greer RB 3rd. Surgery as a team sport. Am J Orthop (Belle Mead NJ). 1995;24(8):582.
27. Filho E, Tenenbaum G, Yang Y. Cohesion, team mental models, and collective efficacy: towards an integrated framework of team dynamics in sport. J Sports Sci. 2015;33(6):641–53.
28. Wergin VV, Mallett CJ, Mesagno C, Zimanyi Z, Beckmann J. When you watch your team fall apart—coaches' and sport psychologists' perceptions on causes of collective sport team collapse. Front Psychol. 2019;10:1331.
29. Wergin VV, Zimanyi Z, Mesagno C, Beckmann J. When suddenly nothing works anymore within a team—causes of collective sport team collapse. Front Psychol. 2018;9:2115.
30. Pendleton D, Schofield T, Tate P, Havelock P. The consultation: an approach to learning and teaching. Oxford: Oxford University Press; 1984.
31. Mullis BH, Siegel J. Now that I'm in charge: what do I do? J Orthop Trauma. 2015;29(Suppl 11):S12–4.
32. Joint Commission on Accreditation of Healthcare Organizations. Sentinel events: evaluating cause and planning improvement. Oakbrook Terrace, IL: Joint Commission on Accreditation of Healthcare Organizations; 1998.
33. Rosen MA, DiazGranados D, Dietz AS, et al. Teamwork in healthcare: key discoveries enabling safer, high-quality care. Am Psychol. 2018;73(4):433–50.
34. Institute of Medicine Committee on Quality of Health Care in America. To err is human: building a safer health system. Washington, DC: National Academies Press (US); 1999.
35. Daugherty Biddison EL, Paine L, Murakami P, Herzke C, Weaver SJ. Associations between safety culture and employee engagement over time: a retrospective analysis. BMJ Qual Saf. 2016;25(1):31–7.
36. Bowers L, Nijman H, Simpson A, Jones J. The relationship between leadership, teamworking, structure, burnout and attitude to patients on acute psychiatric wards. Soc Psychiatry Psychiatr Epidemiol. 2011;46(2):143–8.
37. Seys D, Scott S, Wu A, et al. Supporting involved health care professionals (second victims) following an adverse health event: a literature review. Int J Nurs Stud. 2013;50(5):678–87.
38. Stalhandske E, Bagian JP, Gosbee J. Department of Veterans Affairs patient safety program. Am J Infect Control. 2002;30(5):296–302.
39. Khuri SF, Daley J, Henderson W, et al. The Department of Veterans Affairs' NSQIP: the first

national, validated, outcome-based, risk-adjusted, and peer-controlled program for the measurement and enhancement of the quality of surgical care. National VA Surgical Quality Improvement Program. Ann Surg. 1998;228(4):491–507.
40. Khuri SF. The NSQIP: a new frontier in surgery. Surgery. 2005;138(5):837–43.
41. Sax HC. Building high-performance teams in the operating room. Surg Clin North Am. 2012;92(1):15–9.
42. Kazory A, Zaidi Z. Team-based learning activities for first-year medical students: perception of the learners. South Med J. 2018;111(9):525–9.
43. Richard K, Noujaim M, Thorndyke LE, Fischer MA. Preparing medical students to be physician leaders: a leadership training program for students designed and led by students. MedEdPORTAL. 2019;15:10863.
44. Robertson B, Kaplan B, Atallah H, Higgins M, Lewitt MJ, Ander DS. The use of simulation and a modified TeamSTEPPS curriculum for medical and nursing student team training. Simul Healthc. 2010;5(6):332–7.
45. Meier AH, Boehler ML, McDowell CM, et al. A surgical simulation curriculum for senior medical students based on TeamSTEPPS. Arch Surg. 2012;147(8):761–6.
46. Chole RA, Ogden MA. Predictors of future success in otolaryngology residency applicants. Arch Otolaryngol Head Neck Surg. 2012;138(8):707–12.
47. Spitzer AB, Gage MJ, Looze CA, Walsh M, Zuckerman JD, Egol KA. Factors associated with successful performance in an orthopaedic surgery residency. J Bone Joint Surg Am. 2009;91(11):2750–5.
48. Greenberg CC, Regenbogen SE, Studdert DM, et al. Patterns of communication breakdowns resulting in injury to surgical patients. J Am Coll Surg. 2007;204(4):533–40.
49. Leonard M, Graham S, Bonacum D. The human factor: the critical importance of effective teamwork and communication in providing safe care. Qual Saf Health Care. 2004;13(Suppl 1):i85–90.
50. Rogers SO Jr, Gawande AA, Kwaan M, et al. Analysis of surgical errors in closed malpractice claims at 4 liability insurers. Surgery. 2006;140(1):25–33.
51. Price SH. The sinking of the "captain of the ship". Reexamining the vicarious liability of an operating surgeon for the negligence of assisting hospital personnel. J Leg Med. 1989;10(2):323–56.
52. Murphy EK. "Captain of the ship" doctrine continues to take on water. AORN J. 2001;74(4):525–8.
53. Chand M, Qureshi T. Evolution in surgical training: what can we learn from professional coaches and elite athletes? J R Soc Med. 2014;107(7):290–2.
54. Aggarwal R, Grantcharov T, Moorthy K, Milland T, Darzi A. Toward feasible, valid, and reliable video-based assessments of technical surgical skills in the operating room. Ann Surg. 2008;247(2):372–9.
55. Gawande A. The coach in the operating room. Annals of Medicine, 2011.
56. Vande Walle KG, Greenberg C. Surgical coaching. https://www.facs.org/education/division-of-education/publications/rise/articles/surg-coaching. Accessed 15 Sept 2020.
57. Bonrath EM, Dedy NJ, Gordon LE, Grantcharov TP. Comprehensive surgical coaching enhances surgical skill in the operating room: a randomized controlled trial. Ann Surg. 2015;262(2):205–12.
58. Hu YY, Peyre SE, Arriaga AF, et al. Postgame analysis: using video-based coaching for continuous professional development. J Am Coll Surg. 2012;214(1):115–24.
59. Nakada SY, Hedican SP, Bishoff JT, Shichman SJ, Wolf JS Jr. Expert videotape analysis and critiquing benefit laparoscopic skills training of urologists. JSLS. 2004;8(2):183–6.
60. Singh P, Aggarwal R, Tahir M, Pucher PH, Darzi A. A randomized controlled study to evaluate the role of video-based coaching in training laparoscopic skills. Ann Surg. 2015;261(5):862–9.
61. The Academy for Surgical Coaching. 2020. https://surgicalcoaching.org/. Accessed 25 Sept 2020.
62. Leape LL. Error in medicine. JAMA. 1994;272(23):1851–7.
63. Paige JT, Garbee DD, Kozmenko V, et al. Getting a head start: high-fidelity, simulation-based operating room team training of interprofessional students. J Am Coll Surg. 2014;218(1):140–9.
64. Gillespie BM, Gwinner K, Chaboyer W, Fairweather N. Team communications in surgery—creating a culture of safety. J Interprof Care. 2013;27(5):387–93.
65. Arriaga AF, Gawande AA, Raemer DB, et al. Pilot testing of a model for insurer-driven, large-scale multicenter simulation training for operating room teams. Ann Surg. 2014;259(3):403–10.
66. Makary MA, Sexton JB, Freischlag JA, et al. Operating room teamwork among physicians and nurses: teamwork in the eye of the beholder. J Am Coll Surg. 2006;202(5):746–52.
67. Mills P, Neily J, Dunn E. Teamwork and communication in surgical teams: implications for patient safety. J Am Coll Surg. 2008;206(1):107–12.
68. Pronovost PJ. Learning accountability for patient outcomes. JAMA. 2010;304(2):204–5.
69. Achor TS, Ahn J. Becoming the "captain of the ship" in the OR. J Orthop Trauma. 2014;28(Suppl 9):S18–9.
70. Anthony SD, Eyring M, Gibson L. Mapping your innovation strategy. Harv Bus Rev. 2006;84(5):104–13, 157.
71. World Alliance for Patient Safety. Safe surgery saves lives. Geneva: World Health Organization; 2008.
72. Keebler JR, Lazzara EH, Patzer BS, et al. Meta-analyses of the effects of standardized handoff protocols on patient, provider, and organizational outcomes. Hum Factors. 2016;58(8):1187–205.
73. Singer SJ, Molina G, Li Z, et al. Relationship between operating room teamwork, contextual factors, and safety checklist performance. J Am Coll Surg. 2016;223(4):568–580.e562.

74. de Vries EN, Prins HA, Crolla RM, et al. Effect of a comprehensive surgical safety system on patient outcomes. N Engl J Med. 2010;363(20):1928–37.
75. Haynes AB, Weiser TG, Berry WR, et al. A surgical safety checklist to reduce morbidity and mortality in a global population. N Engl J Med. 2009;360(5):491–9.
76. Neily J, Mills PD, Young-Xu Y, et al. Association between implementation of a medical team training program and surgical mortality. JAMA. 2010;304(15):1693–700.
77. Pronovost PJ, Freischlag JA. Improving teamwork to reduce surgical mortality. JAMA. 2010;304(15):1721–2.
78. Salas E, DiazGranados D, Klein C, et al. Does team training improve team performance? A meta-analysis. Hum Factors. 2008;50(6):903–33.
79. Lundberg PW, Korndorffer JR Jr. Using simulation to improve systems. Surg Clin North Am. 2015;95(4):885–92.
80. Wolf FA, Way LW, Stewart L. The efficacy of medical team training: improved team performance and decreased operating room delays: a detailed analysis of 4863 cases. Ann Surg. 2010;252(3):477–83; discussion 483–5.
81. King HB, Battles J, Baker DP, et al. TeamSTEPPS: team strategies and tools to enhance performance and patient safety. In: Henriksen K, Battles JB, Keyes MA, Grady ML, editors. Advances in patient safety: new directions and alternative approaches, Performance and tools, vol. Vol. 3. Rockville, MD, Agency for Healthcare Research and Quality; 2008.
82. Lee SH, Khanuja HS, Blanding RJ, et al. Sustaining teamwork behaviors through reinforcement of TeamSTEPPS principles. J Patient Saf. 2017; https://doi.org/10.1097/PTS.0000000000000414.
83. Weaver SJ, Rosen MA, DiazGranados D, et al. Does teamwork improve performance in the operating room? A multilevel evaluation. Jt Comm J Qual Patient Saf. 2010;36(3):133–42.
84. Weld LR, Stringer MT, Ebertowski JS, et al. TeamSTEPPS improves operating room efficiency and patient safety. Am J Med Qual. 2016;31(5):408–14.
85. Fischer MM, Tubb CC, Brennan JA, Soderdahl DW, Johnson AE. Implementation of TeamSTEPPS at a level-1 military trauma center: the San Antonio military medical center experience. US Army Med Dep J. 2015:75–9.
86. Tibbs SM, Moss J. Promoting teamwork and surgical optimization: combining TeamSTEPPS with a specialty team protocol. AORN J. 2014;100(5):477–88.
87. Mayer CM, Cluff L, Lin WT, et al. Evaluating efforts to optimize TeamSTEPPS implementation in surgical and pediatric intensive care units. Jt Comm J Qual Patient Saf. 2011;37(8):365–74.
88. Armour Forse R, Bramble JD, McQuillan R. Team training can improve operating room performance. Surgery. 2011;150(4):771–8.
89. Thomas L, Galla C. Building a culture of safety through team training and engagement. BMJ Qual Saf. 2013;22(5):425–34.
90. Subcommittee A. Advanced trauma life support (ATLS) student course manual. 10th ed. Chicago: American College of Surgeons; 2018.
91. Dennis BM, Vella MA, Gunter OL, et al. Rural Trauma Team Development Course decreases time to transfer for trauma patients. J Trauma Acute Care Surg. 2016;81(4):632–7.
92. American College of Surgeons. Rural trauma team development course. https://www.facs.org/quality%20programs/trauma/education/rttdc. Accessed 1 Sept 2020.
93. American College of Surgeons. Trauma evaluation and management. https://www.facs.org/quality-programs/trauma/atls/team. Accessed 27 Sept 2020.
94. Capella J, Smith S, Philp A, et al. Teamwork training improves the clinical care of trauma patients. J Surg Educ. 2010;67(6):439–43.
95. Fitzgerald M, Reilly S, Smit V, et al. The World Health Organization trauma checklist versus trauma team time-out: a perspective. Emerg Med Australas. 2019;31(5):882–5.
96. Fiedler AG, Lewis EE, Hermsen JL. We agree: cardiopulmonary bypass is a team sport. Ann Thorac Surg. 2020;110:1437–8.
97. Cook C, Alreshidan M, Salman M, et al. It's a team sport. Semin Thorac Cardiovasc Surg. 2019;31(3):442–3.
98. Lawton JS. Commentary: "Isn't cardiac surgery a team sport?". J Thorac Cardiovasc Surg. 2019; https://doi.org/10.1016/j.jtcvs.2019.03.021.
99. Wahr JA, Prager RL, Abernathy JH 3rd, et al. Patient safety in the cardiac operating room: human factors and teamwork: a scientific statement from the American Heart Association. Circulation. 2013;128(10):1139–69.
100. Likosky DS, Dickinson TA, Paugh TA. Blood conservation-a team sport. J Extra Corpor Technol. 2016;48(3):99–104.
101. Hollingsworth JM, Funk RJ, Garrison SA, et al. Association between physician teamwork and health system outcomes after coronary artery bypass grafting. Circ Cardiovasc Qual Outcomes. 2016;9(6):641–8.
102. Dahl AB, Ben Abdallah A, Maniar H, et al. Building a collaborative culture in cardiothoracic operating rooms: pre and postintervention study protocol for evaluation of the implementation of teamSTEPPS training and the impact on perceived psychological safety. BMJ Open. 2017;7(9):e017389.
103. Dalia AA, Ortoleva J, Fiedler A, Villavicencio M, Shelton K, Cudemus GD. Extracorporeal membrane oxygenation is a team sport: institutional survival benefits of a formalized ECMO team. J Cardiothorac Vasc Anesth. 2019;33(4):902–7.
104. Cotza M, Carboni G, Ballotta A, et al. Modern ECMO: why an ECMO programme in a tertiary care hospital. Eur Heart J Suppl. 2016;18(Suppl E):E79–85.

105. Coppola CP, Tyree M, Larry K, DiGeronimo R. A 22-year experience in global transport extracorporeal membrane oxygenation. J Pediatr Surg. 2008;43(1):46–52; discussion 52.
106. Nwozuzu A, Fontes ML, Schonberger RB. Mobile extracorporeal membrane oxygenation teams: the North American versus the European experience. J Cardiothorac Vasc Anesth. 2016;30(6):1441–8.
107. Moll V, Teo EY, Grenda DS, et al. Rapid development and implementation of an ECMO program. ASAIO J. 2016;62(3):354–8.
108. Read MD, Nam JJ, Biscotti M, et al. Evolution of the United States military extracorporeal membrane oxygenation transport team. Mil Med. 2020;185:e2055–60.
109. Unbeck M, Dalen N, Muren O, Lillkrona U, Harenstam KP. Healthcare processes must be improved to reduce the occurrence of orthopaedic adverse events. Scand J Caring Sci. 2010;24(4):671–7.
110. Panesar SS, Carson-Stevens A, Mann BS, Bhandari M, Madhok R. Mortality as an indicator of patient safety in orthopaedics: lessons from qualitative analysis of a database of medical errors. BMC Musculoskelet Disord. 2012;13:93.
111. Caprari E, Porsius JT, D'Olivo P, et al. Dynamics of an orthopaedic team: insights to improve teamwork through a design thinking approach. Work. 2018;61(1):21–39.
112. Khanuja HS, Naseer ZA, Jones LC, Ficke JR, Burney DW III. Implementation of TeamSTEPPS in orthopaedic surgery. Instr Course Lect. 2017;66:635–45.
113. LeBlanc J, Donnon T, Hutchison C, Duffy P. Development of an orthopedic surgery trauma patient handover checklist. Can J Surg. 2014;57(1):8–14.
114. Makhni EC, Bozic KJ. Team approach: clinical outcome collection, done practically. JBJS Rev. 2018;6(9):e5.
115. Kehlet H. Fast-track colorectal surgery. Lancet. 2008;371(9615):791–3.
116. Ban KA, Berian JR, Ko CY. Does implementation of enhanced recovery after surgery (ERAS) protocols in colorectal surgery improve patient outcomes? Clin Colon Rectal Surg. 2019;32(2):109–13.
117. Varadhan KK, Neal KR, Dejong CH, Fearon KC, Ljungqvist O, Lobo DN. The enhanced recovery after surgery (ERAS) pathway for patients undergoing major elective open colorectal surgery: a meta-analysis of randomized controlled trials. Clin Nutr. 2010;29(4):434–40.
118. Forsmo HM, Pfeffer F, Rasdal A, et al. Compliance with enhanced recovery after surgery criteria and preoperative and postoperative counselling reduces length of hospital stay in colorectal surgery: results of a randomized controlled trial. Color Dis. 2016;18(6):603–11.
119. Cima R, Dankbar E, Lovely J, et al. Colorectal surgery surgical site infection reduction program: a national surgical quality improvement program—driven multidisciplinary single-institution experience. J Am Coll Surg. 2013;216(1):23–33.
120. Nagle D, Pare T, Keenan E, Marcet K, Tizio S, Poylin V. Ileostomy pathway virtually eliminates readmissions for dehydration in new ostomates. Dis Colon Rectum. 2012;55(12):1266–72.
121. Iqbal A, Raza A, Huang E, Goldstein L, Hughes SJ, Tan SA. Cost effectiveness of a novel attempt to reduce readmission after ileostomy creation. JSLS. 2017;21(1):e2016.00082.
122. Hardiman KM, Reames CD, McLeod MC, Regenbogen SE. Patient autonomy-centered self-care checklist reduces hospital readmissions after ileostomy creation. Surgery. 2016;160(5):1302–8.
123. van Loon YT, Poylin VY, Nagle D, Zimmerman DDE. Effectiveness of the ileostomy pathway in reducing readmissions for dehydration: does it stand the test of time? Dis Colon Rectum. 2020;63(8):1151–5.
124. Shaffer VO, Owi T, Kumarusamy MA, et al. Decreasing hospital readmission in ileostomy patients: results of novel pilot program. J Am Coll Surg. 2017;224(4):425–30.
125. Gonella F, Valenti A, Massucco P, et al. A novel patient-centered protocol to reduce hospital readmissions for dehydration after ileostomy. Updat Surg. 2019;71(3):515–21.
126. Ahmed M, Sevdalis N, Paige J, Paragi-Gururaja R, Nestel D, Arora S. Identifying best practice guidelines for debriefing in surgery: a tri-continental study. Am J Surg. 2012;203(4):523–9.
127. Santora TA, Trooskin SZ, Blank CA, Clarke JR, Schinco MA. Video assessment of trauma response: adherence to ATLS protocols. Am J Emerg Med. 1996;14(6):564–9.
128. Hoyt DB, Shackford SR, Fridland PH, et al. Video recording trauma resuscitations: an effective teaching technique. J Trauma. 1988;28(4):435–40.
129. Townsend RN, Clark R, Ramenofsky ML, Diamond DL. ATLS-based videotape trauma resuscitation review: education and outcome. J Trauma. 1993;34(1):133–8.
130. Knobel A, Overheu D, Gruessing M, Juergensen I, Struewer J. Regular, in-situ, team-based training in trauma resuscitation with video debriefing enhances confidence and clinical efficiency. BMC Med Educ. 2018;18(1):127.
131. Scherer LA, Chang MC, Meredith JW, Battistella FD. Videotape review leads to rapid and sustained learning. Am J Surg. 2003;185(6):516–20.
132. Green JL, Suresh V, Bittar P, Ledbetter L, Mithani SK, Allori A. The utilization of video technology in surgical education: a systematic review. J Surg Res. 2019;235:171–80.
133. Ahmet A, Gamze K, Rustem M, Sezen KA. Is video-based education an effective method in surgical education? A systematic review. J Surg Educ. 2018;75(5):1150–8.

134. Soucisse ML, Boulva K, Sideris L, Drolet P, Morin M, Dube P. Video coaching as an efficient teaching method for surgical residents-a randomized controlled trial. J Surg Educ. 2017;74(2):365–71.
135. McQueen S, McKinnon V, VanderBeek L, McCarthy C, Sonnadara R. Video-based assessment in surgical education: a scoping review. J Surg Educ. 2019;76(6):1645–54.
136. Hamad GG, Brown MT, Clavijo-Alvarez JA. Postoperative video debriefing reduces technical errors in laparoscopic surgery. Am J Surg. 2007;194(1):110–4.
137. Gawande AA, Zinner MJ, Studdert DM, Brennan TA. Analysis of errors reported by surgeons at three teaching hospitals. Surgery. 2003;133(6):614–21.
138. Muller M, Jurgens J, Redaelli M, Klingberg K, Hautz WE, Stock S. Impact of the communication and patient hand-off tool SBAR on patient safety: a systematic review. BMJ Open. 2018;8(8):e022202.

Sepsis Resuscitation

34

Christopher A. Guidry and Robert G. Sawyer

Case Presentation

You are the surgical intensivist covering the SICU overnight. One of your patients is a 65-year-old, 80 kg female with a history of diabetes and congestive heart failure who is now 4 h status post a sigmoid colectomy with end colostomy for perforated diverticulitis. She is intubated, sedated, in sinus tachycardia, with hypotension on escalating doses of two vasoactive agents to maintain a mean arterial pressure of 65 mmHg. Her hemoglobin level is 8.0 g/dL, INR is 1.8, with a lactate of 4.2 mmol/L. She was given approximately 2 L of crystalloid during the operation. The resident asks you if the patient might benefit from additional volume resuscitation.

C. A. Guidry (✉)
Department of Surgery, Division of Acute Care Surgery, Trauma, and Surgical Critical Care, University of Kansas Medical Center, Kansas City, KS, USA
e-mail: cguidry2@kumc.edu

R. G. Sawyer
Department of Surgery, Western Michigan University Homer Stryker M.D. School of Medicine, Kalamazoo, MI, USA

Department of Engineering, Western Michigan University College of Engineering and Applied Sciences, Kalamazoo, MI, USA
e-mail: Robert.Sawyer@med.wmich.edu

Diagnosis of Sepsis and Septic Shock

Evolving Definitions

For over 20 years, sepsis was defined as existing on a clinical spectrum beginning with systemic inflammatory response syndrome (SIRS) and ending with septic shock [1, 2]. Using these criteria, sepsis was defined as SIRS plus an infectious source, severe sepsis was defined as sepsis with organ dysfunction, and septic shock was defined as severe sepsis with persistent arterial hypotension despite adequate resuscitation [2].

In 2016, the Third Consensus Definition for Sepsis and Septic Shock re-defined sepsis as "life-threatening organ dysfunction caused by a dysregulated host response to infection" [3]. The consensus task force acknowledges that this definition is somewhat vague and that there remains no standardized clinical measure of a dysregulated host response [3]. Septic shock is the subset of sepsis with profound circulatory and metabolic abnormalities, clinically identifiable by the need for vasopressors to maintain a mean arterial pressure of 65 mmHg, and a serum lactate >2 mmol/L in the absence of hypovolemia [3].

In the current definitions, organ dysfunction is operationalized as an increase of ≥2 in the Sequential Organ Failure Assessment (SOFA) score [3]. SOFA has been validated as a marker

M. D. Zielinski, O. Guillamondegui (eds.), *The Acute Management of Surgical Disease*,
https://doi.org/10.1007/978-3-031-07881-1_34

of organ dysfunction related to mortality in multiple patient populations [4, 5]. The term "severe sepsis" is still occasionally used but is no longer a part of the current definitions.

There are several limitations to the application of these definitions in current practice which affect treatment. It is important to note that the SOFA score is a maker of mortality related to organ dysfunction, not the presence or absence of infection [6]. Because SOFA describes organ dysfunction, trauma patients with significant injury often present with elevated SOFA scores on admission. SEPSIS-3 defines infection-related organ dysfunction as an increase in the SOFA score of ≥2, some patients may have trouble meeting this formal definition, as trauma patients frequently have lower SOFA scores at the time of infection compared with admission [7]. Additionally, the Quick Sequential Organ Failure Assessment (qSOFA) score is not well-validated and appears to perform poorly in ICU populations [5].

Initial Assessment of Volume Resuscitation

The goal of volume resuscitation in sepsis is to improve cardiac output and, as a result, improve perfusion and oxygen delivery thereby reducing organ dysfunction [8]. Conceptually, this is straightforward, however, in practice providing the "right" amount of fluid is difficult to assess. Patients with sepsis can present with varying degrees of hypovolemia due to volume loss from several sources (e.g., gastrointestinal loss or fever), and relative hypovolemia due to vasodilation and endothelial leak. These states are compounded by the patient's comorbidities resulting in varying degrees of responsiveness to volume resuscitation [8, 9].

Current practice involves initial empiric fluid administration followed by ongoing assessments of the patient's response to therapy and need for additional fluid. There is no "one-size-fits-all" approach and there can be a fine line between appropriate volume replacement and over resuscitation.

History and Physical Exam

The assessment of the septic patient begins with the history and physical exam. A patient who has been struggling at home with diminished intake for several days may have more profound volume requirements than one whose symptoms began a few hours ago. Moreover, a history of significant or ongoing volume loss such as vomiting or diarrhea should alert the clinician to the need for volume resuscitation. Classic findings such as dry mucus membranes or decreased skin turgor may also be found in the septic patient, although these findings may be affected by the duration of symptoms, comorbidities, and the patient's baseline intake. Vital signs such as tachycardia and hypotension are also classically considered reliable markers of volume status; unfortunately, they are not specific and are subject to the patient's comorbidities [10]. Using vital signs alone to predict shock-appropriate treatment is not reliable; clinicians are poor at predicting the type of shock-appropriate treatment using vitals alone [11]. Most of the literature on vital signs and physical exam makers of volume status are in patients with heart failure or those with acute blood loss limiting their generalizability to patients with sepsis or septic shock [12]. While it remains important to elucidate a proper history and physical exam, in practice, physical exam has limited utility in the assessment of intravascular volume and volume responsiveness [13].

A review of physical exam findings in hypovolemic patients found that a dry axilla was associated with an increased likelihood of hypovolemia (positive likelihood ratio: 2.8; 95% CI: 1.5–5.4) while moist mucus membranes and a tongue without furrows did not support hypovolemia (negative likelihood ratio: 0.3; 95% CI 0.1–0.6). Skin turgor, mild postural dizziness, and capillary refill were not associated with volume status in this study [14]. Significant postural hypotension was sensitive (97%; 95% CI: 91–100%) and specific (98%; 95% CI: 97–99%) for hypovolemia to large volume blood loss, but not due to hypovolemia by other causes [14]. The authors point out that in the absence of acute blood loss, most exam findings are unreliable [12, 14].

Most of the literature relating physical exam findings with volume overload comes from heart failure patients. While sepsis and septic shock are vasodilatory states generally resulting in functional volume depletion, hypervolemia can exist concurrently in sepsis, particularly after several days of resuscitation and/or in the setting cardiac or renal failure. Findings such as pitting edema and dyspnea are not specific for intravascular volume and can be caused by a variety of mechanisms. One review of patients presenting to the emergency department with dyspnea found that paroxysmal nocturnal dyspnea, a third heart sound (S3 gallop), and atrial fibrillation to be the history and exam elements most correlated with the presence of heart failure [15]. The absence of rales or dyspnea were the exam findings that suggested that heart failure was not the cause of the patient's dyspnea [15]. While heart failure is generally associated with hypervolemia, caution should be taken when applying these findings to patients with potential sepsis.

Early Goal-Directed Therapy

In 2001, Rivers et al. published the first major study of early goal-directed therapy (EGDT) in severe sepsis and septic shock [16]. In this study, 263 patients with two or more SIRS criteria, a systolic blood pressure of ≤90 mmHg (after a 20–30 cc/kg fluid bolus), and/or a lactate ≥4 mmol/L were randomized to either "standard therapy" or early goal-directed therapy. In this study, EGDT was a standardized sepsis resuscitation algorithm that consists of placement of a central line to measure central venous pressure (CVP) and central venous oxygen saturation ($ScvO_2$). Volume was given in 500 cc increments to achieve a CVP of 8–12 mmHg and vasoactive agents are given to maintain a mean arterial pressure (MAP) of greater than 65 mmHg. In EGDT, blood was also administered to achieve a hematocrit of at least 30% if the $ScvO_2$ was less than 70%. In this initial study, in-hospital mortality was significantly lower in the group that received EGDT compared to standard therapy (30.5% vs. 46.5%; *p*-value = 0.009) [16]. Based on the success of this trial and others, early goal-directed therapy was incorporated into the Surviving Sepsis Guidelines [17].

Since publication of the Rivers trial, there have been several large randomized trials that have challenged early-goal-directed therapy. In contrast to the single-site Rivers trial, the ProCESS, ARISE, and ProMISe trials enrolled over 4200 patients in aggregate across 138 centers, with each trial having a minimum of 1260 patients [18–20]. None of these three trials were able to replicate the findings of the Rivers trial. A subsequent meta-analysis also failed to identify a mortality benefit to protocolized sepsis resuscitation as outlined by early goal-directed therapy algorithms [21]. Early goal-directed therapy also was found to be less cost-effective than standard treatment [20, 21].

Empiric Fluid Administration Goals

Fluids are commonly given empirically during the initial assessment of a patient with suspected sepsis or septic shock. The Surviving Sepsis Campaign recommends an empiric fluid administration of 30 mL/kg over the first 3 h for all patients with sepsis or septic shock [22]. The ProCESS and ARISE trials both averaged approximately 30 mL/kg before randomization [18, 19, 22]. A recent retrospective study identified that patients who were elderly, male, obese, had end-stage renal disease, heart failure, or documented "fluid overload" were less likely to achieve the SCC's fluid goal by 3 h [23]. While concerns for limiting over-resuscitation are appropriate and valid, failure to meet this initial fluid resuscitation goal of 30 mL/kg by 3 h has been associated with increased mortality (OR 1.52; 95% CI: 1.03–2.24) [23]. Another retrospective analysis identified that patients who received at least 0.25 mL/kg/min infusion rates to meet the 30 mL/kg goal had higher proportions of shock resolution (HR: 1.22; 95% CI: 1.06–1.41), shorter median times to shock resolution, and lower mortality rates at 28 days (HR: 0.71, 95% CI: 0.60–0.85) than those with lower infusion rates [24]. Even patients with a history of congestive heart failure, who are typically considered more at risk from high-volume resuscitation, have been found to have improved mortality in sepsis when they meet the 30 mL/kg within 3 h goal [25].

Over Resuscitation

While initial empiric fluid administration of 30 mL/kg within the first 3 h is associated with improved outcomes, "more" is not "better." Several observational studies have demonstrated poor outcomes with increased fluid balance [26–29]. One retrospective analysis of Vasopressin in Septic Shock Trial (VASST) data demonstrated that a positive fluid balance and elevated central venous pressure was associated with increased mortality [26]. Another retrospective study of 2632 ICU patients with sepsis suggests that for every 1 L of cumulative fluid balance at 72 h, hospital mortality increased by 6% (OR 1.06%, 95% CI: 1.04–1.08) [27]. A recent meta-analysis found that fluid overload at any time point was associated with an adjusted relative risk for mortality of 2.79 (95% CI: 1.55–5.00) [30]. Another study of 23,513 patients with sepsis and septic shock found that patients who received >5 L of fluid on the first hospital day had increased mortality [31]. Fluid overload has also been associated with a decreased slope in the recovery of the SOFA score in septic patients following initial resuscitation suggesting prolonged organ dysfunction in that subset of patients [32]. Not surprisingly, increased fluid balance has also been associated with acute kidney injury and respiratory failure [33].

Dynamic Measures of Volume Responsiveness

Protocolized volume resuscitation is not associated with improved outcomes; however, achieving 30 mL/kg within the first 3 h does appear to reduce mortality. Further complicating resuscitation is cumulative fluid balance and fluid overload being associated with increased mortality. For up to 50% of hemodynamically unstable patients, additional fluid may not result in improved hemodynamics [31]. Given these seemingly conflicting viewpoints, what information can be used to guide ongoing resuscitation measures? Current management following initial empiric volume resuscitation has transitioned to using measures of volume responsiveness to guide resuscitation efforts beyond initial empiric fluid administration. The use of these markers of fluid responsiveness, particularly dynamic tests, has been associated with reduced mortality and fewer complications compared to standard therapy [33, 34].

Fluid Challenge

In practical terms, the fluid challenge may be the most common method of assessing volume responsiveness. The approach is simple enough: give fluid and see if the patient's hemodynamics improve. While the results are easy to interpret, this method clearly predisposes to over resuscitation. However, with close cardiac output monitoring (via thermodilution, bioimpedance, or pulse contour analysis) smaller volumes of fluid (100 mL) can be given very rapidly over about 1 min and changes to stroke volume can be quickly assessed. Using this method of low-volume rapid infusion, fluid responsiveness can be directly tested while minimizing the risk of volume overload. A recent meta-analysis found that the pooled sensitivity and specificity of the "mini" fluid challenge for predicting volume responsiveness in sedated, mechanically ventilated patients without arrhythmia was 82% (95% CI: 76–88%) and 83% (95% CI: 77–89%) [35].

Passive Leg Raise

The passive leg-raise (PLR), or modified fluid challenge, is a straightforward way to assess whether a fluid bolus will result in improved stroke volume. The procedure is performed by lying the patient flat in bed. Both legs are then simultaneously raised to 45° angle. Venous blood that had been pooling in the lower extremities is then quickly transferred to the central venous system increasing preload. An increase in stroke volume of 10–15% or more is considered a positive test and is associated with volume responsiveness. The benefits of this maneuver are that the increased volume is relatively small (250–300 mL) and it is completely and rapidly reversible. Additionally, the PLR is useful in both mechanically ventilated and spontaneously breathing patients as well as those with cardiac arrhythmias [8]. A large meta-analysis demonstrated that PLR had a pooled sensitivity of 86% (95% CI: 79–92%) and specificity of 92% (95% CI: 88–96%) for predicting volume responsiveness [36]. Frequently, an increase in pulse pressure of 10–15% or more on an arterial line tracing is used as a surrogate for stroke volume or cardiac output. Using pulse pressure variation as a surrogate in this setting is associated with reduced sensitivity (58%; 95% CI: 44–70) and specificity (83%; 95% CI: 68–92%) of PLR [36]. A recent randomized controlled trial found that the use of PLR (with response measured via NICOM bioresistance device) was associated with lower cumulative fluid balance as well as lower rates of renal and respiratory failure when compared to traditional fluid management relying on vital signs [33]. Notably, this test should not be used in those with spine, pelvic, or lower extremity injuries.

End-Expiratory Occlusion Test

Preload varies naturally with inspiration. Many of the tests discussed in this chapter make use of that fact. In patients who are deeply sedated and mechanically ventilated, the ventilator can be used to exploit this relationship and provide a temporary and completely reversible fluid "bolus" to assess volume responsiveness similar to the passive leg raise. Left-sided cardiac preload decreases with inspiration, therefore performing a 15-s end-expiratory hold should prevent this inspiration-associated drop in preload. An increase in arterial pulse pressure of >5 mmHg is considered a positive test [37]. In one recent meta-analysis the EEOT had the highest pooled sensitivity (86%; 95% CI: 74–94%) and specificity (91%; 95% CI: 85–95%) of all the methods assessed [35].

Pulse Pressure and Stroke Volume Variation

Pulse pressure is the difference between the systolic and diastolic blood pressures as determined by arterial waveform analysis. These values vary naturally over the course of the respiratory cycle as changes in intrathoracic pressure influence preload. Pulse pressure variation (PPV) is defined as the maximum pulse pressure (PPmax) minus the minimum pulse pressure (PPmin) divided by the average of these two values (PPavg). This ratio is multiplied by 100 to represent a percentage of variation with respect to the mean [PPV = (PPmax − PPmin/PPavg) × 100]. Pulse pressure variation of 12% or more is considered consistent with fluid responsiveness [37]. A large meta-analysis identified a pooled sensitivity of 88% (95% CI: 81–92%) and a specificity of 89% (95% CI: 84–92%) for predicting fluid responsiveness in a population of critically ill mechanically ventilated patients receiving at least 8 mL/kg tidal volumes [38].

Like pulse pressure variation, stroke volume naturally varies across the respiratory cycle. Using pulse waveform analysis (via FloTrac or PiCCO) the stroke volume can be estimated. Stroke volume variation can be measured using the analogous formula to that used for PPV. A stroke volume variation of 13% or more is considered consistent with volume responsiveness [37]. In critically ill mechanically ventilated patients receiving at least 8 mL/kg tidal volumes, SVV has a sensitivity of 81% (95% CI: 77–85%) and specificity of 80% (95% CI: 68–89%) for predicting fluid responsiveness [39].

The PPV and SVV measurements share many of the same limitations. Both require an invasive arterial line with SVV requiring additional devices for practical use. They are both validated for intubated patients receiving large tidal volumes (8–10 mL/kg) who are not spontaneously breathing and have no cardiac arrhythmias [37]. In practice, most patients may not meet these criteria. One prospective study found that only 2% of the patients they evaluated met the criteria for accurate use of PPV [40]. The tidal volume limitation can be overcome by incorporating a "Tidal Volume Challenge" where the PPV and/or SVV measurements are taken, the tidal volumes are temporarily increased to 8–10 mL/kg and the measurement are then repeated. A change in the PPV of at least 3.5% between the lower and higher tidal volume states (2.5% for SVV) is associated with fluid responsiveness [41].

Systolic Blood Pressure Variation

Respiratory variation in systolic blood pressure (SPV) is occasionally and inappropriately used interchangeably with pulse pressure variation in clinical settings. Pulse pressure variation follows the measurement and calculation described. Measuring systolic blood pressure variation involves establishing the baseline systolic blood pressure during a short end-expiratory pause on the ventilator and then using an arterial waveform to measure respiratory changes in systolic blood pressure both above ("delta up" or "dUP") and below ("delta down" or "dDown") this baseline [37]. One study of cardiac surgery patients found that the overall systolic pressure variation threshold of >8.5 mmHg had a sensitivity of 82% and specificity of 86% for predicting volume responsiveness. The delta down component, with a threshold of >5 mmHg, had a sensitivity of 86% and sensitivity of 86%. In this series, both the overall variation in SPV and the delta down component were both inferior to PPV in predicting fluid responsiveness [42]. Another small series of patients with sepsis-induced hypotension found that delta down component of SPV >5 mmHg had a positive predictive value of 95% and a negative predictive value of 93% for predicting volume responsiveness [43]. As with PPV and SVV, accurate SPV measurements require that the patient be mechanically ventilated without spontaneous respiration. Additionally, the patient should be without any cardiac arrhythmias [37].

Inferior Vena Cava Index

Respiratory variation in the IVC diameter is an increasingly common method of evaluating fluid responsiveness. The M mode on the ultrasound is used to measure the maximum and minimum IVC diameters across the respiratory cycle; ideally at about 1 cm caudal to the hepatic veins. The threshold for volume responsiveness is a change in IVC diameter of 40–50% in spontaneously breathing patients and 12–18% in mechanically ventilated patients [44]. One meta-analysis found an overall sensitivity of 63% (95% CI: 56–69%) and specificity of 73% (95% CI: 67–78%) for volume responsiveness. This same study found that the sensitivity and specificity for non-ventilated patients was 52% (95% CI: 42–62%) and 77% (95% CI: 68–84%) respectively while the sensitivity and specificity of the IVC index in mechanically ventilated patients was 67% (95% CI: 58–75%) and 68% (95% CI: 60–76%) respectively [44]. Another recent meta-analysis found that the pooled sensitivity and specificity for predicting volume responsiveness in mechanically ventilated patients was 69% (95% CI: 51–83%) and 80% (95% CI: 66–89%) respectively [45].

There are several benefits to the IVC index that have made it popular. It is a completely non-invasive test that can be repeated as many times as needed without the requirements for invasive monitoring or expensive cardiac output devices. The only mechanical requirement is a capable ultrasound machine which is found in almost all modern intensive care settings. Additionally, the visual information garnered by the ultrasound provides intuitive gross information about the patient's volume status. However, like the CVP measurement (discussed below) the IVC diameter, and therefore IVC index, is influenced by several factors that will affect its interpretation. Tidal volumes, heart failure, tricuspid regurgitation, pericardial tamponade, pneumothorax, COPD, intra-abdominal hypertension, and pericardial disease can all affect the central venous pressure, which may then alter the diameter of the IVC [37, 44]. Using the IVC index as opposed to the IVC diameter should minimize, but not negate these confounding factors as it provides a more functional assessment rather than a static value. Additionally, while calculating the IVC index is straightforward, it is operator dependent. Visualization of the IVC can also be affected by factors such as retained pneumoperitoneum from recent surgery, gastric or colonic distension, or body habitus.

Static Measures of Volume Responsiveness

Static predictors of volume responsiveness are generally considered to be less accurate than dynamic measures which is why they are not recommended by clinical guidelines [22]. Most of the static assessments below represent estimates of preload without any indication of myocardial contractility. Since the steep slope of the Frank-Starling curve is dependent on contractility, and the relationship between preload and stroke volume is non-linear, static preload estimates often fail to provide an accurate assessment of volume responsiveness [46].

Central Venous Pressure

Central venous pressure (CVP) has long been known to have no correlation with intravascular blood volume [47]. However, largely due to early goal-directed therapy protocols, titrating volume to a goal CVP of 8–12 mmHg remained a mainstay of sepsis resuscitation until recently. Central venous pressure is thought to represent right ventricular end-diastolic volume and is used as a marker of pre-load. However, a variety of conditions can result in an elevated CVP including, but not limited to, right heart failure, tricuspid regurgitation, pulmonary embolism, pulmonary hypertension, tension pneumothorax, renal failure, cardiac tamponade, and increased intrathoracic pressure from positive pressure ventilation [48, 49]. Left heart failure may present with an increased or decreased CVP [49]. In fact, for patients with cardiac dysfunction, a falling CVP is more likely to indicate improved stroke volume and cardiac function rather than hypovolemia [49]. While hypovolemia and venous dilation remain common causes of a decreased CVP in surgical patients, the high prevalence of other comorbidities complicates the interpretation of the CVP measurement and therefore make it an unreliable marker of volume responsiveness. One large meta-analysis demonstrated no correlation between CVP measurements and volume responsiveness in either the ICU or intra-operative setting demonstrating an AUC of 0.56 [50].

Pulmonary Artery Occlusion Pressure

The use of pulmonary artery catheters in the diagnosis and treatment of septic shock is largely historical. Much of the information gathered from these devices is now collected via non-invasive or minimally invasive means. These catheters carry a significant risk of complication including arrhythmias, pulmonary artery rupture, and entanglement [51]. The pulmonary artery occlusion (or wedge) pressure (PAOP) was thought to be a reliable measure of left ventricular preload [37]. However, in practice, PAOP is subject to many other conditions unrelated to volume status that can alter the measurement and decrease its accuracy, including left ventricular compliance, right ventricular function, pericarditis, and intrathoracic volume [37]. One review found that in 7 out of 9 studies, there was no correlation between PAOP and volume responsiveness [52].

Inferior Vena Cava Diameter

Measurement of the inferior vena cava diameter is assumed to correlate with right atrial pressure and therefore serve as a marker of preload. Assessment of the IVC diameter via bedside ultrasound is relatively straightforward but is highly operator-dependent. Additionally, factors such as the presence of residual pneumoperitoneum after surgery, pneumothorax, dilated stomach or colon, and body habitus can make the visualization of the vena cava difficult. In essence, static measurement of the IVC diameter is a visual representation of the central venous pressure and is subject to the same limitations [53].

Left Ventricular End-Diastolic Area

Bedside echocardiography has increased in popularity in the ICU setting. Measuring the left ventricular end-diastolic area (LVDA) has been proposed as a measure of volume responsiveness. In practical use, bedside echocardiography is highly operator-dependent and requires more skill than ultrasound assessment of the IVC diameter. The LVDA is measured in the four-chamber view using a transthoracic or transesophageal approach and is expected to be low in hypovolemic patients and increase with volume loading [37]. The LVDA can be assessed before and after volume loading to provide a LVDA index. This step, however, can only be performed after the volume is already given and is therefore of little utility when trying to avoid over resuscitation. LVDA has been found to have a lower AUROC than systolic pressure variation [43].

Choice of Fluid

Crystalloid

Crystalloid solutions are the most prescribed form of volume expander in septic patients with normal saline (0.9% saline solution) being the most commonly used historically. Recently the paired SALT-ED and SMART cluster randomized trials compared normal saline administration to balanced crystalloid solutions (lactated Ringer's solution or Plasma-lyte A) [54, 55]. The SALT-ED trial was focused on non-critically ill patients and evaluated a primary outcome of hospital-free alive days with a secondary composite outcome of death, new renal-replacement therapy, or persistent renal dysfunction. Across 13,347 patients there was no difference in the number of hospital-free alive days based on the fluid given. However, patients receiving balanced crystalloids had a lower rate of the composite secondary outcome (4.7% vs. 5.6%; $p = 0.01$) compared to those receiving saline [54]. The SMART trial focused on critically ill patients and had a primary composite outcome of death, new renal-replacement therapy, or persistent renal dysfunction censored at 30 days. Similar to SALT-ED, of the 15,802 patients that were enrolled in the SMART trial, those that received balanced crystalloid solution had lower rates of the composite outcome compared to those that received saline (14.3% vs 15.4%; $p = 0.04$) [55]. A subgroup analysis of the SMART trial found that septic patients also had lower rates of the composite outcome as well as lower overall mortality when receiving balanced crystalloid solution (supplemental appendix) [55].

Concerns for new or worsening hyperkalemia when using balanced crystalloid solutions also appear unfounded. Two randomized trials of lactated Ringer's solution versus normal saline in renal transplant recipients both found that those receiving normal saline were more likely to have hyperkalemic episodes than those receiving lactated Ringer's solution [56, 57].

Colloid

Despite minimal evidence of clinical benefit, colloids remain an often-suggested resuscitative fluid. Multiple prospective clinical trials have demonstrated no difference in mortality between albumin (or other colloids) versus crystalloids for patients in a variety of shock states [58, 59]. Patients with sepsis were included as subgroup analyses in both the SAFE and CRISTAL studies and demonstrated no difference in mortality [58, 59]. A cost-effectiveness analysis using these studies demonstrated that albumin, but not hydroxyethyl starch, was cost-effective compared to crystalloid [60]. The 2014 ALBIOS study found that during the first 7 days, mean arterial pressure was higher, heart rates were lower, and net fluid balance was lower in patients who received albumin. However, there was no difference in organ failure or mortality rates between the groups [61]. Interestingly, a post-hoc analysis of patients in septic shock, demonstrated a relative risk of mortality of 0.87 (95%

CI: 0.77–0.99) [61]. A retrospective analysis of the ALBIOS cohort failed to identify a significant mortality difference based on albumin administration (48.7% vs 54.9%; $p = 0.11$) when the new SEPSIS-3 criteria for septic shock were applied [62].

Blood Products

Transfusion of blood products, particularly packed red blood cells (PRBCs), were a key component of early-goal-directed therapy protocols [16, 18–20]. However, PRBC transfusion has been associated with adverse outcomes such as immune suppression, increased infection rates, and increased rates of cancer recurrence [63–71]. The TRICC trial established that a restrictive transfusion threshold of 7.0 g/dL was safe and effective in stable critically ill patients [72]. The TRISS trial further evaluated transfusion thresholds in patients with septic shock and again found no difference in outcomes [73]. There is some data to suggest that oncologic patients in septic shock may benefit from a liberal transfusion threshold [74]. For patients with sepsis or septic shock, who are not bleeding acutely or displaying symptomatic anemia, we recommend a restrictive transfusion threshold of 7.0 g/dL.

In recent years, plasma-heavy resuscitations have demonstrated improved outcomes in the setting of trauma and major abdominal surgery [75–77]. Fresh frozen plasma (FFP) has demonstrated improved survival in animal models of sepsis [78]. While FFP is clearly beneficial in the correction of coagulopathy, there is currently limited data on its use as a resuscitative fluid in septic patients [79].

Resuscitation Endpoints

Serum Lactate

Since the current sepsis definitions use serum lactate, and not hemodynamics, as the primary determinate of septic shock, it should come as no surprise that normalization of serum lactate is considered an endpoint of resuscitation [3]. While not a direct measure of tissue hypoperfusion, the Surviving Sepsis Campaign nevertheless recommends correction of serum lactate to normal levels as the primary resuscitation endpoint [22]. Lactate is the byproduct of anaerobic glycolysis in the setting of tissue hypoperfusion. Multiple trials have demonstrated benefit in resuscitation strategies based on lactate clearance [80–84]. Recently the ANDROMEDA-SHOCK trial compared resuscitation protocols aimed at lactate clearance of at least 20% every 2 h to another protocol based on normalization of capillary refill time. While there was a trend toward increased mortality in the lactate clearance arm that did not meet statistical significance, organ dysfunction rates were also higher at 72 h in the lactate clearance arm [85].

Base Deficit

Base deficit is often mentioned as another potential endpoint of resuscitation, as abnormal values are associated with poor outcomes in patients with shock. Larger negative values (below −3 mmol) are associated with metabolic acidosis and generally considered to be a marker of metabolic acidosis. However, despite being associated with outcomes, base deficit is affected by many other common clinical entities such as hypothermia, renal failure, CO_2 retention, alcohol consumption, and sodium bicarbonate administration to name a few [86]. These confounding factors limit the use of base deficit as a reliable endpoint of resuscitation.

Empiric Antimicrobials

Timing

The Surviving Sepsis Campaign guidelines recommend aggressive initiation of antimicrobials within the first hour of recognition of sepsis or septic shock [22]. Recently, these recommendations have come under scrutiny as a growing body of evidence indicates that a more nuanced approach to antimicrobial initiation may be warranted [87–89]. A number of prospective observational studies have identified no association between the timing of antimicrobials and patient outcomes [90–95], while others have demonstrated a mortality benefit only for those patients presenting with septic shock. For example, a recent study of mandated sepsis care in New York State demonstrated that overall delays in antibiotic administration increased mortality by 4% per hour [96]. However, when analyzed separately, only patients with septic shock had a higher mortality rate with delays in initiation while those presenting without shock had no benefit from earlier antibiotic administration [97]. A large study by the Surviving Sepsis Campaign reported that patients for whom antibiotics were started within 3 h of sepsis recognition had improved survival rates [98]. However, patients with and without shock were not analyzed separately.

In 2018, Alam et al. published their prospective randomized trial of antimicrobial initiation in patients suspected of sepsis. In their study, patients en route to the hospital who were suspected of having sepsis were randomized to either have antibiotics started hyper-aggressively while in the ambulance before arrival at the hospital versus having them initiated after initial evaluation in the emergency department. They randomized 2672 patients and had a differential time to antibiotic administration of 96 min between groups. There was no difference in 28-day or 90-day mortality between the groups. More importantly, there was no difference based on severity of illness, including those presenting with septic shock [99]. To date this remains the only randomized trial on this topic.

Current guidelines recommend aggressive initiation of antimicrobials in cases of suspected sepsis. While we also recommend aggressive initiation in those patients presenting with septic shock, we believe the current literature supports selective initiation of antibiotics in cases without shock where sepsis is suspected but not yet confirmed. The clinician must weigh the risks and benefits of antimicrobial initiation versus watchful waiting in each patient individually.

Empiric Agents

Once the choice to start empiric antimicrobials is made, it is important to choose agents most likely to cover the expected pathogens. The Surviving Sepsis Campaign recommends that one or more agents be initiated to cover all likely pathogens with daily assessment for possible de-escalation [22]. Clinicians must strike a balance between prescribing inappropriately broad antibiotics for the clinical situation, and inadequate antimicrobial coverage since inadequate coverage is associated with poor outcomes in sepsis [100–102].

Source Control

Surgical elimination of the infectious focus whenever possible is a core tenet of sepsis care. One prospective study of critically ill patients with sepsis found that the timing of source control less than 6 h from presentation was the most important predictor of outcomes in patients requiring surgical intervention [90]. In this study, even the timing or adequacy of antibiotics was not associated with improved outcomes when controlling for the timing of source control [90]. We recommend aggressive surgical source control as soon as feasible.

Case Conclusion

We do not advocate using a single isolated piece of information to guide resuscitation. Rather, we would evaluate the patient using a number of techniques and use the prevailing evidence to guide fluid administration. Our goal is to provide adequate volume resuscitation as long as the patient is volume responsive and correct her lactic acidosis, but not necessarily to liberate the patient from vasopressors initially.

In this case, a bedside ultrasound demonstrates a collapsible inferior vena cava as well as an underfilled left ventricle. Pulse pressure variation is calculated at 15%. A passive leg raise is also performed which demonstrates a 12% increase in pulse pressure. An additional 1.5 L of balanced crystalloid solution is given. After volume resuscitation, her vasopressor requirements are decreasing, her lactate is now almost normalized, and her pulse pressure variation only 9%. The patient is no longer volume responsive so further resuscitation is held.

References

1. Bone RC, Balk RA, Cerra FB, Dellinger RP, Fein AM, Knaus WA, et al. Definitions for sepsis and organ failure and guidelines for the use of innovative therapies in sepsis. The ACCP/SCCM Consensus Conference Committee. American College of Chest Physicians/Society of Critical Care Medicine. Chest. 1992;101(6):1644–55.
2. Levy MM, Fink MP, Marshall JC, Abraham E, Angus D, Cook D, et al. 2001 SCCM/ESICM/ACCP/ATS/SIS international sepsis definitions conference. Intensive Care Med. 2003;29(4):530–8.
3. Singer M, Deutschman CS, Seymour CW, Shankar-Hari M, Annane D, Bauer M, et al. The third international consensus definitions for sepsis and septic shock (Sepsis-3). JAMA. 2016;315(8):801–10.
4. Lee MA, Choi KK, Yu B, Park JJ, Park Y, Gwak J, et al. Acute physiology and chronic health evaluation II score and sequential organ failure assessment score as predictors for severe trauma patients in the intensive care unit. Korean J Crit Care Med. 2017;32(4):340–6.
5. Raith EP, Udy AA, Bailey M, McGloughlin S, MacIsaac C, Bellomo R, et al. Prognostic accuracy of the SOFA score, SIRS criteria, and qSOFA score for in-hospital mortality among adults with suspected infection admitted to the intensive care unit. JAMA. 2017;317(3):290–300.
6. Krebs ED, Hassinger TE, Guidry CA, Berry PS, Elwood NR, Sawyer RG. Non-utility of sepsis scores for identifying infection in surgical intensive care unit patients. Am J Surg. 2019;218(2):243–7.
7. Eguia E, Cobb AN, Baker MS, Joyce C, Gilbert E, Gonzalez R, et al. Risk factors for infection and evaluation of Sepsis-3 in patients with trauma. Am J Surg. 2019;218(5):851–7.
8. Brown RM, Semler MW. Fluid management in sepsis. J Intensive Care Med. 2019;34(5):364–73.
9. Leisman DE, Doerfler ME, Schneider SM, Masick KD, D'Amore JA, D'Angelo JK. Predictors, prevalence, and outcomes of early crystalloid responsiveness among initially hypotensive patients with sepsis and septic shock. Crit Care Med. 2018;46(2):189–98.
10. Stephan F, Flahault A, Dieudonne N, Hollande J, Paillard F, Bonnet F. Clinical evaluation of circulating blood volume in critically ill patients—contribution of a clinical scoring system. Br J Anaesth. 2001;86(6):754–62.
11. Eisenberg PR, Jaffe AS, Schuster DP. Clinical evaluation compared to pulmonary artery catheterization in the hemodynamic assessment of critically ill patients. Crit Care Med. 1984;12(7):549–53.
12. Kalantari K, Chang JN, Ronco C, Rosner MH. Assessment of intravascular volume status and volume responsiveness in critically ill patients. Kidney Int. 2013;83(6):1017–28.
13. Scott MC, Mallemat H. Assessing volume status. Emerg Med Clin N Am. 2014;32(4):811–22.
14. McGee S, Abernethy WB 3rd, Simel DL. The rational clinical examination. Is this patient hypovolemic? JAMA. 1999;281(11):1022–9.
15. Wang CS, FitzGerald JM, Schulzer M, Mak E, Ayas NT. Does this dyspneic patient in the emergency department have congestive heart failure? JAMA. 2005;294(15):1944–56.
16. Rivers E, Nguyen B, Havstad S, Ressler J, Muzzin A, Knoblich B, et al. Early goal-directed therapy in the treatment of severe sepsis and septic shock. N Engl J Med. 2001;345(19):1368–77.
17. Weisberg A, Park P, Cherry-Bukowiec JR. Early goal-directed therapy: the history and ongoing impact on management of severe sepsis and septic shock. Surg Infect. 2018;19(2):142–6.
18. Pro CI, Yealy DM, Kellum JA, Huang DT, Barnato AE, Weissfeld LA, et al. A randomized trial of protocol-based care for early septic shock. N Engl J Med. 2014;370(18):1683–93.
19. ARISE Investigators, ANZICS Clinical Trials Group, Peake SL, Delaney A, Bailey M, Bellomo R, et al. Goal-directed resuscitation for patients with early septic shock. N Engl J Med. 2014;371(16):1496–506.
20. Mouncey PR, Osborn TM, Power GS, Harrison DA, Sadique MZ, Grieve RD, et al. Trial of early, goal-directed resuscitation for septic shock. N Engl J Med. 2015;372(14):1301–11.
21. PRISM Investigators, Rowan KM, Angus DC, Bailey M, Barnato AE, Bellomo R, et al. Early, goal-directed therapy for septic shock—a patient-level meta-analysis. N Engl J Med. 2017;376(23):2223–34.
22. Rhodes A, Evans LE, Alhazzani W, Levy MM, Antonelli M, Ferrer R, et al. Surviving sepsis campaign: international guidelines for management of sepsis and septic shock: 2016. Crit Care Med. 2017;45(3):486–552.
23. Kuttab HI, Lykins JD, Hughes MD, Wroblewski K, Keast EP, Kukoyi O, et al. Evaluation and predictors of fluid resuscitation in patients with severe sepsis and septic shock. Crit Care Med. 2019;47(11):1582–90.
24. Hu B, Chen JCY, Dong Y, Frank RD, Passe M, Portner E, et al. Effect of initial infusion rates of fluid resuscitation on outcomes in patients with septic shock: a historical cohort study. Crit Care. 2020;24(1):137.
25. Taenzer AH, Patel SJ, Allen TL, Doerfler ME, Park TR, Savitz LA, et al. Improvement in mortality with early fluid bolus in sepsis patients with a history of congestive heart failure. Mayo Clin Proc Innov Qual Outcomes. 2020;4(5):537–41.
26. Boyd JH, Forbes J, Nakada TA, Walley KR, Russell JA. Fluid resuscitation in septic shock: a positive fluid balance and elevated central venous pressure are associated with increased mortality. Crit Care Med. 2011;39(2):259–65.

27. Neyra JA, Li X, Canepa-Escaro F, Adams-Huet B, Toto RD, Yee J, et al. Cumulative fluid balance and mortality in septic patients with or without acute kidney injury and chronic kidney disease. Crit Care Med. 2016;44(10):1891 900.
28. van Mourik N, Geerts BF, Binnekade JM, Veelo DP, Bos LDJ, Wiersinga WJ, et al. A higher fluid balance in the days after septic shock reversal is associated with increased mortality: an observational cohort study. Crit Care Explor. 2020;2(10):e0219.
29. Sivayoham N, Blake LA, Tharimoopantavida SE, Chughtai S, Hussain AN, Rhodes A. Treatment variables associated with outcome in emergency department patients with suspected sepsis. Ann Intensive Care. 2020;10(1):136.
30. Messmer AS, Zingg C, Muller M, Gerber JL, Schefold JC, Pfortmueller CA. Fluid overload and mortality in adult critical care patients—a systematic review and meta-analysis of observational studies. Crit Care Med. 2020;48:1862–70.
31. Marik PE, Linde-Zwirble WT, Bittner EA, Sahatjian J, Hansell D. Fluid administration in severe sepsis and septic shock, patterns and outcomes: an analysis of a large national database. Intensive Care Med. 2017;43(5):625–32.
32. Chapalain X, Vermeersch V, Egreteau PY, Prat G, Alavi Z, Vicaut E, et al. Association between fluid overload and SOFA score kinetics in septic shock patients: a retrospective multicenter study. J Intensive Care. 2019;7:42.
33. Douglas IS, Alapat PM, Corl KA, Exline MC, Forni LG, Holder AL, et al. Fluid response evaluation in sepsis hypotension and shock: a randomized clinical trial. Chest. 2020;158(4):1431–45.
34. Dubin A, Loudet C, Kanoore Edul VS, Osatnik J, Rios F, Vasquez D, et al. Characteristics of resuscitation, and association between use of dynamic tests of fluid responsiveness and outcomes in septic patients: results of a multicenter prospective cohort study in Argentina. Ann Intensive Care. 2020;10(1):40.
35. Messina A, Dell'Anna A, Baggiani M, Torrini F, Maresca GM, Bennett V, et al. Functional hemodynamic tests: a systematic review and a metanalysis on the reliability of the end-expiratory occlusion test and of the mini-fluid challenge in predicting fluid responsiveness. Crit Care. 2019;23(1):264.
36. Cherpanath TG, Hirsch A, Geerts BF, Lagrand WK, Leeflang MM, Schultz MJ, et al. Predicting fluid responsiveness by passive leg raising: a systematic review and meta-analysis of 23 clinical trials. Crit Care Med. 2016;44(5):981–91.
37. Jalil BA, Cavallazzi R. Predicting fluid responsiveness: a review of literature and a guide for the clinician. Am J Emerg Med. 2018;36(11):2093–102.
38. Yang X, Du B. Does pulse pressure variation predict fluid responsiveness in critically ill patients? A systematic review and meta-analysis. Crit Care. 2014;18(6):650.
39. Zhang Z, Lu B, Sheng X, Jin N. Accuracy of stroke volume variation in predicting fluid responsiveness: a systematic review and meta-analysis. J Anesth. 2011;25(6):904–16.
40. Mahjoub Y, Lejeune V, Muller L, Perbet S, Zieleskiewicz L, Bart F, et al. Evaluation of pulse pressure variation validity criteria in critically ill patients: a prospective observational multicentre point-prevalence study. Br J Anaesth. 2014;112(4):681–5.
41. Myatra SN, Monnet X, Teboul J-L. Use of 'tidal volume challenge' to improve the reliability of pulse pressure variation. Crit Care. 2017;21(1):60.
42. Preisman S, Kogan S, Berkenstadt H, Perel A. Predicting fluid responsiveness in patients undergoing cardiac surgery: functional haemodynamic parameters including the respiratory systolic variation test and static preload indicators. Br J Anaesth. 2005;95(6):746–55.
43. Tavernier B, Makhotine O, Lebuffe G, Dupont J, Scherpereel P. Systolic pressure variation as a guide to fluid therapy in patients with sepsis-induced hypotension. Anesthesiology. 1998;89(6):1313–21.
44. Long E, Oakley E, Duke T, Babl FE, Paediatric Research in Emergency Departments International C. Does respiratory variation in inferior vena cava diameter predict fluid responsiveness: a systematic review and meta-analysis. Shock. 2017;47(5):550–9.
45. Huang H, Shen Q, Liu Y, Xu H, Fang Y. Value of variation index of inferior vena cava diameter in predicting fluid responsiveness in patients with circulatory shock receiving mechanical ventilation: a systematic review and meta-analysis. Crit Care. 2018;22(1):204.
46. Huang CC, Fu JY, Hu HC, Kao KC, Chen NH, Hsieh MJ, et al. Prediction of fluid responsiveness in acute respiratory distress syndrome patients ventilated with low tidal volume and high positive end-expiratory pressure. Crit Care Med. 2008;36(10):2810–6.
47. Shippy CR, Appel PL, Shoemaker WC. Reliability of clinical monitoring to assess blood volume in critically ill patients. Crit Care Med. 1984;12(2):107–12.
48. Shojaee M, Sabzghabaei A, Alimohammadi H, Derakhshanfar H, Amini A, Esmailzadeh B. Effect of positive end-expiratory pressure on central venous pressure in patients under mechanical ventilation. Emerg (Tehran). 2017;5(1):e1.
49. Berlin DA, Bakker J. Starling curves and central venous pressure. Crit Care. 2015;19:55.
50. Marik PE, Cavallazzi R. Does the central venous pressure predict fluid responsiveness? An updated meta-analysis and a plea for some common sense. Crit Care Med. 2013;41(7):1774–81.
51. Armstrong BAGC, May AK. Surgical complications in the ICU. In: Britt LDPA, Barie PS, Jurkovich GJ, editors. Acute care surgery. Philadelphia: Lippincott Williams & Wilkins; 2019. p. 743–58.
52. Michard F, Teboul J-L. Predicting fluid responsiveness in ICU patients: a critical analysis of the evidence. Chest. 2002;121(6):2000–8.
53. Ciozda W, Kedan I, Kehl DW, Zimmer R, Khandwalla R, Kimchi A. The efficacy of sono-

graphic measurement of inferior vena cava diameter as an estimate of central venous pressure. Cardiovasc Ultrasound. 2016;14(1):33.
54. Self WH, Semler MW, Wanderer JP, Wang L, Byrne DW, Collins SP, et al. Balanced crystalloids versus saline in noncritically ill adults. N Engl J Med. 2018;378(9):819–28.
55. Semler MW, Self WH, Wanderer JP, Ehrenfeld JM, Wang L, Byrne DW, et al. Balanced crystalloids versus saline in critically ill adults. N Engl J Med. 2018;378(9):829–39.
56. O'Malley CM, Frumento RJ, Hardy MA, Benvenisty AI, Brentjens TE, Mercer JS, et al. A randomized, double-blind comparison of lactated Ringer's solution and 0.9% NaCl during renal transplantation. Anesth Analg. 2005;100(5):1518–24, table of contents.
57. Khajavi MR, Etezadi F, Moharari RS, Imani F, Meysamie AP, Khashayar P, et al. Effects of normal saline vs. lactated ringer's during renal transplantation. Ren Fail. 2008;30(5):535–9.
58. Finfer S, Bellomo R, Boyce N, French J, Myburgh J, Norton R, et al. A comparison of albumin and saline for fluid resuscitation in the intensive care unit. N Engl J Med. 2004;350(22):2247–56.
59. Annane D, Siami S, Jaber S, Martin C, Elatrous S, Declere AD, et al. Effects of fluid resuscitation with colloids vs crystalloids on mortality in critically ill patients presenting with hypovolemic shock: the CRISTAL randomized trial. JAMA. 2013;310(17):1809–17.
60. Farrugia A, Bansal M, Balboni S, Kimber MC, Martin GS, Cassar J. Choice of fluids in severe septic patients—a cost-effectiveness analysis informed by recent clinical trials. Rev Recent Clin Trials. 2014;9(1):21–30.
61. Caironi P, Tognoni G, Masson S, Fumagalli R, Pesenti A, Romero M, et al. Albumin replacement in patients with severe sepsis or septic shock. N Engl J Med. 2014;370(15):1412–21.
62. Vasques F, Duscio E, Romitti F, Pasticci I, Caironi P, Meessen J, et al. Septic shock-3 vs 2: an analysis of the ALBIOS study. Crit Care. 2018;22(1):237.
63. Claridge JA, Sawyer RG, Schulman AM, McLemore EC, Young JS. Blood transfusions correlate with infections in trauma patients in a dose-dependent manner. Am Surg. 2002;68(7):566–72.
64. Karcutskie CA, Meizoso JP, Ray JJ, Horkan DB, Ruiz XD, Schulman CI, et al. Mechanism of injury May influence infection risk from early blood transfusion. Surg Infect. 2017;18(2):83–8.
65. Teng Z, Zhu Y, Liu Y, Wei G, Wang S, Du S, et al. Restrictive blood transfusion strategies and associated infection in orthopedic patients: a meta-analysis of 8 randomized controlled trials. Sci Rep. 2015;5:13421.
66. Horvath KA, Acker MA, Chang H, Bagiella E, Smith PK, Iribarne A, et al. Blood transfusion and infection after cardiac surgery. Ann Thorac Surg. 2013;95(6):2194–201.
67. Tai YH, Wu HL, Mandell MS, Tsou MY, Chang KY. The association of allogeneic blood transfusion and the recurrence of hepatic cancer after surgical resection. Anaesthesia. 2020;75(4):464–71.
68. Qiu L, Wang DR, Zhang XY, Gao S, Li XX, Sun GP, et al. Impact of perioperative blood transfusion on immune function and prognosis in colorectal cancer patients. Transfus Apher Sci. 2016;54(2):235–41.
69. Pushan Z, Manbiao C, Sulai L, Jun L, Ruidong Z, Hanshen Y. The impact of perioperative blood transfusion on survival and recurrence after radical prostatectomy for prostate cancer: a systematic review and meta-analysis. J Cancer Res Ther. 2018;14(Supplement):S701–S7.
70. Dellinger EP, Anaya DA. Infectious and immunologic consequences of blood transfusion. Crit Care. 2004;8(Suppl 2):S18–23.
71. Wei S, Gonzalez Rodriguez E, Chang R, Holcomb JB, Kao LS, Wade CE, et al. Elevated Syndecan-1 after trauma and risk of sepsis: a secondary analysis of patients from the pragmatic, randomized optimal platelet and plasma ratios (PROPPR) trial. J Am Coll Surg. 2018;227(6):587–95.
72. Hebert PC, Wells G, Blajchman MA, Marshall J, Martin C, Pagliarello G, et al. A multicenter, randomized, controlled clinical trial of transfusion requirements in critical care. Transfusion Requirements in Critical Care Investigators, Canadian Critical Care Trials Group. N Engl J Med. 1999;340(6):409–17.
73. Holst LB, Haase N, Wetterslev J, Wernerman J, Guttormsen AB, Karlsson S, et al. Lower versus higher hemoglobin threshold for transfusion in septic shock. N Engl J Med. 2014;371(15):1381–91.
74. Bergamin FS, Almeida JP, Landoni G, Galas F, Fukushima JT, Fominskiy E, et al. Liberal versus restrictive transfusion strategy in critically ill oncologic patients: the transfusion requirements in critically ill oncologic patients randomized controlled trial. Crit Care Med. 2017;45(5):766–73.
75. Holcomb JB, Fox EE, Wade CE, PROMMTT Study Group. The PRospective Observational Multicenter Major Trauma Transfusion (PROMMTT) study. J Trauma Acute Care Surg. 2013;75(1 Suppl 1):S1–2.
76. Holcomb JB, Tilley BC, Baraniuk S, Fox EE, Wade CE, Podbielski JM, et al. Transfusion of plasma, platelets, and red blood cells in a 1:1:1 vs a 1:1:2 ratio and mortality in patients with severe trauma: the PROPPR randomized clinical trial. JAMA. 2015;313(5):471–82.
77. Saxena A, Chua TC, Fransi S, Liauw W, Morris DL. Effectiveness of early and aggressive administration of fresh frozen plasma to reduce massive blood transfusion during cytoreductive surgery. J Gastrointest Oncol. 2013;4(1):30–9.
78. Chang R, Holcomb JB, Johansson PI, Pati S, Schreiber MA, Wade CE. Plasma resuscitation improved survival in a cecal ligation and puncture rat model of sepsis. Shock. 2018;49(1):53–61.

79. Reiter N, Wesche N, Perner A. The majority of patients in septic shock are transfused with fresh-frozen plasma. Dan Med J. 2013;60(4):A4606.
80. Jansen TC, van Bommel J, Schoonderbeek FJ, Sleeswijk Visser SJ, van der Klooster JM, Lima AP, et al. Early lactate-guided therapy in intensive care unit patients: a multicenter, open-label, randomized controlled trial. Am J Respir Crit Care Med. 2010;182(6):752–61.
81. Jones AE, Shapiro NI, Trzeciak S, Arnold RC, Claremont HA, Kline JA, et al. Lactate clearance vs central venous oxygen saturation as goals of early sepsis therapy: a randomized clinical trial. JAMA. 2010;303(8):739–46.
82. Lyu X, Xu Q, Cai G, Yan J, Yan M. [Efficacies of fluid resuscitation as guided by lactate clearance rate and central venous oxygen saturation in patients with septic shock]. Zhonghua Yi Xue Za Zhi. 2015;95(7):496–500.
83. Tian HH, Han SS, Lv CJ, Wang T, Li Z, Hao D, et al. [The effect of early goal lactate clearance rate on the outcome of septic shock patients with severe pneumonia]. Zhongguo Wei Zhong Bing Ji Jiu Yi Xue. 2012;24(1):42–5.
84. Yu B, Tian HY, Hu ZJ, Zhao C, Liu LX, Zhang Y, et al. [Comparison of the effect of fluid resuscitation as guided either by lactate clearance rate or by central venous oxygen saturation in patients with sepsis]. Zhonghua Wei Zhong Bing Ji Jiu Yi Xue. 2013;25(10):578–83.
85. Hernandez G, Ospina-Tascon GA, Damiani LP, Estenssoro E, Dubin A, Hurtado J, et al. Effect of a resuscitation strategy targeting peripheral perfusion status vs serum lactate levels on 28-day mortality among patients with septic shock: the ANDROMEDA-SHOCK randomized clinical trial. JAMA. 2019;321(7):654–64.
86. Cestero RF, Dent DL. Endpoints of resuscitation. Surg Clin N Am. 2015;95(2):319–36.
87. Prescott HC, Iwashyna TJ. Improving sepsis treatment by embracing diagnostic uncertainty. Ann Am Thorac Soc. 2019;16(4):426–9.
88. Rhee C, Strich JR, Klompas M, Yealy DM, Masur H. SEP-1 has brought much needed attention to improving sepsis care... But now is the time to improve SEP-1. Crit Care Med. 2020;48(6):779–82.
89. Rhee C, Chiotos K, Cosgrove SE, Heil EL, Kadri SS, Kalil AC, et al. Infectious Diseases Society of America position paper: recommended revisions to the national severe sepsis and septic shock early management bundle (SEP-1) sepsis quality measure. Clin Infect Dis. 2020; https://doi.org/10.1093/cid/ciaa059.
90. Bloos F, Thomas-Ruddel D, Ruddel H, Engel C, Schwarzkopf D, Marshall JC, et al. Impact of compliance with infection management guidelines on outcome in patients with severe sepsis: a prospective observational multi-center study. Crit Care. 2014;18(2):R42.
91. Abe T, Ogura H, Shiraishi A, Kushimoto S, Saitoh D, Fujishima S, et al. Characteristics, management, and in-hospital mortality among patients with severe sepsis in intensive care units in Japan: the FORECAST study. Crit Care. 2018;22(1):322.
92. de Groot B, Ansems A, Gerling DH, Rijpsma D, van Amstel P, Linzel D, et al. The association between time to antibiotics and relevant clinical outcomes in emergency department patients with various stages of sepsis: a prospective multi-center study. Crit Care. 2015;19:194.
93. Kaasch AJ, Rieg S, Kuetscher J, Brodt HR, Widmann T, Herrmann M, et al. Delay in the administration of appropriate antimicrobial therapy in Staphylococcus aureus bloodstream infection: a prospective multicenter hospital-based cohort study. Infection. 2013;41(5):979–85.
94. van Zanten AR, Brinkman S, Arbous MS, Abu-Hanna A, Levy MM, de Keizer NF, et al. Guideline bundles adherence and mortality in severe sepsis and septic shock. Crit Care Med. 2014;42(8):1890–8.
95. Hranjec T, Rosenberger LH, Swenson B, Metzger R, Flohr TR, Politano AD, et al. Aggressive versus conservative initiation of antimicrobial treatment in critically ill surgical patients with suspected intensive-care-unit-acquired infection: a quasi-experimental, before and after observational cohort study. Lancet Infect Dis. 2012;12(10):774–80.
96. Seymour CW, Gesten F, Prescott HC, Friedrich ME, Iwashyna TJ, Phillips GS, et al. Time to treatment and mortality during mandated emergency care for sepsis. N Engl J Med. 2017;376(23):2235–44.
97. Seymour CW, Gesten F, Prescott HC, Friedrich ME, Iwashyna TJ, Phillips GS, et al. Time to treatment and mortality during mandated emergency care for sepsis (supplemental appendix). N Engl J Med. 2017;376(23):2235–44.
98. Levy MM, Rhodes A, Phillips GS, Townsend SR, Schorr CA, Beale R, et al. Surviving sepsis campaign: association between performance metrics and outcomes in a 7.5-year study. Crit Care Med. 2015;43(1):3–12.
99. Alam N, Oskam E, Stassen PM, Exter PV, van de Ven PM, Haak HR, et al. Prehospital antibiotics in the ambulance for sepsis: a multicentre, open label, randomised trial. Lancet Respir Med. 2018;6(1):40–50.
100. Kumar A, Ellis P, Arabi Y, Roberts D, Light B, Parrillo JE, et al. Initiation of inappropriate antimicrobial therapy results in a fivefold reduction of survival in human septic shock. Chest. 2009;136(5):1237–48.
101. Ibrahim EH, Sherman G, Ward S, Fraser VJ, Kollef MH. The influence of inadequate antimicrobial treatment of bloodstream infections on patient outcomes in the ICU setting. Chest. 2000;118(1):146–55.
102. Paul M, Shani V, Muchtar E, Kariv G, Robenshtok E, Leibovici L. Systematic review and meta-analysis of the efficacy of appropriate empiric antibiotic therapy for sepsis. Antimicrob Agents Chemother. 2010;54(11):4851–63.

Surgical Approach to Cirrhotic Patients

35

Zachary R. Bergman and Greg J. Beilman

Case Report

A 69-year-old female with a history of hepatitis C/alcoholic cirrhosis (MELD 16) presented to an outside hospital with an umbilical hernia. She reports she had the hernia for years. She had noticed some skin changes for several months with an acute onset of leakage of fluid. She reported that within the past several days, she had increasing output from the hernia site that had been leaking through her clothes. She denied any bleeding, fevers, chills, nausea or vomiting, diarrhea or constipation, or shortness of breath.

The patient was transferred to the Emergency Department where basic laboratory work and a CT scan of the abdomen were obtained. She was found to be anemic (hemoglobin 8.2), leukopenic (WBC 3.2), and thrombocytopenic (platelet count of 26). Computed tomography of the abdomen demonstrated nodular liver cirrhosis with splenomegaly and mild amount of perihepatic ascites (Fig. 35.1). There was a small umbilical hernia with associated fluid collection. On exam, she was found to have umbilical hernia with swollen attenuated skin full of clear fluid with continuous leakage of clear fluid at a slow rate as well as a suture at the site of leakage on the hernia sac that was placed at the outside hospital prior to transfer.

The patient was admitted to the general surgery service and underwent urgent open suture hernia repair to avoid peritonitis. At the time of the operation a 19 french round fluted drain was placed in the peritoneum to avoid leakage of ascites across the repair. She tolerated the procedure without complication.

The drain was removed on post-operative day 3. Paracentesis was performed on a frequent basis (every day or every-other-day) while in the hospital to prevent ascites build-up and breakdown of the operative site. She was discharged on post-operative day 6 with ongoing outpatient paracentesis scheduled. She was also scheduled for a transjugular intrahepatic portosystemic shunt (TIPS) procedure to manage her ascites long-term.

Z. R. Bergman
Department of Surgery, University of Minnesota, Minneapolis, MN, USA
e-mail: zbergman@umn.edu

G. J. Beilman (✉)
M Health-Fairview Health System, Minneapolis, MN, USA

Department of Surgery, University of Minnesota, Minneapolis, MN, USA
e-mail: beilman@umn.edu

M. D. Zielinski, O. Guillamondegui (eds.), *The Acute Management of Surgical Disease*,
https://doi.org/10.1007/978-3-031-07881-1_35

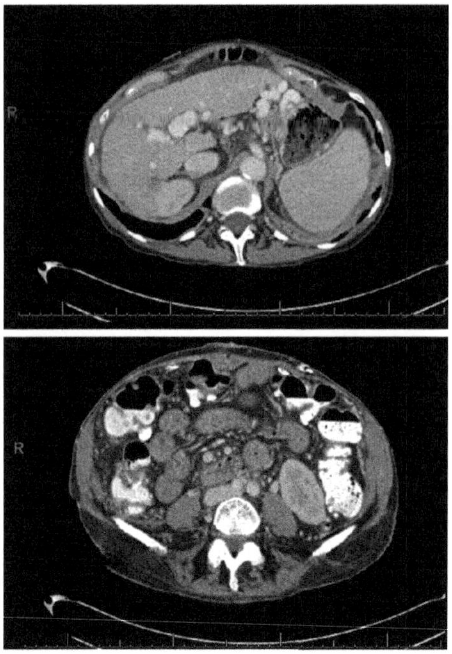

Fig. 35.1 Computed tomography of the abdomen of a 69-year-old female who presented with ruptured umbilical hernia that demonstrates nodular liver cirrhosis with splenomegaly and mild amount of perihepatic ascites (left) as well as an umbilical fascia defect with associated fluid collection and intraperitoneal air (right)

Introduction

Patients with liver disease, and those with cirrhosis in particular, have long been among the most complex and difficult to manage for healthcare providers of all specialties. For surgeons, this diagnosis alone can be enough to cause even the most aggressive to take pause when considering operative intervention. Unfortunately, this all-too-common affliction is ever-present and often exacerbates other underlying conditions to the point of needing surgical intervention. In the past, it has been estimated that one in ten patients with liver disease will need surgery during their final 2 years of life [1, 2]. As the incidence of liver disease and cirrhosis has increased, so has the severity of hepatic disease, as patients continue to live longer with improved medical management [3].

In the setting of Acute Care Surgery and non-hepatic operations, it is well-established that liver disease and cirrhosis have a drastic impact on morbidity and mortality. It is therefore understandable and appropriate that surgeons should have an appreciation for the complexities associated with the care of these patients. However, with appropriate perioperative planning and with meticulous post-operative management, surgeons can successfully navigate this subset of patients through the perils of this crucial period to provide beneficial and life-saving interventions. In the subsequent chapter, we will review the causes of cirrhosis, predictors of mortality, and pre-operative, intraoperative, and post-operative considerations to ensure the best possible outcomes for Acute Care Surgeons.

Causes of Cirrhosis

Important to successful perioperative management of cirrhosis is an understanding of the liver's function and where and when processes go awry during the progression of liver disease. Liver disease is common, affecting almost 800 million people worldwide, and is the underlying cause of approximately 2 million deaths per year [4]. Within the United States, the incidence of cirrhosis specifically is estimated to be 0.3%, accounting for nearly 600,000 patients [5]. There are a wide range of causes of liver disease including infectious, dietary, substance abuse, autoimmune diseases, and hereditary diseases.

The most common causes of liver disease worldwide are chronic hepatotropic viruses, primarily hepatitis B—which is the most common risk factor in Asia—and hepatitis C [4]. These infections are closely followed by excessive alcohol consumption as a global etiology. In the Western Hemisphere, diet that is heavily composed of high-fat foods has contributed to the increased incidence of non-alcoholic fatty liver disease (NAFLD). Trailing these environmental and social causes are less frequent causes of liver disease such as autoimmune and hereditary diseases. Among the most common autoimmune diseases are primary biliary cirrhosis (PBC), primary sclerosing cholangitis (PSC), and autoimmune hepatitis. Hereditary diseases of note include Wilson's disease, hemochromatosis, and alpha-1 antitrypsin deficiency.

Despite the frequent incidence of liver disease worldwide, there are prominent geographic differences in the most common cause of cirrhosis. In western countries, diet and lifestyle are the primary contributors. The top three causes of liver disease in Europe and the United States are non-alcoholic fatty liver disease, recently replacing alcoholic liver disease as the most common, and thirdly hepatitis C [6]. In comparison, hepatitis B remains the most common cause of liver disease in Asian-Pacific countries with alcoholic liver disease the second most common [7].

Anatomy of the Liver

There are a wide range of etiologies for hepatic cirrhosis, but the underlying pathophysiology follows a common pathway. This pathway consists of an initial insult that leads to degeneration of hepatocytes, resulting in cell apoptosis. The liver parenchyma is then replaced by fibrotic tissues and regenerative nodules, thereby leading to loss of liver function. Understanding the histologic cell types within the liver helps clarify the process of cirrhosis. There are two primary cell types, hepatocytes and non-parenchymal cells. Both contribute to the fibrosis of the liver in the setting of inflammation.

Hepatocytes form the parenchyma of the liver. They are the main target of the majority of hepatotoxic agents including viruses, alcohol, and bile acids. When injured, they trigger apoptosis, which stimulates release of pro-inflammatory cytokines from Kupffer cells causing activation of hepatic stellate cells. This is exacerbated by the additional release of reactive oxygen species that continue to promote localized inflammation. As liver injury progresses to fibrosis (the underlying mechanism of cirrhosis) the functional capacity of the liver decreases. The primary functions of the hepatocytes, including glucose metabolism, detoxification, and protein synthesis, suffer derangements corresponding to the severity of liver injury and cirrhosis [8–10]. Understanding where these biological processes fail is crucial to caring for the clinical manifestations of liver failure.

Non-parenchymal cells are composed of hepatic stellate cells, liver sinusoidal stellate cells, and Kupffer cells. Hepatic stellate cells are present in the sinusoidal walls. Their primary function is storage of vitamin A and other retinoids. In the setting of persistent inflammation, these cells are activated and begin to deposit collagen, the irreversible progression toward liver fibrosis (Fig. 35.2). Liver sinusoidal stellate cells form the structure of the sinusoidal wall providing endothelial filtration. They exchange fluids and nutrients between sinusoidal blood and hepatocytes. Inflammation causes increased production of extracellular matrix, which decreases the

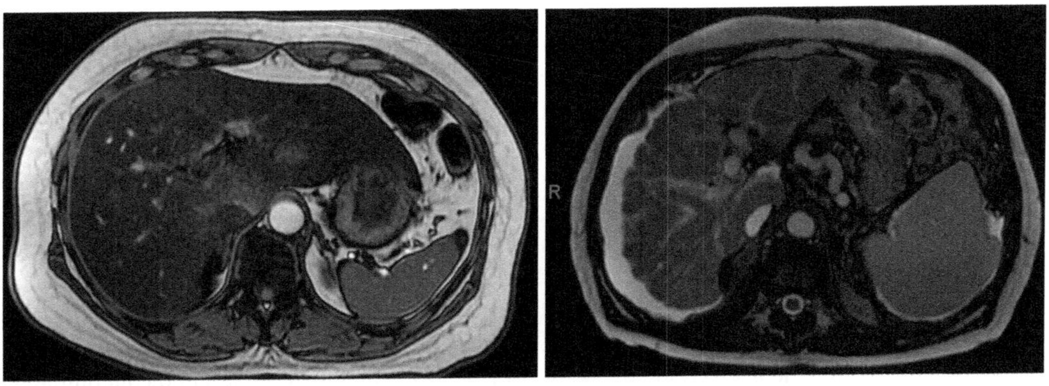

Fig. 35.2 Abdominal MRI in T1 weighted images demonstrating healthy liver parenchyma (left) and micronodular cirrhosis and ascites (right)

filter function of the sinusoidal wall. This leads to impaired substrate exchange, thereby increasing hepatic pressure. Healthy liver sinusoidal stellate cells can promote deactivation of hepatic stellate cells and halt progression of fibrosis of the liver. Kupffer cells are specialized macrophages located within the lining of the sinusoidal wall. They are activated in the setting of liver injury, release cytokines that promote destruction of hepatocytes and worsen liver injury and fibrosis. Kupffer cells are involved in the activation of hepatic stellate cells, driving fibrosis through cyclic inflammation [7–10].

As the focus of this chapter is acute care surgery and cirrhosis, we will not include an extensive description of liver anatomy as it is detailed in many other surgical texts; however, it is important to understand the basic principles. The liver is the largest intra-abdominal organ, accounting for 2–3% of total body weight. The internal anatomy of the liver was initially described in detail by Claude Couinaud in 1957 [11]. It was based on vascular and biliary relationships as opposed to surface anatomy that had been the mainstay of descriptive anatomy. The division of 8 functional segments is based on their relationship to the hepatic veins and it remains the most commonly used anatomical system for surgical resection. Important to the understanding of cirrhosis is that all segments are affected equally.

Lastly, and most importantly, is understanding the functional roles of the liver and the changes in physiology that arise when these functions fail. The primary functions that are essential to grasp for perioperative care are the metabolism and coagulation functions of the liver. Metabolism within the liver is a complex process. The liver plays a key role in processing, portioning, and storing of nutrients. Key among these is the storage of glucose in the form of glycogen. It also has a critical role in the processing of amino acids. The liver secretes the majority of amino acids into the blood and is the primary producer of albumin, which serves as a marker for nutritional status. Finally, hepatocytes detoxify many of the byproducts of the biologic pathways in the body, most importantly, disposing of nitrogenous waste through the Urea cycle [8, 9].

The clotting cascade is highly dependent on liver function. Liver parenchymal cells produce all of the coagulation factors involved in the generation of a fibrin clot with the exception of Factor VIII, which is primarily synthesized by the hepatic endothelium and extrahepatic endothelial cells [10]. When this process starts to falter, there is a complex cascade of clotting derangements. Identifying where the primary derangements in the coagulation cascade lie is essential in the perioperative period and will be discussed extensively in the next sections of the chapter.

Severity of Cirrhosis

How far along the path to end-stage liver disease a patient has progressed and, as a result, the severity of their cirrhosis, has profound effects on the outcomes for patients who undergo surgery. There have been many attempts to create scoring systems to estimate the severity of liver disease. These scoring systems do not capture the entire clinical picture, but they are useful tools for clinicians in assessing risk. As a result, there has been exhaustive research to establish an association of scoring systems and outcomes of nearly all surgical procedures including Trauma and Acute Care operations. The primary scoring systems that are utilized, and the two we will focus on for this chapter, are Child-Turcotte-Pugh (CTP) and Model for End-Stage Liver Disease (MELD) and the subsequent variations thereafter.

The Child-Turcotte-Pugh scoring system was initially proposed in 1964 as a predictor of surgical mortality [12]. It underwent revision in 1972 and is now widely used to determine prognosis in liver disease, focusing primarily on cirrhosis. It is a scoring system based on a combination of lab values (total bilirubin, serum albumin, prothrombin time (PTT), and international normalized ratio (INR) and clinical evaluation (presence of ascites and hepatic encephalopathy)). Scores of 1–3 are assigned for each factor and total scores are given a grade A–C with C suggesting the most severe disease [13]. Higher or worse grades have been shown extensively to be associated with worse prognosis. Child scores were used as the primary scoring system for many of the early studies of outcomes associated with liver function in surgery. For this reason, it remains a helpful predictor for surgical decision making.

The Model for End-Stage Liver Disease (MELD) scoring system was developed in 2000 to predict outcomes in liver disease using a series of patients undergoing transhepatic intrajugular porto-systemic (TIPS) placement [14]. However, it was quickly appreciated as a tool for assigning need for liver transplantation. Unlike the Child score, MELD is calculated using a formula that considers only a patient's lab values (serum bilirubin, creatinine, and INR) to produce a score. Similar to Child score, higher MELD scores are associated with increased mortality at 3 months following operative intervention [15].

For non-hepatic operations specifically, increased severity of score in either system is associated with increased risk of perioperative mortality. In the setting of elective surgery, mortality increases steeply with worsening liver function. The 30-day mortality in the setting of Child class A is 10%, Child class B is 30%, and class C is 80%. This often means that class C cirrhotic patients' risk of operative intervention is prohibitively high and non-operative management should be the primary goal whenever possible. MELD score follows a similar trend with 5.7% 30-day mortality in patients with MELD less than 8 and just over 50% in patients with MELD greater than 20 [16–19] (Table 35.1).

Table 35.1 30-Day mortality associated with elective surgical procedures stratified by cirrhosis severity score

Scoring system	Mortality (%) [16–19]
Child-Turcotte-Pugh	
Class A	10
Class B	30
Class C	76–82
Model for End-Stage Liver Disease (MELD)	
Score <8	5.7
Score >20	>50

Liver disease is often accompanied by other risk factors that have their own independent effects on surgical risk. Other considerations include portal hypertension, age, and comorbidities. Portal hypertension in the setting of cirrhosis is an independent risk factor that doubles perioperative mortality [20]. Advanced age has also been shown to represent an independent risk factor for gallstone symptom development in patients with hepatic cirrhosis [21]. Comorbidities including malnutrition, renal failure, and coagulopathies are frequent in cirrhotic patients and will be addressed in future sections of this chapter.

An important distinction that does not fit within a scoring system but is based on clinical picture is **compensated** versus **decompensated** cirrhosis. Compensated cirrhosis is defined as liver failure in which non-invasive parameters such as hepatic function tests and INR all may be normal. This is frequently diagnosed on imaging, but liver biopsy is the gold standard for diagnosis. Patients with compensated cirrhosis are, by definition, asymptomatic. Overall, the median survival time for these patients is 10–12 years. Patients with decompensated cirrhosis have had at least one complication including ascites, jaundice, variceal hemorrhage, or hepatic encephalopathy. Once progression occurs to decompensated cirrhosis, mortality drastically increases. At this stage, overall median survival time is 2–5 years [22, 23].

Acute Care Surgery

As the focus of this textbook is Acute Care Surgery, we will concentrate on non-hepatic operations—primarily urgent and emergent operations. It should be noted that a large portion of the surgical outcomes research comes from elective operations and some extrapolation is required to apply it to the Acute Care Surgery setting.

Cirrhotic patients who undergo non-hepatic operations demonstrate increased in-hospital mortality of 8–25% compared to 1.1% mortality in non-cirrhotic patients [24, 25]. This includes elective procedures. When focusing on strictly

Table 35.2 Morbidity and mortality associated with common Acute Care Surgery operations

	Morbidity (%)		Mortality (%)	
Type of surgery	+ Cirrhosis	– Cirrhosis	+ Cirrhosis	– Cirrhosis
Gall bladder [27, 57]				
Laparoscopic	13–33	0–3.2	<1	<1
Open	30–47.7	3.6	0–7.7	0.5–1
Abdominal wall hernia [28, 29]				
Umbilical	7–20	2.2	2–11	<1
Inguinal	6.3–10.9	6.8	0.8–2.7	0.7
Gastric [16, 24, 25]	53.3–67.7	20–24	23–64	17–18
Appendix [33, 34]				
Laparoscopic	2.1	0.7	0.5	0.3
Open	20.8	1.8	3.2–9	0.7
Colon—diverticular disease [37, 38]	46–51	32.6	13–23	5
Trauma laparotomy [40, 41]	**45**	**23**	40–45	15–24

urgent and emergent operations, the mortality risk is likely higher. The increased mortality is thought to be due, in large part, to acute decompensation of cirrhosis and increased risk of infection. As discussed previously, the underlying severity of cirrhosis, as well as the surgical procedure being performed, are important determinants of post-operative outcomes.

Cardiac and open abdominal operations carry the highest associated risks [24]. Open abdominal operations are thought to have increased risk secondary to hepatic ischemia [25]. Portal hypertension—if present—greatly increases the risk of perioperative hemorrhage [18]. Postoperative morbidity and mortality rates vary greatly depending on severity of the cirrhosis and the surgical procedure (Table 35.2). For this reason, it is crucial to consider both the patient's clinical picture as well as the indicated procedure when determining surgical risk. This section will address Acute Care operations that are likely to arise in cirrhotic patients with a focus on special considerations to help improve outcomes and pitfalls to avoid.

Gallstone Disease

Gallbladder pathology is the most likely surgical disease encountered in this patient population. Gallstone disease has an increased incidence in the setting of liver cirrhosis, 17–46% compared to 10–20% in the general population [20, 26]. Unlike the general population where cholesterol stones are the primary source of gallstone disease, pigment gallstones are the most frequent type in cirrhotics. Cholesterol stones represent about 15% of all stones in this patient population. The increased rate of pigment gallstones is thought to be due to increased secretion of unconjugated bilirubin, increased hydrolysis of conjugated bilirubin in the bile, and reduced secretion of bile acids and phospholipids in bile [18].

Presence of gallstones alone does not cause gallstone disease. Stones are common in the general population and cirrhotic patients alike, with up to 80% of patients with gallstones experiencing no symptoms [26]. Cirrhotic patients likely have increased detection rates of asymptomatic stones given the routine use of right upper quadrant ultrasound to monitor their liver disease. Expectant management for patients with asymptomatic gallstones is appropriate in the general population and this approach should be more highly favored with cirrhotic patients given their higher operative risk [20].

In the setting of right upper quadrant pain with concern for gallstone disease, the clinical workup remains relatively unchanged for cirrhotic patients. Right upper quadrant ultrasound and basic hematology and hepatic labs should always be obtained. It is important to note that hepatic function labs, primarily bilirubin, may be elevated in patients with liver disease and therefore additional imaging such as a HIDA scan or MRCP may be necessary to rule out choledocholithiasis if there is concern on the ultrasound or clinical suspicion.

Once diagnosed, treatment of cholecystitis requires evaluation of the severity of the patient's liver disease. Cholecystectomy is often appropriate and will frequently be necessary. This procedure is the most common non-hepatic operation performed in the setting of cirrhosis. Laparoscopic cholecystectomy is the preferred operative approach in patients with Child A or B classification. Perioperative mortality of laparoscopic cholecystectomy in this group of patients is ~1% compared to 2–7% for open cholecystectomy. Overall complications are much lower for laparoscopic removal (17.6%) versus open (47.7%). As liver disease increases in severity, perioperative mortality of cholecystectomy may be prohibitively high, with Child C patients demonstrating mortality of 23–50% [27]. Consensus treatment for this group is medical management with antibiotics. In the setting of failed medical management of pyocholecysitis, percutaneous drainage via Interventional Radiology should be the invasive treatment of choice.

Management changes in the setting of choledocholithiasis. The presence of a common bile duct stone increases the morbidity and mortality associated with gallstone disease. Gastroenterology should be involved early, as improved survival has been demonstrated with endoscopic sphincterotomy followed by laparoscopic cholecystectomy versus surgery for common bile duct stones. In the setting of Child C cirrhosis, mortality can still be as high as 7% with endoscopic sphincterotomy [24] and many centers now propose endoscopic balloon dilation versus sphincterotomy to avoid any incisions with resultant bleeding in this high-risk patient population.

Abdominal Wall Hernias

As with gallstone disease, abdominal wall hernias are another surgical problem that is more common in cirrhotic patients. The incidence is 16% in cirrhotic patients but increases to 24% in the setting of ascites. Over half of these abdominal wall hernias are umbilical hernias and the risk of umbilical hernia is over four times higher in the setting of cirrhosis [28]. There are many factors that contribute to the development of umbilical hernia. These patients have increased intra-abdominal pressure from ascites, poor nutritional status leading to weakness of the abdominal fascia and muscle wasting, and the pre-existent supra-umbilical fascial opening in patients with portal hypertension due to a dilated umbilical vein.

Historically, overall mortality associated with umbilical hernia repair was approximately 5%. However, the clinical presentation has a drastic impact on outcomes: there is an 11% mortality with emergent operations for obstruction or rupture versus 2% for elective repairs [24, 25, 27]. There seem to be substantial improvements with perioperative management of this disease as multiple studies have demonstrated zero perioperative mortalities when umbilical hernia repair is performed at quaternary centers [24].

The use of mesh in umbilical hernia repair in cirrhotic patients has long been debated. The concern for placement of mesh in this patient population is a theoretical increased risk of mesh infection. A recent randomized control trial, however, evaluated the placement of permanent mesh for umbilical hernia repair with encouraging results. Hernia recurrence was significantly less in the mesh hernioplasty group. No mesh exposure or fistulae were experienced. There was no need to remove any of the placed mesh prostheses [28]. Additional studies need to be performed to confirm the safety of mesh placement, however, early results are promising.

The incidence of inguinal hernia in patients with cirrhosis has not been fully established, though as with other hernias, it is thought to be increased in this patient population. Historical studies have demonstrated 5% mortality and 8% recurrence rates in Child A and B patients [24, 25]. A more recent prospective trial demonstrated complications, mortality, and recurrence rates were not significantly higher in elective inguinal hernia repairs when compared to the general population [29]. Overall, inguinal hernia repair conveys the lowest risk amongst non-hepatic operations in the setting of cirrhosis. It is reasonable to repair these electively and incarcerated or strangulated hernias should be approached in a similar fashion to non-cirrhotic patients.

As with inguinal hernias, the incidence of incisional hernias is not well described in the cirrhotic patient population. However, there should be consideration of repair electively when these hernias are discovered if not limited by severe liver disease. A recent study demonstrated increased mortality, recurrence, and seroma formation rate in patients who underwent urgent repair compared to those who underwent elective repair in the setting of cirrhosis [30].

Gastric

Cirrhotic patients also have an increased incidence of peptic ulcer disease (PUD), estimated to be 8–20% [31]. The mortality for emergent surgery for PUD (e.g., perforation or bleeding) is extremely high, ranging from 23% to 64% [19, 32]. As with other operations, increased severity of cirrhosis and presence of ascites are both associated with worse outcomes. There has been a recent decrease in mortality with improvement in endoscopic management of bleeding ulcers and laparoscopic suture repair for perforations in combination with proton pump inhibitor treatment. It is therefore recommended that bleeding ulcers treatment first be attempted via endoscopy. Apart from limited case reports, there are no studies evaluating laparoscopic repair of perforated ulcers compared to open repair in cirrhotic patients. Given the increased mortality associated with open operations for cirrhotic patients and the proven safety and efficacy of laparoscopic perforated peptic ulcer repair overall, a minimally invasive approach should be attempted prior to open repair when possible.

Appendix

Unlike many other surgical diseases, there does not seem to be an increased incidence of appendicitis in the setting of cirrhosis. As a result, the effect of cirrhosis on mortality rate is not well described in this patient population. A large database review examined outcomes with patients who underwent appendectomy in the setting of no cirrhosis, compensated cirrhosis, and decompensated cirrhosis. Compensated cirrhosis and control groups had similar outcomes while patients with decompensated cirrhosis had significantly higher mortality, higher cost, and longer hospital length of stay. Laparoscopic appendectomy was superior across all groups as it demonstrated higher survival, lower cost, shorter duration of hospitalization, and lower incidence of complications [33]. Multiple studies support the use of laparoscopic compared to open appendectomy in cirrhotic patients as laparoscopic appendectomy has been associated with improved post-operative pain and decreased operative complication versus open appendectomy [33, 34]. Larger studies are suggesting treatment of uncomplicated appendicitis may be possible with antibiotics alone [35]. In patients with decompensated cirrhosis it is reasonable to consider this approach and in patients with end-stage liver disease (CTP class C) this should be the first-line treatment given the almost prohibitively high surgical risk.

Colon

Diverticular disease and colorectal cancer are the two most common reasons for operative intervention on the colon. Mortality for colon operations in the setting of cirrhosis is 13–23% with 46–51% morbidity [36]. As with other operations, higher MELD or Child scores, presence of ascites, and emergency surgery are all associated with worse outcomes. Given the high risk of emergent surgery in this patient population, endoscopic intervention in the form of colonic stenting for obstruction and cauterization for bleeding is recommended when available.

Acute Care Surgery is most often concerned with the management of diverticular disease. Multiple large database studies have examined diverticulitis in cirrhotic patients. The mortality rate of diverticulitis increases more than two-fold if cirrhosis is present. This impact comes in large part from patients with decompensated cirrhosis, as patients with compensated cirrhosis did not have significantly higher mortality. However, patients with compensated cirrhosis underwent significantly fewer operations than the general public [37]. This is likely due to surgeons' apprehension with this population and the known surgical risk factors. Overall, patients with diverticulitis and cirrhosis were found to have increased cost of stay and length of hospitalization compared to the general population [37].

Understandably, surgeons often try to manage diverticular disease conservatively when possible. However, when an operation is indicated as in the setting of diverticulitis resulting in peritonitis, there is evidence to support the superiority of laparoscopic versus open colon resection. In a large database review, laparoscopic colectomy for acute diverticulitis was accompanied by shorter hospital length of stay, lower costs, and significantly decreased mortality rate compared with open colectomy in compensated and decompensated cirrhotic patients. There was marked increase in mortality, hospital length of stay, and cost observed for decompensated cirrhotic patients regardless of the type of treatment [38]. The success of this operation, it should be noted, is also dependent on the surgeon's comfort level with advanced laparoscopic technique.

Trauma

Not unexpectedly, the presence of liver disease directly impacts outcomes in trauma. In a prospective study of a level 1 trauma registry, the overall in-hospital mortality after trauma for cirrhotic patients is nearly three times that of non-cirrhotic controls (20% versus 7%) [39]. A retrospective review found similar results, with 12% mortality in cirrhotic trauma patients compared to non-cirrhotic controls. They also found cirrhotic patients were more likely to develop acute respiratory distress syndrome (ARDS), coagulopathy, and sepsis. When analyzing only those patients with cirrhosis who underwent emergent exploratory laparotomy, the mortality rate increased to 40%, compared to 15% in patients without cirrhosis [40]. Similar mortality was reported in another matched retrospective study: 45% mortality in cirrhotics compared to 24% in matched controls [41].

This prominent effect on survival extends to minor trauma (defined as Injury Severity Score <16) as well, with a mortality rate in cirrhotic patients of 29%. When examining only blunt trauma, a MELD score greater than 16 was associated with a significantly higher mortality rate compared to patients with lower MELD scores [41]. Given the emergent nature of trauma surgery, it is unlikely that pre-operative adjustments can be made to improve outcomes, so improvements must be made in the perioperative care that as discussed in the coming sections of this chapter.

Preoperative Optimization

There is frequently limited time for preoperative optimization for urgent or emergent operative indications. However, whenever possible patients with cirrhosis benefit from minimal interventions that may have important downstream effects on mortality. Many of the manifestations of liver failure—and their needed corrections—are evident on standard laboratory values obtained during diagnosis and workup in the Emergency Department. When identified, they should be corrected, if possible, prior to surgery. Other manifestations may require slightly more investigation from the surgeon but should be equally appreciated and evaluated when time allows (Table 35.3).

Coagulopathy

The liver plays an important role in production of factors of the coagulation cascade. INR is a poor marker for clinical bleeding risk as it is unable to truly assess for the balance of the coagulation pathway, especially when liver function is impacted. However, this test continues to be used for pre-operative planning given the ease of test-

Table 35.3 Perioperative evaluation and management of common complications of cirrhosis

Complication	Etiology	Presentation	Evaluation	Management strategies
Coagulopathy	Decreased synthetic liver function	Bleeding, thrombocytopenia	Complete blood count, INR, thromboelastography	– INR correction with FFP, vitamin K, cryoprecipitate – Transfusion to maintain platelet count >50,000 – DDAVP and tranexamic acid
Hepatic encephalopathy	Build-up of nitrogenous waste	Altered mental status	Clinical assessment, BUN level	– Lactulose and rifaximin – Treat infections – Correct electrolyte derangements
Ascites	Increased portal pressure	Increased drain output, wound breakdown	Clinical exam, abdominal ultrasonography	– Salt and water restriction – Diuresis – Large volume paracentesis – Fluid removal through surgical drain, if present – TIPS for refractory ascites
Renal failure	Hypovolemia leading to poor renal perfusion and ATN	Decreased urine output	Fluid overload on clinical exam, close monitoring of I/Os, creatinine, glomerular filtration rate	– Avoid nephrotoxic drugs and contrast agents – Albumin in the setting of hepatorenal syndrome – Early dialysis with constant renal replacement when indicated
Pulmonary failure	Transfer of ascites into the pleural space	Pleural effusions, increasing oxygen requirements	Monitor oxygen requirements, chest imaging (XR or CT)	– Incentive spirometry – Ascites management – Thoracentesis in the setting of pulmonary failure
Malnutrition	Protein calorie malnutrition, glycogen storage depletion	Muscle wasting, decreased wound healing, decreased mobility	Serum albumin, lean body mass	– High carbohydrate and lipid diet – Early enteral nutrition as needed – Thiamine and folate in alcoholic liver disease
Electrolyte derangements	Fluid balance disturbances	Electrolyte disturbances	Complete metabolic panel, blood glucose	– Replete electrolytes – Manage fluid overload – Maintain normoglycemia

ing. When INR is abnormal, coagulopathy due to decreased synthesis of coagulation components in the liver cannot be corrected with vitamin K supplements. However, if the operation in question is not urgent or emergent, vitamin K administration should still be implemented in case malabsorption has contributed to coagulopathy [42].

A more precise evaluation of coagulation deficiencies can be provided by utilizing thromboelastography (TEG). In the perioperative setting, it has been shown to reduce unnecessary transfusions and their related complications [43]. When available, TEG should be utilized to determine which coagulation derangements require correction (Fig. 35.3). The primary intervention for correcting these derangements should be transfusion with fractioned blood products. These include [42]:

Fresh Frozen Plasma

- Used to correct elevated INR.
- INR of FFP is approximately 1.6–1.7 and cannot improve INR past this value.
- FFP transfusion can be large volume and lead to fluid overload and pulmonary congestion.

Cryoprecipitate

- Concentrated solution of clotting factors including large amount of fibrinogen and vWB factor as well as Factors VIII and XIII.
- In the setting of fluid overload, cryoprecipitate is preferred to FFP.

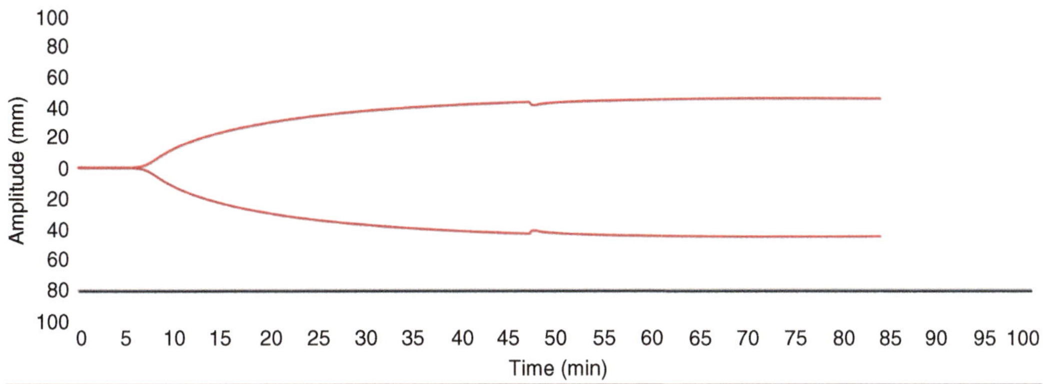

	R (min)	K (min)	ANGLE (deg)	MA (mm)	LY30 (%)
K	7.2 4.0 – 9.0	6.1 1.0 – 3.0	36.5 59.0 – 74.0	41.7 55.0 – 74.0	0.0 0.0 – 8.0

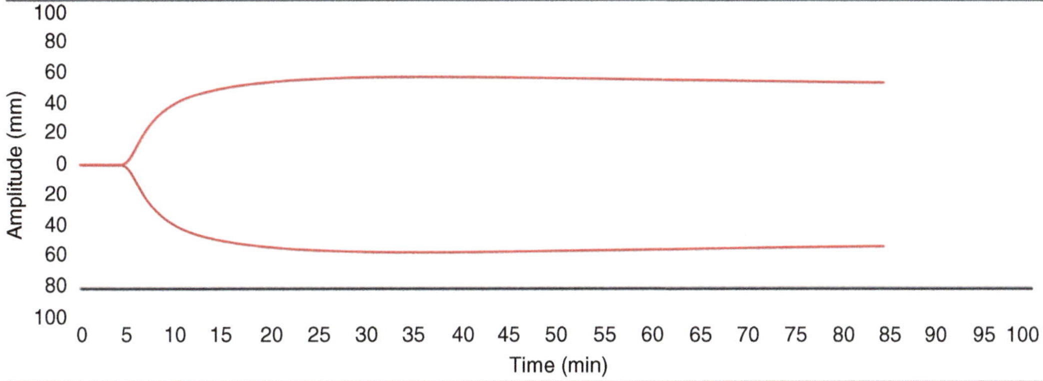

	R (min)	K (min)	ANGLE (deg)	MA (mm)	LY30 (%)
CK	4.8 5.0 –10.0	1.8 1.0 – 3.0	66.6 53.0 – 72.0	56.1 50.0 – 70.0	0.0 0.0 – 8.0

Fig. 35.3 A 45-year-old male with history of alcoholic liver cirrhosis (MELD 29) who underwent orthotopic liver transplantation. Thromboelastography (TEG) just prior to transplantation (above) demonstrates increased K time (time to appropriate clot strength), decreased angle, and decreased maximum amplitude (MA). This combination is due to decreased synthetic liver function and thrombocytopenia. TEG from the same patient on post-operative day 10 (below) demonstrates a normalized curve following improvement in synthetic liver function and resolution of thrombocytopenia

Platelets

- Thrombocytopenia is a common complication of cirrhosis with portal hypertension due to the sequestration and consumption of platelets secondary to splenomegaly.
- Platelet transfusion is indicated for operative intervention in the setting of thrombocytopenia <50,000 plts/mm^3.

There are pharmacological methods for correcting coagulation that can be used in supplementing transfusion or if blood products cannot be given. The two to consider are desmopressin and tranexamic acid. Desmopressin stimulates the release vWB from vascular endothelium and can be used as an alternative to FFP. Tranexamic acid is an anti-fibrinolytic agent. It should be considered if fibrinolysis time is decreased on TEG.

Hepatic Encephalopathy

Hepatic encephalopathy (HE) occurs in liver failure from a build-up of nitrogenous waste in the blood that the liver fails to detoxify. HE can cause extensive problems post-operatively including aggressive and uncooperative patient behavior interfering with delivery of important treatment measures and nursing care, immobility, aspiration pneumonia, and at times a complex and invasive work-up for delirium. Subtle HE not detected prior to operative intervention can lead to overt HE post-operatively. Neuropsychiatric testing may need to be pursued to detect subtle HE. A low protein diet and avoidance of certain medications are recommended post-operatively to avoid exacerbation of HE [44].

Ascites

It is important to identify the presence of ascites as this can have a profound impact on perioperative care. Often operative intervention can exacerbate ascites production, which can result in fluid and electrolyte imbalances. In the setting of elective procedures, medical management of ascites may improve the Child-Turcotte-Pugh class, and surgery may become feasible in some patients if it was previously contraindicated due to ascites. Refractory ascites may need transjugular, intrahepatic portosystemic shunting (TIPS) as a rescue measure prior to surgery. Post-operatively, a low sodium diet should be continued to prevent re-accumulation of ascites. Discussion of post-operative management of ascites is addressed in the next section and is critical to wound-healing, especially in the setting of hernia repair.

Renal Function

As with coagulopathy, lab values associated with renal function can be difficult to interpret. Glomerular filtration rate is often overestimated in cirrhotic patients as creatinine is often lower secondary to decreased lean body mass from malnutrition. As the severity of liver failure progresses, the incidence of renal failure increases, with up to 24% of outpatients with cirrhosis developing some type of renal failure within 1 year of the first episode of ascites [45]. Multiple studies have demonstrated that life expectancy decreases significantly with the diagnosis of renal failure in the setting of decompensated liver failure [45, 46].

For cirrhotic patients with renal failure, pre-operative management includes close monitoring of fluid status and avoidance of nephrotoxic medications. Diuretics should be avoided. This is particularly true when the patient has refractory ascites because several drugs can induce acute kidney injury. If paracentesis for uncontrolled ascites is indicated, albumin should be replaced intravenously at a rate of 6–8 g/L of ascites removed to maintain adequate renal perfusion [20].

Pulmonary Function

Pleural effusions in the setting of ascites are common though rarely cause pulmonary complications. Only moderate to large pleural effusions that are causing clinical pulmonary restriction should be considered for drainage via thoracentesis. More concerning is the presence of hepatopulmonary syndrome that is defined as: hypoxia as a result of pulmonary vasculature abnormalities in the setting of cirrhosis. If patients have hepatopulmonary syndrome and are in need of urgent or emergent surgery, the risk of prolonged pulmonary compromise as well as embolic stroke should be explained. Non-surgical management should be attempted when possible [42].

Infection

Cirrhosis can increase the risk of infection as the innate immune system is impaired by the disruption of the hepatic cellular organization, damage to the reticulo-endothelial system, and decreased liver protein synthesis. This causes a weakened immune surveillance capacity of the liver as well as decreased synthesis of innate immunity proteins. Pre-operative work-up should include thorough infectious evaluation as untreated infections in patients with cirrhosis have increased morbidity and mortality compared to non-cirrhotic patients. There is also an increased incidence of multidrug-resistant organisms in this patient population. Broad-spectrum antibiotics that cover organisms associated with spontaneous bacterial peritonitis (SBP) are recommended in the setting of low-protein ascites (<1.5 g/dL), advanced cirrhosis, and prior history of SBP [47]. If these conditions are not present, surgical prophylactic antibiotics are the same for cirrhotic and non-cirrhotic patients [48].

Nutrition

Nutrition plays a pivotal role in liver disease that is often overlooked. Liver disease can drive many factors leading to malnutrition and poor nutrition alone can worsen liver disease. The incidence of malnutrition is severely elevated in cirrhotic patients, with up to 80% suffering from at least mild deficiencies [49]. Multiple factors contribute to worsening nutrition including increased catabolism, impaired absorption of nutrients, and poor oral intake. Severity of malnutrition is independently associated with decreased survival in the setting of cirrhosis.

Evaluation of lean body mass and serum albumin are quick surrogates for nutritional status. Hypoalbuminemia is a predictor of mortality following surgery and should be evaluated when timing allows. A low serum albumin level (≤2.1 g/dL) when compared with normal range serum albumin level (≥4.6 g/dL) was associated with drastically increased mortality of 29% vs 1%. There was also a higher morbidity of 65% vs 10% [50]. Of note, albumin is a negative acute phase reactant and is unreliable in the setting of post-operative inflammation. Therefore, when possible this should be measured pre-operatively. Intravenous albumin supplementation has been shown to have no effect on mortality and is not indicated for hypoalbuminemia alone.

If adequately considered and addressed, liver function can be optimized by improving nutritional status. Perioperative nutrition is an essential component, and improvement in perioperative nutritional status may be associated with improved outcomes. A nutritional consult and perioperative supplementation should always be considered in the setting of cirrhosis. If adequate oral intake cannot be achieved by the patient, enteral feeding access and supplemental tube feeds should be considered at the earliest possible time point.

Managing Cirrhosis Intra- and Post-operatively

The most crucial and difficult management of cirrhotic patients occurs post-operatively. The stress of surgery and anesthesia can often push the patient from compensated to decompensated liver failure. This has effects on multiple organ systems and requires close clinical monitoring.

Anesthesia

Although it is not managed by the Acute Care Surgeon, it is important to understand the impact that anesthesia can have on liver function. General anesthesia can lead to acute liver decompensation, likely secondary to hypotension and decreased hepatic blood flow. It is important to understand the common drugs that depend on hepatic metabolism and therefore require dose reduction. The primary drugs to be aware of are propofol, dexmedetomidine, midazolam, and morphine (discussed in detail in the Pain Management Section).

Critical Care

The close clinical monitoring required post-operatively is most effectively achieved in the Intensive Care Unit (ICU). Fluid management is often among the most difficult to manage as these patients can appear to be total volume up, but still be intravascularly depleted. Crystalloid solution is recommended initially for volume resuscitation. Albumin has been shown to be beneficial in three scenarios: Spontaneous bacterial peritonitis (SBP), large volume paracentesis, and type 1 hepatorenal syndrome [20]. Fluid management in cirrhotic patients requires careful monitoring of volume status. Non-invasive parameters such as trends in serum lactate (though this may have delayed clearance due to decreased metabolism in the liver) should be attempted first. However, invasive monitoring such as Swan-Ganz catheters may need to be used if there are ongoing questions about fluid status. Persistent hypotension should be treated with vasoactive drugs such as norepinephrine or vasopressin followed by a trial of steroids.

Serum Chemistry

Electrolyte imbalances (hypokalemia, hypocalcemia, hypomagnesemia, and dilutional hyponatremia) are common and should be monitored and corrected when identified. A high index of suspicion for malnutrition and micronutrient deficiencies (folate, vitamins A, D, E, K, and complex B) needs to be maintained. Cirrhosis causes deficiencies in gluconeogenesis and therefore post-operative hypoglycemia is common. Blood glucose status should be closely monitored and corrected appropriately as needed. If there is concern for alcohol dependence, thiamine in combination with glucose should be administered to avoid progression of Wernicke encephalopathy.

Ascites Management

The most common manifestation of decompensated liver cirrhosis post-operatively is the new development of ascites. Large-volume ascites after abdominal surgery increases the risk of abdominal wall dehiscence and herniation. It also has pulmonary implications as it increases the risk of atelectasis, aspiration, and pneumonia. Fluid shifts might precipitate electrolyte imbalances, hypovolemia, and acute kidney injury. Management is based on sodium restriction and judicious use of diuretics, with close monitoring of electrolytes and renal function. There are multiple options for management for ascites post-operatively.

Use of intra-abdominal drains to help control postoperative ascites and prevent surgical wound complications is a controversial topic. The safety of post-operative drains in the context of cirrhosis remains poorly explored. The rationale to drain placement is better control of postoperative ascites and the potential associated surgical wound complications; however, the risk of contamination of ascites and increased postoperative fluid shifts should be taken into account. In the setting of hepatic resection, prophylactic drain placement has not been favored in recent literature [51]. However, there are little data in the realm of Acute Care Surgery for proper management of post-operative ascites. If a drain is placed, it should be removed by post-operative days 5–7 to reduce infectious complications, if possible [52]. It is likely that with ongoing high ascites output from the drain that additional paracentesis will be required.

Supplemental large-volume paracentesis can be utilized for ascites management as well, or as back-up therapy following surgical drain removal. Therapeutic paracentesis should be reserved for refractory cases and limited to symptomatic relief. If paracentesis is performed, replacement of the fluid should be routinely performed with albumin as described previously. For ascites refractory to repeat paracentesis, a final option to consider is an Interventional Radiology-placed drain. This allows for the placement of a cuffed drain to minimize infectious risk. It also prevents repeat interventions in the setting of high bleeding risk.

Renal Function

Renal function is an important prognostic indicator post-operatively as the renal and hepatic systems are vitally linked. Studies evaluating the effect of acute kidney injury (AKI) in the setting of cirrhosis are limited to hepatic resections and have not been thoroughly evaluated in the general post-operative population. However, in non-surgical patient the presence of renal failure in cirrhotic patients is associated with a significant increase in mortality with 50% mortality at 1 month and 80% mortality at 6 months [53]. Post-operative AKI is multifactorial primarily driven by hypoperfusion from depletion of intravascular volume and reduced systemic vascular resistance causing acute tubular necrosis. The severity of AKI can be exacerbated by ongoing bleeding, infection, or unregulated inflammatory response.

When AKI is identified post-operatively, management should focus on prevention of renal failure by maintaining adequate systemic blood pressure, prompt identification and treatment of infections and judicious use of contrast agents, because once established, the prognosis is considerably poorer. If an AKI progresses to the point of renal failure, early treatment of renal failure is imperative. Early use of continuous renal replacement therapy, rather than intermittent hemodialysis or hemofiltration, which provides a hemodynamically stable approach in such patients [20]. Unfortunately, progression to renal failure requiring dialysis carries a poor prognosis.

Nutrition

Again, it is crucial to highlight the importance of adequate perioperative nutrition. As with preoperative management, enteral supplementation should be utilized early if there is any indication that oral intake will be delayed or inadequate. There is minimal evidence regarding the use of parenteral nutrition in emergency surgery; however, there are studies that support its use following liver transplantation [54]. Parenteral nutrition and early enteral nutrition were comparable in their ability to maintain a healthy nutritional state. The infectious complications appear to be higher with the use of parenteral nutrition and this approach should therefore be reserved for cases when enteral feeding is not feasible.

DVT Prophylaxis

Coagulation disorders of cirrhosis confer an increased risk of both venous thromboembolism and hemorrhage. This makes deep vein thrombosis (DVT) prophylaxis decisions much more complex. Conventional coagulation tests do not reflect these risks, and an increased INR is not necessarily protective for thromboembolic events. Although detailed guidelines remain unavailable, thromboprophylaxis is recommended in most patients, and certainly in high-risk situations. In the setting of cirrhosis and renal failure, unfractionated heparin should be utilized for DVT prophylaxis as opposed to low-molecular-weight heparin owing to its shorter half-life and decreased risk in the setting of potential renal failure.

Pain Management [55]

Post-operative pain management for cirrhotic patients can seem daunting to many clinicians as the metabolic and detoxification properties of the liver are diminished. This can affect the safety of entire classes of therapeutics and even those that can still be safely used may have dramatic changes in their acceptable dosages. Importantly, uncontrolled post-operative pain can incite mental status changes that prevent proper monitoring of many of the other post-operative complications. For this reason, a multimodal approach is key to obtaining adequate control.

The metabolism of opioids varies greatly between different formulations and it is difficult to provide overarching recommendations for the category as a whole. The simplest way to approach opioid use in the setting of cirrhosis is with an understanding that half-life can often be prolonged and extended-release versions should be avoided while spacing out the dosing interval with immediate-release formulations. It is important to know how each opioid is metabolized when determining their safety for patients with liver failure. Below is a summary of the most commonly used opioids and recommendations for their use in this patient population.

Oxycodone

- Diminished first-pass metabolism results in prolonged half-life.
- Decreased dosage of 5 mg every 6 h recommended as a starting point.

Hydrocodone

- Minimal effect on the metabolism by the liver, however, it is often formulated in combination with acetaminophen and therefore should be closely evaluated to ensure that acetaminophen dosing does not exceed recommended levels in cirrhotic patients.
- Decreased dosage of 5 mg every 6 h recommended as a starting point.

Morphine

- Morphine is metabolized into two major metabolites: one with analgesic properties (morphine-6-glucuronide) and the other (morphine-3-glucuronide) with neurotoxic side effects such as confusion, seizures, and respiratory depression.
- In the setting of renal failure, the neurotoxic metabolites are poorly excreted. As cirrhotic patients often have concomitant renal failure, this should be taken into consideration.
- Decreased oral dosage of 5 mg every 6 h recommended as a starting point.

Hydromorphone

- Metabolized exclusively by glucuronidation and therefore unaffected by liver and renal function.
- Should be considered the first line opioid of choice in the setting of cirrhosis and renal failure.
- Decreased dosage of 1 mg every 6 h recommended as a starting point.

Tramadol

- Metabolism independent of liver function.
- It can decrease the seizure threshold and can cause serotonin syndrome when used in combination with SSRIs or TCAs.

Multimodal pain control with non-opioid medications is recommended in all post-operative patients. However, just as with opioids, the metabolism of these therapeutics is often diminished in patients with liver failure. Non-steroidal anti-inflammatory drugs (NSAIDs) have multiple concerning features for patients with cirrhosis. In the setting of cirrhosis there is increased bioavailability, which can precipitate acute renal failure and gastrointestinal bleeding due to prostaglandin inhibition. There is increased risk for thrombocytopenia, which can further increase the risk for variceal and nonvariceal gastrointestinal bleeding. NSAIDs can promote sodium retention, thereby worsening ascites and edema. The recommendation is that this class of drugs should therefore be avoided in this patient population. For acetaminophen or Tylenol, it is a common misconception that patients with cirrhosis should avoid this drug entirely. However, in lower doses, it remains a safe and effective analgesic. Daily dosage should not exceed 2–3 g/day.

For more directed therapy, it is reasonable to consider regional anesthesia as this is generally safe in cirrhotic patients. The surgeon should consider administration of directed local anesthesia such as a transversus abdominal plane (TAP) block at the time of surgery to decrease post-operative opioid use. Post-operatively, topical lidocaine patches demonstrate minimal systemic absorption and can be safely utilized in the setting of cirrhosis.

Finally, epidurals may be considered if there is adequate time pre-operatively. Coagulopathy is a contraindication to epidural anesthesia due to the risk of epidural hematoma. In a recent study, the risk of epidural hematoma after removal in the setting of coagulopathy was 0.3%, compared to 0.01–0.03% in baseline population [56]. Patients with liver disease with normal coagulation factors, platelet count, and pre-procedure TEG are good candidates for epidural anesthesia. Catheter removal should be evaluated with the same coagulopathy work-up and can be removed safely after normalization of parameters.

References

1. Jackson FC, Christophersen EB, Peternel WW, Kirimli B. Preoperative management of patients with liver disease. Surg Clin North Am. 1968;48(4):907–30. https://doi.org/10.1016/s0039-6109(16)38591-7.
2. Patel T. Surgery in the patient with liver disease. Mayo Clin Proc. 1999;74(6):593–9. https://doi.org/10.4065/74.6.593.

3. Propst A, Propst T, Zangerl G, Ofner D, Judmaier G, Vogel W. Prognosis and life expectancy in chronic liver disease. Dig Dis Sci. 1995;40(8):1805–15. https://doi.org/10.1007/BF02212706.
4. Parola M, Pinzani M. Liver fibrosis: pathophysiology, pathogenetic targets and clinical issues. Mol Asp Med. 2019;65:37–55. https://doi.org/10.1016/j.mam.2018.09.002.
5. Scaglione S, Kliethermes S, Cao G, et al. The epidemiology of cirrhosis in the United States: a population-based study. J Clin Gastroenterol. 2015;49(8):690–6. https://doi.org/10.1097/MCG.0000000000000208.
6. Smith A, Baumgartner K, Bositis C. Cirrhosis: diagnosis and management. Am Fam Physician. 2019;100(12):759–70.
7. Zhou W-C, Zhang Q-B, Qiao L. Pathogenesis of liver cirrhosis. World J Gastroenterol. 2014;20(23):7312–24. https://doi.org/10.3748/wjg.v20.i23.7312.
8. Abdel-Misih SRZ, Bloomston M. Liver anatomy. Surg Clin North Am. 2010;90(4):643–53. https://doi.org/10.1016/j.suc.2010.04.017.
9. Trefts E, Gannon M, Wasserman DH. The liver. Curr Biol. 2017;27(21):R1147–51. https://doi.org/10.1016/j.cub.2017.09.019.
10. Schuppan D, Afdhal NH. Liver cirrhosis. Lancet (London, England). 2008;371(9615):838–51. https://doi.org/10.1016/S0140-6736(08)60383-9.
11. Couinaud C. Le foie. Études anatomiques et chirurgicales. Paris: Masson; 1957.
12. Child CG, Turcotte JG. Surgery and portal hypertension. Major Probl Clin Surg. 1964;1:1–85.
13. Pugh RN, Murray-Lyon IM, Dawson JL, Pietroni MC, Williams R. Transection of the oesophagus for bleeding oesophageal varices. Br J Surg. 1973;60(8):646–9. https://doi.org/10.1002/bjs.1800600817.
14. Malinchoc M, Kamath PS, Gordon FD, Peine CJ, Rank J, ter Borg PC. A model to predict poor survival in patients undergoing transjugular intrahepatic portosystemic shunts. Hepatology. 2000;31(4):864–71. https://doi.org/10.1053/he.2000.5852.
15. Cholongitas E, Papatheodoridis GV, Vangeli M, Terreni N, Patch D, Burroughs AK. Systematic review: the model for end-stage liver disease—should it replace Child-Pugh's classification for assessing prognosis in cirrhosis? Aliment Pharmacol Ther. 2005;22(11–12):1079–89. https://doi.org/10.1111/j.1365-2036.2005.02691.x.
16. de Goede B, Klitsie PJ, Lange JF, Metselaar HJ, Kazemier G. Morbidity and mortality related to non-hepatic surgery in patients with liver cirrhosis: a systematic review. Best Pract Res Clin Gastroenterol. 2012;26(1):47–59. https://doi.org/10.1016/j.bpg.2012.01.010.
17. Mansour A, Watson W, Shayani V, Pickleman J. Abdominal operations in patients with cirrhosis: still a major surgical challenge. Surgery. 1997;122(4):730–6. https://doi.org/10.1016/s0039-6060(97)90080-5.
18. Teh SH, Nagorney DM, Stevens SR, et al. Risk factors for mortality after surgery in patients with cirrhosis. Gastroenterology. 2007;132(4):1261–9. https://doi.org/10.1053/j.gastro.2007.01.040.
19. Garrison RN, Cryer HM, Howard DA, Polk HCJ. Clarification of risk factors for abdominal operations in patients with hepatic cirrhosis. Ann Surg. 1984;199(6):648–55. https://doi.org/10.1097/00000658-198406000-00003.
20. Hickman L, Tanner L, Christein J, Vickers S. Non-hepatic abdominal surgery in patients with cirrhotic liver disease. J Gastrointest Surg. 2019;23(3):634–42. https://doi.org/10.1007/s11605-018-3991-7.
21. Acalovschi M. Gallstones in patients with liver cirrhosis: incidence, etiology, clinical and therapeutical aspects. World J Gastroenterol. 2014;20(23):7277–85. https://doi.org/10.3748/wjg.v20.i23.7277.
22. D'Amico G, Garcia-Tsao G, Pagliaro L. Natural history and prognostic indicators of survival in cirrhosis: a systematic review of 118 studies. J Hepatol. 2006;44(1):217–31. https://doi.org/10.1016/j.jhep.2005.10.013.
23. Samonakis DN, Koulentaki M, Coucoutsi C, et al. Clinical outcomes of compensated and decompensated cirrhosis: a long term study. World J Hepatol. 2014;6(7):504–12. https://doi.org/10.4254/wjh.v6.i7.504.
24. Bhangui P, Laurent A, Amathieu R, Azoulay D. Assessment of risk for non-hepatic surgery in cirrhotic patients. J Hepatol. 2012;57(4):874–84. https://doi.org/10.1016/j.jhep.2012.03.037.
25. Lopez-Delgado JC, Ballus J, Esteve F, et al. Outcomes of abdominal surgery in patients with liver cirrhosis. World J Gastroenterol. 2016;22(9):2657–67. https://doi.org/10.3748/wjg.v22.i9.2657.
26. Stinton LM, Shaffer EA. Epidemiology of gallbladder disease: cholelithiasis and cancer. Gut Liver. 2012;6(2):172–87. https://doi.org/10.5009/gnl.2012.6.2.172.
27. Laurence JM, Tran PD, Richardson AJ, Pleass HCC, Lam VWT. Laparoscopic or open cholecystectomy in cirrhosis: a systematic review of outcomes and meta-analysis of randomized trials. HPB (Oxford). 2012;14(3):153–61. https://doi.org/10.1111/j.1477-2574.2011.00425.
28. Ammar SA. Management of complicated umbilical hernias in cirrhotic patients using permanent mesh: randomized clinical trial. Hernia. 2010;14(1):35–8. https://doi.org/10.1007/s10029-009-0556-4.
29. Oh H-K, Kim H, Ryoo S, Choe EK, Park KJ. Inguinal hernia repair in patients with cirrhosis is not associated with increased risk of complications and recurrence. World J Surg. 2011;35(6):1229–33; discussion 1234. https://doi.org/10.1007/s00268-011-1007-9.
30. Licari L, Salamone G, Ciolino G, et al. The abdominal wall incisional hernia repair in cirrhotic patients. G Chir. 2018;39(1):20–3. https://doi.org/10.11138/gchir/2018.39.1.020.
31. Rabinovitz M, Schade RR, Dindzans V, Van Thiel DH, Gavaler JS. Prevalence of duodenal ulcer in cirrhotic males referred for liver transplantation. Does

the etiology of cirrhosis make a difference? Dig Dis Sci. 1990;35(3):321–6. https://doi.org/10.1007/BF01537409.
32. Lehnert T, Herfarth C. Peptic ulcer surgery in patients with liver cirrhosis. Ann Surg. 1993;217(4):338–46. https://doi.org/10.1097/00000658-199304000-00005.
33. Garcia M, Gerber A, Zakhary B, et al. Management and outcomes of acute appendicitis in the presence of cirrhosis: a Nationwide analysis. Am Surg. 2019;85(10):1129–33.
34. Tsugawa K, Koyanagi N, Hashizume M, et al. A comparison of an open and laparoscopic appendectomy for patients with liver cirrhosis. Surg Laparosc Endosc Percutan Tech. 2001;11(3):189–94.
35. Salminen P, Tuominen R, Paajanen H, et al. Five-year follow-up of antibiotic therapy for uncomplicated acute appendicitis in the APPAC randomized clinical trial. JAMA. 2018;320(12):1259–65. https://doi.org/10.1001/jama.2018.13201.
36. Gervaz P, Pak-art R, Nivatvongs S, Wolff BG, Larson D, Ringel S. Colorectal adenocarcinoma in cirrhotic patients. J Am Coll Surg. 2003;196(6):874–9. https://doi.org/10.1016/S1072-7515(03)00117-0.
37. Kruger AJ, Mumtaz K, Anaizi A, et al. Cirrhosis is associated with increased mortality in patients with diverticulitis: a Nationwide cross-sectional study. Dig Dis Sci. 2017;62(11):3149–55. https://doi.org/10.1007/s10620-017-4782-9.
38. Kazi A, Finco TB, Zakhary B, et al. Acute colonic diverticulitis and cirrhosis: outcomes of laparoscopic colectomy compared with an open approach. J Am Coll Surg. 2020;230(6):1045–53. https://doi.org/10.1016/j.jamcollsurg.2020.03.016.
39. Talving P, Lustenberger T, Okoye OT, et al. The impact of liver cirrhosis on outcomes in trauma patients: a prospective study. J Trauma Acute Care Surg. 2013;75(4):699–703. https://doi.org/10.1097/TA.0b013e31829a2c19.
40. Georgiou C, Inaba K, Teixeira PGR, et al. Cirrhosis and trauma are a lethal combination. World J Surg. 2009;33(5):1087–92. https://doi.org/10.1007/s00268-009-9923-7.
41. Demetriades D, Constantinou C, Salim A, Velmahos G, Rhee P, Chan L. Liver cirrhosis in patients undergoing laparotomy for trauma: effect on outcomes. J Am Coll Surg. 2004;199(4):538–42. https://doi.org/10.1016/j.jamcollsurg.2004.06.017.
42. Abbas N, Makker J, Abbas H, Balar B. Perioperative care of patients with liver cirrhosis: a review. Health Serv Insights. 2017;10:1178632917691270. https://doi.org/10.1177/1178632917691270.
43. De Pietri L, Bianchini M, Montalti R, et al. Thrombelastography-guided blood product use before invasive procedures in cirrhosis with severe coagulopathy: a randomized, controlled trial. Hepatology. 2016;63(2):566–73. https://doi.org/10.1002/hep.28148.
44. Bleszynski MS, Bressan AK, Joos E, Morad Hameed S, Ball CG. Acute care and emergency general surgery in patients with chronic liver disease: how can we optimize perioperative care? A review of the literature. World J Emerg Surg. 2018;13:32. https://doi.org/10.1186/s13017-018-0194-1.
45. Montoliu S, Ballesté B, Planas R, et al. Incidence and prognosis of different types of functional renal failure in cirrhotic patients with ascites. Clin Gastroenterol Hepatol. 2010;8(7):616–22; quiz e80. https://doi.org/10.1016/j.cgh.2010.03.029.
46. Bittencourt PL, Farias AQ, Terra C. Renal failure in cirrhosis: emerging concepts. World J Hepatol. 2015;7(21):2336–43. https://doi.org/10.4254/wjh.v7.i21.2336.
47. Jalan R, Fernandez J, Wiest R, et al. Bacterial infections in cirrhosis: a position statement based on the EASL Special Conference 2013. J Hepatol. 2014;60(6):1310–24. https://doi.org/10.1016/j.jhep.2014.01.024.
48. Douard R, Lentschener C, Ozier Y, Dousset B. Operative risks of digestive surgery in cirrhotic patients. Gastroenterol Clin Biol. 2009;33(6–7):555–64. https://doi.org/10.1016/j.gcb.2009.03.012.
49. Bunchorntavakul C, Supanun R, Atsawarungruangkit A. Nutritional status and its impact on clinical outcomes for patients admitted to hospital with cirrhosis. J Med Assoc Thail. 2016;99(Suppl 2):S47–55.
50. Gibbs J, Cull W, Henderson W, Daley J, Hur K, Khuri SF. Preoperative serum albumin level as a predictor of operative mortality and morbidity: results from the National VA Surgical Risk Study. Arch Surg. 1999;134(1):36–42. https://doi.org/10.1001/archsurg.134.1.36.
51. Arita J, Sakamaki K, Saiura A, et al. Drain placement after uncomplicated hepatic resection increases severe postoperative complication rate: a Japanese multi-institutional randomized controlled trial (ND-trial). Ann Surg. 2021;273(2):224–31. https://doi.org/10.1097/SLA.0000000000004051.
52. Diaz KE, Schiano TD. Evaluation and management of cirrhotic patients undergoing elective surgery. Curr Gastroenterol Rep. 2019;21(7):32. https://doi.org/10.1007/s11894-019-0700-y.
53. Ginès P, Schrier RW. Renal failure in cirrhosis. N Engl J Med. 2009;361(13):1279–90. https://doi.org/10.1056/NEJMra0809139.
54. Wicks C, Somasundaram S, Bjarnason I, et al. Comparison of enteral feeding and total parenteral nutrition after liver transplantation. Lancet (London, England). 1994;344(8926):837–40. https://doi.org/10.1016/s0140-6736(94)92824-x.
55. Rakoski M, Goyal P, Spencer-Safier M, Weissman J, Mohr G, Volk M. Pain management in patients with cirrhosis. Clin Liver Dis. 2018;11(6):135–40. https://doi.org/10.1002/cld.711.
56. Gulur P, Tsui B, Pathak R, Koury KM, Lee H. Retrospective analysis of the incidence of epidural haematoma in patients with epidural catheters and abnormal coagulation parameters. Br J Anaesth. 2015;114(5):808–11. https://doi.org/10.1093/bja/aeu461.
57. Girard RM, Morin M. Open cholecystectomy: its morbidity and mortality as a reference standard. Can J Surg. 1993;36(1):75–80.

Nutrition Considerations in Emergency Surgery

36

Molly J. Douglas, Muhammad Khurrum, and Bellal Joseph

Case Study

Mr. M is a 64 y/o man with a prior hiatal hernia repair, who presented with abdominal pain, nausea, and emesis. CT demonstrated a recurrent paraesophageal hernia containing small bowel and colon, with evidence of large bowel obstruction within the hernia sac. He was taken to the OR and underwent open reduction of the hernia and primary repair of the diaphragmatic defect with absorbable mesh reinforcement. Post-operatively, he initially did well and had his nasogastric (NG) tube removed on post-op day 1. After 4 days of poor oral intake, however, he developed bilious emesis and the NG was replaced. CT with enteral contrast demonstrated early post-op small bowel obstruction with a transition point in the mid-abdomen. This was managed non-operatively, and by post-op day 9 he was able to resume oral intake. However, in the meantime, he developed a partial midline fascial dehiscence and a stage II sacral decubitus ulcer.

Could malnutrition have played a role in these complications?

Importance of Nutrition

The answer to the above question is yes! Nutrition is a fundamental component of overall health. Adequate nutrition contributes to normal immune function, appropriate stress response, adequate wound healing, resistance to non-communicable illness, and greater longevity [1–4].

Malnutrition, on the other hand, occurs when the nutrients provided to the body are in some way inadequate to meet its many physiologic needs. This may occur from inadequate calories, inadequate protein, or deficiencies of particular vitamins, minerals, or essential fatty acids. Further, increased metabolic demands in times of acute surgical stress or systemic inflammatory response place patients at increased risk of nutritional deficits, particularly if the level of nourishment is not escalated to meet the increased demand.

M. J. Douglas · M. Khurrum · B. Joseph (✉)
Division of Trauma, Critical Care, Burns, and Emergency Surgery, Department of Surgery, University of Arizona College of Medicine, Tucson, AZ, USA
e-mail: mjdouglas@surgery.arizona.edu; khurrum@surgery.arizona.edu; bjoseph@surgery.arizona.edu

M. D. Zielinski, O. Guillamondegui (eds.), *The Acute Management of Surgical Disease*,
https://doi.org/10.1007/978-3-031-07881-1_36

Table 36.1 Benefits of nutrition in emergency surgery patients

Benefits of early and adequate nutrition
– Lower mortality
– Preserved gut mucosal barrier function
– Preserved immune response
– Fewer infections
– More rapid wound healing
– Maintenance of lean body mass
– Fewer decubitus ulcers
– Shorter length of stay
– Enhanced patient comfort

Inadequate nutrition has been associated with a multitude of complications in hospitalized patients, including impaired immune function and higher risk of infection [5–10], delayed wound healing and formation of pressure ulcers [11, 12], wasting of lean muscle mass and an accordingly slower functional recovery [13], as well as longer length of stay [14]. In particular, in general surgery patients requiring ICU care, malnutrition at the time of ICU admission is associated with significantly increased mortality [15, 16]. Provision of adequate nutrition can reduce these complications (Table 36.1).

Assessing Baseline Nutrition Status

An assessment of nutritional status is key to identify pre-existing or impending malnutrition, to monitor changes in the adequacy of nourishment over time, and to guide nutritional interventions. In the United States, the Joint Commission has mandated nutritional screening within 24 h of hospital admission since 1995, although the choice of nutrition assessment method is left to the institution [17]. In the emergency surgery patient, the combination of increased physiologic demand and frequently decreased capacity for intake mandates special consideration [18]. It is generally accepted that no single metric provides a perfect indicator of nutritional status. Methods of nutritional status assessment range from simple bedside exams to invasive procedures, and several common methods are described below.

Anthropometric Measurements

Anthropometric measures is a non-invasive and widely used tool for nutritional assessment. Such measures can be performed at the bedside or in ambulatory settings and may include an individual's weight, height, body mass index (BMI), body circumference (arm, waist, hip, calf), waist to hip ratio (WHR), and triceps skinfold thickness. The BMI is perhaps the most widely used crude measure of nutrition status, and is calculated from an individual's height and weight as follows:

$$\text{BMI} = \frac{\text{Weight in kg}}{(\text{Height in meters})^2} \quad (36.1)$$

The National Institutes of Health define normal BMI as 18.5–24.5 kg/m^2, while <18.5 is termed underweight and BMIs greater than 25 are termed overweight. While a markedly underweight status may reliably reflect under-nutrition, BMI's lack of accounting for body composition limits interpretation of numbers at the larger end of the BMI spectrum [19]. With the exception of the BMI, most anthropometric measurements are operator dependent, and inter-observer variability combined with normal variations in individual proportions makes these metrics unreliable indicators of nutritional status [19].

Subjective Global Assessment

Subjective global assessment (SGA) is one of the few clinically reproducible methods of accessing a patient's nutritional status based on history and physical examination. The factors considered in arriving at the SGA are detailed in Fig. 36.1. The assessment takes into account weight change, changes in dietary intake, gastrointestinal symptoms, functional capacity, and diagnoses that may impact nutritional needs. The physical examination component looks for loss of subcutaneous fat, muscle wasting, edema, and ascites as potential markers of malnutrition. After assessing these factors, the examiner is instructed to "subjectively" combine them into a categorization for the patient as well-nourished, moderately

SUBJECTIVE GLOBAL ASSESSMENT

History:

Weight change Overall weight loss in past 6 months: amount in kg and % loss Change in past 2 weeks: Increase, No change, Decrease

Dietary intake change (relative to normal), No, change, Change, duration in weeks type: sub-optimal solid diet, full liquid diet hypocaloric liquids, starvation

Gastrointestinal symptoms (that persisted for >2 weeks): None, Nausea, Vomiting, Diarrhea, Anorexia

Functional capacity No dysfunction (e.g., full capacity); Dysfunction: Duration in weeks, Type: working suboptimally, ambulatory, bedridden

Disease and its relation to nutritional requirements Primary diagnosis (specify), Metabolic demand (stress): No stress, Low stress. Moderate stress, High stress

Physical:
(for each: 0 = normal, 1+ = mild, 2+ = moderate, 3+ = severe)

Loss of subcutaneous fat (triceps, chest)

Muscle wasting (quadriceps, deltoids)

Ankle edema

Sacral edema

Ascites

SGA rating: Select based on subjective combination of a history and physical factors

A = Well-nourished

B = Moderately (or suspected of being) malnourished

C = Severely malnourished

Fig. 36.1 Subjective global assessment of nutritional status. (Adapted from [20])

malnourished, or severely malnourished. Developed in the 1980s, the method outperformed more objective measures (anthropomorphic and laboratory metrics) of nutritional status in its ability to predict postoperative infections [20–24]. Further, high inter-observer agreement was found, despite the subjective nature of the assessment [22, 23], making this an attractive bedside tool for baseline nutritional assessment.

It is important to note that numerous other history and physical-based or combined nutritional scoring systems have been developed over the years. A more comprehensive review is provided by Reber and colleagues [25].

Albumin

Albumin is the most prevalent plasma protein, and plays key roles in maintaining plasma oncotic pressure, antioxidant activity, and substrate binding and transport (e.g., bilirubin, long-chain fatty acids, calcium, magnesium, and many drugs) [26]. In healthy subjects, it is produced in the liver at a rate of 10–15 g/day, and has a long turnover time of approximately 25 days [26, 27].

Albumin has historically been cast as a marker of nutritional status, most likely because Kwashiorkor (protein malnutrition in the setting of adequate carbohydrate caloric intake) is associated with profound hypoalbuminemia [26, 28]. However, albumin's ability to reliably reflect malnutrition has been called into question, as examinations of marasmus (total calorie malnutrition), severe anorexia nervosa, and controlled starvation studies find that serum albumin levels are generally maintained at near-normal despite significant energy deficits [26, 28–30]. Further, nutritional supplementation in ill patients does not reliably increase albumin levels, despite weight gain and positive nitrogen balance [31, 32].

Nevertheless, hypoalbuminemia, variably defined as serum albumin concentration <3.0–3.5 mg/dL, has been shown to be a strong predictor of surgical complications. A notable 1999 analysis of greater than 54,000 patients from the Veterans Administration (VA) Surgical Risk Study database found that post-op mortality increased nearly exponentially with change in albumin concentration from 4.6 g/dL (<1% mortality) to <2.1 g/dL (28% mortality) [33]. Hypoalbuminemia has been associated with anastomotic leak, surgical site infection, mortality, and length of stay in other studies [34–36]. A retrospective review of 1.7 million life insurance applicants further demonstrated a striking inverse correlation between serum albumin concentration and all-cause mortality [37].

As albumin is highly associated with post-op complications and mortality, yet not clearly associated with nutritional status, another mediator must be at play. Recent literature indicates this mediator is most likely acute and chronic inflammation. Elevation of inflammatory cytokines, particularly TNF-α, IL-1, and IL-6, results in reduced albumin synthesis [26, 27] and increased protein breakdown [26, 38]. Increased vascular permeability, which permits leak of albumin out of the intravascular space, is also implicated in the rapid decline in albumin concentration seen in sepsis or acute injury [26].

Thus, a low albumin level may still be considered an important marker of pre-operative surgical risk, but should be interpreted as an indicator of underlying systemic disease (and should prompt a search for the source of such an illness, if time and patient condition permit). However, albumin should not be relied upon as an indicator of nutritional status or as a marker of the need for nutrition therapy.

Prealbumin

Prealbumin has also been held up as a marker of malnutrition, yet more recent data shows that this protein, like albumin, is a reliable marker of systemic disease and a very poor indicator of nutritional status.

Prealbumin is a protein synthesized mainly in the liver, but also in smaller amounts in the choroid plexus and retina. It plays a role in the transport of thyroxine as well as vitamin A (retinol), which explains its alternate name transthyretin (**trans**ports **thyr**oxine and **retin**ol) [39].

A 1972 Lancet paper initially correlated prealbumin with malnutrition in Kwashiorkor patients [40]. Whereas albumin turns over approximately every 20 days, prealbumin has a much shorter turnover time of just 2–3 days, which historically has made it attractive for monitoring the response to nutritional therapy [40]. Prealbumin is well known to drop rapidly in acute stress states [41], which may correlate with times of poor appetite and decreased nutritional intake, furthering the myth of hepatic proteins as nutritional markers. However, a 2015 systematic review including more than 1000 subjects by Lee and colleagues found that in the absence of systemic disease, caloric restriction (due to decreased access or psychiatric conditions), prealbumin levels are preserved within the normal range (>20 mg/dL) until severe and obvious clinical starvation (e.g., BMI <12 kg/m^2) has occurred. Notably, average prealbumin remained normal even among 62 individuals with average BMI of 12.9 kg/m^2 [30].

Nitrogen Balance

Nitrogen balance, defined as the difference between nitrogen intake and nitrogen losses, quantifies the relationship between protein anabolism and catabolism. It is estimated as [42]:

$$\text{Nitrogen balance} = \frac{\text{Protein intake}}{6.25} - (24\ \text{h urine urea nitrogen} + 4) \tag{36.2}$$

where nitrogen balance, dietary protein, urea nitrogen, and the constant "4" are in grams, and 6.25 is the commonly accepted conversion factor for grams of protein per gram of nitrogen [43]. This assumes a constant 4 g of non-urinary nitrogen losses per day, although some studies find that GI and integumentary losses may be higher in acute illness, for example, in cases of diarrhea or burns [44]. Clearly, estimation of nitrogen balance by this method requires collection and laboratory assessment of the urine over 24 h, as well as strict quantification of all protein consumed. Given these logistical challenges, it is uncommonly used in routine clinical practice outside of a research setting.

Adequate protein intake helps to protect against excessive tissue breakdown and loss of lean muscle mass, particularly when overall calories are also adequate [45, 46]. Unlike albumin and prealbumin levels, positive nitrogen balance appears to reliably correlate with increased protein administration [47, 48], and provision of protein in excess of nitrogen losses has also been associated with increased protein synthesis (anabolism) [45]. Although large trials are lacking, limited evidence supports a correlation between positive nitrogen balance and improved outcome in critical illness [49, 50]. Nitrogen balance however does not reliably reflect the adequacy of non-protein calorie delivery [51].

Limitations to the use of nitrogen balance include patients with end-stage renal disease requiring dialysis, for whom nitrogen losses to the dialysate fluid must be quantified in addition to urinary measurements [52]. Further, for patients with an open abdomen (or those undergoing large-volume paracentesis for other reasons) nitrogen losses via the abdominal fluid must also be considered. While the nitrogen content of this fluid may be measured directly, a reasonable estimate is 2 g of nitrogen loss per liter of peritoneal fluid drained [53].

Thus, nitrogen balance is a reasonable metric of whether protein delivery is adequate to meet tissue turnover demands, but does not quantify the adequacy of non-protein calories, and its accurate calculation requires close attention to all sources of nitrogen input and output.

How Much Nutrition (Energy) Do Patients Need?

Awareness of the nutritional requirements of surgical patients is essential, because the provision of inadequate or excess calories can adversely affect outcome. Caloric needs may be ascertained through bedside measurements (e.g., indirect calorimetry), or through mathematical estimations. Computational prediction of energy needs is challenging, however, as demands may vary considerably from individual to individual, and also change over time for any given patient based on physiologic condition and activity level. Numerous techniques and formulas have been proposed to predict caloric requirements [54]. Several of the best-studied are discussed below.

Direct Calorimetry

Direct calorimetry is the measurement of heat emitted from a system, e.g., a device, animal, or human being. Animal calorimetry was first documented in eighteenth-century France, and involved placing a guinea pig in an ice-lined, snow-insulated box, and measuring the water accumulated from ice melt due to heat generated by the animal over a period of time. As a homeostatic mammal will maintain a constant body temperature, all energy processed by the animal is ultimately dissipated as heat. In these early experiments, knowing the specific heat of water allowed calculation of the heat evolved. Further, the investigators also measured CO_2 produced by the guinea pig, which permitted development of conversion factors for how much heat was generated per mole of CO_2 exhaled [55]. In the modern day, whole-room calorimeters for measuring heat loss from humans have been constructed. Although it is equipment-intensive, direct calorimetry is considered the gold standard against which all other measures of metabolism are assessed [55].

Indirect Calorimetry

Indirect calorimetry (IC) is the quantification of energy use (heat production) via the measurement of O_2 consumed and CO_2 produced. This is enabled by these relationships having been quantified via direct calorimetry studies. IC equipment now exists in a bedside form, commonly called a "metabolic cart." In using a metabolic cart, the patient is connected to the device via a tight-fitting face mask or via their existing mechanical ventilator circuit. Expired oxygen and carbon dioxide volumes are recorded until a steady state is reached [56]. The metabolic rate is then calculated as follows [56, 57]:

$$M = 3.91 \cdot VO_2 + 1.1 \cdot VCO_2 - 2.17 \cdot \mathrm{UN} \tag{36.3}$$

where M is the metabolic rate in kcal/min, and VO_2 and VCO_2 are the L/min of oxygen and carbon dioxide consumed and expired, respectively. UN is urinary nitrogen excretion in g/day, and helps to adjust the metabolic rate for the effects for protein metabolism [57]. The result can be multiplied by the number of minutes in 24 h (1440) to obtain the energy expenditure in the more familiar kcal/day.

Although significantly more accessible than direct calorimetry, indirect calorimetry remains somewhat equipment and time-intensive, and is not readily available at all centers. Given the limitations of predictive formulas (discussed below), periodic use of IC to guide nutrition therapy in critically ill patients is recommended by both the European (ESPEN) and American (ASPEN) Societies for Parenteral and Enteral Nutrition [58, 59]. However, IC has not reliably been correlated with enhanced patient outcomes [59]. Significantly, IC does lay the groundwork for deriving predictive equations that non-invasively estimate caloric needs.

Harris-Benedict Equations

The Harris-Benedict equations were originally published in 1918 after analysis of indirect calorimetry data for 136 men and 100 women in good health and ranging in age from 21 to 70 years [60]. Measurements were done with subjects completely at rest to quantify a resting or "basal" energy expenditure. A later validation study with data from a small number of additional subjects suggested good accuracy [61]. The Harris-Benedict equations remain among the most widely used formulas for estimating resting energy expenditure, or basal metabolic rate (BMR), which is calculated as follows [60]:

For men:

$$\begin{aligned} \mathrm{BMR} = {} & 66.5 + 13.6 \cdot \mathrm{weight} + 5.00 \cdot \mathrm{height} \\ & - 6.76 \cdot \mathrm{age} \end{aligned} \tag{36.4}$$

For women:

$$\begin{aligned} \mathrm{BMR} = {} & 655 + 9.56 \cdot \mathrm{weight} + 1.85 \cdot \mathrm{height} \\ & - 4.68 \cdot \mathrm{age} \end{aligned} \tag{36.5}$$

where BMR is in kilocalories (kcal)/day, weight is in kilograms (kg), height is in centimeters (cm), and age is in years.

As emergency general surgery patients generally face increased metabolic demand due to physiologic stress, in contrast to the state of complete rest assumed in the Harris-Benedict calculations, multiplication by stress or activity factors is needed. The total daily caloric requirement is equal to the BMR multiplied by the relevant stress factor. Typically, stress factors range from 1.2 to 1.7 depending upon the severity of illness [62].

Multiple studies have investigated the accuracy of stress factors for use with the Harris-Benedict equation, across a range of stressors including hospitalization, mechanical ventilation, comorbidities, surgical procedures, and burns. Barak et al. [62] reviewed a heterogeneous group of >500 hospitalized patients who underwent indirect calorimetry, and found that the average stress factor (measured energy expenditure divided by the Harris-Benedict equation's predicted energy expenditure) across the cohort was 1.25. The subgroup of general surgery patients showed average stress factors of 1.2–1.4, and this was higher for burn patients at 1.5–1.6 [62]. Notably, the investigators found that similar stress factors held true in the underweight and overweight populations, when actual body weight was used for calculation in the underweight group, and when an adjusted body weight consisting of the "ideal" weight plus 50% of the difference between the actual and "ideal" weight was used in the overweight group.

Heterogeneity in appropriate stress factors has been found in the critically ill population. A 2003 review 76 mechanically ventilated patients found that a stress factor of 1.6 produced energy expenditure estimates within 20% of that measured by indirect calorimetry in 80% of cases [63], yet a 2020 study of another critically ill cohort found a stress factor of only 1.25 to accurately predicted energy expenditure to within 35% of indirect calorimetry measurements [64]. It is likely that the variation in applicability of different stress factor stems from differences in the severity of illness in the underlying populations, which may be poorly quantified by blanket labels such as "critically ill" or "surgical patients."

Mifflin-St Jeor Equations

Concerns about nutrition and obesity in America in the late twentieth century fueled further research seeking quantify human energy needs. Mifflin and colleagues performed indirect calorimetry on 498 healthy adults, approximately evenly split between men and women, and also split between the "obese" and "non-obese" categories. In 1990, they published the following formulas, which utilized the same input measures as the classic Harris-Benedict equations, but on average predicted slightly (50–100 kcal/day) lower energy needs [65]. The authors suggested the observed differences from Harris and Benedict's work might be related, and an older and larger body-size cohort was used for their derivations.

For men:

$$\begin{aligned}\text{BMR} = 10 \cdot \text{weight} + 6.25 \cdot \text{height} \\ - 5 \cdot \text{age} + 5\end{aligned} \tag{36.6}$$

For women:

$$\begin{aligned}\text{BMR} = 10 \cdot \text{weight} + 6.25 \cdot \text{height} \\ - 5 \cdot \text{age} - 161\end{aligned} \tag{36.7}$$

where, again, BMR is in kcal/day, weight is in kg, height is in cm, and age is in years. As with Harris-Benedict, the Mifflin-St Jeor formulas predict only resting energy expenditure, and for stressed patients the actual daily caloric needs must be adjusted upward.

Swinamer Equation

In 1990, Swinamer and colleagues sought to address the issue of predicting caloric needs accurately in the critically ill. They analyzed indirect calorimetry from 112 mechanically ventilated patients (a mixture of trauma and non-trauma patients, with a slight male predominance), and arrived at a predictive formula based on body surface area, age, temperature, respiratory rate, and tidal volume. The equation, shown below, out-performed Harris-Benedict for estimating energy expenditure in this population [63, 66]

$$\begin{aligned}\text{EE} = 945 \cdot \text{BSA} - 6.4 \cdot \text{age} + 108 \cdot \text{temp} \\ + 24.2 \cdot \text{RR} + 81.7 \cdot \text{TV} - 4349\end{aligned} \tag{36.8}$$

where EE is energy expenditure in kcal/day, BSA is body surface area is in m^2, age is in years, temp is temperature in °C, RR is respiratory rate in breaths/min, and TV is tidal volume in L.

Several studies have explored the predictive accuracy of the Swinamer equation in mechanically ventilated patients. In a study of critically ill patients with body mass index <30 kg/m^2, MacDonald et al. found that the Swinamer equation predicted measured energy expenditure to within 10% of indirect calorimetry values in approximately half of cases, and to within 20%

of indirect calorimetry values 88% of the time [63]. A study of a mixed hospitalized population (ICU and non-ICU) found similar results, with the Swinamer equation predicting energy expenditure to within 10% of measured values in 45% of cases [67]. Further, a recent prospective observational study compared resting energy expenditure estimated by 15 different predictive equations against indirect calorimetry at different phases of critical illness (acute ≤5 days, late 6–10 days, and chronic ≥11 days). It was shown that the Swinamer equation was the most accurate predictive equation during all three phases of ICU stay [64].

Penn State and Modified Penn State Equations

The Penn State equation was developed to improve accuracy of energy expenditure prediction in the critically ill. It was based on data from 169 mixed-ICU patients, and first appeared in book form in 1998. The formula uses Harris-Benedict the BMR calculation as a starting point, then effectively computes the "stress factor" based on minute ventilation and body temperature [68, 69]:

$$\begin{aligned} EE = 1.1 \cdot BMR_{HB} + 32 \cdot MV \\ + 140 \cdot T_{max} - 5340 \end{aligned} \tag{36.9}$$

where EE is energy expenditure in kcal/day, BMR_{HB} is basal metabolic rate as calculated by the Harris-Benedict equations, MV is minute ventilation in L, and T_{max} is the maximum temperature in °C observed over 24 h.

Of note, a 2003 update to the Penn State formula recommended the use of actual rather than adjusted body weight, where adjust body weight is ideal body weight + 0.25 · (actual – ideal body weight), to avoid under-estimation of needs in larger-bodied patients [70].

Validation study showed up to 79% accuracy of the Penn State formula in predicting energy expenditure to within 10% of measured values in non-obese patients. However, accuracy was only to 61% in the small group of patients with BMI >30 [70]. The lower accuracy in the latter population prompted creation of the modified Penn State formula, intended for patients over age 60 with BMI >30 [71]:

$$\begin{aligned} EE = 0.71 \cdot BMR_{MSJ} + 85 \cdot T_{max} \\ + 64 \cdot MV - 3085 \end{aligned} \tag{36.10}$$

In this modification, BMR is calculated using actual body weight according to the Mifflin-St Jeor rather than Harris-Benedict equations, and the constants are also modified from the original Penn State formula.

Validation of this formula on a group of predominantly non-trauma surgical patients, all of the target population (age >60, BMI >30), showed 70% accuracy in predicting energy expenditure to within 10% of measured.

Which Formula to Use?

Despite decades of study, systematic reviews find that each of these formulas may over or underestimate the caloric requirement by 200 to >500 kcal/day [54]. In critically ill patients, predictive equations accurately predict energy expenditure to within 10% of direct calorimetry measurements only half of the time [72]. American Society for Parenteral and Enteral Nutrition (ASPEN) guidelines state that no formula clearly outperforms the others, even in critically ill patients. Further, daily recalculation of energy needs based on fever curve and ventilator parameters may be cumbersome, particularly when it is unclear if the added precision improves outcomes. For every day use outside of a research setting, a simplistic weight-based formula is easy to apply and provides a clinically acceptable estimation of energy expenditure [59]:

$$EE = 20 - 30\,\text{kcal}/\text{kg}/\text{day} \tag{36.11}$$

where the higher end of the calorie range should be used for patients under greater physiologic stress.

Estimating Protein Needs

Adequate protein is a key driver of response to nutritional intervention (see below: Permissive Underfeeding). Protein intake requirements to prevent catabolism can be estimated by calculating the nitrogen losses, as described in the previous section. Much like total calories, however a simple weight-based, stress-adjusted formula remains the standard for day-to-day estimation of protein requirements [59]:

$$\text{Protein required} = 1.2 - \text{g}/\text{kg}/\text{day} \quad (36.12)$$

where the higher end of the protein range should be used for patients under greater physiologic stress.

The Role of Permissive Underfeeding

The premise of permissive underfeeding, or providing fewer calories than required based on the methods of estimation detailed above, has its roots in several beliefs. First, hyperglycemia, which is known to be associated with infectious complications, may be exacerbated by feeding during acute illness and its associated increased insulin resistance—leading some to conclude feeding should be curtailed [73]. Second, autophagy, the autodigestion of stressed or dysfunctional cells and proteins, may be an important part of the immune response in the early phase of illness, and may be suppressed by the provision of nutrients [73].

Recent trials have compared early underfeeding to "standard" nutritional therapy in mixed ICU populations. Several studies that initially showed benefit were limited by the confounding factor that adequate protein (>1 g/kg/day) was delivered *only* in the hypocaloric group [74, 75]. A large-scale multicenter RCT published in 2015, the PermiT Trial [76], compared hypocaloric (40–60% of estimated caloric needs) to standard nutrition (70–100% of estimated needs) over 14 days, while maintaining 1.2–1.5 g/kg/day of protein administration in both groups. This revealed no significant difference in the primary endpoint of 90-day mortality, and no difference in infectious complications or length of stay. However, significantly less hyperglycemia and lower insulin requirements were observed in the hypocaloric group. A post-hoc analysis of the study comparing subgroups of high and low nutritional risk also showed no difference in mortality in the hypocaloric vs standard feeding groups [77].

The available evidence suggests that adequate protein is a key driver of outcome in response to nutritional interventions, and that as long as adequate protein administration is preserved, patients tolerate a short-term caloric deficit quite well. Further study is needed to determine the optimal timing and quantity of feeding, particularly in the critically ill.

Risk of Overfeeding

Although adequate nutrition is well-established to be beneficial, provision of calories in excess of metabolic demands has been associated with significant complications. These include hyperglycemia, hepatic steatosis, hypertriglyceridemia, and hypercapnia [78]. Hyperglycemia is readily mitigated with strict insulin protocols. Hepatic steatosis however, which has been reproduced in animal models of overfeeding [79, 80], is associated with potentially severe long-term complications including cirrhosis, liver failure, and hepatocellular carcinoma [81].

Hypercapnia may result from excessive carbohydrate or total calorie administration. As both the carbon content and the metabolic pathways for carbohydrates, fats, and proteins vary, their metabolism yields differing amounts of CO_2 production. This is described by the respiratory quotient, defined as the molar quantity of CO_2 evolved per mole of O_2 used. The respiratory quotient for pure carbohydrate metabolism is 1.0, whereas for protein and fat it is 0.8 and 0.7 respectively [82]. A respiratory quotient of >1.0 suggests overfeeding of carbohydrates or overall calories. Further, the bulk of CO_2 produced must be cleared through the respiratory system. Thus, greater CO_2 production mandates a higher minute ventilation to maintain homeostasis. In critically ill patients, this may result in difficulty with liberating from the ventilator.

Choice of Nutritional Route

In emergency surgery patients, enteral nutrition is always preferable to parenteral nutrition due to the documented significant morbidity and mortality risk associated with parenteral nutrition [83–85]. Despite the significant risk of morbidity and mortality with parenteral nutrition, the most recent advances in the management of surgical patients have significantly mitigated the risk. Multiple studies have shown that there was no significant increase in the risk of morbidity and mortality with parenteral nutrition compared to enteral nutrition [86, 87]. An issue with relying solely on enteral nutrition is that, due to a partly functional gastrointestinal tract or side effects associated with enteral feedings, it is difficult to attain caloric targets in emergency general surgery patients. European guidelines recommend early initiation of parenteral nutrition to minimize nutritional deficits, while North American guidelines favor hypocaloric enteral nutrition for up to 1 week in patients with a good nutritional baseline before considering TPN [59, 88]. Also, there is an increasing trend of using parenteral nutrition as a supplement to, rather than replacement for enteral nutrition. However, the results are non-uniform across the literature and this remains the topic of debate [89–93].

Enteral

Enteral nutrition is the provision of nutrients via the GI tract. This is preferable to parenteral nutrition, in the presence of functioning bowel. Enteral nutrition promotes the maintenance of an intact brush border and intercellular tight junctions, which helps to minimize bacterial translocation, reduces the risk of infection, and stimulates gut motility. Enteral feeding has been consistently associated with fewer infections, reduced cost, earlier gut function, and reduced length of stay when compared to parenteral nutrition [94].

Oral Nutrition

Oral nutrition is the natural choice for patients who are awake with a functioning GI tract and adequate swallowing mechanics. A key advantage of oral nutrition is that it requires no instrumentation of the patient, and therefore risks such as enteral tube malposition or venous catheter infection are not incurred. Eating by mouth allows self-regulation of intake based on normal thirst, hunger, and fullness cues, and simply being allowed to eat provides a sense of both satisfaction and normalcy to most individuals.

Non-oral Enteral Nutrition

Non-oral enteral feeds may be needed for patients who are intubated or otherwise have impaired swallowing mechanics, or who require bypass of non-functioning portions of the GI tract. Feeds are delivered by tube, most commonly to the stomach or post-pyloric small intestine; either the duodenum or jejunum may be reached. A discussion of long-term feeding access options, e.g., trans-abdominal gastric and jejunal tubes, is outside the scope of this chapter, and we will focus instead on short-term, naso-enteral, and oro-enteral feeding equipment.

Gastric vs Post-pyloric Feeding

Debates over the relative safety of gastric versus post-pyloric feedings are longstanding, with proponents of post-pyloric feedings arguing that the more distal location should logically reduce regurgitation, aspiration and events, and associated pneumonia. However, this has not been borne out by evidence. A 2003 systematic review [95] found no difference in rates of pneumonia, mortality, or calorie delivery between critically ill patients fed by the gastric versus post-pyloric route. Further, gastric residual volume (GRV, the volume of gastric contents that can be suctioned back out of the stomach for measurement after a period of feeding) appears to be a poor marker for risk of aspiration or feeding complications [96]. Montejo and colleagues found that allowing a residual volume of up to 500 mL vs the more traditional 200 mL was not associated with any increase in pneumonia, ICU length of stay, or GI complications. The higher GRV tolerance was associated with a reduced need for supplemental TPN [96]. Further, a multicenter randomized controlled trial in France found no increase in ventilator-associated pneumonia when gastric residual volumes were simply not checked at all, and that patients without GRV checks were more likely to reach their caloric intake goals [97]. Overall, checking and limiting nutrition delivery based on gastric residual volume appears to do more harm than good, and should not be part of routine care [98]. Additionally, the stomach, unlike the small intestine, can tolerate bolus feeding. This may be particularly helpful for volume-based feeding protocols in which periods of "missed" tube feeding are delivered later at higher rates or bolus volumes to prevent accumulation of a significant caloric deficit [99].

Gastric vs Post-pyloric Feeding: Equipment

The gastric vs post-pyloric routes differ in the type of equipment required and the ease tube of placement. Nasogastric (NG), or in sedated patient orogastric, tubes are readily placed into the stomach without imaging guidance. Placement can be confirmed by auscultating for air insufflation over the left upper quadrant and by aspiration of gastric-appearing contents. Depending on institutional policy and level of clinical concern, an X-ray may also be obtained to ensure the tube tip is below the diaphragm. A Salem-sump type tube is a common choice, as its larger bore facilitates the administration of crushed medications as well as feeds, while the air intake port combined with tube size allows suctioning of the stomach if decompression is needed (Fig. 36.2). Common sizes are 12–16 French.

Reaching the duodenum or jejunum, by contrast, often requires a longer tube that takes advantage of gut motility. The Dobhoff tube (Fig. 36.3) is thin (commonly 8–10 French) and flexible with a weighted metal tip, intended to help the GI tract mobilize it into the small intestine by peristalsis. The Tiger Tube (Cook Medical) is another option which has cilia-like projections that help it to be propelled by peristalsis. An X-ray or other imaging study is needed to confirm post-pyloric tube location. The fact that these tubes may take some time to pass beyond the stomach helps to explain why post-pyloric feeding has been associated with a delay in initiating enteral nutrition [95]. Bedside technology to help with post-pyloric tube placement, either with video-transmitting tube tips or electromagnetic guidance systems, is used in some institutions to improve speed and accuracy of post-pyloric tube placement.

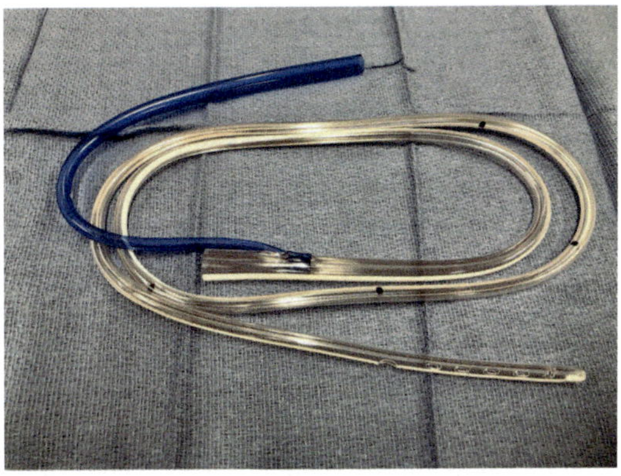

Fig. 36.2 Salem Sump NG tube: Note the multiple side holes, as well as the blue vent (air intake lumen), which allows air to be pulled through the system to reduce clogging

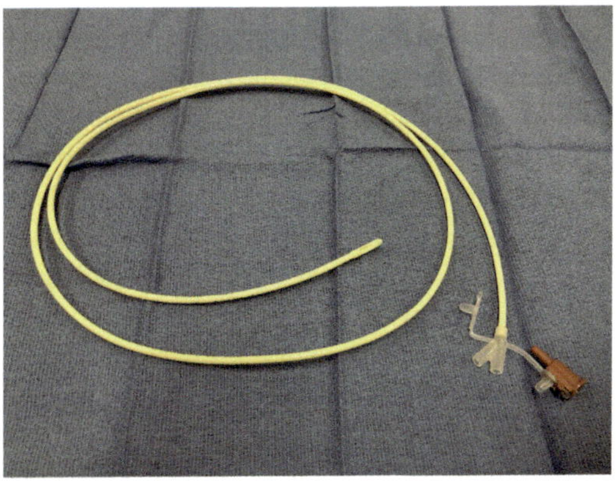

Fig. 36.3 Dobhoff post-pyloric feeding tube: Note the small caliber for patient comfort and the single feeding lumen

Complications of Feeding Tubes

All feeding tubes have the potential to cause complications. Intrapulmonary placement can occur due to the passage of the tube down the trachea rather than the esophagus. If not promptly recognized, this can result in bronchial perforation with pneumothorax or bronchopleural fistula, as well as intrathoracic or intrapulmonary administration of tube feeds, any of which may prove fatal [100, 101]. Life-threatening nasopharyngeal and pulmonary hemorrhages as a result of nasoenteral tube placement have also been observed [102]. Clinical signs of correct GI tract placement such as absence of coughing are not highly reliable, especially in an obtunded patient [103]. Given this, the use of an objective confirmatory test to improve patient safety is advisable. Options include capnography, in which absence of CO_2 detection confirms a non-pulmonary tube location, use of video-tipped tubes which allow visual confirmation GI mucosa rather than tracheal rings, and X-ray protocols such as that originally described by Roubenoff and Ravich [103, 104]. In this protocol, a tube is inserted only to 30 cm and a chest X-ray is taken. If this X-ray shows the tube in the midline of the thorax below the level of the carina (rather than tracking out along the right or left mainstem bronchus), then the tube is assumed to be intra-esophageal and is advanced to the desired depth at which point a second confirmatory X-ray can be taken. Otherwise, the tube is withdrawn and the process is restarted [104].

Parenteral

Parenteral nutrition (PN) is the provision of nutrients directly into the bloodstream, rather than via the GI tract. Developed in its modern form in the 1960s [105], it is potentially life-saving when the GI tract is non-functional.

Total parenteral nutrition (TPN) refers to meeting all nutrient requirements by vein, whereas partial parenteral nutrition (PPN) implies the intravenous nutrition is supplementary to another source of intake. Peripheral parenteral nutrition should be limited to <900 mOsm/L to prevent phlebitis [106]. Thus, central venous administration, where higher osmolarity is tolerated, is required to meet daily caloric needs without exceeding a patient's fluid needs by several-fold [105, 106].

PN Indications

With modern enhanced recovery after surgery (ERAS) pathways, indications for perioperative PN are highly selective, as most patients, including those undergoing GI surgery, can generally resume an oral diet within 1–3 days of operation [107]. Notable exceptions are surgical diseases in which GI continuity cannot be immediately restored, e.g., due to intestinal ischemia or high output intestinal fistula, or when there is persistent obstruction or prolonged post-op ileus.

In these cases, the baseline nutritional assessment and the expected time to regaining GI function should guide the timing of PN. ASPEN and ESPEN recommend that patients who are well-nourished before surgery should have PN started if they are unable to meet their needs enterally by 7–10 days post-op, and those with baseline malnutrition should be considered for earlier PN [108, 109].

PN Complications

The recommended delays in PN initiation when EN is not an option are intended to balance the risks of PN delivery against the risks of prolonged malnutrition. Central venous catheterization for infusion carries risks of vessel injury, thrombosis, and bloodstream infection. These risks can be mitigated through ultrasound-guided catheter placement and line insertion bundles that promote sterility. After line insertion, catheter site care and infusion set maintenance are critical to prolonging the infection-free life of the line [110].

Hyperglycemia is another potential PN complication, and is associated with both underlying physiologic stress and also with higher glucose infusion rates [111]. Avoidance of hyperglycemia exceeding 180 mg/dL has become a perioperative quality metric, as elevated blood glucose is associated with increased infections and longer length of stay [112]. PN-associated hyperglycemia can be mitigated by limiting the dextrose load to <150–200 g/day, and making use of subcutaneous or intravenous insulin protocols to treat hyperglycemia when it occurs [111].

Liver dysfunction may also occur with PN. Bypassing the alimentary tract is associated with cholestasis, oxidative stress, hepatocyte dysfunction, and liver fibrosis [113, 114]. The exact mechanisms for this are still being elucidated, but PN administration and the absence of gut stimulation result in disruption of the enterohepatic circulation triggering a number of hormonal, microbiome, and visceral hemodynamic changes which may contribute to the liver injury [115].

What Are the Barriers to Providing Enteral Nutrition in Emergency Surgery Patients?

There are multiple potential barriers to providing nutrition to emergency surgery patients, as summarized in Table 36.2 and discussed below.

Physiologic Barriers

Ileus

Paralytic ileus is a condition of disorganized or absent gut peristalsis that impairs normal movement of substrates through the GI tract. Although the mechanisms are not fully understood, ileus appears to arise from reactions to surgical stress and in particular to handling of the bowel. Initial surgical stress triggers an adrenergic response, which results in acute, intraoperative inhibition of peristalsis. This is further driven by neurohumoral signaling pathways via hypothalamic and pontine-medullary nuclei, promoting inhibitory vagal and sympathetic outflow to splanchnic and mesenteric nerves [116]. However, the more prolonged and clinically significant inhibition of GI function, lasting hours to days, appears to be an immune-mediated inflammatory response. Research shows that peritoneal mast cells become activated with manipulation of the bowel, and this in turn activates intestinal wall macrophages. A signaling cascade is initiated with the release of cytokines and chemokines, and an influx of leukocytes to the affected area occurs. This alone has been shown to reduce GI muscle reactivity to a stimulus in-vitro. It is thought that this inflammatory response further triggers neural inhibition of motility at both the location of the insult and also remote areas of the intestine [116].

Table 36.2 Common barriers to enteral feeding in emergency surgery patients

Barriers to feeding	Approaches to mitigation of barriers
NPO after midnight	NPO after midnight was never an evidence-based recommendation; it was largely a convenience for staff Current evidence and ASA guidelines support – NPO from clears for 2 h pre-op – NPO from solid foods for 6–8 h pre-op
Ileus	Ongoing ileus precludes enteral feeding The following may reduce ileus occurrence and duration – Avoid volume overload and bowel wall edema – Opiate-sparing analgesia – Early mobilization – Early PO intake as soon as the patient is not nauseated – NG only if vomiting or significant distention occur
Obstruction	Ongoing obstruction precludes enteral feeding Perform early assessment for resolution, by symptoms and/or water-soluble contrast study If obstruction persists, pursue early surgical correction of the obstruction (within 72 h of presentation)
Pancreatitis	The historical concern that enteral feeds may worsen the pancreatitis has been largely debunked Enteral feeding (versus parenteral nutrition) decreases infectious complications in pancreatitis With severe inflammation, duodenal obstruction may occur; passage of a distal feeding tube may allow enteral feeding to continue
Enteroatmospheric fistula	Adequate pouching and skin protection systems are a prerequisite for enteral nutrition With good skin protection, most patients can be partially or fully supported with enteral nutrition Localization of the fistula within the GI tract can facilitate feeding of the longest intact segment

(continued)

Table 36.2 (continued)

Barriers to feeding	Approaches to mitigation of barriers
Hemodynamic instability	Tube-feed induced intestinal ischemia is extremely rare Even for patients on pressors, enteral feeding has been shown to enhance intestinal blood flow Feeding should be attempted in most patients on stable or decreasing doses of vasopressors Hemodynamic thresholds beyond which enteral feeding should be avoided have not been defined
Perceived intolerance due to elevated gastric residual volume	Monitoring gastric residual volumes (GRV) and withholding feeds for elevated GRV have not been shown to reduce pneumonia Withholding feeds based on GRV alone may prevent patients from meeting their enteral nutrition goals without benefit. There is no need to monitor GRV routinely
Sentiment that nutrition is not as important as the patient's other active problems	Adequate nutrition is critical to homeostasis and recovery from stress Daily checklists and involvement of dieticians may both help to ensure feeding is not forgotten Providing nutrition is a relatively easy way to improve patient outcome—it is an opportunity that should not be overlooked

Ileus may occur from non-mechanical physiologic disruptions as well, such as critical illness, opiate administration, and non-GI surgery. Ogilvie's syndrome, also known as acute colonic pseudo-obstruction, is one well-known form of this.

Lack of gut motility effectively precludes adequate enteral intake, and attempts to eat will usually result in nausea, bloating, and emesis. Thus, the prevention and treatment of post-operative ileus has been the subject of much investigation. Enhanced Recovery After Surgery (ERAS) programs have shown significant promise in reducing ileus duration, through a multi-modal strategy of judicious IV fluid administration which may decrease bowel wall edema, narcotic-sparing pain regimens to minimize the anti-motility complications of opiates, early oral intake, and early mobilization [117]. Typical post-op ileus is thought to last about 24 h for small intestine, 1–2 days for the stomach, and 1–3 days for the colon. However, the widespread success of ERAS programs suggests that most patients can self-regulate, and that allowing oral intake as long as the patient is not nauseated results in faster recovery than does withholding oral intake until more objective measures of GI function such as flatus or a bowel movement occur [118]. When ileus does occur, supportive care and reversal of any underlying physiologic derangements are the mainstays of treatment. In cases of vomiting, placement of a nasogastric tube should be considered to reduce the likelihood of aspiration. Depending on the patient's pre-operative nutritional status, parenteral nutrition support may be needed if the ileus last longer than 5–7 days.

Obstruction

Bowel obstruction is a common condition managed by general surgeons. Obstructions involving a closed loop or bowel ischemia require urgent surgical management as discussed elsewhere in this text. Excluding these surgical emergencies, the key to bowel obstructions from a nutritional standpoint is to differentiate those that will be self-resolving from those that will not, and for the latter category, to operate within 48–72 h, before the patient becomes significantly nutritionally compromised. A water-soluble contrast challenge is helpful in making this distinction. Multiple institutional protocols exist, but in essence oral contrast is administered by mouth or by NG tube, and its progress is followed with serial abdominal radiographs every 4–8 h until 24 h after contrast consumption. Visualization of contrast in the colon by 24 h has shown specificity of up to 98% for resolution of the obstruction non-operatively [119]. Patients that fail to pass contrast through to the colon in this time frame should be strongly considered for operative management.

A special form of complete obstruction that may occur in emergency surgery patients is GI tract discontinuity. The benefits of damage control surgery for critically ill patients have been recognized in recent years [120, 121], and accordingly patients may undergo resection of one or more segments of intestine, but remain too unstable for GI continuity to be re-established at the initial operation. Questionable viability of bowel, as may occur with mesenteric ischemia, may also render anastomosis at the index operation unsafe. Thus, patients may transition to the ICU with their GI tract blind-ending at one or more points, and an open abdomen, for ongoing resuscitation. It is important that all parties caring for these patients are aware of the GI discontinuity, and that enteral feeds are not given. NG or OG decompression should be continued to reduce distention and the risk of perforation. As with other forms of obstruction, relieving the "blockage" by re-establishing GI continuity (via anastomosis or ostomy formation) should be done as soon as possible, and enteral feeds can be considered thereafter.

Pancreatitis

Concerns about pancreatic exocrine stimulation, and therefore worsening pancreatic inflammation, historically limited the use of enteral nutrition in pancreatitis. More recent literature, however, has shown this to be unfounded. A 2008 systematic review showed significantly reduced mortality with any (enteral or parenteral) nutritional support vs no nutrition in pancreatitis. Further, the same review found a 60% reduction in infectious complications with the use of enteral versus parental nutrition, with no statistically significant mortality difference [122]. The decrease in infections may be mediated by enhanced gut mucosal immunity with enteral nutrition, as well as avoidance of infections associated with the central venous access required for parenteral nutrition.

Gastric feeding has been shown to be safe in pancreatitis [122], and there is no need for routine post-pyloric feeding. However, severe peripancreatic inflammation may result in mechanical duodenal obstruction and therefore intolerance to oral and gastric feeding. In such cases, continuation of enteral nutrition can be achieved by passage of small bore tube beyond the area of obstruction, in conjunction with nasogastric decompression.

Enteroatmospheric Fistula

Enteroatmospheric (or enterocutaneous) fistulae present a complex set of problems requiring multidisciplinary management, and adequacy of nutritional support is one of the key drivers of a good outcome [123]. Fistulas are routinely classified as high (>500 mL/day) or low (<500 mL/day) output. Low output fistulas are easier to manage in terms of pouching and skin protection, and their lesser fluid and electrolyte losses are better tolerated by patients. Output quantity depends largely on fistula location within the GI tract, type and quantity of enteral intake, and response to pharmacologic measures such as octreotide and antidiarrheals. While most patients with enteroatmospheric (EA) fistula require a period of parenteral nutrition early in their course, adequate resuscitation, infectious source control, mapping of fistula anatomy, and functioning wound management systems allow the majority of patients to be transitioned partially or fully to EN [123, 124]. With eating, fistula effluent tends to increase somewhat, so adequate skin protection and attention to electrolyte and volume status are crucial.

Means to localize the fistula within the GI tract include assessment of output quality, fistulograms, small bowel fluoroscopy, and CT scan. Defining the anatomy facilitates the utilization of the longest intact segment for EN. This may be achieved through an oral diet, or via tube access to the distal fistula limb for infusion of feeds. Re-feeding of proximal effluent into the distal limb is also an option, and may be particularly helpful in mitigating dehydration and electrolyte derangements if the output is high, or in supporting a patient in an environment where PN is not an option [123].

Hemodynamic Instability

Hemodynamically unstable patients supported with vasopressors may present a conundrum, given concerns that feeding will increase GI tract oxygen demand and potentially precipitate bowel ischemia, particularly when other end-organ perfusion is already compromised. Bowel ischemia as a result of enteral nutrition is extremely rare, with large case series placing the incidence at around 0.2% for gastric feeds, and 0.3–3.8% for small bowel feeds [125]. EN has been shown to actually increase intestinal blood flow, even in most hemodynamically unstable patients [125, 126]. In a large, propensity-matched retrospective review of patients requiring vasopressor support, early (within 48 h of intubation) initiation of EN was associated with significantly lower ICU mortality (22.5% vs 28.3%) than delayed EN, and the benefit was more pronounced in the sickest patients requiring multiple pressors [126]. Despite numerous investigations [127], the question of how much pressor is "too much" to safely initiate enteral feeds remains unanswered. Further, the question of safety for EN is likely more nuanced than defining a single dose number, and depends on patient comorbidities, underlying disease process, and the adequacy of volume resuscitation. 2016 ASPEN guidelines recommend delaying EN until patients are well-resuscitated and on a stable or decreasing dose of vasopressors [59]. If clear signs of intolerance such as significant bloating, pain, or emesis occur, the feeds will need to be stopped until symptoms subside.

Damage Control Laparotomy and the Open Abdomen

The concept of damage control laparotomy originated in trauma, but its use has expanded to the emergency general surgery population. Its principles are immediate control of hemorrhage and contamination, with delay of definitive reconstructions until the patient's physiology is stabilized by further resuscitation and time. The duration of the index operation is minimized, to avoid unnecessary blood loss and hypothermia and their downstream effects. This generally results in leaving the abdomen open with a temporary dressing, and returning to the OR in 24–48 h for a repeat operation for definitive management [121].

Despite instinctive concerns about feeding patients with an open abdomen, the indications and contraindications for enteral nutrition should be no different from those for other surgical patients. Acute GI discontinuity, as discussed above, is a contraindication to feeding, and the proximal segment should remain decompressed with NG or OG suction. Hemodynamic instability may be present in patients requiring damage control surgery, and high-dose pressors are an indication for caution around enteral feeds as previously discussed. Baring these concerns, the bulk of evidence shows that providing enteral nutrition to patients with an open abdomen is safe, and may even decrease infectious complications [128–130]. In open-abdomen patients with sepsis and enterocutaneous fistulae, enteral feeds are associated with improved rates of abdominal closure and decreased mortality [131].

Cultural and Logistical Barriers

The Dogma of "NPO After Midnight"

The notion of "nil per os" or NPO after midnight prior to surgery (regardless of the time of day of the procedure) had been a standard from the 1960s until quite recently [132], and is still the default in many hospital order sets. In acute surgical patients who may require serial operations, procedures, and episodes of sedation or general anesthesia, however, adherence to this tradition can result in accrual of a significant calorie deficit [133]. Further, substantial evidence supports the safety of the intake of solid foods until 6–8 h prior to anesthesia, and of clear liquids until just 2 h prior [134–140]. Indeed, since the early 2000s, this has been the guideline recommendation of the American Society of Anesthesiologists (ASA) for patients undergoing elective surgery [141, 142]. Further, a carbohydrate drink shortly before surgery is an established component of many ERAS protocols [143].

There are multiple ways to mitigate practices of excessive perioperative fasting. In outpatients with planned surgery, ASA guideline-based instructions are usually given. For hospitalized patients well enough for oral intake, orders may simply be changed to permit eating and drinking until closer to the procedure. This would be facilitated by graded pre-operative diet orders, allowing providers to specify the expected procedure time, and the associated times for ceasing solid and liquid intake accordingly. However, such order sets are not widely in use, so "NPO after midnight" may become a convenient but unfortunate default. In the critically ill and tube-fed population, volume-based feeding protocols have shown significant promise. The essence of these protocols is that a target volume of feeding formula is determined for an entire 24 h period, and the hourly rate is then adjusted dynamically to deliver that target volume despite potential interruptions. This results in meeting a greater percentage of caloric needs, without observed ill effects [99, 100, 144, 145].

Many centers treat intubated or post-pylorically fed patients differently in terms of anesthetic aspiration risk, and may feed up to and even through surgery [146–149]. However, no national guideline or consensus yet exits on which patients, with which types of feeding tubes and airways in place, may routinely forgo any preoperative fast.

Nutrition Is "Less Important" Than Other Issues in the Acutely Ill Patient

For the reasons outlined earlier in this chapter, nutrition plays a major role in healing and patient outcomes. As such, steps should be taken to ensure nutrition is not overlooked among the multitude of other issues that may need to be addressed. Daily checklists that include nutrition, and team-based rounding involving dietitians are both helpful.

How Do I Calculate TPN?

In the inpatient setting, TPN prescriptions are often calculated by a dedicated nutrition support team. However, the core concepts for prescribing TPN should be familiar to providers. TPN is composed of a combination of the three macronutrients—carbohydrates (dextrose), fat (generally as a soy bean or olive oil emulsion), and protein (delivered as an amino acid emulsion), plus electrolyte, trace mineral additives, and enough fluid to dilute the components and meet volume needs. A safe and appropriate adult TPN prescription can be arrived at using the following steps [109, 150]. A 70 kg patient with moderately severe illness is used as an example.

1. Calculate non-nitrogen energy needs as 20–30 kcal/kg/day. Higher energy requirements are appropriate for those with baseline malnutrition or severe systemic illness. Ex:

   70 kg × 25 kcal/kg/day = 1750 kcal/day

2. Divide the non-nitrogen energy requirement between carbohydrate (dextrose) and fat, to calculate the number of dextrose and lipid grams needed in 24 h. Either a 70/30 or 60/40 dextrose/lipid split is acceptable. Dextrose contains 3.4 kcal/g, and lipid contains 9 kcal/g. Ex:

   - $$\mathit{Dextrose}: 1750\ \text{kcal} \times 0.7 \times \frac{1\ \text{g}}{3.4\ \text{kcal}} = \mathbf{360\ g\ dextrose}$$

   - $$\mathit{Lipid}: 1750\ \text{kcal} \times 0.3 \times \frac{1\ \text{g}}{9\ \text{kcal}} = \mathbf{58\ g\ lipid}$$

3. Calculate the protein requirements as 1–2.5 g/kg/day. Patients with more severe illness and stress requiring more protein. Ex:

   70 kg × 1.5 g/day = **105 g protein**
4. Utilizing standard electrolyte and trace mineral additives is reasonable, unless there is a known deficiency or excess. Twenty-four-hour requirements include sodium and potassium (1–2 mEq/kg), calcium (10–15 mEq), magnesium (8–20 mEq), phosphorus (20–40 mmol), and chloride or acetate as needed to electrically balance the cations. Trace minerals may include B vitamins, folic acid, biotin, and vitamins C, A, D, E, and K. Many order sets have these additives pre-populated, but they may be changed as needed.
5. Calculate the minimum fluid volume needed to deliver the nutrients. The exact minimum is dictated by the concentrations of the off-the-shelf components used. Dextrose is usually provided as D50 (0.5 g/mL), whereas amino acids are generally provided as a 10–15% solution (0.1–0.15 g/mL). Lipids are commonly provided as a 20% solution, or 0.2 g/mL. Therefore:

   - $$\mathit{Dextrose}: 360\ \text{g} \times \frac{1\ \text{mL}}{0.5\ \text{g}} = 720\ \text{mL}$$

- *Lipid*: $58\ \text{g} \times \frac{1\ \text{mL}}{0.2\ \text{g}} = 290\ \text{mL}$
- *Protein*: $105\ \text{g} \times \frac{1\ \text{mL}}{0.15\ \text{g}} = 700\ \text{mL}$
- *Total minimum volume*: 720 mL + 290 mL + 700 mL = **1710 mL**

6. Calculate the TPN rate in mL/h from the total volume. Ex:
   1710 mL ÷ 24 h = 71.25 mL/h
   Additional volume may always be added, depending on the patient's fluid needs. In this case, we may wish to simply round the hourly rate to 75 mL/h, for a total daily volume of **1800 mL**.
7. Combine the above into a single TPN prescription. Ex:
   360 g dextrose, 58 g lipid, 105 g protein with standard additives in a total volume of 1800 mL, to be run at 75 mL/h over 24 h.

Micronutrients and Immunonutrition

Micronutrients

Whereas macronutrients include the major categories of energy-containing molecules—carbohydrates, fats, and proteins—the term micronutrients refers to the trace minerals and vitamins that are required to maintain normal cellular function. Complete tables of estimated daily needs of such nutrients are widely available [151]. Here, we will discuss several that are particularly critical to wound healing and recovery in surgical patients.

Vitamin C

Vitamin C is a necessary cofactor for the hydroxylation of proline during collagen synthesis. Thus, it plays a critical function in wound healing, and its deficiency results in the soft tissue disorder scurvy [152]. Vitamin C acts in numerous other metabolic pathways, with mounting evidence demonstrating its role as an antioxidant for free radical scavenging, a cofactor for catecholamine and steroid synthesis, and a factor which improves endothelial barrier function and leukocyte phagocytosis [153]. Supra physiologic Vitamin C supplementation (e.g., 50–200 mg/kg IV/day, as opposed to the USDA recommended daily value of 75–90 mg/day for adults [151]) is an area of active investigation, with animal models suggesting benefit in reducing fluid resuscitation needs in burn injury and reducing end-organ dysfunction in hemorrhagic shock. Small-scale human studies have also shown promise for improved outcomes in sepsis [154, 155]. Vitamin C deficiency should be avoided in the emergency general surgery population, although in those without a clinical deficiency, the optimal dose and indication for vitamin C supplementation is still unknown.

Vitamin A

Vitamin A also has diverse physiologic roles, including in fetal development, growth and cell differentiation, vision and immune function, in addition to its crucial in wound healing [156]. Vitamin A promotes collagen cross-linking, and also increases the robustness of the inflammatory phase of wound healing by accentuating chemotaxis of phagocytes [152]. Of particular significance for surgical patients, high-dose vitamin A largely reverses the inhibitory effects of steroids on wound healing [152, 156]. For mitigation of steroid effects, administration of 15,000–20,000 international units of vitamin A orally for 2–3 weeks has been recommended [157].

Zinc

Zinc is a mineral needed in small amounts (8–10 mg/day) which acts in numerous pathways including phagocyte function, keratinocyte migration, and wound auto-debridement via zinc-dependent matrix metal-loproteases [152, 158]. It has gained particular attention for its role in wound healing. True zinc deficiency can be challenging to diagnose, as serum levels fluctuate with meals and circadian rhythm, and blood levels may also be maintained in a normal range despite tissue deficiencies [159]. Clinical signs of deficiency include anorexia, diarrhea, ataxia, hair loss, dermatitis, depression, and delayed wound healing [158]. Zinc is primarily absorbed in the duodenum and proximal jejunum, and thus may be deficient in patients who have undergone removal or bypass of these regions of the GI tract. Studies of oral zinc supplementation, in the absence of overt deficiency, have failed to consistently demonstrate any benefit to wound healing [158, 159].

Topical zinc preparations, however, including in Unna boots for venous stasis ulcers and zinc oxide creams, are frequently used for chronic wounds and have repeatedly shown benefit in reducing time to wound closure. The antimicrobial properties of topical zinc may contribute to this benefit [158].

Selenium

Although less rigorously investigated to date than the above nutrients, selenium has a plausible role in tissue healing via its antioxidant effects. Animal studies have suggested a benefit to wound healing with selenium supplementation [160, 161], and a small human randomized controlled trial of parenteral supplementation of selenium combined with zinc and copper found benefit in time to wound closure and reduction of infections [162].

Immunonutrition

Immunonutrition can be defined as the targeted supplementation of specific nutrients in greater than normal dietary quantities, with the goal of improving immune system function and clinical outcomes. This may occur at the level of gut mucosal barrier function, cellular defense, or the local and systemic inflammatory response [163]. Although the micronutrients discussed above each may play a regulatory role in the immune response, several amino acids and fatty acids have been specifically investigated for their immune-modulating properties in recent decades. Below we provide a brief overview of these key nutrients, followed by a discussion of the evidence.

Glutamine

Glutamine is a conditionally essential amino acid during physiologic stress [164]. It serves as a key source of fuel for rapidly dividing cells, including enterocytes and leukocytes. This has contributed to enthusiasm for its supplementation in critical illness, when the catabolic stress response may deplete glutamine stores, resulting in a weakened immunocyte response and impaired gut mucosal barrier function [165].

Arginine

Arginine is another conditionally essential amino acid during stress. It is required for proline formation for collagen synthesis, as well as normal B-cell, T-cell, and macrophage function. It can be metabolized to nitric oxide to mediate blood flow and vascular tone. It also plays a role in metabolic homeostasis by stimulating the release of growth hormone, glucagon, and insulin [164].

Omega-3 Polyunsaturated Fatty Acids

Omega-3 polyunsaturated fatty acids, particularly eicosapentaenoic acid (EPA) and docosahexaenoic acid (DHA), have anti-inflammatory properties. Adequate intake of omega-3s may suppress the production of the more inflammatory omega-6 fatty acid arachidonic acid, which is the precursor for multiple immune mediators including prostaglandins, leukotrienes, and thromboxanes [164]. Increasing omega-3 levels can shift the ratio of omega-3 to omega-6 fatty acids in cell membranes toward omega-3, thereby reducing cell responsiveness to pro-inflammatory stimuli. Omega-3s have also been shown to modulate leukocyte adhesion and chemotaxis through the down-regulation of E-selectin and other intercellular adhesion molecules [59, 165, 166]. Omega-3 intake may also synergistically improve arginine availability, through increased delivery and decreased degradation [164]. Limited evidence suggests adults require 2 g/day of omega-3 fatty acids to realize these immune benefits [166].

Nucleotides

Nucleotides, the building blocks of DNA and RNA, are also considered conditionally essential in times of rapid cell proliferation [165]. In particular, inadequate intake of nucleotides has been shown to impair the function of T-cells and natural killer cells, reduce gut mucosal integrity, and suppress lymphocyte proliferation [163]. While there are normal dietary sources of nucleotides [167], these compounds are generally lacking in standard tube feed formulas [164], which has led to a market for nucleotide-supplemented formulations.

Evidence for Immunonutrition

A key limitation in interpreting the literature on immunonutrition is the significant heterogeneity of trials, both in terms of study population and also in terms of the varied doses and combinations of nutrients utilized. Data to clearly delineate the effects and therapeutic dose of individual nutrients remains lacking [164, 165]. Nevertheless, individual studies and meta-analyses have consistently suggested a benefit to immunonutrition in infection reduction for elective and emergency surgery patients, SICU populations, and those with significant trauma or burns [59]. These benefits were found in studies examining combination supplementation with omega-3 fatty acids and arginine [168–170], and the effects were more pronounced when supplementation was started pre-operatively [170]. No reductions in mortality were seen, however. ASPEN/SCCM 2016 guidelines support the use of fatty-acid and arginine supplemented formulas for SICU and post-operative patients requiring enteral nutrition support [59]. Routine glutamine supplementation is no longer recommended due to a lack of clear benefit [59, 165], and no immunonutrition is routinely recommended for mixed ICU or MICU populations [59].

Summary

Adequate nutrient intake is key to maintaining homeostasis and allowing optimal recovery from surgical stress. Assessment of baseline nutritional status and ongoing protein and energy needs facilitates adequate feeding. However, it is important to note that historically relied-upon hepatic proteins may reflect systemic inflammation more than nutritional state.

Despite the many potential barriers to feeding in emergency general surgery patients, current evidence supports the safety and superiority of early post-operative enteral feeding, unless there are clear contraindications such as GI discontinuity. Parenteral nutrition can be used when enteral feeding is not possible. Adequate protein intake is key, and patients tolerate a total calorie deficit with adequate protein much better than a combined protein-calorie deficit. Supplementation of specific micronutrients or "immunonutrients" may improve wound healing and reduce infections, particularly in high-risk populations.

In summary, when in doubt—consider feeding the patient.

References

1. McClave SA. Drivers of oxidative stress in acute pancreatitis: the role of nutrition therapy. J Parenter Enter Nutr. 2012;36(1):24–35.
2. Azizi F, Rahmani M, Emami H, Mirmiran P, Hajipour R, Madjid M, Ghanbili J, Ghanbarian A, Mehrabi J, Saadat N, et al. Cardiovascular risk factors in an iranian urban population: Tehran lipid and glucose study (phase 1). Soz Praventivmed. 2002;47(6):408–26.
3. Ekmekcioglu C. Nutrition and longevity—from mechanisms to uncertainties. Crit Rev Food Sci Nutr. 2019:1–20. https://doi.org/10.1080/10408398.2019.1676698.
4. Childs CE, Calder PC, Miles EA. Diet and immune function. Basel: MDPI; 2019.
5. Pham NV, Cox-Reijven PLM, Greve JW, Soeters PB. Application of subjective global assessment as a screening tool for malnutrition in surgical patients in Vietnam. Clin Nutr. 2006;25(1):102–8.
6. Hulsewe KWE, van Acker BAC, von Meyenfeldt MF, Soeters PB. Nutritional depletion and dietary manipulation: effects on the immune response. World J Surg. 1999;23(6):536–44.
7. Schneider SM, Veyres P, Pivot X, Soummer A-M, Jambou P, Filippi J, van Obberghen E, Hebuterne X. Malnutrition is an independent factor associated with nosocomial infections. Br J Nutr. 2004;92(1):105–11.
8. Rubinson L, Diette GB, Song X, Brower RG, Krishnan JA. Low caloric intake is associated with nosocomial bloodstream infections in patients in the medical intensive care unit. Crit Care Med. 2004;32(2):350–7.
9. Dhaliwal R, Heyland DK. Nutrition and infection in the intensive care unit: what does the evidence show? Curr Opin Crit Care. 2005;11(5):461–7.

10. Villet S, Chiolero RL, Bollmann MD, Revelly J-P, Cayeux R N M-C, Delarue J, Berger MM. Negative impact of hypocaloric feeding and energy balance on clinical outcome in ICU patients. Clin Nutr. 2005;24(4):502–9.
11. Eachempati SR, Hydo LJ, Barie PS. Factors influencing the development of decubitus ulcers in critically ill surgical patients. Crit Care Med. 2001;29(9):1678–82.
12. Haydock DA, Hill GL. Impaired wound healing in surgical patients with varying degrees of malnutrition. J Parenter Enter Nutr. 1986;10(6):550–4.
13. Lennmarken C, Larsson J. Skeletal muscle function and energy metabolites in malnourished surgical patients. Acta Chir Scand. 1986;152:169–73.
14. Braga M, Gianotti L, Nespoli L, Radaelli G, Di Carlo V. Nutritional approach in malnourished surgical patients: a prospective randomized study. Arch Surg. 2002;137(2):174–80.
15. Havens JM, Columbus AB, Seshadri AJ, Olufajo OA, Mogensen KM, Rawn JD, Salim A, Christopher KB. Malnutrition at intensive care unit admission predicts mortality in emergency general surgery patients. J Parenter Enter Nutr. 2018;42(1):156–63.
16. Havens JM, Olufajo O, Mogensen KM, Rawn JD, Salim A, Christopher KB. Emergency general surgery, malnutrition and outcomes in critical illness. Intensive Care Med Exp. 2015;3(1):1–2.
17. Patel V, Romano M, Corkins MR, DiMaria-Ghalili RA, Earthman C, Malone A, Miller S, Sabino K, Wooley J, Guenter P, et al. Nutrition screening and assessment in hospitalized patients: a survey of current practice in the united states. Nutr Clin Pract. 2014;29(4):483–90.
18. Kudsk KA, Reddy SK, Sacks GS, Lai H-C. Joint commission for accreditation of health care organizations guidelines: too late to intervene for nutritionally at-risk surgical patients. J Parenter Enter Nutr. 2003;27(4):288–90.
19. Nevill AM, Stewart AD, Olds T, Holder R. Relationship between adiposity and body size reveals limitations of BMI. Am J Phys Anthropol. 2006;129(1):151–6. eprint: https://onlinelibrary.wiley.com/doi/pdf/10.1002/ajpa.20262.
20. Detsky AS, McLaughlin JR, Baker JP, Johnston N, Whittaker S, Mendelson RA, Jeejeebhoy KN. What is subjective global assessment of nutritional status? JPEN J Parenter Enter Nutr. 1987;11(1):8–13.
21. Detsky AS, Baker JP, Mendelson RA, Wolman SL, Wesson DE, Jeejeebhoy KN. Evaluating the accuracy of nutritional assessment techniques applied to hospitalized patients: methodology and comparisons. JPEN J Parenter Enter Nutr. 1984;8(2):153–9.
22. Baker JP, Detsky AS, Whitwell J, Langer B, Jeejeebhoy KN. A comparison of the predictive value of nutritional assessment techniques. Hum Nutr Clin Nutr. 1982;36(3):233–41.
23. Baker JP, Detsky AS, Wesson DE, Wolman SL, Stewart S, Whitewell J, Langer B, Jeejeebhoy KN. Nutritional assessment: a comparison of clinical judgement and objective measurements. N Engl J Med. 1982;306(16):969–72.
24. Persson MD, Brismar KE, Katzarski KS, Nordenström J, Cederholm TE. Nutritional status using mini nutritional assessment and subjective global assessment predict mortality in geriatric patients. J Am Geriatr Soc. 2002;50(12):1996–2002.
25. Reber E, Gomes F, Vasiloglou MF, Schuetz P, Stanga Z. Nutritional risk screening and assessment. J Clin Med. 2019;8(7):1065.
26. Levitt DG, Levitt MD. Human serum albumin homeostasis: a new look at the roles of synthesis, catabolism, renal and gastrointestinal excretion, and the clinical value of serum albumin measurements. Int J Gen Med. 2016;9:229.
27. Chojkier M. Inhibition of albumin synthesis in chronic diseases: molecular mechanisms. J Clin Gastroenterol. 2005;39(4):S143–6.
28. Friedman AN, Fadem SZ. Reassessment of albumin as a nutritional marker in kidney disease. JASN. 2010;21(2):223–30.
29. Keys A, Brozek J, Henschel A, Mickelsen O, Taylor HL. The biology of human starvation. Minneapolis, MN: Minnesota Press; 1950.
30. Lee JL, Oh ES, Lee RW, Finucane TE. Serum albumin and pre-albumin in calorically restricted, nondiseased individuals: a systematic review. Am J Med. 2015;128(9):1023.e1–22.
31. Carlson DE, Cioffi WG, Mason AD, McManus WF, Pruitt BA. Evaluation of serum visceral protein levels as indicators of nitrogen balance in thermally injured patients. JPEN J Parenter Enter Nutr. 1991;15(4):440–4.
32. Gray GE, Meguid MM. Can total parenteral nutrition reverse hypoalbuminemia in oncology patients? Nutrition. 1990;6(3):225–8.
33. Gibbs J, Cull W, Henderson W, Daley J, Hur K, Khuri SF. Preoperative serum albumin level as a predictor of operative mortality and morbidity: results from the National VA Surgical Risk Study. Arch Surg. 1999;134(1):36–42.
34. Testini M, Margari A, Amoruso M, Lissidini G, Bonomo GM. The dehiscence of colorectal anastomoses: the risk factors. Ann Ital Chir. 2000;71(4):433–40.
35. Delgado-Rodríguez M, Medina-Cuadros M, Gómez-Ortega A, Martínez-Gallego G, Mariscal-Ortiz M, Martinez-Gonzalez MA, Sillero-Arenas M. Cholesterol and serum albumin levels as predictors of cross infection, death, and length of hospital stay. Arch Surg. 2002;137(7):805–12.
36. Detsky AS, Baker JP, O'Rourke K, Johnston N, Whitwell J, Mendelson RA, Jeejeebhoy KN. Predicting nutrition-associated complications for patients undergoing gastrointestinal surgery. J Parenter Enter Nutr. 1987;11(5):440–6.
37. Fulks M, Stout RL, Dolan VF. Albumin and all-cause mortality risk in insurance applicants. J Insur Med. 2010;42(1):11–7.

38. Malafarina V, Uriz-Otano F, Iniesta R, Gil-Guerrero L. Sarcopenia in the elderly: diagnosis, physiopathology and treatment. Maturitas. 2012;71(2):109–14.
39. Bartalena L, Piantanida E. Serum thyroid hormone-binding proteins. In: Huhtaniemi I, Martini L, editors. Encyclopedia of endocrine diseases. 2nd ed. Oxford: Academic Press; 2019. p. 442–7.
40. Ingenbleek Y, De Visscher M, De Nayer P. Measurement of prealbumin as index of protein-calorie malnutrition. Lancet. 1972;2(7768):106–9.
41. Boosalis MG, Ott L, Levine AS, Slag MF, Morley JE, Young B, McClain CJ. Relationship of visceral proteins to nutritional status in chronic and acute stress. Crit Care Med. 1989;17(8):741–7.
42. Mackenzie TA, Clark NG, Bistrian BR, Flatt JP, Hallowell EM, Blackburn GL. A simple method for estimating nitrogen balance in hospitalized patients: a review and supporting data for a previously proposed technique. J Am Coll Nutr. 1985;4(5):575–81.
43. Mariotti F, Tomé D, Mirand PP. Converting nitrogen into protein—beyond 6.25 and jones' factors. Crit Rev Food Sci Nutr. 2008;48(2):177–84.
44. Dickerson RN. Nitrogen balance and protein requirements for critically ill older patients. Nutrients. 2016;8(4):226.
45. Tomé D, Bos C. Dietary protein and nitrogen utilization. J Nutr. 2000;130(7):1868S–73S.
46. Cerra FB, Lehmann S, Konstantinides N, Dzik J, Fish J, Konstantinides F, LiCari JJ, Holman RT. Improvement in immune function in ICU patients by enteral nutrition supplemented with arginine, RNA, and menhaden oil is independent of nitrogen balance. Nutrition. 1991;7(3):193–9.
47. Danielis M, Lorenzoni G, Azzolina D, Iacobucci A, Trombini O, De Monte A, Gregori D, Beltrame F. Effect of protein-fortified diet on nitrogen balance in critically ill patients: results from the OPINiB trial. Nutrients. 2019;11(5):972.
48. Singer P. High-dose amino acid infusion preserves diuresis and improves nitrogen balance in non-oliguric acute renal failure. Wien Klin Wochenschr. 2007;119(7):218–22.
49. Felicetti-Lordani CR, Eckert RG, Valério NMP, Lordani TVA, Jorge AC, Duarte PAD. Nitrogen balance in nutritional monitoring of critically ill adult patients: a prospective observational study. Yŏgun Bakım Derg. 2017;8(3):59–64.
50. Badjatia N, Monahan A, Carpenter A, Zimmerman J, Schmidt JM, Claassen J, Connolly ES, Mayer SA, Karmally W, Seres D. Inflammation, negative nitrogen balance, and outcome after aneurysmal subarachnoid hemorrhage. Neurology. 2015;84(7):680.
51. Mancusi-Ungaro HR, Van Way CW, McCool C. Caloric and nitrogen balances as predictors of nutritional outcome in patients with burns. J Burn Care Rehabil. 1992;13(6):695–702.
52. Salame C, Eaton S, Grimble G, Davenport A. Protein losses and urea nitrogen underestimate total nitrogen losses in peritoneal dialysis and hemodialysis patients. J Ren Nutr. 2018;28(5):317–23.
53. Cheatham ML, Safcsak K, Brzezinski SJ, Lube MW. Nitrogen balance, protein loss, and the open abdomen. Crit Care Med. 2007;35(1):127–31.
54. Parker EA, Feinberg TM, Wappel S, Verceles AC. Considerations when using predictive equations to estimate energy needs among older, hospitalized patients: a narrative review. Curr Nutr Rep. 2017;6(2):102–10.
55. Kenny GP, Notley SR, Gagnon D. Direct calorimetry: a brief historical review of its use in the study of human metabolism and thermoregulation. Eur J Appl Physiol. 2017;117(9):1765–85.
56. Mtaweh H, Tuira L, Floh AA, Parshuram CS. Indirect calorimetry: history, technology, and application. Front Pediatr. 2018;6:257.
57. Weir JBDV. New methods for calculating metabolic rate with special reference to protein metabolism. J Physiol. 1949;109(1–2):1–9.
58. Singer P, Blaser AR, Berger MM, Alhazzani W, Calder PC, Casaer MP, Hiesmayr M, Mayer K, Montejo JC, Pichard C, et al. Espen guideline on clinical nutrition in the intensive care unit. Clin Nutr. 2019;38(1):48–79.
59. McClave SA, Taylor BE, Martindale RG, Warren MM, Johnson DR, Braunschweig C, McCarthy MS, Davanos E, Rice TW, Cresci GA, Gervasio JM, Sacks GS, Roberts PR, Compher C, Society of Critical Care Medicine, American Society for Parenteral and Enteral Nutrition. Guidelines for the provision and assessment of nutrition support therapy in the adult critically ill patient: Society of Critical Care Medicine (SCCM) and American Society for Parenteral and Enteral Nutrition (A.S.P.E.N.). JPEN J Parenter Enter Nutr. 2016;40(2):159–211.
60. Arthur Harris J, Benedict FG. A biometric study of human basal metabolism. Proc Natl Acad Sci U S A. 1918;4(12):370–3.
61. Roza AM, Shizgal HM. The Harris benedict equation reevaluated: resting energy requirements and the body cell mass. Am J Clin Nutr. 1984;40(1):168–82.
62. Barak N, Wall-Alonso E, Sitrin MD. Evaluation of stress factors and body weight adjustments currently used to estimate energy expenditure in hospitalized patients. J Parenter Enter Nutr. 2002;26(4):231–8.
63. MacDonald A, Hildebrandt L. Comparison of formulaic equations to determine energy expenditure in the critically ill patient. Nutrition. 2003;19(3):233–9.
64. Tah PC, Lee Z-Y, Poh BK, Majid HA, Hakumat-Rai V-R, Nor MBM, Kee CC, Zaman MK, Hasan MS. A single-center prospective observational study comparing resting energy expenditure in different phases of critical illness: Indirect calorimetry versus predictive equations. Crit Care Med. 2020;48(5):e380–90.
65. Mifflin MD, St Jeor ST, Hill LA, Scott BJ, Daugherty SA, Koh YO. A new predictive equation for resting energy expenditure in healthy individuals. Am J Clin Nutr. 1990;51(2):241–7.
66. Swinamer DL, Grace MG, Hamilton SM, Jones RL, Roberts P, King EG. Predictive equation for assessing

energy expenditure in mechanically ventilated critically ill patients. Crit Care Med. 1990;18(6):657–61.
67. Boullata J, Williams J, Cottrell F, Hudson L, Compher C. Accurate determination of energy needs in hospitalized patients. J Am Diet Assoc. 2007;107(3):393–401.
68. Matarese LE, Gottschlich MM, editors. Contemporary nutrition support practice: a clinical guide. Philadelphia, PA: WB Saunders; 1998.
69. Frankenfield D, Hise M, Malone A, Russell M, Gradwell E, Compher C, Evidence Analysis Working Group. Prediction of resting metabolic rate in critically ill adult patients: results of a systematic review of the evidence. J Am Diet Assoc. 2007;107(9):1552–61.
70. Frankenfield D, Smith JS, Cooney RN. Validation of 2 approaches to predicting resting metabolic rate in critically ill patients. JPEN J Parenter Enter Nutr. 2004;28(4):259–64.
71. Frankenfield D. Validation of an equation for resting metabolic rate in older obese, critically ill patients. JPEN J Parenter Enter Nutr. 2011;35(2):264–9.
72. Tatucu-Babet OA, Ridley EJ, Tierney AC. Prevalence of underprescription or overprescription of energy needs in critically ill mechanically ventilated adults as determined by indirect calorimetry: a systematic literature review. J Parenter Enter Nutr. 2016;40(2):212–25.
73. Patel JJ, Martindale RG, McClave SA. Controversies surrounding critical care nutrition: an appraisal of permissive underfeeding, protein, and outcomes. J Parenter Enter Nutr. 2018;42(3):508–15. eprint: https://onlinelibrary.wiley.com/doi/pdf/10.1177/0148607117721908.
74. Allingstrup MJ, Esmailzadeh N, Knudsen AW, Espersen K, Jensen TH, Wiis J, Perner A, Kondrup J. Provision of protein and energy in relation to measured requirements in intensive care patients. Clin Nutr. 2012;31(4):462–8.
75. Rugeles S-J, Rueda J-D, Díaz C-E, Rosselli D. Hyperproteic hypocaloric enteral nutrition in the critically ill patient: a randomized controlled clinical trial. Indian J Crit Care Med. 2013;17(6):343–9.
76. Arabi YM, Aldawood AS, Haddad SH, Al-Dorzi HM, Tamim HM, Jones G, Mehta S, McIntyre L, Solaiman O, Sakkijha MH, Sadat M, Afesh L. Permissive underfeeding or standard enteral feeding in critically ill adults. N Engl J Med. 2015;372(25):2398–408. https://doi.org/10.1056/NEJMoa1502826.
77. Arabi YM, Aldawood AS, Al-Dorzi HM, Tamim HM, Haddad SH, Jones G, McIntyre L, Solaiman O, Sakkijha MH, Sadat M, et al. Permissive underfeeding or standard enteral feeding in high- and low-nutritional-risk critically ill adults. Post hoc analysis of the permit trial. Am J Respir Crit Care Med. 2017;195(5):652–62.
78. Klein CJ, Stanek GS, Wiles CE III. Overfeeding macronutrients to critically ill adults: metabolic complications. J Am Diet Assoc. 1998;98(7):795–806.
79. Deng Q-G, She H, Cheng JH, French SW, Koop DR, Xiong S, Tsukamoto H. Steatohepatitis induced by intragastric overfeeding in mice. Hepatology. 2005;42(4):905–14.
80. Baumgardner JN, Shankar K, Hennings L, Badger TM, Ronis MJJ. A new model for nonalcoholic steatohepatitis in the rat utilizing total enteral nutrition to overfeed a high-polyunsaturated fat diet. Am J Physiol Gastrointest Liver Physiol. 2008;294:G27–8.
81. Golabi P, Sayiner M, Fazel Y, Koenig A, Henry L, Younossi ZM. Current complications and challenges in nonalcoholic steatohepatitis screening and diagnosis. Expert Rev Gastroenterol Hepatol. 2016;10(1):63–71.
82. Chen L-L, Stralovich-Romani A. Chapter 7—Nutrition in critically ill patients. In: Parsons PE, Wiener-Kronish JP, editors. Critical care secrets. 4th ed. Philadelphia: Mosby; 2007. p. 39–46.
83. Arenas Márquez H, Prieto Chávez E, Hernández Higareda LA, Gutiérrez de la Rosa JL, De Mucha Mora R. Morbidity, mortality, and total parenteral nutrition in esophageal and gastric surgery for benign pathology. Rev Invest Clin. 1993;45(2):139–43.
84. Tamiya H, Yasunaga H, Matusi H, Fushimi K, Akishita M, Ogawa S. Comparison of short-term mortality and morbidity between parenteral and enteral nutrition for adults without cancer: a propensity-matched analysis using a national inpatient database. Am J Clin Nutr. 2015;102(5):1222–8.
85. Abunnaja S, Cuviello A, Sanchez JA. Enteral and parenteral nutrition in the perioperative period: state of the art. Nutrients. 2013;5(2):608–23.
86. Pacelli F, Bossola M, Papa V, Malerba M, Modesti C, Sgadari A, Bellantone R, Doglietto GB. Enteral vs parenteral nutrition after major abdominal surgery: an even match. Arch Surgery. 2001;136(8):933–6.
87. Harvey SE, Parrott F, Harrison DA, Bear DE, Segaran E, Beale R, Bellingan G, Leonard R, Mythen MG, Rowan KM. Trial of the route of early nutritional support in critically ill adults. N Engl J Med. 2014;371(18):1673–84.
88. Singer P, Berger MM, Van den Berghe G, Biolo G, Calder P, Forbes A, Griffiths R, Kreyman G, Leverve X, Pichard C. Espen guidelines on parenteral nutrition: intensive care. Clin Nutr. 2009;28(4):387–400.
89. Bost RBC, Tjan DHT, van Zanten ARH. Timing of (supplemental) parenteral nutrition in critically ill patients: a systematic review. Ann Intensive Care. 2014;4(1):31.
90. Singer P, Anbar R, Cohen J, Shapiro H, Shalita-Chesner M, Lev S, Grozovski E, Theilla M, Frishman S, Madar Z. The tight calorie control study (ticacos): a prospective, randomized, controlled pilot study of nutritional support in critically ill patients. Intensive Care Med. 2011;37(4):601–9.
91. Kutsogiannis J, Alberda C, Gramlich L, Cahill NE, Wang M, Day AG, Dhaliwal R, Heyland DK. Early use of supplemental parenteral nutrition in critically ill patients: results of an international

multicenter observational study. Crit Care Med. 2011;39(12):2691–9.
92. Heidegger CP, Berger MM, Graf S, Zingg W, Darmon P, Costanza MC, Thibault R, Pichard C. Optimisation of energy provision with supplemental parenteral nutrition in critically ill patients: a randomised controlled clinical trial. Lancet. 2013;381(9864):385–93.
93. Casaer MP, Mesotten D, Hermans G, Wouters PJ, Schetz M, Meyfroidt G, Van Cromphaut S, Ingels C, Meersseman P, Muller J, et al. Early versus late parenteral nutrition in critically ill adults. N Engl J Med. 2011;365(6):506–17.
94. Seres DS, Valcarcel M, Guillaume A. Advantages of enteral nutrition over parenteral nutrition. Ther Adv Gastroenterol. 2013;6(2):157–67.
95. Marik PE, Zaloga GP. Gastric versus post-pyloric feeding: a systematic review. Crit Care. 2003;7(3):R46–51.
96. Montejo JC, Miñambres E, Bordeje L, Mesejo A, Acosta J, Heras A, Ferre M, Fernandez-Ortega F, Vaquerizo CI, Manzanedo R. Gastric residual volume during enteral nutrition in ICU patients: the REGANE study. Intensive Care Med. 2010;36(8):1386–93.
97. Reignier J, Mercier E, Le Gouge A, Boulain T, Desachy A, Bellec F, Clavel M, Frat J-P, Plantefeve G, Quenot J-P, Lascarrou J-B, Clinical Research in Intensive Care and Sepsis (CRICS) Group. Effect of not monitoring residual gastric volume on risk of ventilator-associated pneumonia in adults receiving mechanical ventilation and early enteral feeding: a randomized controlled trial. JAMA. 2013;309(3):249–56.
98. Diamond SJ, Medici V, Rice TW, Miller K. Should we stop using gastric residual volumes? Curr Nutr Rep. 2015;4(3):236–41.
99. Brierley-Hobson S, Clarke G, O'Keeffe V. Safety and efficacy of volume-based feeding in critically ill, mechanically ventilated adults using the 'protein & energy requirements fed for every critically ill patient every time' (PERFECT) protocol: a before-and-after study. Crit Care. 2019;23(1):105.
100. Abidali A, Mangram A, Shirah GR, Wilson W, Abidali A, Moeser P, Dzandu JK. Bilateral pneumothoraces in a trauma patient after Dobhoff tube insertion. Am J Case Rep. 2018;19:244–8.
101. Smith MD, McCall J, Plank L, Herbison PG, Soop M, Nygren J. Preoperative carbohydrate treatment for enhancing recovery after elective surgery [systematic review]. Cochrane Database Syst Rev. 2014;(8):CD009161.
102. Smith AL, Santa Ana CA, Fordtran JS, Guileyardo JM. Deaths associated with insertion of nasogastric tubes for enteral nutrition in the medical intensive care unit: clinical and autopsy findings. Proc (Bayl Univ Med Cent). 2018;31(3):310–6.
103. Pillai JB, Vegas A, Brister S. Thoracic complications of nasogastric tube: review of safe practice. Interact Cardiovasc Thorac Surg. 2005;4(5):429–33.
104. Roubenoff R, Ravich WJ. Pneumothorax due to nasogastric feeding tubes: report of four cases, review of the literature, and recommendations for prevention. Arch Intern Med. 1989;149(1):184–8
105. Dudrick SJ. History of parenteral nutrition. J Am Coll Nutr. 2009;28(3):243–51.
106. Boullata JI, Gilbert K, Sacks G, Labossiere RJ, Crill C, Goday P, Kumpf VJ, Mattox TW, Plogsted S, Holcombe B, American Society for Parenteral and Enteral Nutrition. A.S.P.E.N. clinical guidelines: parenteral nutrition ordering, order review, compounding, labeling, and dispensing. JPEN J Parenter Enter Nutr. 2014;38(3):334–77.
107. Ljungqvist O, Scott M, Fearon KC. Enhanced recovery after surgery: a review. JAMA Surg. 2017;152(3):292–8.
108. ASPEN. Clinical guidelines for the use of parenteral and enteral nutrition in adult and pediatric patients, 2009. J Parenter Enter Nutr. 2009;33(3):255–9. eprint: https://onlinelibrary.wiley.com/doi/pdf/10.1177/0148607109333115.
109. Braga M, Ljungqvist O, Soeters P, Fearon K, Weimann A, Bozzetti F. ESPEN guidelines on parenteral nutrition: surgery. Clin Nutr. 2009;28(4):378–86.
110. Pittiruti M, Hamilton H, Biffi R, MacFie J, Pertkiewicz M. ESPEN guidelines on parenteral nutrition: central venous catheters (access, care, diagnosis and therapy of complications). Clin Nutr. 2009;28(4):365–77.
111. Gosmanov AR, Umpierrez GE. Management of hyperglycemia during enteral and parenteral nutrition therapy. Curr Diab Rep. 2013;13(1):155–62.
112. Duggan EW, Carlson K, Umpierrez GE. Perioperative hyperglycemia management: an update. Anesthesiology. 2017;126(3):547–60.
113. Naini BV, Lassman CR. Total parenteral nutrition therapy and liver injury: a histopathologic study with clinical correlation. Hum Pathol. 2012;43(6):826–33.
114. Cai W, Jiang W, Hong L, Yuanfei X, Tang Q, Shi C. Oxidative injury and hepatocyte apoptosis in total parenteral nutrition–associated liver dysfunction. J Pediatr Surg. 2006;41(10):1663–8.
115. Jain AK, Teckman JH. Newly identified mechanisms of total parenteral nutrition related liver injury. Adv Hepatol. 2014;2014:621380.
116. Boeckxstaens GE, de Jonge WJ. Neuroimmune mechanisms in postoperative ileus. Gut. 2009;58(9):1300–11.
117. Barbieux J, Hamy A, Talbot MF, Casa C, Mucci S, Lermite E, Venara A. Does enhanced recovery reduce postoperative ileus after colorectal surgery? J Visc Surg. 2017;154(2):79–85.
118. Greer N, Sultan S, Shaukat A, Dahm P, Lee A, MacDonald R, McKenzie L, Ercan-Fang D, editors. Enhanced recovery after surgery (ERAS) programs for patients undergoing colorectal surgery. Executive summary. Washington, DC: Department of Veterans Affairs (US); 2017.

119. Branco BC, Barmparas G, Schnüriger B, Inaba K, Chan LS, Demetriades D. Systematic review and meta-analysis of the diagnostic and therapeutic role of water-soluble contrast agent in adhesive small bowel obstruction. Br J Surg. 2010;97(4):470–8. eprint: https://onlinelibrary.wiley.com/doi/pdf/10.1002/bjs.7019.
120. Stawicki SP, Brooks A, Bilski T, Scaff D, Gupta R, Schwab CW, Gracias VH. The concept of damage control: extending the paradigm to emergency general surgery. Injury. 2008;39(1):93–101.
121. Becher RD, Peitzman AB, Sperry JL, Gallaher JR, Neff LP, Sun Y, Miller PR, Chang MC. Damage control operations in non-trauma patients: defining criteria for the staged rapid source control laparotomy in emergency general surgery. World J Emerg Surg. 2016;11(1):1–8.
122. Petrov MS, Pylypchuk RD, Emelyanov NV. Systematic review: nutritional support in acute pancreatitis. Aliment Pharmacol Therap. 2008;28(6):704–12. eprint: https://onlinelibrary.wiley.com/doi/pdf/10.1111/j.1365-2036.2008.03786.x.
123. Polk TM, William Schwab C. Metabolic and nutritional support of the enterocutaneous fistula patient: a three-phase approach. World J Surg. 2012;36(3):524–33.
124. Yin J, Wang J, Yao D, Zhang S, Mao Q, Kong W, Ren L, Li Y, Li J. Is it feasible to implement enteral nutrition in patients with enteroatmospheric fistulae? A single-center experience. Nutr Clin Pract. 2014;29(5):656–61. eprint: https://onlinelibrary.wiley.com/doi/pdf/10.1177/0884533614536587.
125. McClave SA, Chang W-K. Feeding the hypotensive patient: does enteral feeding precipitate or protect against ischemic bowel? Nutr Clin Pract. 2003;18(4):279–84.
126. Khalid I, Doshi P, DiGiovine B. Early enteral nutrition and outcomes of critically ill patients treated with vasopressors and mechanical ventilation. Am J Crit Care. 2010;19(3):261–8.
127. Es Covello LHS, Gava-Brandolis MG, Castro MG, Dos Santos Netos MF, Manzanares W, Toledo DO. Vasopressors and nutrition therapy: safe dose for the outset of enteral nutrition? Crit Care Res Pract. 2020;2020:1095693.
128. Dissanaike S, Pham T, Shalhub S, Warner K, Hennessy L, Moore EE, Maier RV, O'Keefe GE, Cuschieri J. Effect of immediate enteral feeding on trauma patients with an open abdomen: protection from nosocomial infections. J Am Coll Surg. 2008;207(5):690–7.
129. Collier B, Guillamondegui O, Cotton B, Donahue R, Conrad A, Groh K, Richman J, Vogel T, Miller R, Diaz J Jr. Feeding the open abdomen. J Parenter Enter Nutr. 2007;31(5):410–5.
130. Bansal V, Coimbra R. Nutritional support in patients following damage control laparotomy with an open abdomen. Eur J Trauma Emerg Surg. 2013;39(3):243.
131. Yuan Y, Ren J, Guosheng G, Chen J, Li J. Early enteral nutrition improves outcomes of open abdomen in gastrointestinal fistula patients complicated with severe sepsis. Nutr Clin Pract. 2011;26(6):688–94.
132. Roger Maltby J. Fasting from midnight—the history behind the dogma. Best Pract Res Clin Anaesthesiol. 2006;20(3):363–78.
133. Douglas MJ, Ciraulo D. Variability in perioperative fasting practices negatively impacts nutritional support of critically ill intubated patients. Am Surg. 2017;83(8):895–900.
134. Agarwal A, Chari P, Singh H. Fluid deprivation before operation. The effect of a small drink. Anaesthesia. 1989;44(8):632–4.
135. Hutchinson A, Maltby JR, Reid CR. Gastric fluid volume and pH in elective inpatients. Part I: coffee or orange juice versus overnight fast. Can J Anaesth. 1988;35(1):12–5.
136. McGrady EM, Macdonald AG. Effect of the preoperative administration of water on gastric volume and pH. Br J Anaesth. 1988;60(7):803–5.
137. Phillips S, Hutchinson S, Davidson T. Preoperative drinking does not affect gastric contents. Br J Anaesth. 1993;70(1):6–9.
138. Read MS, Vaughan RS. Allowing pre-operative patients to drink: effects on patients' safety and comfort of unlimited oral water until 2 hours before anaesthesia. Acta Anaesthesiol Scand. 1991;35(7):591–5.
139. Sutherland AD, Maltby JR, Sale JP, Reid CR. The effect of preoperative oral fluid and ranitidine on gastric fluid volume and pH. Can J Anaesth. 1987;34(2):117–21.
140. Yagci G, Can MF, Ozturk E, Dag B, Ozgurtas T, Cosar A, Tufan T. Effects of preoperative carbohydrate loading on glucose metabolism and gastric contents in patients undergoing moderate surgery: a randomized, controlled trial. Nutrition. 2008;24(3):212–6.
141. American Society of Anesthesiologists Committee. Practice guidelines for preoperative fasting and the use of pharmacologic agents to reduce the risk of pulmonary aspiration: application to healthy patients undergoing elective procedures: an updated report by the American Society of Anesthesiologists Committee on Standards and Practice Parameters. Anesthesiology. 2011;114(3):495–511.
142. American Society of Anesthesiologists. Practice guidelines for preoperative fasting and the use of pharmacologic agents to reduce the risk of pulmonary aspiration: application to healthy patients undergoing elective procedures: an updated report by the American Society of Anesthesiologists Task Force on Preoperative Fasting and the use of pharmacologic agents to reduce the risk of pulmonary aspiration. Anesthesiology. 2017;126(3):376–93.
143. Rawlinson A, Kang P, Evans J, Khanna A. A systematic review of enhanced recovery protocols

in colorectal surgery. Ann R Coll Surg Engl. 2011;93(8):583–8.
144. McClave SA, Saad MA, Esterle M, Anderson M, Jotautas AE, Franklin GA, Heyland DK, Hurt RT. Volume-based feeding in the critically ill patient. J Parenter Enter Nutr. 2015;39(6):707–12. eprint: https://onlinelibrary.wiley.com/doi/pdf/10.1177/0148607114540004.
145. Krebs ED, O'Donnell K, Berry A, Guidry CA, Hassinger TE, Sawyer RG. Volume-based feeding improves nutritional adequacy in surgical patients. Am J Surg. 2018;216(6):1155–9.
146. Parent BA, Mandell SP, Maier RV, Minei J, Sperry J, Moore EE, O'Keefe GE. Safety of minimizing pre-operative starvation in critically-ill and intubated trauma patients. J Trauma Acute Care Surg. 2016;80(6):957–63.
147. Imeokparia F, Johnson M, Thakkar RK, Giles S, Capello T, Fabia R. Safety and efficacy of uninterrupted perioperative enteral feeding in pediatric burn patients. Burns. 2018;44(2):344–9.
148. Kratzing C. Pre-operative nutrition and carbohydrate loading. Proc Nutr Soc. 2011;70(3):311–5.
149. Segaran E, Lovejoy TD, Proctor C, Bispham WL, Jordan R, Jenkins B, O'Neill E, Harkess SEJ, Terblanche M. Exploring fasting practices for critical care patients—a web-based survey of UK intensive care units. J Intensive Care Soc. 2018;19(3):188–95.
150. American Society for Parenteral and Enteral Nutrition. Appropriate dosing for parenteral nutrition: ASPEN recommendations, 2019.
151. U.S. Department of Agriculture. Vitamins and minerals | Food and Nutrition Information Center | NAL | USDA.
152. Chow O, Barbul A. Immunonutrition: role in wound healing and tissue regeneration. Adv Wound Care. 2013;3(1):46–53.
153. Nabzdyk CS, Bittner EA. Vitamin C in the critically ill-indications and controversies. World J Crit Care Med. 2018;7(5):52.
154. Marik PE, Khangoora V, Rivera R, Hooper MH, Catravas J. Hydrocortisone, vitamin c, and thiamine for the treatment of severe sepsis and septic shock: a retrospective before-after study. Chest. 2017;151(6):1229–38.
155. Fowler AA, Syed AA, Knowlson S, Sculthorpe R, Farthing D, DeWilde C, Farthing CA, Larus TL, Martin E, Brophy DF, Gupta S, Medical Respiratory Intensive Care Unit Nursing, Fisher BJ, Natarajan R. Phase I safety trial of intravenous ascorbic acid in patients with severe sepsis. J Transl Med. 2014;12:32.
156. Polcz ME, Barbul A. The role of vitamin a in wound healing. Nutr Clin Pract. 2019;34(5):695–700.
157. Zinder R, Cooley R, Vlad LG, Molnar JA. Vitamin a and wound healing. Nutr Clin Pract. 2019;34(6):839–49.
158. Lansdown ABG, Mirastschijski U, Stubbs N, Scanlon E, Agren MS. Zinc in wound healing: theoretical, experimental, and clinical aspects. Wound Repair Regen. 2007;15(1):2–16.
159. Wilkinson EAJ. Oral zinc for arterial and venous leg ulcers. Cochrane Database Syst Rev. 2014;(9):CD001273.
160. Gümüstekin K, Seven B, Karabulut N, Aktas O, Gürsan N, Aslan S, Keles M, Varoglu E, Dane S. Effects of sleep deprivation, nicotine, and selenium on wound healing in rats. Int J Neurosci. 2004;114(11):1433–42.
161. Stephen AO, James O, Ikoojo ER, Sunday AO. Effects of selenium treatment on healing of acetic acid induced gastric ulcer in albino wistar rats. Am J Biomed Res. 2016;4(1):18–22.
162. Berger MM, Baines M, Raffoul W, Benathan M, Chiolero RL, Reeves C, Revelly J-P, Cayeux M-C, Śeñechaud I, Shenkin A. Trace element supplementation after major burns modulates antioxidant status and clinical course by way of increased tissue trace element concentrations. Am J Clin Nutr. 2007;85(5):1293–300.
163. Suchner U, Kuhn KS, P. Fürst. The scientific basis of immunonutrition. Proc Nutr Soc. 2000;59(4):553–63.
164. Roehl K. Immunonutrition in 2016: benefit, harm or neither? Pract Gastro. 2016;XL(8). practicalgastro.com.
165. McCarthy MS, Martindale RG. Immunonutrition in critical illness: what is the role? Nutr Clin Pract. 2018;33(3):348–58.
166. Calder PC. Omega-3 polyunsaturated fatty acids and inflammatory processes: nutrition or pharmacology? Br J Clin Pharmacol. 2013;75(3):645–62.
167. Dancey CP, Attree EA, Brown KF. Nucleotide supplementation: a randomised double-blind placebo controlled trial of IntestAidIB in people with irritable bowel syndrome [ISRCTN67764449]. Nutr J. 2006;5:16.
168. Drover JW, Dhaliwal R, Weitzel L, Wischmeyer PE, Ochoa JB, Heyland DK. Perioperative use of arginine-supplemented diets: a systematic review of the evidence. J Am Coll Surg. 2011;212(3):385–99, 399.e1.
169. Marimuthu K, Varadhan KK, Ljungqvist O, Lobo DN. A meta-analysis of the effect of combinations of immune modulating nutrients on outcome in patients undergoing major open gastrointestinal surgery. Ann Surg. 2012;255(6):1060–8.
170. Osland E, Belal Hossain M, Khan S, Memon MA. Effect of timing of pharmaconutrition (immunonutrition) administration on outcomes of elective surgery for gastrointestinal malignancies: a systematic review and meta-analysis. JPEN J Parenter Enter Nutr. 2014;38(1):53–69.

Geriatrics/Frailty and End of Life Care

37

Mohana Karlekar and Myrick C. Shinall Jr

Case Example

Mr. S was a 78-year-old man who was brought to the emergency room by his son for complaints of abdominal pain and altered mental status over the past 24 h. He lived at home with his son who helped him buy groceries and manage his finances, but he was independent for the rest of his daily activities. He had been hospitalized twice in the past 6 months for exacerbations of chronic medical problems and had lost 15 pounds over that time which his son attributed to the patient's disinterest in eating and poor appetite. On exam he was tachycardic with focal peritonitis. CT scan was notable for pneumatosis in the right colon and portal venous gas. Labs revealed a leukocytosis and mild lactic acidosis. The Acute Care Surgery team recommended exploration with possible bowel resection and had a lengthy discussion with the patient and his son about the operation. They also discussed what non-operative management would entail and the implications of poor outcomes after either decision to operate or not. After this discussion, the patient was taken to the OR.

On exploration, the surgeons discovered an ischemia extending from the cecum to the mid-transverse colon. There was a palpable pulse in the root of the mesentery although there had been no evidence on CT scan of arterial or venous occlusion. The surgeons performed an extended right colectomy with end ileostomy. When the patient aroused from anesthesia, his mentation was clearer than prior and the son reported he was back to his baseline mentally. The patient initially recovered without incident but acutely developed delirium on post-operative day 4. Work-up revealed pneumonia, presumably from aspiration. With antibiotic treatment, the patient slowly recovered, but remained severely debilitated and required nursing home placement at the conclusion of his hospitalization.

Over the next month, the patient was readmitted several times with dehydration from excessive ileostomy output that resulted in acute kidney injury as well as recurrent pneumonia. He continued to lose

M. Karlekar (✉)
Section of Palliative Care, Division of General Internal Medicine and Public Health, Department of Medicine, Vanderbilt University, Nashville, TN, USA
e-mail: mohana.b.karlekar@vumc.org

M. C. Shinall Jr
Surgery and Medicine, Vanderbilt University Medical Center, Nashville, TN, USA

M. D. Zielinski, O. Guillamondegui (eds.), *The Acute Management of Surgical Disease*,
https://doi.org/10.1007/978-3-031-07881-1_37

weight over this period and was not regaining strength despite maximal efforts to improve his nutrition and functioning. He was very discouraged by his frequent readmissions and inability to return home. During one of his readmissions, the palliative care team was consulted to discuss his goals of care. After a family meeting involving the patient, his son, the palliative care physicians, and the surgeon, it became clear that the patient's primary goal was to return home, and he was unwilling to continue life-prolonging measures he felt were burdensome, which included inpatient admissions. In conjunction with his primary care physician, the palliative care team helped him enroll in hospice, which provided care for him at home. He lived at home for 2 months before developing pneumonia and dying.

Introduction

Older patients like Mr. S pose particular challenges for the Acute Care Surgeon. Evaluating and caring for these patients requires the surgeon to be familiar with the various age-related conditions that impact their tolerance of the physiologic strain of an operation and post-operative complications. Moreover, making decisions about whether to operate and how to manage serious complications requires the surgeon to understand the patient's goals and how these goals can best be achieved. This chapter will review the complexities of the perioperative management of older patients along with the palliative care skills necessary to ensure challenging treatment decisions are congruent with patients' goals.

Frailty and Geriatric Syndromes

Surgeons face many challenges providing care for older patients. Many conditions that can complicate recovery from surgery (such as malignancy, cardiovascular disease, and chronic organ failure) increase in incidence and severity with increasing age. Moreover, older patients suffer from multi-system, overlapping geriatric syndromes that impact their outcomes from surgery and make perioperative management more complex.

Frailty is a syndrome of increased vulnerability to physiologic stressors resulting from age-related depletion of reserve across multiple organ systems [1, 2]. Frail patients have high risk of serious or fatal illness even after minor inciting events such as infections or low-energy trauma. Frail patients also often have high levels of debility and comorbidities. Frail surgical patients are high-risk operative patients, regardless of the intensity of the procedure [3]. They suffer higher rates of post-operative complications along with more failure to rescue when complications occur, leading to higher post-operative mortality when compared to non-frail cohorts [4]. Moreover, frail patients and those with pre-existing debility are at high risk for post-operative decreases in functional status and independence, both of outcomes patients consistently rate as very important [5].

Age is also a risk factor for delirium, an acute form of brain dysfunction marked by waxing and waning level of consciousness. Older adults have higher rates of several risk factors for delirium including higher rates of underlying cognitive dysfunction or dementia, more use of deliriogenic medications, and higher rates of visual and auditory deficits that make unfamiliar environments more disorienting. Delirium can be the presenting symptom for a range of non-neurologic disorders in the elderly, from minor conditions such as uncomplicated urinary tract infection to major life-threatening conditions such as sepsis. Hospitalized patients who suffer delirium have higher mortality rates than non-delirious patients, and delirium is also a risk factor for subsequent cognitive dysfunction [6, 7].

Older patients also often have high risk for falls due to more difficulties with balance, greater loss of strength, lower visual acuity, more orthostasis, and more confusion related to delirium and/or dementia. Moreover, osteoporosis, use of antithrombotic or anticoagulant medications, and overall frailty place seniors who do fall at higher risk of serious injury from intracranial hemorrhage and fractures.

Dysphagia is also increasingly recognized as a geriatric syndrome [8]. The complex neuromotor mechanisms required for effective swallowing slow with aging, resulting in difficulty swallowing for a significant number of people as they age. Additionally, weakness related to sarcopenia, impaired cognition, and deteriorating dentition can all contribute to dysphagia and are all more common as we age. Dysphagia places older adults at higher risk of malnutrition and aspiration.

Finally, older patients tend to take more medication, and polypharmacy may be an independent driver of poor outcomes. In both general medical and surgical populations, polypharmacy is associated with increased risk of mortality. It is not clear to what degree polypharmacy is simply a proxy for the underlying risk factor of multimorbidity vs. an independent causal factor in poor outcomes [9]. Nevertheless, many drugs are risk factors for geriatric syndromes and post-operative complications: psychoactive medications increase the risk of delirium and falls, anti-hypertensives increase risk of falls from orthostasis, and anti-platelet and anti-coagulant medications increase bleeding risk both from surgery and low-energy trauma such as falls from standing.

Management of the Older EGS Patient

Preoperative

The American College of Surgeons and the American Geriatrics Association have developed a checklist of preoperative evaluations that should be completed for older patients [10]. Recommendations include screening for frailty, cognitive impairment, impaired functional status and falls, cardiac and pulmonary risk factors, depression, alcohol and substance dependence, and nutritional status. It is rarely feasible to perform formal screening for these conditions in the emergency setting, but focused attention to these issues while taking the history can alert the surgeon to the particular vulnerabilities of the patient. Cognitive status can be especially challenging to evaluate because older surgical patients are also more vulnerable to delirium as they present with an acute surgical problem. Without corroboration from those who know the patient, it can be impossible to determine to what extent the patient with altered mental status is suffering from delirium vs. chronic cognitive dysfunction and dementia. Finding an informant of the patient's baseline mental status, such as family, friends, or staff at a long-term living facility, is highly desirable as the surgeon formulates the treatment plan.

Ideally, the treatment plan is developed through a process of shared decision making between the surgeon and the patient or the patient's surrogate if the patient lacks capacity. This shared decision-making process can be conceptualized as comprising four steps: (1) providing information on the acute surgical condition in the context of the patient's overall health status; (2) presenting the viable treatment options and their likely outcomes; (3) eliciting patient preferences and values; and (4) helping decide the course of treatment most congruent with the patient's preferences and values [11].

The first step, presenting information on the acute surgical condition in the context of the patient's overall health status, can be challenging for an acute care surgeon who has never met the patient before and may not be an expert in the patient's other disease processes. However, most chronic, life-threatening illnesses follow one of three trajectories that are fairly easy to recognize. The first pattern is typical of cancer, where patients typically maintain a very high or normal level of functioning for most of the disease course and then suffer a fairly rapid (weeks to months) decline to death. The second pattern occurs in chronic organ failure (e.g., chronic obstructive pulmonary disease, chronic heart failure, cirrhosis) which cause the patient to suffer acute exacerbations with recovery to baseline, at least initially. As the disease progresses, exacerbations become more frequent and severe, and recovery does not reach the pre-exacerbation baseline until an exacerbation eventually ends the patient's life. Finally, frailty and dementia tend to follow a trajectory of insidious but nearly continuous decline in function until the patient experiences a stressor from which they cannot recover. Questions about changes in functional status over the past 6 months, weight loss, and frequency of hospitalizations can give the surgeon an idea of where the patient currently sits on these trajectories and the likelihood that addressing the acute surgical problem will alter the patient's long-term course.

Once the surgeon and the patient/surrogate have a shared understanding of how the acute surgical problem fits into the patient's overall illness trajectory, the surgeon can discuss the various treatment options and their likely outcomes. One particularly helpful method for this discussion is the best case/worst case paradigm [12]. In this method, the surgeon lays out the viable options for treatment (usually operative vs. non-operative management). For each option the surgeon describes what the best reasonable outcome would look like from the patient's perspective, what the worst outcome would look like, and where in between these two extremes the surgeon thinks the patient is most likely to end up if that treatment option is chosen. This method helps the surgeon present information about the treatment options that patients can readily understand.

The next aspect of the shared decision-making model is for the surgeon to elicit patient preferences. The goal for this step is for the surgeon to learn enough about the patient's values and preferences to make informed recommendations about which treatment option best fits the patient's values. Asking open-ended questions about who and what are important to the patient are helpful ways of getting this information. Alternatively asking what the patient would be unwilling to live without (e.g., the ability to do a hobby, independence in activities of daily living, ability to live at home, ability to interact with loved ones) can also help the patient articulate preferences. After this discussion, the patient (or surrogate) should have enough information about the medical facts and the surgeon should have enough information about the patient's values that together they can agree on the treatment plan that fits the patient best.

As the treatment plan is being developed and implemented, several other pieces of information can be helpful for further care. Determining the patient's preferences regarding code status, who the patient's preferred surrogate is, and whether the patient has any advance care planning documentation should occur as soon as possible. It is also especially helpful to probe for evidence of pre-existing mild cognitive dysfunction, history of falls, difficulty swallowing, and urinary or fecal incontinence in addition to typical information in the past medical history.

Intraoperative

The acute care surgeon must remain aware of several issues while operating on the older patient. As mentioned above, resuscitation of the older patient is challenging, and frequent communication between the operative and anesthesia teams is critical to keeping the patient stable. There are also operative choices that age-related patient factors influence. If the operation involves disrupting colonic continuity, careful consideration of reconstruction is warranted. An anastomotic leak will be harder for an older frailer patient to tolerate than for a younger patient. A colostomy is more likely to be permanent in an older patient, but if the patient has problems with fecal incontinence or immobility at baseline, a permanent colostomy can be advantageous and improve quality of life. If a diverting ileostomy is considered, thought should be given to the patient's ability to tolerate high output, especially if the patient has compromised cardiovascular or renal function. In performing major abdominal surgery on an older patient, the surgeon should also consider intraoperative placement of enteral access. A history of dysphagia or dementia or anticipation of prolonged endotracheal intubation should prompt the surgeon to consider placing either a nasoenteric tube or a feeding gastrostomy or jejunostomy depending on their best estimate of whether post-operative dysphagia may be temporary or long lasting.

Post-operative

In addition to the routine issues faced by all patients as they recover from an emergent operation, older patients face issues related to the geriatric syndromes discussed earlier in the chapter. Due to the frequent convergence of several predisposing factors, older post-operative patients often have high risk of delirium. There is no proven pharmacologic agent to prevent or treat delirium, so management focuses on minimizing or eliminating precipitating factors. The mnemonic "DR. DRE" can provide a framework for thinking about ameliorating these precipitating factors. First is "Disease Remediation," which involves searching for an underlying medical cause of delirium, which in the post-operative patient is often a complication. Delirium can be the first sign of a complication, and it should trigger a search for physical signs and laboratory evidence of an underlying complication. Disease remediation also includes treating distressing symptoms, such as pain, which can also be precipitating factors for delirium.

While the work-up for potential complications is ongoing, the surgeon should also attend to the next steps of delirium management, "Drug Removal" and the "Environment." The patient's current medication list should be scrutinized for any deliriogenic medications whose doses could be reduced or eliminated. The surgeon should also attend to the possibility of withdrawal from alcohol or medications as causing the delirium. Finally, any steps that could normalize the patient's relationship to their environment should be taken, including removing unnecessary indwelling devices (such as bladder catheters or nasogastric tubes), minimizing monitoring alarms and other interruptions of the patient's sleep, and ensuring that the patient has ready access to any needed sensory aids, such as glasses or hearing aids.

The older post-operative patient may also be at high risk for falling. Mobilizing after an operation is crucial for regaining function as quickly as possible and speeding recovery. Nevertheless, care must be taken so that ambulation can be accomplished safely. Most fall prevention efforts focus on arranging the physical layout of the patient's room to minimize hazards for falling and on ensuring adequate assistance from staff when the patient is out of bed. The physician team can help prevent falls by attention to medical issues that make patients more susceptible to falling. Delirium increases the risk for falling, so prompt recognition of delirium and modification of precipitating factors can help reduce fall risk. Similarly, orthostasis can predispose older patients to falling, especially in the post-operative context when fluid shifts are occurring. Patients on home anti-hypertensive regimens warrant special attention in this regard.

The post-operative environment also increases the risk of dysphagia and aspiration for older patients. Rates of post-operative aspiration increase rapidly with increasing age [13]. In addition to underlying difficulties swallowing, additional risk factors include the intra-operative or post-operative placement of devices across the oropharynx (such as endotracheal tubes, nasogastric tubes, and transesophageal echocardiogram probes) as well as post-operative ileus. Patients at risk for aspiration should have precautions in place that include elevation of the head of the bed especially during and after eating and consultation with a speech therapist to recommend the safest consistency diet.

Surgical Outcomes

Frail older patients bear significant burdens of morbidity and mortality after emergent operations. One study in the veteran population found that frail patients experience a 6-month post-operative mortality of 23% after even moderate intensity emergent operations, such as laparoscopic cholecystectomy [14]. In addition to mortality, these frail patients suffer significant morbidity post-operatively. One study found that in the year after emergency general surgery, frail older patients had more hospital encounters and spent over a month less time at home than non-frail patients [15]. Screening patients for frailty in the emergent setting can be difficult, but increasing evidence shows psoas muscle volume on CT scan provides a proxy for frailty and similarly predicts poor post-operative outcomes [16]. Automated evaluation for sarcopenia on axial imaging may in the future provide surgeons a valuable clinical tool for identifying at risk emergent surgical patients.

Older surgical patients can also suffer reductions in their functional status after surgery. Maintaining physical and cognitive functioning is frequently valued more highly than survival among older patients undergoing treatment for a chronic illness [17]. Thus, post-operative loss of functional independence can negatively impact quality of life for many older patients. Unfortunately, post-operative declines in functional status are common among older patients. One study found that patients 80 and older had declines in functional status at 30 days post-operatively in about 20% of cases. Of those with functional decline, over half were no longer able to live at home [5].

These stark results make proper pre-operative counseling essential for older patients with emergent surgical conditions. The risks of morbidity, mortality, and loss of independence may not change the patient's decision to undergo a potentially life-saving operation, but these risks may inform decision making in the event of a complication that renders full recovery unlikely.

Palliative Care

Although many clinicians practice palliative care principles within their own practice, palliative care (PC) as a unique specialty is relatively new. PC grew out of the hospice movement almost 25 years ago and became a recognized subspecialty in medicine in 2012. The Center to Advance Palliative care defines palliative care as "specialized medical care for people living with a serious illness." This type of care is focused on providing relief from the symptoms and stress of a serious illness. PC improves quality of life for both the patient and the family" [18]. PC programs have grown dramatically over the last decade across the nation and are accessible in some form in most large acute care hospitals. Dumanovsky et al. reported in 2016 that 96% of hospitals with 300 beds or more have a palliative care program [19].

Primary Palliative Care vs. Specialty Palliative Care

Palliative care is classified into primary palliative care (PPC) and specialty palliative care (SPC). PPC is the clinical knowledge and skill set that all health care providers be versed in when caring for patients faced with a serious illness. In contrast, SPC is provided by clinicians with specialized training in PC. As a result of their additional training, SPC clinicians are able to meet the more complex and difficult needs of the patients and families requiring specialty care [20, 21].

Acute Care Surgeons may provide either PPC or SPC [20]. This will depend on many factors including time, training, and comfort level. There is a growing recognition and emphasis that all surgeons master the basic PC skills [22–24]. As a result, current surgical house staff receive more formal training on PC topics [24]. There remain no clearly identified triggers for referral to SPC for patients cared for by EGS. Despite the American College Surgeons' recommendation that PC be integrated into the care of all surgical patients with poor prognosis, referral to SPC in this population remains underutilized [25, 26].

Goals of Care

Older adults undergoing emergent surgical procedures are at high risk of complications. Navigating patient expectations in the context of the medical reality can be challenging [27]. Suboptimal communication can lead to treatment without benefit [28]. PC teams excel in communication and can be a valuable partner to the EGS in order to provide goal concordant care [29, 30]. Goals of care (GOC) conversations are the cornerstone in providing quality care. Stanek describes GOC as "desired health expectations that are formulated through the thoughtful interaction between a human being seeking medical care and the healthcare team in the healthcare system and are appropriate, agreed on, documented and communicated." She adds that the "development of clear goals of care can increase patient satisfaction and quality of care while decreasing costs, hospital length of stay and hospital readmission" [31].

Shared Decision Making

All older adults undergoing emergent surgical procedures should undergo a GOC conversation [32]. In most of these cases, a shared decision-making approach is the preferred model [28]. A shared decision approach by definition assumes that the patient and healthcare provider together develop a common understanding and plan of care based on a patient's goals [33, 34]. The patient under the guidance of their healthcare provider will select the treatment choice that best fits his or her values [35]. A shared decision-making approach can empower the surgeon to effectively communicate and offer only those procedures that are helpful and not offer futile procedures [35]. It is important to note however that some patients facing surgical emergencies may not have any treatment options. In these cases, the prognosis may be grim, and death is certain. In these cases, it is the EGS's responsibility to clearly communicate prognosis and plan of care [27].

A Framework to Navigate GOC Conversations

There exist many approaches to explore a patient's GOC; there is no single correct framework. Most effective methods are predicated on "sharing prognostic information, eliciting decision-making preferences, understanding fears and goals, exploring views on trade-offs and impaired function, and wishes for family involvement [36]." REMAP a mnemonic coined by Vitaltalks™ has been utilized in the cancer population, is an easy to use framework that can easily be applied in the emergency surgery population (see Table 37.1) [37].

Table 37.1 Examples of clinician statements to guide conversations regarding goals of care

REMAP	Physician statement
Reframe	"You've worked very hard with all the treatments over the years, and I hear that now you're feeling more tired and it's harder for you to do the things you enjoy. I'm seeing that you're in a different place now. Further treatments may be too hard on you."
Emotion	"What worries you most about this?" "It's understandable that you would feel sad when thinking about these things." "This is hard to talk about." "It is OK to talk about what this all means for the future?"
Map	"Tell me about some of the things you enjoy doing." "What's most important to you given that time is limited?"
Align	"From what I'm hearing from you, the most important thing for you is to have time at home, sitting on the porch with your family. You feel like at this point you've spent too much time in the hospital, and you wouldn't want to come back if it could only extend your life a few days or week."
Propose a plan	"Given what you've told me, I'd propose that we do everything to help you spent time at home with your family. I don't think more cancer treatment is likely to help with that. I think getting hospice involved would help you do what you want to do with the time you have. What do you think?"

Step 1: Involves reframing the condition from the patient's perspective and exploring the patient's understanding of his or her condition. The reframe allows the individual patient to put their illness in the context of the big picture. This can be overwhelming for the patient, as it can trigger a patient to rethink their personal goals knowing what he or she had hoped for may no longer be possible [38].

Step 2: Is to expect emotion. This is often a consequence of step one, once a patient has understood the bigger picture. In this step it is important to respond to the emotion. The response could be empathetic listening, a statement acknowledging how difficult this must be or even an invitation to continue talking.

Step 3: The physician will map out the patients' values using open-ended questions. This is a dynamic conversation where the physician and patient dialogue about the patient's values and ultimately the physician helps the patient prioritize which values are most important.

Step 4: The physician repeats back their understanding of the patient's values to the patient and describes what this would look like in the medical context of the patient's illness, in other words align the plan of care with patient's values.

Step 5: The physician recommends a medical plan of care that is both medically feasible and likely to successfully achieve a patients' prioritized goals and values [37].

Advance Care Planning

Sudore and colleagues defines advance care planning as a "process that supports adults at any age or stage of health in understanding and sharing their personal values, life goals, and preferences regarding future medical care." She goes on to state that "the goal of advance care planning is to help ensure that people receive medical care that is consistent with their values, goals and preferences during serious and chronic illness, and for many people, this process may include choosing and preparing another trusted person or persons to make medical decisions in the event the person can no longer make his or her own decisions [39]." Advance care planning has many benefits to the patient, healthcare team and healthcare system. Benefits include a "decrease in life-sustaining treatments, reduction in inappropriate hospitalizations, increased use of hospice and palliative care services," decreased patient and family distress and decreased cost of inpatient care [40–43].

There are many barriers to the successful completion and implementation of advance care directives [44]. Advance care directives can vary from state to state and are often subject to clinician interpretation. The selection of advance care directive may vary depending on the patient's capacity to make medical decisions. It is important for the clinician to both understand and use the appropriate directive depending on clinical setting. Some directives are appropriate only in the outpatient setting, while others applicable in the hospitalized patient. Finally, all completed directives should be reviewed for accuracy. Unfortunately, a great many directives are deemed invalid as are filled out incorrectly [45].

Advance Care Directives

There are three major directives, the living will (LW), healthcare power of attorney (HPOA), and "informal statue or preferences [42]." The living will is a legal document that takes effect *in the future*. Here, the individual patient describes in a legal written document his or her preferences on treatments and or quality of life at the end of life. In order to complete a living will, the patient must have the capacity to make complex medical decisions as determined by their healthcare provider. There are many different types of living wills. Individual documents vary from state to state. Not all states honor a directive completed in a different state, so it is important to be familiar with the standards of care at one's own institution and state.

The HPOA is the individual legally named by the patient to make decisions on his or her behalf. The HPOA may make decisions on a patient's behalf only if the individual patient lacks capacity to make his or her own decisions. Healthcare providers should counsel their patients when selecting a HPOA to pick someone who is reasonably available, shows care and compassion and is willing and able to make decisions based on the patient's own preferences using substituted judgment [46]. Finally, informal preferences or statues or are either written or verbal statements made by the patient to their friends, family or healthcare providers that describe their healthcare preferences [42].

Resuscitation Orders

In the acute care setting, it is assumed that all patients want an attempt at cardio-pulmonary resuscitation even if this is not accurate. Any patient who declines cardio-pulmonary resuscitation should have a code status order or do not resuscitate orders (DNR) placed. It is important to distinguish the fact that resuscitation orders speak only to whether a patient will have resuscitative care attempted in the event of a cardiac arrest. These orders do not speak to patient's broader treatment preferences and or desires on quality of life. For example, it is perfectly appropriate for a patient with a DNR order to transition care to the intensive care unit for vasopressors and escalation of care, as long as it is consistent with a patient's goals of care.

In the community setting, resuscitation orders are reflected in an out-of-hospital DNR order or order for life-sustaining treatment. The names of these documents vary from state to state (physician order for scope of treatment, medical order for life-sustaining treatment…) and not all states have these documents codified into law [44]. It is important for clinicians to become familiar with their local state's practices.

Family Meetings

PC specialists often refer to the family meeting (FM) as the procedure that defines this specialty [47]. FM should be thought of as any clinical procedure, with clear indications, aims and a clear stepwise process to follow when executing [48, 49]. Indications for FM include to assess a patient/family's understanding of an illness or injury, discuss prognosis, review treatment options, elicit GOC, and facilitate end of life planning [50–52].

FM can benefit both the patient/family and the clinical team. FM encourages more patient involvement and "may provide additional and valued opportunities for patients and families to express mutual concerns, deliver messages of comfort and appreciation, and prepare for death [53]." Clinicians can better connect with their patients and family members through compassionate communication [54].

Timing of family meetings varies depending on the situation and acuity of illness. Because FM generally are thought to improve communication, they can be helpful when communicating a new serious diagnosis, a change in condition/functional status, and in complex medical conditions and transitions to end of life care [50, 51, 55].

There are many models described in the literature on how to conduct a family meeting [48, 56, 57]. All models are predicated on the same basic principles. Regardless of the approach chosen, it is important to ensure that the framework chosen is followed.

Family meetings are composed of three major components, the pre-meeting, the meeting, and post-meeting. The pre-meeting consists of all of the *preparatory work* done prior to the actual meeting. The meeting includes all components of the interaction during the meeting itself. The post-meeting includes the action items to be completed at the conclusion of the actual meeting.

The Pre-Meeting: This is the *work done prior to the meeting* including the following items [49, 58–60]:

1. Review the patient information so the history and salient medical issues are clear to all clinicians participating in the family meeting.
2. Determine the purpose of the meeting.
3. Clarify what information is to be conveyed. If there is disagreement among clinicians on how to answer these questions, a consensus must be reached *prior to* the actual meeting between clinicians.
4. Determine who should be invited from the clinical team and patient/family and what does the patient/family understand and how are they coping?
5. Identify who will lead the meeting?
6. Ensure a private location and convenient time is chosen for the actual meeting itself with enough lead time for all participants to be able to attend.

The Meeting [37, 61–64]:

1. Find a comfortable and private space and then make introductions. Allow everyone to introduce themselves and what their role is. This includes family members. Discuss the purpose of the meeting.

2. Determine what the patient/family understand by using open-ended questions such as "Tell me what your understanding of Mr. X's illness is?
3. Request permission to share information. Ask the patient/family if it is ok for the clinical team to explain the patient's condition in more detail; specifically, what led up to the diagnosis, the salient active issues, and what to expect with this particular diagnosis.
4. Respond to emotion and allow for silence.
5. Encourage the patient/family to ask questions and ask them to repeat back what they understand.
6. Summarize the meeting and discuss next steps. This includes determining if another meeting is indicated and if so when.

The Post-Meeting [37]:

1. Debrief the family meeting to ensure no one has any questions or there is ambiguity in the plan of care.
2. Communicate the salient aspects of the meeting to healthcare providers such as nursing, patients' primary care provider, etc.
3. Document the key aspects of the meeting.

What Can Go Wrong?

Most all clinicians have participated in a FM that has not gone well. This can be the result of a variety of reasons. Families may become confused or angry if information is not communicated compassionately or messaging is inconsistent [62, 65]. Patients and families may become overwhelmed if too much information is shared, or clinicians use too much medical jargon [61]. Finally, patients and or families may be overwhelmed to make decisions if they were not prepared to receive difficult news [60].

Dying with Dignity

Facilitating a "good death" involves careful planning, collaboration, and attention to detail much like any surgical procedure. The good death is patient-centered and affords our patients dignity, privacy, emotional support, optimal symptom management, and access to hospice care. In addition, the good death offers our patients the opportunity to know when death is near, to be able to say goodbye, and to have control in who is present and where one dies [66].

Optimizing Pain and Symptom Management

Many patients worry about needlessly suffering at the end of life not knowing that the great majority of symptoms can be addressed effectively [67]. Common symptoms in the last hours to days of life include pain, dyspnea, delirium, and terminal secretions. Optimizing end of life symptoms first requires that we appropriately recognize that death is near and then complete a thorough assessment of our patient to determine which symptoms are causing distress [68]. There are numerous papers published in the literature guiding clinicians on best practices of treatment of dyspnea, pain, terminal secretions, and delirium [67, 69–71]. The authors would recommend that clinicians become familiar with the management of these conditions and utilize best practices and or guides to when treating symptoms at the end of life.

Withdrawing Life Support

Withdrawal of life support should be considered a procedure with a logical set of steps that should be undertaken in a sequential manner that requires foresight and collaboration. The language in how we communicate with patients and their families "withdrawal of support" also matters. We should avoid terms like "withdrawing care" or "stopping everything" and instead use language that clearly indicates a transition of care but that emphasizes that we are still providing care. Examples of preferable language include "transitioning our care to comfort, withdrawing life support, and/or focusing on comfort".

Before initiating withdrawal of life support, the goals of care must be clear about expectations. Is the goal to allow a natural dying process and stop all measures that are extending life or is the goal to transition to comfort with withdrawal of life support but continue supportive care measures that offer quality of life even if this adds time? If the goals are not clear, then one has to re-engage the patient/family to ensure clarification prior.

The process of withdrawing support can be broken down into three broad sub-categories:

Prework

The prework involves a careful assessment of the patient's condition, values and beliefs, life expectancy and what potential symptom he/she may experience. Clinicians should determine which therapies are prolonging life, and which therapies are providing comfort, as ultimately one wants to know which therapies can be withdrawn safely without untoward sequelae and which therapies should be continued from a quality of life/optimal symptom management perspective [72, 73].

1. Assess your patient and determine which therapies will be stopped, when and in what order.
2. Huddle with the team. During huddle, providers should alert bedside nurses to which medications/doses they will be required and order these ordered in advance.
3. Communicate with your clinical team the specifics on the plan for withdrawal. Which therapies will be withdrawn and in what order?
4. Meet with family and explain process of life support withdrawal. Specifically ask/address with families:
   (a) What date/time withdrawal will be scheduled?
   (b) Who should be present (from the family)?
   (c) Will the family be in the room or outside?
   (d) Would the patient/family like a spiritual advisor/chaplain to visit?
   (e) Always address what the plan is for artificial hydration and nutrition prior to withdrawal.
   (f) Explain to family, what to expect in terms of time and symptoms and how the team will optimize symptoms to minimize distress.

The Withdrawal of Life Support Therapy

1. Clinical team enters room and asks family if anyone has questions about process. If no, family is asked to step out of room ideally with a social worker, spiritual advisor, or chaplain to support them.
2. Bedside nurse and provider dose medications prior if medically appropriate, and remove life support/therapies per plan communicated earlier.
3. Symptoms are optimized, patient is groomed, bedding adjusted, chairs assembled around bed and family is invited back into room.
4. Healthcare provider explains how process went, what to expect and allow family private time with patient.

Post Withdrawal Support to Clinical Team, Patient, and Family

1. Provider should review with bed side nurse what to expect and plan for addressing symptoms. In addition, he/she should share his/her contact information with bedside.
2. Bedside nurse to dose medications asking for guidance as appropriate.
3. Provider should check in to reevaluate patient within the hour to see if the family has questions and assess/treat symptoms.
4. Bedside nurse and provider should complete all appropriate documentation into the medical record.

Hospice Care

Medicare created the hospice benefit over 30 years ago. The goals of hospice care are to support patients and their families at the end of life when the primary clinician feels life expectancy is less than 6 months and the goals are comfort. It may be challenging to determine when hospice care is medically appropriate and possible for the EGS patient given that the acuity of these patients is high and life expectancy can be short. Collaboration with palliative care teams and local hospice agencies is recommended for these patients to determine what is best/possible for the patient. The literature supports the use of hospice care to benefit not just patients and families but healthcare institutions as well. Its use has been associated with "reduced hospital care and Medicare expenditures [74]."

References

1. Fried LP, Tangen CM, Walston J, Newman AB, Hirsch C, Gottdiener J, Seeman T, Tracy R, Kop WJ, Burke G, McBurnie MA, Cardiovascular Health Study Collaborative Research Group. Frailty in older adults: evidence for a phenotype. J Gerontol A Biol Sci Med Sci. 2001;56:M146–56.
2. Rockwood K, Song X, MacKnight C, Bergman H, Hogan DB, McDowell I, Mitnitski A. A global clinical measure of fitness and frailty in elderly people. CMAJ. 2005;173:489–95.
3. Shinall MC Jr, Arya S, Youk A, Varley P, Shah R, Massarweh NN, Shireman PK, Johanning JM, Brown AJ, Christie NA, Crist L, Curtin CM, Drolet BC, Dhupar R, Griffin J, Ibinson JW, Johnson JT, Kinney S, LaGrange C, Langerman A, Loyd GE, Mady LJ, Mott MP, Patri M, Siebler JC, Stimson CJ, Thorell WE, Vincent SA, Hall DE. Association of preoperative patient frailty and operative stress with postoperative mortality. JAMA Surg. 2020;155:e194620.
4. Shah R, Attwood K, Arya S, Hall DE, Johanning JM, Gabriel E, Visioni A, Nurkin S, Kukar M, Hochwald S, Massarweh NN. Association of frailty with failure to rescue after low-risk and high-risk inpatient surgery. JAMA Surg. 2018;153:e180214.
5. Zhang LM, Hornor MA, Robinson T, Rosenthal RA, Ko CY, Russell MM. Evaluation of postoperative functional health status decline among older adults. JAMA Surg. 2020;155:950–8.
6. Rockwood K, Cosway S, Carver D, Jarrett P, Stadnyk K, Fisk J. The risk of dementia and death after delirium. Age Ageing. 1999;28:551–6.
7. Robinson TN, Raeburn CD, Tran ZV, Angles EM, Brenner LA, Moss M. Postoperative delirium in the elderly: risk factors and outcomes. Ann Surg. 2009;249:173–8.
8. Baijens LW, Clave P, Cras P, Ekberg O, Forster A, Kolb GF, Leners JC, Masiero S, Mateos-Nozal J, Ortega O, Smithard DG, Speyer R, Walshe M. European Society for Swallowing Disorders—European Union Geriatric Medicine Society white paper: oropharyngeal dysphagia as a geriatric syndrome. Clin Interv Aging. 2016;11:1403–28.
9. Fried TR, O'Leary J, Towle V, Goldstein MK, Trentalange M, Martin DK. Health outcomes associated with polypharmacy in community-dwelling older adults: a systematic review. J Am Geriatr Soc. 2014;62:2261–72.
10. Chow WB, Rosenthal RA, Merkow RP, Ko CY, Esnaola NF, American College of Surgeons National Surgical Quality Improvement Program, American Geriatrics Society. Optimal preoperative assessment of the geriatric surgical patient: a best practices guideline from the American College of Surgeons National Surgical Quality Improvement Program and the American Geriatrics Society. J Am Coll Surg. 2012;215:453–66.
11. Taylor LJ, Johnson SK, Nabozny MJ, Tucholka JL, Steffens NM, Kwekkeboom KL, Brasel KJ, Campbell TC, Schwarze ML. Barriers to goal-concordant care for older patients with acute surgical illness: communication patterns extrinsic to decision aids. Ann Surg. 2018;267:677–82.
12. Taylor LJ, Nabozny MJ, Steffens NM, Tucholka JL, Brasel KJ, Johnson SK, Zelenski A, Rathouz PJ, Zhao Q, Kwekkeboom KL, Campbell TC, Schwarze ML. A framework to improve surgeon communication in high-stakes surgical decisions: best case/worst case. JAMA Surg. 2017;152:531–8.
13. Kozlow JH, Berenholtz SM, Garrett E, Dorman T, Pronovost PJ. Epidemiology and impact of aspiration pneumonia in patients undergoing surgery in Maryland, 1999-2000. Crit Care Med. 2003;31:1930–7.
14. Shinall MC Jr, Youk A, Massarweh NN, Shireman PK, Arya S, George EL, Hall DE. Association of preoperative frailty and operative stress with mortality after elective vs emergency surgery. JAMA Netw Open. 2020;3:e2010358.
15. Lee KC, Streid J, Sturgeon D, Lipsitz S, Weissman JS, Rosenthal RA, Kim DH, Mitchell SL, Cooper Z. The impact of frailty on long-term patient-oriented outcomes after emergency general surgery: a retrospective cohort study. J Am Geriatr Soc. 2020;68:1037–43.
16. Rangel EL, Rios-Diaz AJ, Uyeda JW, Castillo-Angeles M, Cooper Z, Olufajo OA, Salim A, Sodickson AD. Sarcopenia increases risk of long-term mortality in elderly patients undergoing emergency abdominal surgery. J Trauma Acute Care Surg. 2017;83:1179–86.
17. Fried TR, Bradley EH, Towle VR, Allore H. Understanding the treatment preferences of seriously ill patients. N Engl J Med. 2002;346:1061–6.
18. https://www.capc.org/about/palliative-care/.
19. Dumanovsky T, Augustin R, Rogers M, Lettang K, Meier DE, Morrison RS. The growth of palliative care in U.S. hospitals: a status report. J Palliat Med. 2016;19:8–15.
20. Miner TJ. Understanding the core principles of primary and specialty surgical palliative care. J Am Coll Surg. 2020;231:185–6.

21. Quill TE, Abernethy AP. Generalist plus specialist palliative care—creating a more sustainable model. N Engl J Med. 2013;368:1173–5.
22. Brasel KJ, Weissman DE. Palliative care education for surgeons. J Am Coll Surg. 2004;199:495–9.
23. Huffman JL. Educating surgeons for the new golden hours: honing the skills of palliative care. Surg Clin North Am. 2005;85:383–91.
24. Bradley CT, Brasel KJ. Core competencies in palliative care for surgeons: interpersonal and communication skills. Am J Hosp Palliat Care. 2007;24:499–507.
25. Dunn GP. Surgery, palliative care, and the American College of Surgeons. Ann Palliat Med. 2015;4:5–9.
26. Evans BA, Turner MC, Gloria JN, Pickett LC, Galanos AN. Palliative care consultation is underutilized in critically ill general surgery patients. Am J Hosp Palliat Care. 2020;37:149–53.
27. Desserud KF, Veen T, Soreide K. Emergency general surgery in the geriatric patient. Br J Surg. 2016;103:e52–61.
28. Cooper Z, Courtwright A, Karlage A, Gawande A, Block S. Pitfalls in communication that lead to nonbeneficial emergency surgery in elderly patients with serious illness: description of the problem and elements of a solution. Ann Surg. 2014;260:949–57.
29. Tilden LB, Williams BR, Tucker RO, MacLennan PA, Ritchie CS. Surgeons' attitudes and practices in the utilization of palliative and supportive care services for patients with a sudden advanced illness. J Palliat Med. 2009;12:1037–42.
30. Mosenthal AC, Murphy PA. Interdisciplinary model for palliative care in the trauma and surgical intensive care unit: Robert Wood Johnson Foundation demonstration project for improving palliative care in the intensive care unit. Crit Care Med. 2006;34:S399–403.
31. Stanek S. Goals of care: a concept clarification. J Adv Nurs. 2017;73:1302–14.
32. Aucoin S, McIsaac DI. Emergency general surgery in older adults: a review. Anesthesiol Clin. 2019;37:493–505.
33. de Mik SML, Stubenrouch FE, Balm R, Ubbink DT. Systematic review of shared decision-making in surgery. Br J Surg. 2018;105:1721–30.
34. Wancata LM, Hinshaw DB. Rethinking autonomy: decision making between patient and surgeon in advanced illnesses. Ann Transl Med. 2016;4:77.
35. Morris RS, Ruck JM, Conca-Cheng AM, Smith TJ, Carver TW, Johnston FM. Shared decision-making in acute surgical illness: the surgeon's perspective. J Am Coll Surg. 2018;226:784–95.
36. Bernacki RE, Block SD, American College of Physicians High Value Care Task Force. Communication about serious illness care goals: a review and synthesis of best practices. JAMA Intern Med. 2014;174:1994–2003.
37. Childers JW, Back AL, Tulsky JA, Arnold RM. REMAP: a framework for goals of care conversations. J Oncol Pract. 2017;13:e844–50.
38. Zier LS, Burack JH, Micco G, Chipman AK, Frank JA, White DB. Surrogate decision makers' responses to physicians' predictions of medical futility. Chest. 2009;136:110–7.
39. Sudore RL, Lum HD, You JJ, Hanson LC, Meier DE, Pantilat SZ, Matlock DD, Rietjens JAC, Korfage IJ, Ritchie CS, Kutner JS, Teno JM, Thomas J, McMahan RD, Heyland DK. Defining advance care planning for adults: a consensus definition from a multidisciplinary Delphi panel. J Pain Symptom Manag. 2017;53:821–832.e1.
40. Bond WF, Kim M, Franciskovich CM, Weinberg JE, Svendsen JD, Fehr LS, Funk A, Sawicki R, Asche CV. Advance care planning in an accountable care organization is associated with increased advanced directive documentation and decreased costs. J Palliat Med. 2018;21:489–502.
41. Brinkman-Stoppelenburg A, Rietjens JA, van der Heide A. The effects of advance care planning on end-of-life care: a systematic review. Palliat Med. 2014;28:1000–25.
42. Perez Mdel V, Macchi MJ, Agranatti AF. Advance directives in the context of end-of-life palliative care. Curr Opin Support Palliat Care. 2013;7:406–10.
43. Houben CHM, Spruit MA, Groenen MTJ, Wouters EFM, Janssen DJA. Efficacy of advance care planning: a systematic review and meta-analysis. J Am Med Dir Assoc. 2014;15:477–89.
44. Tran M, Grant M, Clayton J, Rhee J. Advance care decision making and planning. Aust J Gen Pract. 2018;47:753–7.
45. Mirarchi FL, Juhasz K, Cooney TE, Puller J, Kordes T, Weissert L, Lewis ML, Intrieri B, Cook N. TRIAD XII: are patients aware of and agree with DNR or POLST orders in their medical records. J Patient Saf. 2019;15:230–7.
46. Wendler D. The theory and practice of surrogate decision-making. Hast Cent Rep. 2017;47:29–31.
47. Joshi R. Family meetings: an essential component of comprehensive palliative care. Can Fam Physician. 2013;59:637–9.
48. Hudson P, Quinn K, O'Hanlon B, Aranda S. Family meetings in palliative care: multidisciplinary clinical practice guidelines. BMC Palliat Care. 2008;7:12.
49. Curtis JR, Patrick DL, Shannon SE, Treece PD, Engelberg RA, Rubenfeld GD. The family conference as a focus to improve communication about end-of-life care in the intensive care unit: opportunities for improvement. Crit Care Med. 2001;29:N26–33.
50. Machare Delgado E, Callahan A, Paganelli G, Reville B, Parks SM, Marik PE. Multidisciplinary family meetings in the ICU facilitate end-of-life decision making. Am J Hosp Palliat Care. 2009;26:295–302.
51. O'Neill D. Care planning meetings can aid communication with patient and family. BMJ. 2017;359:j5528.
52. Piscitello GM, Parham WM 3rd, Huber MT, Siegler M, Parker WF. The timing of family meetings in the medical intensive care unit. Am J Hosp Palliat Care. 2019;36:1049–56.
53. Sanderson CR, Cahill PJ, Phillips JL, Johnson A, Lobb EA. Patient-centered family meetings in palliative care: a quality improvement project to explore a new

model of family meetings with patients and families at the end of life. Ann Palliat Med. 2017;6:S195–205.
54. Forbat L, Francois K, O'Callaghan L, Kulikowski J. Family meetings in inpatient specialist palliative care: a mechanism to convey empathy. J Pain Symptom Manag. 2018;55:1253–9.
55. Billings JA. The end-of-life family meeting in intensive care part I: indications, outcomes, and family needs. J Palliat Med. 2011;14:1042–50.
56. Gritti P. The family meetings in oncology: some practical guidelines. Front Psychol. 2014;5:1552.
57. Meyer DL, Gershman K, Broberg L, Craigie FC Jr, Antonucci J. Conducting family meetings in nursing homes: resident, nurse, and family perceptions. Fam Med. 1991;23:36–9.
58. Lautrette A, Ciroldi M, Ksibi H, Azoulay E. End-of-life family conferences: rooted in the evidence. Crit Care Med. 2006;34:S364–72.
59. King DA, Quill T. Working with families in palliative care: one size does not fit all. J Palliat Med. 2006;9:704–15.
60. Weiner JS, Roth J. Avoiding iatrogenic harm to patient and family while discussing goals of care near the end of life. J Palliat Med. 2006;9:451–63.
61. Stapleton RD, Engelberg RA, Wenrich MD, Goss CH, Curtis JR. Clinician statements and family satisfaction with family conferences in the intensive care unit. Crit Care Med. 2006;34:1679–85.
62. Quill TE, Townsend P. Bad news: delivery, dialogue, and dilemmas. Arch Intern Med. 1991;151:463–8.
63. Quill TE, Arnold RM, Platt F. "I wish things were different": expressing wishes in response to loss, futility, and unrealistic hopes. Ann Intern Med. 2001;135:551–5.
64. Hashim MJ. Patient-centered communication: basic skills. Am Fam Physician. 2017;95:29–34.
65. Sisk BA, Malone JR. Hope, optimism, and compassionate communication. JAMA Pediatr. 2018;172:311–2.
66. https://www.bgs.org.uk/resources/palliative-care.
67. Albert RH. End-of-life care: managing common symptoms. Am Fam Physician. 2017;95:356–61.
68. Frankenhauser S, Geist MJP, Weigand MA, Bardenheuer HJ, Kessler J. [Interprofessional symptom management at the end of life]. Urologe A. 2018;57:609–20.
69. Vargas-Bermudez A, Cardenal F, Porta-Sales J. Opioids for the management of dyspnea in cancer patients: evidence of the last 15 years—a systematic review. J Pain Palliat Care Pharmacother. 2015;29:341–52.
70. Lokker ME, van Zuylen L, van der Rijt CC, van der Heide A. Prevalence, impact, and treatment of death rattle: a systematic review. J Pain Symptom Manag. 2014;47:105–22.
71. Bobb B. Dyspnea and delirium at the end of life. Clin J Oncol Nurs. 2016;20:244–6.
72. Wiegand DL, Cheon J, Netzer G. Seeing the patient and family through: nurses and physicians experiences with withdrawal of life-sustaining therapy in the ICU. Am J Hosp Palliat Care. 2019;36:13–23.
73. Downar J, Delaney JW, Hawryluck L, Kenny L. Guidelines for the withdrawal of life-sustaining measures. Intensive Care Med. 2016;42:1003–17.
74. Zuckerman RB, Stearns SC, Sheingold SH. Hospice use, hospitalization, and medicare spending at the end of life. J Gerontol B Psychol Sci Soc Sci. 2016;71:569–80.

Index

M. D. Zielinski, O. Guillamondegui (eds.), *The Acute Management of Surgical Disease*,
https://doi.org/10.1007/978-3-031-07881-1

GPSR Compliance

The European Union's (EU) General Product Safety Regulation (GPSR) is a set of rules that requires consumer products to be safe and our obligations to ensure this.

If you have any concerns about our products, you can contact us on ProductSafety@springernature.com

In case Publisher is established outside the EU, the EU authorized representative is:

Springer Nature Customer Service Center GmbH
Europaplatz 3
69115 Heidelberg, Germany

Batch number: 10731383

Printed by Printforce, the Netherlands